RECENT ADVANCES IN THE PATHOGENESIS, PREVENTION AND MANAGEMENT OF TYPE 2 DIABETES AND ITS COMPLICATIONS

Edited by **Mark B. Zimering**

Recent Advances in the Pathogenesis, Prevention and Management of Type 2 Diabetes and its Complications
Edited by Dr Mark B. Zimering

Published by InTech

Janeza Trdine 9, 51000 Rijeka, Croatia

Publishing Process Manager Mirna Cvijic

Technical Editor Teodora Smiljanic

Cover Designer InTech Design Team

Additional hard copies can be obtained from orders@intechopen.com

Recent Advances in the Pathogenesis, Prevention and Management of Type 2 Diabetes and its Complications, Edited by Mark B. Zimering
p. cm.
ISBN 978-953-307-597-6

For EU product safety concerns:
IN TECH d.o.o., Prolaz Marije Krucifikse Kozulić 3, 51000 Rijeka, Croatia,
info@intechopen.com or visit our website at intechopen.com.

Meet the editor

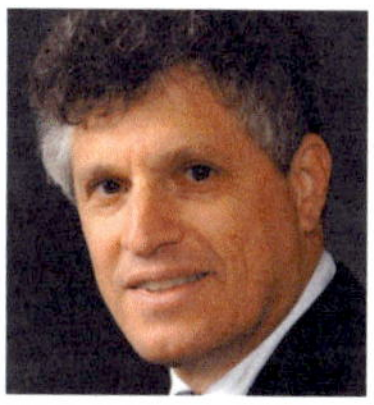

Dr. Mark Zimering is the Chief of Endocrinology at the Department of Veterans Affairs in East Orange, New Jersey and Associate Professor of Medicine Co-Terminous at UMDNJ/Robert Wood Johnson Medical School. Dr. Zimering received his undergraduate training at Harvard College, MD and PhD degrees from the Albert Einstein College of Medicine, and completed an endocrinology fellowship at the NIH. His research has focused on roles for basic fibroblast growth factor (or autoantibodies which mimic or inhibit its effects) in diabetic vascular complications. He reported markedly increased plasma basic fibroblast growth in a subset of obese adult participants from the Veterans Affairs Diabetes Trial having increased coronary heart disease occurrence. His group reported low levels of plasma basic fibroblast growth factor in adult diabetes having a cluster of microvascular complications (macular edema, albuminuria, painful neuropathy) in association with endothelial cell inhibitory autoantibodies which activated the RhoA/Rho kinase signaling pathway in endothelial cells or caused global increases in intracellular calcium in endothelial cells, neurons or cardiomyocytes.

Contents

Preface

Type 2 diabetes mellitus affects nearly 120 million persons worldwide- and according to the World Health Organization this number is expected to double by the year 2030. Owing to a rapidly increasing disease prevalence- the medical, social and economic burdens associated with the microvascular and macrovascular complications of type 2 diabetes are likely to increase dramatically in the coming decades. In this volume, leading contributors to the field review the pathogenesis, treatment and management of type 2 diabetes and its complications. They provide invaluable insight and share their discoveries about potentially important new techniques for the diagnosis, treatment and prevention of diabetic complications.

Neuropathy is the most common microvascular complication in diabetes. In the Section on *Diabetic Neuropathy,* Bjorkman et al. provide evidence for how a novel technique known as 'targeted plasticity' may be useful for stimulating recovery of somatosensory function in diabetic neuropathy affecting the hand. Watanabe and co-workers describe the use of ultrasound of peripheral nerve as a potentially promising new modality for the evaluation of patients having distal polyneuropathy. Thomsen et al summarize the differences in nerve fiber morphology between large vs small fiber neuropathy.

Type 2 diabetes is associated with a two-four- fold increased risk for cardiovascular disease. In the section *Diabetes and Cardiovascular Disease,* Hermans et al. review the evidence supporting atherogenic dyslipidemia as a potentially important component of residual vascular risk in diabetes. Stasko et al. treat the important topic of diabetes and fibrinolysis, including evidence for plasminogen activator inhibitor-1 as a predictor of cardiovascular risk in type 2 diabetes. Yaturu and Mousa discuss evidence for aspirin resistance in diabetes. Ojji reviews the pathogenesis of diabetic cardiomyopathy focusing on the unique contribution of diastolic dysfunction to heart failure in diabetes. Pappone et al summarize the results of a large prospective observational study in which type 2 diabetes was associated with an increased risk for progression from paroxysmal to persistent atrial fibrillation. Silent ischemia is highlighted in an excellent chapter by Emilia and Vlad Babes. Finally, Arce-Esquivel and colleagues review the beneficial effects of exercise on endothelial function.

Hypertension frequently complicates type 2 diabetes contributing to a substantially increased risk for cardiovascular disease or progression of nephropathy. In three excellent chapters written by Carella, Swislocki & Siegel, and Masuo & Lambert the latest advances in treatment of hypertension in type 2 diabetes are summarized. Ertugrul et al review treatment advances in diabetic nephropathy. MacFarlane and colleagues summarize the management of chronic anemia in diabetic nephropathy. Martinez et al describe a rat model which mimics certain key features of human diabetic nephropathy which may be useful for improving understanding and screening potential treatments to prevent this debilitating microvascular complication.

Diabetes is a multi-systemic disease which can affect many different target organs. In a chapter by Nakajima et al, liver, muscle and lung involvement in diabetes are reviewed with a focus on the association between diabetes and restrictive lung disease. Diana Yu and Jamal Mohammad summarize evidence supporting an association between type 2 diabetes and an increased risk for certain types of cancer affecting the gastrointestinal tract. Kamoi summarizes evidence supporting the role for high blood pressure and techniques for improving the predictive value of high blood pressure as an important mediator of microvascular and macrovascular complications in diabetes.

Finally, three excellent chapters by Begum et al, Perez-Martinez et al, and Huang & Liu informatively review aspects of the use of medicinal plants, nutritional therapy and the pharmacogenetics of anti-diabetic drugs in the treatment of type 2 diabetes.

Mark B. Zimering, MD, PhD
Chief, Endocrinology
Veterans Affairs New Jersey Healthcare System
East Orange, New Jersey,
USA
Associate Professor of Medicine
University of Medicine and Dentistry of New Jersey/
Robert Wood Johnson Medical School, New Brunswick, New Jersey,
USA

Part 1

Diabetic Neuropathy

1

New Treatment Strategies in Diabetic Neuropathy

Anders Björkman, Niels Thomsen and Lars Dahlin
Department of Hand Surgery, Skåne University Hospital, Lund University
Sweden

1. Introduction

Diabetes mellitus is associated with complications from a variety of tissues in the human body. Among them, diabetic neuropathy is a devastating complication leading to severe disability and even mortality. Neuropathy is common among type 1 and 2 diabetic patients and may yet be detected at the time of diagnosis among type 2 diabetic patients. The symptoms the patients experience vary from sensory disturbances with pain to muscle wasting. The results of autonomic neuropathy should also be considered as a severe problem in the patients, but will not be discussed in the present chapter.

The possibilities to treat diabetic neuropathy are limited and a strict glycaemic control has mainly been advocated. The pathophysiology of diabetic neuropathy is complex and includes e.g. biochemical disturbances and vascular factors. Of the former, the polyol pathway has been the target for pharmacological attention. Based on the detailed knowledge of the polyol pathway, obtained from experimental models and human studies, that sorbitol accumulates in peripheral nerve trunks, pharmacological substances were developed with the purpose to decrease sorbitol levels. Such aldose reductase inhibitors have in different studies shown promising results (Bril et al., 2009; Hotta et al., 2008; Oates, 2008; Schemmel et al., 2010), but are still at a stage of development. Presently, various strategies are emerging on the management of diabetic neuropathy, where it is stressed that an appropriate diagnosis is crucial and that the condition is not untreatable (Perkins & Krolewski, 2005). In the present chapter, we present a different approach than treatment with pharmacological substances or focusing on the glycaemic level; namely, utilization of the capacity of the brain to adapt to alterations. Thus, our intention is to use the plasticity of the brain as a treatment strategy - i.e. targeted plasticity.

2. Peripheral neuropathy

A peripheral neuropathy in diabetes may affect both the upper and lower extremities, where the latter location is more common and has gained more attention in research on diabetic neuropathy. Up to 50% of patients with diabetes in the United States may have a neuropathy in the lower extremity (Dyck et al., 1993). The prevalence of neuropathy in diabetes may vary from different studies depending on which diabetic population is examined, e.g. differences in Europe and Asia have been reported (Abbott et al., 2010; Rubino et al., 2007). In addition, various techniques, such as electrophysiology, examination of vibrotactile sense, skin and nerve biopsies and monofilament tests, have been used to detect neuropathy in diabetes. However, although the intense research over the years on various aspects of diabetic neuropathy the mechanisms, which include biochemical and vascular components, behind the different types of neuropathies in diabetes are not clarified. The pathophysiology of the neuropathy is multifaceted and not completely elucidated, although peripheral nerve dysfunction and established neuropathy in diabetes seem to be related to the degree of hyperglycaemia (Lehtinen et al., 1989; Malik et al., 1993). Recently, some studies on diabetic neuropathy with long term data on HbA1c levels available have not found any association between glycaemic level and larger fibre neuropathy (vibrotactile sense) (Dahlin et al., 2011). A specific issue in this context is if even impaired glucose tolerance can induce neuropathy, but so far large myelinated nerve fibre neuropathy is probably not associated with impaired glucose tolerance (Dahlin et al., 2008). However, reports indicate that small nerve fibre dysfunction is present in patients with impaired glucose intolerance (Dahlin et al., 2008). The latter condition and the question of possible presence of neuropathy is a complex issue and are beyond the focus of the present chapter.

2.1 Diabetic foot ulcers

A particular problem in diabetes is the diabetic foot ulcer, which induces severe problems for the patients (Bengtsson et al., 2008) and causes tremendous costs for society (Prompers et al., 2008). It has long been known that diabetes may itself play an active part in the causation of perforating foot ulcers (Londahl et al., 2010). Foot ulcers are common in diabetic patients and associated with high morbidity and mortality. The prevalence of diabetic foot ulcer is 1.7 - 2.9% and the annual population based incidence among diabetic patients is 1.9 - 3.6%. Interestingly, the annual incidence rates of foot ulcers in patients with diabetic neuropathy vary from 5 to 7% (Abbott et al., 2010) and the recurrence rate is high. It is estimated that 70% of healed foot ulcers recur within five years (Apelqvist et al., 1993). It is generally accepted that the majority of amputations in diabetes are preceded by foot ulcers on the same leg with a lifetime risk of a foot ulcer estimated to reach 15-25%, where the majority of the ulcers are located to the toes.

The main cause of diabetic foot ulcers are neuropathy and macro- and microvascular disease, but also other factors may increase the risk for an ulceration (Londahl et al., 2010). Patients with loss of sensation in the foot seem to have a sevenfold increased risk of developing foot ulcers as compared to diabetic patients without neuropathy (Young & Harris, 1994). In addition, a defect proprioception due to neuropathy may also cause impaired balance and postural instability contributing to the risk for foot ulceration. In clinical practice, sensory neuropathy is usually evaluated using monofilaments, 128 Hz tune fork or biothesiometer, where the latter is considered to be the most appropriate method (Edmonds, 2004). However, a multifrequency technique to examine vibrotactile sense has not previously been used to evaluate neuropathy in the foot, particularly as related to the risk for recurrence of foot ulcers. It may be an exiting approach in the future to refine detection of neuropathy. Interestingly, adjunct hyperbaric oxygen therapy, used in a multidisciplinary setting, can improve healing of chronic diabetic foot ulcers (Londahl et al., 2010); a therapy that may also beneficial in nerve regeneration after injury.

2.2 Carpal tunnel syndrome in diabetes

Diabetic patients have an increased prevalence of one of the most common peripheral nerve compression lesions, i.e. carpal tunnel syndrome (CTS), which is compression of the median

nerve at wrist level. It has a prevalence of 2-4% in the general population, while in diabetes it may be as high as 15%. Furthermore, if the subject has diabetic neuropathy in the lower extremity, the prevalence of CTS may approach 30% (Perkins et al., 2002). Interestingly, it has been shown that there seems to be an increased general susceptibility to peripheral nerve compression in diabetic rats (Dahlin et al., 2008), which can be related to disturbed axonal transport and a propensity to inhibit such transport in compression of diabetic nerves (Dahlin et al., 1987; Dahlin et al., 1986).
Previously, it has been stated that surgical release of the median nerve in the carpal tunnel has no benefit for the patients and their symptoms from the CTS. Two previous studies showed diverse results (Mondelli et al., 2004; Ozkul et al., 2002), and proper conclusions can be difficult due to definition and selection of patients, extent of neuropathy and many other factors. Recently, we presented a prospective study where the outcome after surgical release of the carpal ligament was examined in diabetic patients with CTS and compared with age- and gender-matched healthy patients with CTS. The overall conclusion was that diabetic patients with CTS do benefit from surgical release of the carpal ligmament. This statement is relevant irrespective of the severity of the compression lesion or if signs of peripheral neuropathy are present (Thomsen et al., 2009). However, our data do not support a general view that any peripheral nerve trunk in diabetic patients should be surgically released.

3. Introduction to brain plasticity

The brain has been seen as a rather static organ until about 20 years ago. It was widely believed by neuroscientists that no new neural connections could be formed in the adult brain (Kandel et al., 2000; Purves, 2004). It was assumed that once connections had been established in foetal life, or in early infancy, they hardly changed later in life. This stability of connections in the adult brain has often been used to explain why there is usually very little functional recovery after damage to the nervous system. On the other hand, memory and learning require that some changes are possible also in the adult brain (Kandel et al., 2000). It has often been assumed that these phenomena are based on small changes at the synaptic level and do not necessarily involve alterations in the basic circuit of the brain.
The picture has changed radically in the last decades. One of the most interesting questions in neuroscience concerns the manner in which the nervous system can modify its organisation and ultimately its function throughout an individuals lifetime based on sensory input, experience, learning and injury (Donoghue, 1996; Kaas, 1991); a phenomenon that is often referred to as brain plasticity (Kandel et al., 2000; Purves, 2004).

3.1 Plasticity in the adult somatosensory pathways

There is a complete somatotopic map of the entire body surface in the somatosensory cortex of primates (Kaas et al., 1983; Merzenich et al., 1983). Merzenich et al (Merzenich et al., 1984) showed that after amputation of the middle finger of adult primates, the area in the cortex corresponding to the amputated digit began, within two months, to respond to touch stimuli presented to the adjacent digits; i.e. this area is "taken over" by sensory input from adjacent digits. Merzenich et al (Merzenich et al., 1984) also showed that if a monkey "used" one finger excessively, for an hour and a half a day, then, after 3 months, the area of cortex corresponding to that finger "expanded" at the expense of adjacent fingers. Furthermore, if a monkey was forced to always use two fingers jointly by suturing two of its fingers together, it was found at seven weeks that single neurons in area 3b in the primary somatosensory cortex had receptive fields that spanned the border separating the two digits. Interestingly, if more than one finger was amputated there was no "take over" beyond about 1 mm of cortex. Merzenich et al (Merzenich et al., 1987) concluded from this that the expansion is probably mediated by arborisation of thalamo-cortical axons that typically do not extend beyond 1 mm. The figure 1 mm has often been cited as the fixed upper limit of reorganization of sensory pathways in adult animals (Calford, 1991). Pons et al (Pons et al., 1991), however, suggested that this view might be incorrect. They found that after long-term (12 years) deafferentation of an upper limb, the cortical area originally corresponding to the hand in the primary somatosensory cortex was taken over by sensory input from the face. The cells in "the cortical hand area" now started to respond to stimuli applied to the lower face region. Since this patch of cortex is more than 1 cm wide, they concluded that sensory reorganisation could occur over at least this distance, i.e. an order of magnitude ten times greater than the original 1 mm limit.

In addition to these long-term changes that are typically seen weeks or months after deprivation or stimulation, Calford and Tweelade (Calford, 1990) reported rapid, short term changes that are based, presumably, on the unmasking of pre-existing connections rather than on anatomical "sprouting". They anaesthetized the middle finger of flying foxes and found that within 20 minutes the cortical neurons in the primary somatosensory cortex that originally responded to the middle finger could then be activated by touching the adjacent digits, indicating that the receptive fields had expanded to include adjacent digits.

Calford and Tweedale (Calford, 1990) also showed that a small unilateral peripheral denervation in adult flying foxes lead to expansion of the cortical receptive field for neighboring skin areas as predicted from the work of Merzenich et al (Merzenich et al., 1984).

Rapid plasticity changes are typically seen minutes after injury or an intervention, and are often based on decreased inhibition. Decreased inhibition would theoretically increase the receptive field size and enable more neurons to be activated by the stimulus. This is sometimes referred to as unmasking of synapses or neural structures.

Surprisingly, the receptive field of the homotopic region in the other hemisphere mirrored the change. In other words, the second hemisphere learned what the first had done; it copied the revised sensory map. Maintaining symmetric sensory representation of the two sides in the cerebral cortex may be important for the control of symmetric bilateral motor activity.

Experience dependent plasticity refers to the ability of the adult brain to adjust itself to changes in environmental conditions. It relates to the learning of special skills that requires special training and it often requires motivation and concentration on the task.

Another example of brain plasticity is the so called cross-modal plasticity. This phenomenon implies that one sensory modality can substitute for another (Bavelier & Neville, 2002). The most well known example is in blind persons where an improved sensory function is noticed. It has also been shown that when a blind person reads Braille activation in the occipital lobe occurs implying that the somatosensory stimuli from reading activates the cortical area responsible for vision (Gizewski et al., 2003).

Another example is persons in whom the lack of sensibility can be substituted with hearing. Through small microphones on the fingers the persons can, after a short training period, listen to what they feel (Lundborg et al., 1999). A crucial element in such cross-modal plasticity seems to be training, in order for a sensory modality to "take over" another sensory modality.

3.2 Mechanisms of plasticity

Several cellular mechanisms by which the adult brain can adjust to changes in the environment or in sensory input have been defined, including the following (Kandel et al., 2000; Purves, 2004).

Decreased inhibition

Many connections between the periphery and the cortex as well as intracortical connections are physiologically "silent" because of inhibitory influences (Wall, 1977). Sensory stimulation of a point on the skin activates neurons in the somatosensory system near the centre of the area of cortical representation and inhibits activity in neurons near the edges. In this way the receptive field appears smaller than its actual size. The inhibition is due to activation of inhibitory interneurons near the edges of the receptive field. Decreased inhibition would theoretically increase the receptive field size and enable more neurons to be activated by the stimulus; this is sometimes referred to as unmasking of synapses or neural structures. Gamma-aminobutyric acid (GABA) is the most important inhibitory neurotransmittor in the brain (Jones, 1993) and evidence is strong that reduction of GABAergic inhibition is crucial in mediating short term plasticity changes (Chen et al., 2002).

Increase in synaptic strength

The effectiveness of synaptic connections is continuously adopted in response to functional demands. Synaptic transmission becomes facilitated in a pathway that is frequently used, while those that lay dormant atrophy. In this way, repeated practice of a task leads to increased speed and accuracy of performance. Increased synaptic strength may be a mechanism for learning and also for recovery from brain injury. Repetitive stimulation results in increased excitability and facilitation of transmission in the synapses. These effects persist for some time after the initial stimulus and subsequently show gradual declines (long term potentiation, LTP). Calcium channels in the neuronal membrane appear to be crucial in this process. LTP is probably one of the major mechanism by which learning and memory consolidation takes place in the brain (Kandel et al., 2000).

Axonal and dendritic sprouting

The sprouting and elongation of new dendrites and axons is a common response to injury and cell loss at all levels in the nervous system. Sprouting can also be seen in response to increased functional demand, such as exposure to conditions requiring more complex motor activity (Kleim et al., 1996). Axons at the edges of a lesion send new axonal branches into the damaged area and re-innervate dendrites that have lost their synaptic input. This leads to new synaptic formation at the point of contact of axonal sprouts with these dendritic trees. This mechanism for recovery has been suggested in, for example, the reaction of the somatosensory cortex to loss of its input from the skin (Merzenich et al., 1984; Pons et al., 1991).

3.3 Targeted plasticity

The primary somatosensory-and motorcortex is organized somatotopically, where different body parts project to different parts of the primary somatosensory-and motor cortex (Figure 1). The somatotopic map does not represent the body in its actual proportions. Instead, larger cortical areas are being assigned to sensitive parts or parts with complex motor demands, such as the hands and face. The cortical representation of different body parts alters constantly, depending on the pattern of afferent nerve impulses, injury and increased or decreased use.

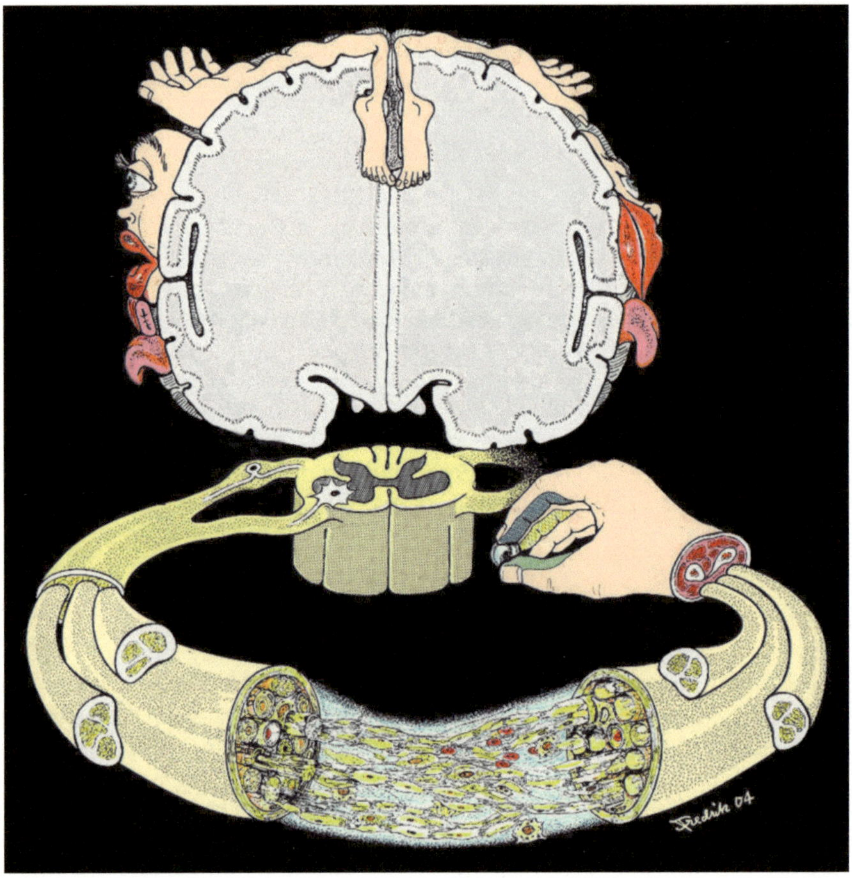

Fig. 1. Sensory information is sent from, in this case, the hand via the peripheral nerve to the dorsal root ganglia, spinal cord and thalamus to the primary somatosensory cortex. Motor information is sent from the primary motor cortex to the spinal cord and the effector muscles.

Both the primary somatosensory and motor cortex are arranged somatotopically. Thus in each hemisphere there is a complete somatotopic map of the body both in the primary somatosensory and motor cortex.

To utilize the central nervous systems' (CNS) ability to change for therapeutic purposes, guided plasticity is an attractive concept with promising results (Duffau, 2006). The potential for cerebral plasticity is, for example, used in treatment of patients to strengthen or promote CNS functions that are lost or weakened. The plastic potential of the brain might be guided using neurosurgical methods, rehabilitation and different pharmacological drugs in order to improve lost or damaged functions (Duffau, 2006). The use of neurosurgical methods is very complicated, sometimes including complex surgical interventions, which limit the usefulness. The use of potent drugs affecting the central nervous system, such as amphetamine (Walker-Batson et al., 2001) and norepinephrine (Plewnia et al., 2004), in order to improve recovery of damaged function, have been described. However, few patients currently benefit from such treatments due to incomplete knowledge of optimal treatment regimes and side effects from the drugs.

Our main objective when starting to develop a treatment regime for diabetic neuropathy was to look for a method more suitable for patient usage, giving a cortical deafferentation "large" enough to induce changes in peripheral function but not unnecessarily large. The method should also be safe with no side effects, pain free, and easy to us for both patient and therapist. Furthermore, it should be specific for sensory functions not affecting the motor function as this would affect the person's ability to perform motor tasks.

It is well known from animal and human experiments that temporary cutaneous anesthesia of one body part leads to cortical re-organization resulting in a corresponding silent area in the sensory cortex. This allows adjacent nearby body parts to rapidly expand at the expense of the silent cortical area this is likely mediated by unmasking of existing synapses.

The forearm is located next to the hand in the somatotopic map and by anaesthetizing the forearm, the cortical hand area can rapidly expand over the forearm area resulted in improved sensory function of the hand in healthy controls (Bjorkman et al., 2009). Thus, more nerve cells can be available for the hand, resulting in improved hand function. In a randomized, controlled trial, sensory re-learning in combination with cutaneous forearm anesthesia, using an anesthetic cream, EMLA® containing 2.5% lidocain and 2.5% prilokain, improved sensory function of the hand compared with sensory re-learning and placebo in patients with ulnar or median nerve repair (Rosen et al., 2006). The participants received treatment twice a week for two consecutive weeks, and the effects lasted 4 weeks after the last EMLA® treatment. These results suggest that sensory recovery is enhanced by temporary anesthesia of adjacent body parts. The long lasting effect indicates that this treatment is clinically useful and relevant.

Recently, the same principle of temporary cutaneous anesthesia as that used for the hand has been applied on the foot in uninjured subjects. In a randomized controlled trial, improvement in sensory function of the foot was observed after EMLA® treatment of the lower leg compared to placebo (Rosen et al., 2009).

There is no specific treatment for neuropathy in diabetes except a strict control of the glycaemic level. However, recent data in healthy subjects and diabetic patients show that the sensory function in the foot and hand, measured by the monofilament test, can be improved by using the central nervous systems ability to change, i.e. brain plasticity. In a recent double blind randomized placebo controlled study male (n=26) or female (n=5) diabetic patients with type 1 (n=30) or type 2 (n=7) with a median duration of diabetes of 35 years, all with insulin treated diabetes, were either treated with EMLA® cream or placebo cream applied to the skin of the lower leg for 1.5 hours (n=18 and n=19, respectively). All the subjects in the EMLA® group with pre-treatment diminished protective sensibility at the first metatarsal head showed improved touch threshold below limits for protective sensibility after 1.5 and 24 hours, while no such changes were observed after the treatment with placebo cream (Fig 2).

Furthermore, the touch thresholds improved at four other assessment sites (third metatarsal head, fifth metatarsal head, pulp of big toe and central of heal) together with increased vibration threshold at 125 Hz. However, the patients observed no subjective improvement, based on examination with a visual analogue scale, after treatment. This new strategy to improve the thresholds of touch creates new possibilities to treat disturbances in sensation of the diabetic foot. Hypothetically, the local anaesthetic cream results in a deafferentation of the lower leg in the primary somatosensory cortex, which allows the foot to expand. Thus, more nerve cells are available for the foot resulting in the observed improved sensory function.

A challenge is to create a long lasting improvement of the sensory function. Studies using cutaneous anaesthesia in the upper extremity in patients with nerve injuries and neuropathy have shown that a lasing improvement of sensibility is possible using repeated sessions with cutaneous anaesthesia (Rosen et al., 2008; Rosen et al., 2006).

In conclusion, treatment of diabetic neuropathy is complicated. However, new knowledge on the effect of a peripheral nerve injury and neuropathy on the central nervous system opens new perspectives to treat neuropathy by targeted plasticity. Cutaneous anaesthesia of the lower leg in diabetic patients is a good example of how targeted plasticity is used in order to improve foot sensibility in patients with diabetic neuropathy. The method is simple, safe, and cost-effective, although future studies are needed to work out the optimal treatment regime for a long lasting or permanent improvement in sensibility.

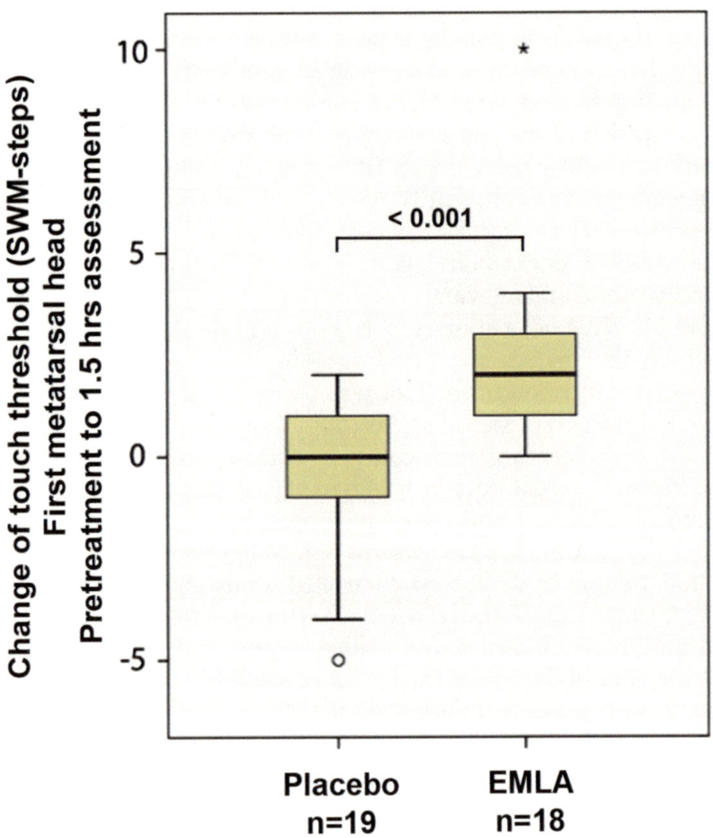

Fig. 2. Change of touch threshold in first metatarsal head in diabetic patients between pre-treatment and after 1.5 h of EMLA® treatment compared with placebo ($P < 0.001$).

4. Acknowledgement

The studies on diabetic neuropathy from our group was supported by the Swedish Research Council (Medicine), Crafoord's Fund for Medical Research, Svenska Diabetesförbundet, Diabetesföreningen Malmö, Konsul Thure Carlsson Fund for Medical Research, Region

Skåne, Stiftelsen Sigurd och Elsa Goljes Minne and Funds from the University Hospital Malmö, Sweden.

5. References

Abbott, CA., Chaturvedi, N., Malik, RA., Salgami, E., Yates, AP., Pemberton, PW., & Boulton, AJ. (2010). Explanations for the lower rates of diabetic neuropathy in Indian Asians versus Europeans. *Diabetes Care,* Vol. 33, No. 6, pp 1325-1330

Apelqvist, J., Larsson, J., & Agardh, C.D. (1993). Long-term prognosis for diabetic patients with foot ulcers. *Journal of Internal Medicine,* Vol. 233, No. 6, pp 485-491

Bavelier, D., & Neville, HJ. (2002). Cross-modal plasticity: where and how? *Nat Rev Neurosci,* Vol. 3, No. 6, pp 443-452

Bengtsson, L., Jonsson, M., & Apelqvist, J., (2008). Wound-related pain is underestimated in patients with diabetic foot ulcers. *Journal of Wound Care,* Vol. 17, No. 10, pp 433-435

Bjorkman, A., Weibull, A., Rosen, B., Svensson, J., & Lundborg, G. (2009). Rapid cortical reorganisation and improved sensitivity of the hand following cutaneous anaesthesia of the forearm. *European Journal of Neuroscience,* Vol. 29, No. 4, pp 837-844

Bril, V., Hirose, T., Tomioka, S., Buchanan, R., & Ranirestat Study Group. (2009). Ranirestat for the management of diabetic sensorimotor polyneuropathy. *Diabetes Care,* Vol. 32, No. 7, pp 1256-1260

Calford, M. (1991). Neurobiology. Curious cortical change. *Nature,* Vol. 352, No. 6338, pp 759-760

Calford, MB., & Tweedale, R. (1990). Interhemispheric transfer of plasticity in the cerebral cortex. *Science,* Vol. 249, pp 805-807

Chen, R., Cohen, LG., & Hallett, M. (2002). Nervous system reorganization following injury. *Neuroscience,* Vol. 111, No. 4, pp 761-773

Dahlin, LB., Archer, DR., & McLean, WG. (1987). Treatment with an aldose reductase inhibitor can reduce the susceptibility of fast axonal transport following nerve compression in the streptozotocin-diabetic rat. *Diabetologia,* Vol. 30, pp 414-418

Dahlin, LB., Granberg, V., Rolandsson, O., Rosen, I., & Dahlin, E. (2011). Disturbed vibrotactile sense in finger pulps in patients with type 1 diabetes - correlations with glycaemic level, clinical examination and electrophysiology. *Diabetic Medicine,* Vol. In press

Dahlin, LB., Meiri, KF., McLean, WG., Rydevik, B., & Sjöstrand, J. (1986). Effects of nerve compression on fast axonal transport in streptozotocin-induced diabetes mellitus. *Diabetologia,* Vol. 29, pp 181-185

Dahlin, LB., Thrainsdottir, S., Cederlund, R., Thomsen, NO., Eriksson, KF., Rosen, I., Speidel, T., & Sundqvist, G. (2008). Vibrotactile sense in median and ulnar nerve innervated fingers of men with Type 2 diabetes, normal or impaired glucose tolerance. *Diabetic Medicine,* Vol. 25, No. 5, pp 543-549

Donoghue, JP., Hess, G., & Sanes, JN. Motor cortical substrates and mechanisms for learning. In: Bloedel JR, Ebner, T.J., Wise, S.P. (ed). *Acquisition of Motor Behaviour in Vertebrates.* Cambridge, MA: MIT; 1996. pp. 363-386.

Duffau, H. (2006). Brain plasticity: from pathophysiological mechanisms to therapeutic applications. *J Clin Neurosci,* Vol. 13, No. 9, pp 885-897

Dyck, PJ., Kratz, KM., Karnes, JL., Litchy, WJ., Klein, R., Pach, JM., Wilson, DM., O'Brien, PC.,

Melton, LJ., 3rd, & Service, FJ. (1993). The prevalence by staged severity of various types of diabetic neuropathy, retinopathy, and nephropathy in a population-based cohort: the Rochester Diabetic Neuropathy Study. *Neurology,* Vol. 43, No. 4, pp 817-824

Edmonds, ME, (2004). The diabetic foot, 2003. *Diabetes/Metabolism Research and Reviews,* Vol. 20 Suppl 1, pp S9-S12

Gizewski, ER., Gasser, T., de Greiff A., Boehm, A., & Forsting, M. (2003). Cross-modal plasticity for sensory and motor activation patterns in blind subjects. *Neuroimage,* Vol. 19, No. 3, pp 968-975

Hotta, N., Kawamori, R., Atsumi, Y., Baba, M., Kishikawa, H., Nakamura, J., Oikawa, S., Yamada, N., Yasuda, H., & Shigeta, Y.; ADCT Study Group. (2008). Stratified analyses for selecting appropriate target patients with diabetic peripheral neuropathy for long-term treatment with an aldose reductase inhibitor, epalrestat. *Diabetic Medicine,* Vol. 25, No. 7, pp 818-825

Jones, EG. (1993). GABAergic neurons and their role in cortical plasticity in primates. *Cerebral Cortex,* Vol. 3, No. 5, pp 361-372

Kaas, J. (1991). Plasticity of sensory and motor maps in adult mammals. *Ann Rev neurosci,* Vol. 14, pp 137-168.

Kaas, JH., Merzenich, MM., Killackey, HP. (1983). The reorganization of somatosensory cortex following peripheral nerve damage in adult and developing mammals. *Annual Review of Neuroscience,* Vol. 6, pp 325-356

Kandel, ER., Schwartz, JH., & Jessel, TM. *Principles of neural science.* McGraw-Hill; 2000.

Kleim JA, Lussnig E, Schwarz ER *et al.,* (1996). Synaptogenesis and Fos expression in the motor cortex of the adult rat after motor skill learning. *Journal of Neuroscience,* Vol. 16, No. 14, pp 4529-4535

Lehtinen, JM., Uusitupa, M., Siitonen, O. & Pyorala, K. (1989). Prevalence of neuropathy in newly diagnosed NIDDM and nondiabetic control subjects. *Diabetes,* Vol. 38, No. 10, pp 1307-1313

Londahl, M., Katzman, P., Hammarlund, C., Nilsson, A., & Landin-Olsson, M. (2010). Relationship between ulcer healing after hyperbaric oxygen therapy and transcutaneous oximetry, toe blood pressure and ankle-brachial index in patients with diabetes and chronic foot ulcers. *Diabetologia,* Vol. 54, No. 1, pp 65-68

Lundborg, G., Rosén, B., & Lindberg, S. (1999). Hearing as substitution for sensation - a new principle for artificial sensibility. *J Hand Surg,* Vol. 24A, pp 219-224

Malik, RA., Tesfaye, S., Thompson, SD., Veves, A., Sharma, AK., Boulton, AJ., & Ward, JD. (1993). Endoneurial localisation of microvascular damage in human diabetic neuropathy. *Diabetologia,* Vol. 36, No. 5, pp 454-459

Merzenich, MM., Kaas, JH., Wall, RJ., Nelson, M., Sur, D., & Felleman, D. (1983). Topographic reorganization of somatosensory cortical areas 3B and 1 in adult monkeys following restricted deafferentation. *Neuroscience,* Vol. 8, pp 33-55

Merzenich, MM., Nelson, RJ., KaasJH., Stryker, MP., Jenkins, WM., Zook, JM., Cynader, MS., & Schoppmann, A. (1987). Variability in hand surface representations in areas 3 b and 1 in adult own and squirrel monkeys. *Journal of Comparative Neurology,* Vol. 258, pp 281-297

Merzenich, MM., Nelson, RJ., Stryker, MS., Cynader, MS., Schoppmann, A., & Zook, JM. (1984). Somatosensory cortical map changes following digit amputation in adult monkeys. *Journal of Comparative Neurology,* Vol. 224, pp 591-605

Mondelli, M., Padua, L., Reale, F., Signorini, AM., & Romano, C. (2004). Outcome of surgical release among diabetics with carpal tunnel syndrome. *Archives of Physical Medicine and Rehabilitation,* Vol. 85, No. 1, pp 7-13

Oates, PJ. (2008). Aldose reductase, still a compelling target for diabetic neuropathy. *Curr Drug Targets,* Vol. 9, No. 1, pp 14-36,1873-5592 (Electronic) 1389-4501 (Linking).

Ozkul, Y., Sabuncu, T., Kocabey, Y., & Nazligul, Y. (2002). Outcomes of carpal tunnel release in diabetic and non-diabetic patients. *Acta Neurologica Scandinavica,* Vol. 106, No. 3, pp 168-172

Perkins, BA., & Krolewski, AS. (2005). Early nephropathy in type 1 diabetes: a new perspective on who will and who will not progress. *Curr Diab Rep,* Vol. 5, No. 6, pp 455-463,

Perkins, BA., Olaleye, D., & Brilm, V. (2002). Carpal tunnel syndrome in patients with diabetic polyneuropathy. *Diabetes Care,* Vol. 25, No. 3, pp 565-569

Plewnia, C., Hoppe, J., Cohen, LG., & Gerloff, C. (2004). Improved motor skill acquisition after selective stimulation of central norepinephrine. *Neurology,* Vol. 62, No. 11, pp 2124-2126

Pons, T., Preston, E., & Garraghty K, (1991). Massive cortical reorganization after sensory deafferentation in adult macaques. *Science,* Vol. 252, pp 1857-1860

Prompers, L., Huijberts, M., Schaper, N., Apelqvist, J., Bakker, K., Edmonds, M., Holstein, P., Jude, E., Jirkovska, A., Mauricio, D., Piaggesi, A., Reike, H., Spraul, M., Van Acker, K., Van Baal, S., Van Merode, F., Uccioli, L., Urbancic, V., & Ragnarson Tennvall, G. (2008). Resource utilisation and costs associated with the treatment of diabetic foot ulcers. Prospective data from the Eurodiale Study. *Diabetologia,* Vol. 51, No. 10, pp 1826-1834

Purves, D., Augustine, GJ., Fitzpatrick, D., Hall, WC., La Mantia AS., McNamara JO., & Williams SM. *Neuroscience (Sinauer Associates Inc. Sunderland, MA, USA, third edition).* 2004.

Rosen, B., Bjorkman A, & Lundborg G, (2008). Improved hand function in a dental hygienist with neuropathy induced by vibration and compression: The effect of cutaneous anaesthetic treatment of the forearm. *Scandinavian Journal of Plastic and Reconstructive Surgery and Hand Surgery,* Vol. 42, No. 1, pp 51-53

Rosen, B., Bjorkman, A., & Lundborg, G. (2006). Improved sensory relearning after nerve repair induced by selective temporary anaesthesia - a new concept in hand rehabilitation. *Journal of Hand Surgery British Volume,* Vol. 31, No. 2, pp 126-132

Rosen, B., Bjorkman, A., Weibull, A., Svensson, J., & Lundborg, G. (2009). Improved sensibility of the foot after temporary cutaneous anesthesia of the lower leg. *Neuroreport,* Vol. 20, No. 1, pp 37 41

Rubino, A., Rousculp, MD., Davis, K., Wang, J., Bastyr, EJ., & Tesfaye, S. (2007). Diagnosis of diabetic peripheral neuropathy among patients with type 1 and type 2 diabetes in France, Italy, Spain, and the United Kingdom. *Prim Care Diabetes,* Vol. 1, No. 3, pp 129-134

Schemmel, KE., Padiyara, RS., & D'Souza, JJ. (2010). Aldose reductase inhibitors in the treatment of diabetic peripheral neuropathy: a review. *Journal of Diabetes and Its Complications,* Vol. 24, No. 5, pp 354-360,1873-460X (Electronic) 1056-8727 (Linking).

Thomsen, NO., Cederlund, R., Rosen, I., Bjork, J., & Dahlin, LB. (2009). Clinical outcomes of surgical release among diabetic patients with carpal tunnel syndrome: prospective follow-up with matched controls. *J Hand Surg Am,* Vol. 34, No. 7, pp 1177-1187

Walker-Batson, D., Curtis, S., Natarajan, R., Ford, J., Dronkers, N., Salmeron, E., Lai, J., & Unwin, DH. (2001). A double-blind, placebo-controlled study of the use of amphetamine in the treatment of aphasia. *Stroke,* Vol. 32, No. 9, pp 2093-2098,1524-4628 (Electronic).

Wall PD. (1977). The presence of ineffective synapses and the circumstances which unmask them. *Philosophical Transactions of the Royal Society of London Series B: Biological Sciences,* Vol. 278, No. 961, pp 361-372

Young, TK., & Harris, SB, (1994). Risk of clinical diabetes in a northern Native Canadian cohort. *Arctic Medical Research,* Vol. 53, No. 2, pp 64-70

2

Sonographic Imaging of the Peripheral Nerves in Patients with Type 2 Diabetes Mellitus

Tsuneo Watanabe, Shin-ichi Kawachi[1] and Toshio Matsuoka
Department of Sports Medicine and Sports Science,
Gifu University Graduate School of Medicine
[1]Departments of Diabetes and Endocrinology,
Gifu University Graduate School of Medicine
Japan

1. Introduction

The World Health Organization estimates that more than 220 million people worldwide have diabetes mellitus (DM). This figure is estimated to more than double by 2030 (Wild et al., 2004). In Japan, the number of diabetic patients has increased to 8 million, and it is assumed that 35% to 45% of diabetic patients have diabetic symmetric polyneuropathy (DPN). Advanced DPN causes serious complications, such as diabetic foot ulcers, gangrene, and Charcot joint, all of which worsen the quality of life of diabetic patients (Ogawa et al., 2006). Therefore, early detection of nerve dysfunction is important to provide appropriate care for patients with DPN (Chudzik et al., 2007). The diagnosis of diabetic neuropathy is based primarily on characteristic symptoms and is confirmed with nerve conduction studies (NCS), which are time-consuming, slightly invasive, and occasionally not well tolerated for repeated evaluations (Colak et al., 2007). In contrast, ultrasonographic examinations can be performed to assess peripheral nerves with less discomfort and have already been used for the evaluation of several disorders of the peripheral nervous system such as carpal tunnel syndrome (Wiesler et al., 2006a; Abe et al., 2004; Jayaraman et al., 2004; Duncan et al., 1999; Lee et al., 1999), cubital tunnel syndrome (Okamoto et al., 2000; Wiesler et al., 2006b), and traumatic nerve lesions (Cartwright., 2007; Peer et al., 2001). High-resolution diagnostic ultrasonography (US) has improved greatly, allowing for evaluation of minute peripheral nerves (Fornage., 1993; Solbiati et al., 1985). We previously showed that the cross-sectional area (CSA) of the median nerve in the carpal tunnel of patients with DPN is greater than that of controls and correlates with NCS (Watanabe et al., 2009). Furthermore, it appears that the percentage of the hypoechoic area of the peripheral nerves was significantly greater in patients with lower motor nerve conduction velocity (MCV) and DM than in controls or patients with higher MCV and DM (Watanabe et al., 2010).
The purpose of this chapter is to review the current knowledge regarding the overview and diagnosis of the most common forms of neuropathy in type 2 DM. Furthermore, our current sonographic technique and preliminary studies are presented for some cases. In this chapter,

we focus mainly on a simple and noninvasive approach to the evaluation of peripheral nerves in patients with type 2 DM. Although the exact mechanisms contributing to our study have not been clearly identified and are not the main focus of this chapter, they will be discussed in brief.

2. Clinical aspects of diabetic neuropathy

Diabetic neuropathy is a neuropathic disorder that is associated with DM. This condition is thought to result from both diabetic microvascular injury involving small blood vessels that supply nerves and macrovascular conditions that can culminate in DM. More than 80% of patients with clinical diabetic neuropathy have a distal, symmetrical form of the disorder (Said., 2007). In general, the symptoms included numbness, burning feet, pins-and-needles sensations, and lightning pains. These symptoms start in the feet go on to affect more proximal parts of the lower limbs, and eventually affect the distal parts of the upper limbs.
The unified clinical criteria and classification for DPN do not represent the international standard because the causes of peripheral nerve disorders associated with DM are complex and probably involve a variety of causative mechanisms. In this chapter, DPN is classified into 3 groups (hyperglycemic neuropathy, symmetric polyneuropathy, and focal and multifocal neuropathy) according to the classification of the Thomas et al (1997). This classfication is the easiest. The most common of these groups seen in the clinical setting is symmetric distal polyneuropathy.

3. Pathology of diabetic neuropathy

Abnormalities reported in diabetic neuropathy include axonal degeneration in nerve fibers, primary demyelination resulting from Schwann cell dysfunction, secondary segmental demyelination related to impairment of axonal control of myelination, remyelination, proliferation of Schwann cells, atrophy of denervated bands of Schwann cells, onion-bulb formations, and hypertrophy of the basal lamina. Early morphological changes include minimal alteration of myelinated and unmyelinated fibers and axonal regeneration (Yagihashi et al., 2007; Said et al., 2007).
The pathophysiology of DPN is multifactorial and involves genetic, environmental, behavioral, metabolic, neurotrophic, and vascular factors (Vink et al., 1999; Oates, 2002; Vincent, et al., 2002; Perkins, et al., 2003). The vascular concept of peripheral diabetic neuropathy implies that diabetes-induced endothelial dysfunction with a resultant decrease in nerve blood flow, vascular reactivity, and endoneurial hypoxia plays a key role in functional and morphological changes in the diabetic nerve (Cameron et al., 2001). Endothelial changes in the vasa nervorum have been attributed to multiple mechanisms, including increased aldose reductase activity, nonenzymatic glycation and glycoxidation, activation of protein kinase C, oxidative–nitrosative stress, and changes in arachidonic acid and prostaglandin metabolism (Cameron et al., 2001). The complex and interrelated effects of hyperglycemia include increased metabolic flux through the polyol pathway with consequent sorbitol and fructose accumulation and reduced sodium-potassium ATPase levels, altered fatty acid metabolism, alterations in the redox state, reduced myoinositol and sodium-potassium ATPase activity, accumulation of advanced glycated end products, accelerated neuronal apoptosis, immunological alterations, changes in blood flow, and

increased oxidative stresses. The exact mechanisms of DPN are uncertain, but may involve activation of the polyol pathway due to hyperglycemia; the polyol pathway is considered to play a major role in diabetic neuropathy (Greene, et al., 1987). Excellent reviews of this information are available in previous publications.

4. NCS

Diagnosis of DPN on clinical grounds alone is not accurate, and it is difficult to detect small alterations in neuropathies (Feldman et al, 1994; Perkins et al, 2001). Therefore, as a surrogate measure, NCS are widely used as an evaluation of DPN. NCS measure the ability of peripheral nerves to conduct electrical signals, and this ability is impaired when pathological changes are present in the myelin, nodes of Ranvier, and axons. Routine NCS include evaluation of the motor function of the median, ulnar, peroneal, and tibial nerves, and evaluation of the sensory function of the median, ulnar, radial, and sural nerves. Velocities are universally reported in meters per second, motor amplitudes in millivolts, and sensory amplitudes in microvolts. These measurements of upper- and lower-limb motor and sensory nerve functions show the presence, distribution, and severity of peripheral nerve disease (Albers, et al., 1995).

The attribution of peripheral nerve dysfunction to either primary demyelination or primary axonal loss is usually based on nerve conduction velocity and action potential amplitude data. In general, demyelination is indicated by a decreased nerve conduction velocity, conduction block, or increased temporal dispersion, whereas axonal loss is indicated by a reduction in the amplitude or area of the sensory nerve action potential (SNAP) or compound muscle action potential (CMAP). However, there has been considerable disagreement in terms of the clinical and the electrophysiological criteria for the diagnosis of DPN.

Recently, various calculated indices such as the residual latency, terminal latency index, and modified F-wave ratio were introduced as more sensitive electrophysiological tools than a conventional NCS in patients with diverse types of peripheral neuropathies (Attarian et al, 2001; Kaplan, et al, 1978; Radziwill et al, 2003).

5. Sonography

5.1 Sonographic features of normal peripheral nerves

US is a widely utilized diagnostic tool for gynecological purposes and examinations of the heart and intra-abdominal and superficial organs. With the advancement of sonographic resolution, normal peripheral nerves also can be clearly demonstrated. US is a useful technique for the investigation of a number of musculoskeletal disorders. Although US has the well-known advantages of low cost, accessibility, portability, noninvasiveness, and multiplanar imaging, one of its most important diagnostic advantages over other techniques is considered to be its real-time imaging capability, allowing for dynamic evaluation of the musculoskeletal field (Khoury et al., 2007).

US can be used to determine the location, extent, type of lesion as well as the presence of nerve swelling and inflammation. Major peripheral nerves in the extremities, such as the median, ulnar, radial, sciatic, and posterior tibial nerves can be seen using conventional US performed with 5- to 12-MHz probes (Stokvis et al., 2009). In controls, peripheral nerves are seen as hypoechoic neuronal fascicles surrounded by echogenic connective tissue (Silvestri et al., 1995). The basic units of the peripheral nerve consist of a neural fiber embedded in the endoneurium. Because the endoneurium is too thin to reflect the sound beam, it is hypoechogenic on the US scan. The neural fascicle consists of several neural fibers and is embedded in a capsule called the perineurium. This capsule consists of connective tissue, vessels, and lymphatic ducts and is thick enough to reflect the sound beam, resulting in hyperechoic lines on the US scan. The trunk of the peripheral nerve consists of several neural fascicles and is embedded in a thicker membrane called the epineurium, which is seen as bold echogenic lines on the US. Therefore, a peripheral nerve is seen as several parallel hyperechoic lines and bold hypoechoic lines on longitudinal images and as a faveolate pattern on transverse images (Fig 1).

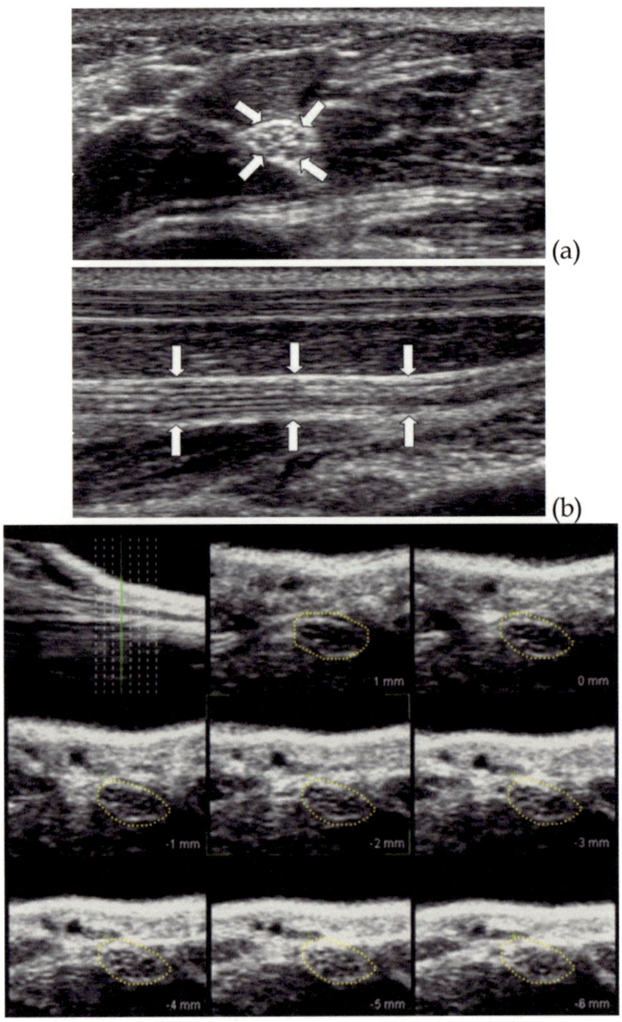

Fig. 1. Sonographic imaging of the median nerve. Transverse sonogram of the median nerve in 5cm proximal to the wrist (a), and longitudinal sonogram of the median nerve (b). Multi-slice views using three-dimensional volumetric ultrasonography images (c). The transverse planes at continuous segment of the median nerves are visualized.

5.2 Sonographic features of the peripheral nerves in patients with type 2 DM

We previuosly reported that peripheral nerves in patients with low MCV and type 2 DM showed enlarged and hypoechoic patterns as compared with those of controls or patients with high MCV and type 2 DM. There are 2 sonographic methods of measuring nerve CSA: the indirect method (ellipsoid formula) and direct method (tracing). Recently, Alemán et al.(2008) reported that median nerve CSA measurements are reproducible by either the direct or indirect method when a standardized ultrasonographic examination protocol is applied. Sernik et al. (2008) also reported a high correlation (r = 0.99) between the areas calculated by the indirect and direct methods.

In patients with DPN, peripheral nerves showed enlarged and hypoechoic patterns. Figure 2 shows sonographic images of several nerves in the controls and in patients with type 2 DM. The CSAs of the median, ulnar, and tibial nerves in patients with DM were significantly larger than those in controls. It is likely that these findings reflect the pathological changes, although the pathogenesis of nerve enlargement and increased percentage of the hypoechoic area in peripheral nerves is uncertain because our study did not include histological evidence. In a 1H-nuclear magnetic resonance study, Suzuki et al. (1994) reported that sorbitol and the sodium accumulation caused by an increase in sorbitol may be major contributors to the increase in intracellular hydration. It has further been hypothesized that peripheral nerves are swollen in individuals with DM because of increased water content related to an increase in the aldose reductase-mediated conversion of glucose to sorbitol. We hypothesize that the increase in the hypoechoic area of peripheral nerves in diabetic patients may be because of increased water content, which is also a cause of enlargement of peripheral nerves.

5.3 Assessment of the internal echo of the peripheral nerves

The ultrasonographic images of the peripheral nerves were saved as JPEG files and transferred to a personal computer for analysis. The monochrome US image was quantized to 8 bits (i.e., 256 gray levels). The brightness of the pixels ranged from 0 (black) to 255 (white). Histogram analysis in US has been expected to offer an objective index for estimating the echo intensity, such as in the diagnosis of fatty liver or hepatitis (Lee et al., 2006; Osawa et al., 1996). The region of interest was set to cover the entire nerve, excluding its hyperechoic rim. We used the percentage of the hypoechoic area as the index after the effects of gain shift on echo intensity in the median nerve were confirmed (Fig. 3).

The normal appearance of a peripheral nerve should be readily recognized. Peripheral nerves consist of multiple hypoechoic bands corresponding to neuronal fascicles, which are separated by hyperechoic lines that correspond to the epineurium. Thus, the value obtained by the discriminant analysis method of Otsu was used as a threshold level for the analysis of the percentage of the hypoechoic area because the echogenicity of peripheral nerves was obtained as a graded echo density from black to white. Otsu's method (1979), which selects a global threshold value by maximizing the separability of the classes in gray levels, is one of the better tequniques for image segmentation. Mathematically, this can be expressed as:

$$p_i = \frac{f_i}{N},\ p_i \geqq 0,\ \sum_{i=1}^{L} p_i = 1. \qquad (1)$$

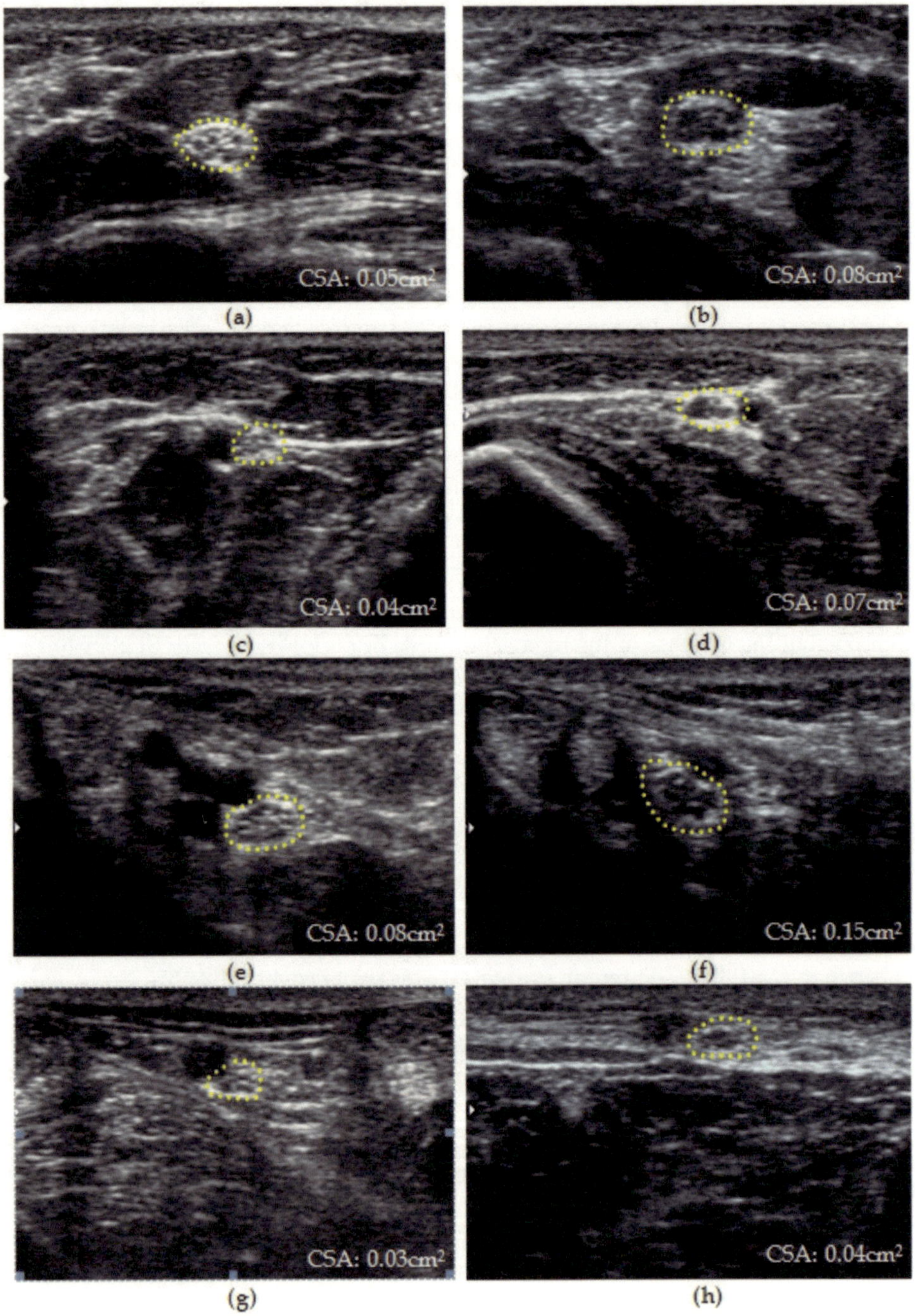

Fig. 2. Comparison of the nerves in controls and in diabetic patients. Transverse image of the median nerve in control' wrist (a), and in diabetic patient's wrist (b). Transverse image of the ulnar nerve in control' wrist (c), and in diabetic patient's wrist (d). Transverse image of the tibial nerve in control' ankle (e), and in diabetic patient's ankle (f). Transverse sonogram of the sural nerve in control' ankle (g), and in diabetic patient's ankle (h).

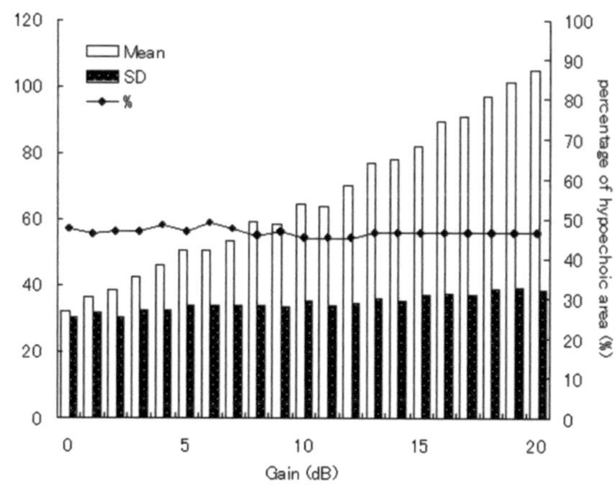

Fig. 3. The effects of the gain shift on the echo intensity in the median nerve. Open bars showed a change of mean, closed bars showed a change of SD, and solid line connecting solid circles showed a change of percentage according to the gain shift.

Assume that the image can be represented in L gray levels (1, 2,…, L). If the number of pixels at level i is denoted by f_i, then the total number of pixels equals $N = f_1 + f_2 + \ldots + f_L$. If an image can be divided into 2 classes (C_1 and C_2) by a threshold at level t, where class C_1 consists of gray levels from 0 to t, and class C_2 contains the other gray levels with $t + 1$ to L, then the cumulative probabilities (w_1 and w_2) and mean levels (μ_1 and μ_2) for classes C_1 and C_2, respectively, are given by

$$w_1 = \sum_{i=1}^{t} p_i , \qquad (2)$$

$$w_2 = \sum_{i=t+1}^{L} p_i , \qquad (3)$$

and

$$\mu_1 = \sum_{i=1}^{t} ip_i / w_1 , \qquad (4)$$

$$\mu_2 = \sum_{i=t+1}^{L} ip_i / w_2 . \qquad (5)$$

Otsu selects an optimal threshold t^* that maximizes the between-class variance σ_B^2 in Eq. (6) based on the discriminant analysis, where μ_T is the mean intensity of the image.

$$t^* = \arg_{1 \le t \le L} \max\{\sigma_B^2(t) \mid \sigma_B^2 = w_1(\mu_1 - \mu_T)^2 + w_2(\mu_2 - \mu_T)^2\} \qquad (6)$$

and

$$\mu_T = \sum_{i=1}^{L} i p_i . \tag{7}$$

The percentage of the hypoechoic area was studied using computer analysis. Using ImageJ software, the amount of the hypoechoic area falling below the threshold echo intensity was calculated. In our computerized method, the flowchart of the echo intensity evaluation process is demonstrated in Figure 4.

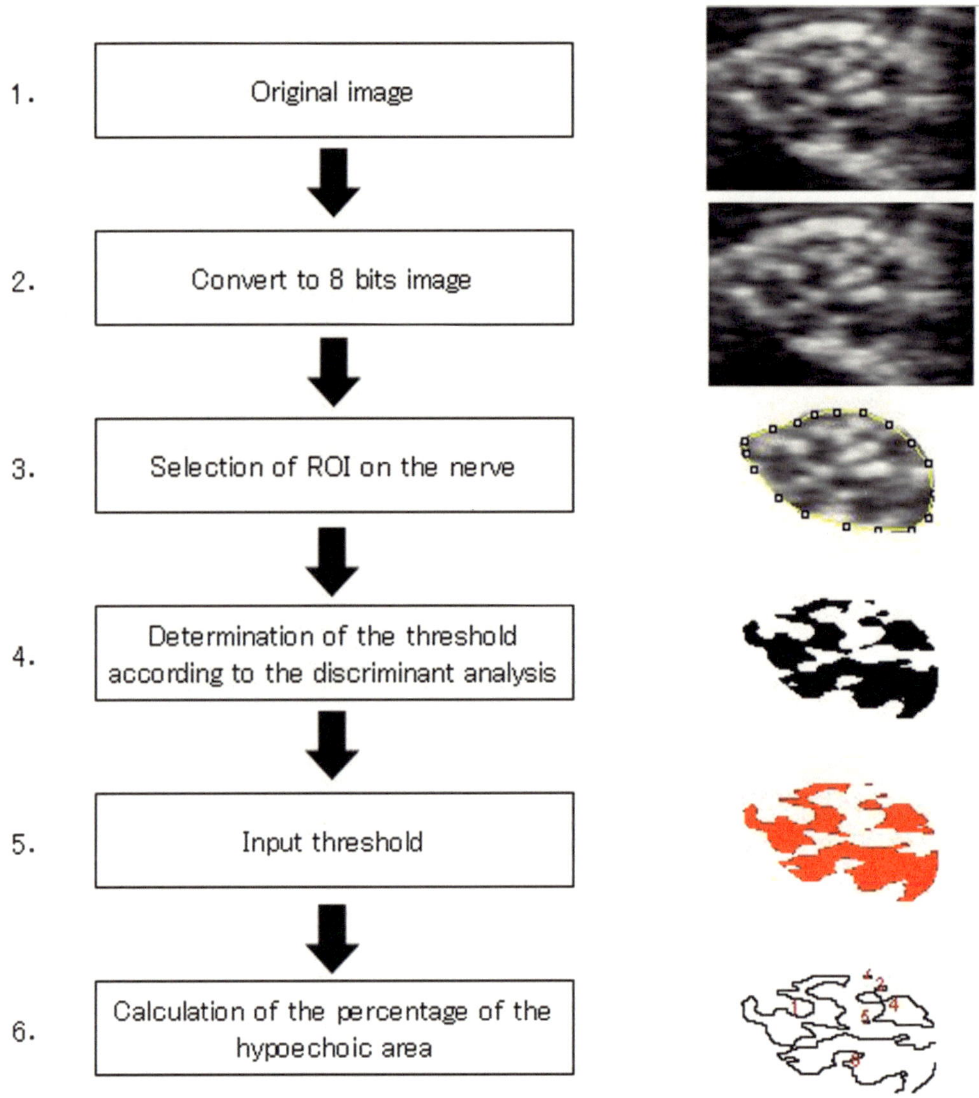

Fig. 4. Illustration of the working flow of the evaluation of the echo intensity.

Representative sonographic images and three-dimensional graphic using ImageJ software of diabetic patients and controls are shown in Fig 5.

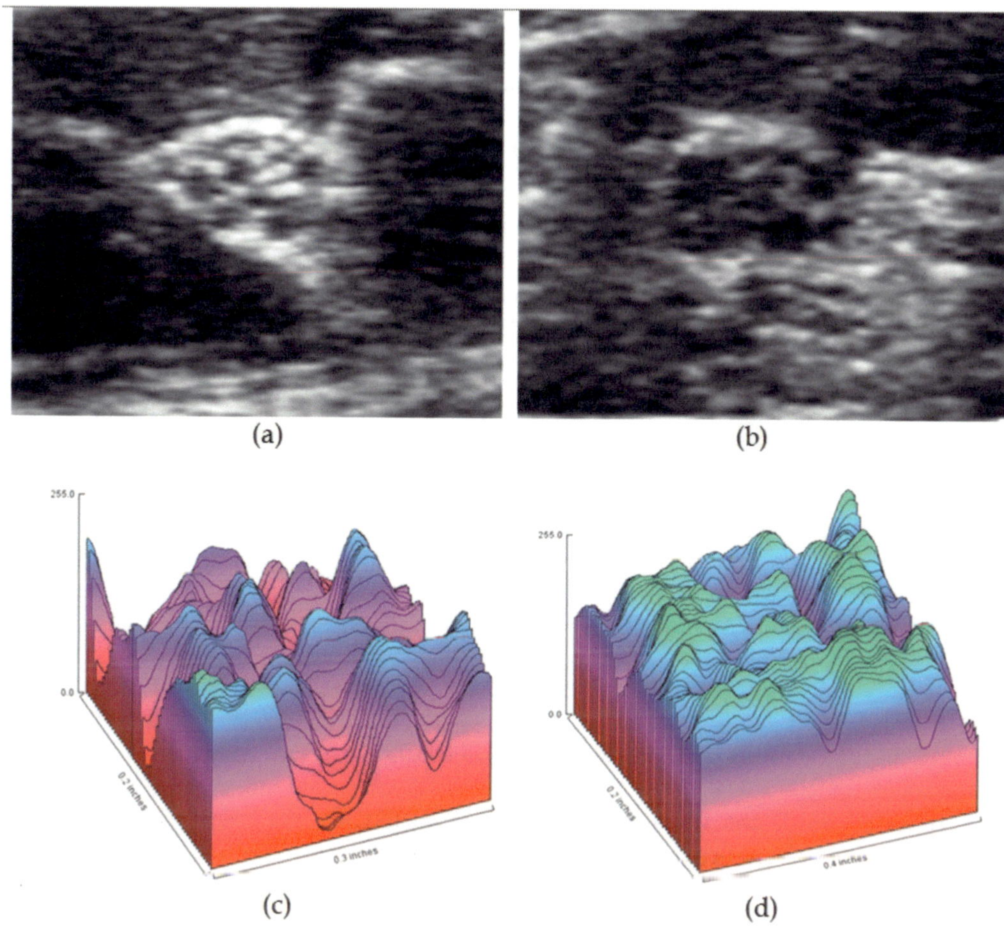

Fig. 5. Distributions of the echo intensity in the median nerve. Transverse sonogram of the median nerve in a control participant's wrist (a). Transverse sonogram of the median nerve in a diabetic patient's wrist (b).Three-dimensional graphic of the distribution of the echo intensity in the control's wrist (c). Three-dimensional graphic of the distribution of the echo intensity in the diabetic patient's wrist (d). Hypoechoic area was displayed "light blue", and hyperechoic area was displayed "pink".

6. Sonography and NCS in patients with type 2 DM

6.1 Relationship between sonography and NCS

We studied 144 peripheral nerves (40 median, 40 ulnar, 40 tibial, and 24 sural nerves) of 40 subjects who underwent both US and NCS (unpublished data). Overall, 20 type 2 diabetes patients [10 men and 10 women; age range, 50-88 years (mean, 68.5 ± 10.7 years)] and 20 healthy volunteers [12 men and 8 women; age range, 26-59 years (mean, 40.0 ± 12.3 years)] were enrolled in this study. All participants whose wrists had symptoms of carpal tunnel syndrome were excluded from the study. This study was approved by the Institutional Review Board of Gifu University Hospital, and informed consent was obtained from all participants.

Ultrasonographic examination was performed by a board-certified sonographer who was blinded to the knowledge of the electrodiagnostic results. A 6.0- to 14.0-MHz linear array probe was used (portable real-time apparatus: Aplio XG; Toshiba Medical Systems, Japan). All subjects were seated on the examination table with their arms on a pillow and fingers semi-extended during examination of the median or ulnar nerves, and in the prone position during examination of the tibial and sural nerves. The CSA of the median nerve was measured at the carpal tunnel (MA) and at 5 cm proximal to the wrist (MB). The CSA of the ulnar nerve was measured at 5 cm proximal to the wrist (UA). The CSA of the tibial nerve was measured at the posterior medial malleolus (TA). The CSA of the sural nerve was measured at the lower third of the crus (SA). US images were quantitatively analyzed using the ImageJ software (National Institutes of Health, USA). We evaluated the relationship between the US and NCS results.

Routine NCS were performed using conventional procedures and standard electromyography (Neuropack MEB-2200; Nihon Kohden Corp., Japan). All examinations were performed in a room with an ambient temperature of 25°C. The skin surface temperature in all cases was 31°C to 34°C. Mann-Whitney *U* test was used to compare data between the 2 groups. Pearson's correlation coefficients were used to investigate the correlation of CSA and the percentage of the hypoechoic area with several NCS parameters. Results are given as mean ± SD, and statistical significance was assessed at $P < 0.05$.

The US and NCS results of diabetic patients and controls are shown in Table 1. The CSAs in the patients with DM group were 0.13 ± 0.05 cm^2 in the MA, 0.09 ± 0.03 cm^2 in the MB, 0.0.7 ± 0.02 cm^2 in the UA, 0.18 ± 0.04 cm^2 in the TA, and 0.05 ± 0.01 cm^2 in the SA. The CSAs in the controls were 0.08 ± 0.02 cm^2 in the MA, 0.07 ± 0.02 cm^2 in the MB, 0.04 ± 0.01 cm^2 in the UA, 0.10 ± 0.03 cm^2 in the TA, and 0.04 ± 0.01 cm^2 in the SA. The CSAs was a significant increase in the diabetic patients compared with that in the controls, with the exception of the sural nerve. The percentage of the hypoechoic area was significantly increased in the diabetic patients compared with that in the controls ($P < 0.05$). The MCV and sensory nerve conduction velocity of all nerves in the diabetic patients showed a significant decrease compared with those in the controls ($P < 0.001$). The CMAP and SNAP of all nerves in the diabetic patients showed a significant decrease compared with those in the controls, with exception of the CMAPs of both the median and tibial nerves ($P < 0.001$). On the other hand, distal latency (DL) was significantly lesser in the diabetic patients than in the controls, with the exception of the sensory ulnar and motor tibial nerves.

The relationships between US findings and NCS parameters are shown in Figure 6. The motor DL period of the median nerve was divided into 3 groups: DL of <3.5 ms; DL of 3.5 to 4.0 ms; and DL of >4.0 ms. The MCV of the median nerve was also divided into 3 groups: MCV of <50 m/s; MCV = 50 to 55 m/s; and MCV of >55 m/s. The categorization of subjects into tertiles of DL yielded 3 separate groups. Compared with the first tertile, the CSAs of the median nerve increased significantly with each tertile. Moreover, after combining tertiles of DL and MCV, even more comprehensive CSA stratification was possible, with all-cause CSA ranging from 0.07 cm^2 in subjects in the lowest tertile of both parameters to 0.17 cm^2 in subjects in the highest tertile (Fig. 6a). The hypoechoic area of the median nerve also increased significantly with each tertile. The hypoechoic area of the median nerve stratification was 52.5% in subjects in the highest tertile of both parameters (Fig. 6b). These results correlated with the electrophysiological severity.

Parameters	Nerve	Controls	Patients with type 2 DM
Sonographic measurements (CSA)			
MA (cm²)	*Median*	0.08 ± 0.02	0.13 ± 0.05***
MB (cm²)	*Median*	0.07 ± 0.02	0.09 ± 0.03**
UA (cm²)	*Ulnar*	0.04 ± 0.01	0.07 ± 0.02***
TA (cm²)	*Tibial*	0.10 ± 0.03	0.18 ± 0.04***
SA (cm²)	*Sural*	0.04 ± 0.01	0.05 ± 0.01
Sonographic measurements (echo intensity)			
MB (%)	*Median*	43.7 ± 5.1	50.0 ± 9.3*
UA (%)	*Ulnar*	43.6 ± 4.1	49.6 ± 10.6*
TA (%)	*Tibial*	44.8 ± 4.5	51.4 ± 7.5*
SA (%)	*Sural*	40.4 ±7.1	48.8 ± 3.7*
Electrophysiologic measurements			
MCV (m/s)	*Median*	59.9 ± 4.4	50.7 ± 5.7***
DL (ms)	*Median*	3.3 ± 0.5	4.5 ± 1.3***
CMAP (mV)	*Median*	11.2 ± 3.7	11.6 ± 4.4
SCV (m/s)	*Median*	69.1 ± 8.6	57.3 ± 5.7***
DL (ms)	*Median*	2.7 ± 0.4	3.3 ± 0.4***
SNAP (uV)	*Median*	38.3 ±11.7	12.5 ± 8.3***
MCV (m/s)	*Ulnar*	64.7± 6.1	52.1± 6.7***
DL (ms)	*Ulnar*	2.5 ± 0.4	2.9 ± 0.5*
CMAP (mV)	*Ulnar*	14.9 ± 3.8	9.4 ± 2.5***
SCV (m/s)	*Ulnar*	72.0 ± 5.4	61.7 ± 10.5***
DL (ms)	*Ulnar*	3.3 ± 0.7	3.9 ± 0.8
SNAP (uV)	*Ulnar*	20.4 ± 10.0	6.3 ± 2.9***
MCV (m/s)	*Tibial*	49.4 ± 2.4	40.3 ± 5.1***
DL (ms)	*Tibial*	3.9 ± 0.5	4.4 ± 0.9
CMAP (mV)	*Tibial*	16.1 ± 5.3	13.1 ± 6.9
SCV (m/s)	*Sural*	55.7± 2.5	49.1± 5.3***
DL (ms)	*Sural*	2.5 ± 0.1	2.9 ± 0.3***
SNAP (uV)	*Sural*	10.3± 4.1	3.6 ± 2.5***

Table 1. US and NCS measurements of controls and patients with type 2 DM (unpublished data).

Mann-Whitney U test: *P<0.05 versus controls; **P<0.01 versus controls; ***P<0.001 versus controls.

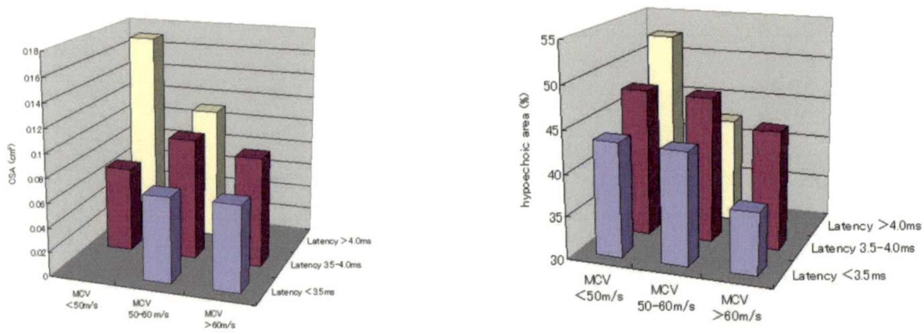

(a) (b)

Fig. 6. Relationships of between US and NCS parameters in the median nerve. Stratification of CSA by combining tertiles of DL and MCV (a). Stratification of hypoechoic area by combining tertiles of DL and MCV (b).

6.2 Comparison of diagnostic ability between US and NCS parameters

NCS are widely used for the diagnosis of DPN. The examinations are deemed to be objective, reliable, and sensitive, and can be used as statistical instruments or surrogate endpoints for neuropathy in large clinical investigations of DPN (Diabetes Control and Complications Trial Research Group., 1995; Cornblath et al., 1999; Dyck et al., 1991). NCS have also been recommended in the medical literature as the "gold standard" with which to evaluate and validate other screening tests that are used to diagnose peripheral neuropathy. We aimed to determine the best diagnostic criterion for diagnosing DPN by US and NCS. A receiver operating characteristic (ROC) curve was generated for each parameter in the US and NCS examinations, and areas under the curve (AUC) were determined. The ROC curves are plots of the true-positive rate (sensitivity) against the false-positive rate (1.0 - specificity) for the different possible cutoff points of a diagnostic test. To determine the accuracy of detection of DPN, we calculated and compared the sensitivity and specificity of both US and NCS.

In our preliminary study, the CSA at TA in the tibial nerve had the best diagnostic accuracy for DPN of all the sonographic examinations. The ROC curves of the CSA at TA revealed that the AUC was 0.919 ($P < 0.001$) with an optimal cutoff value of 0.145 cm^2, yielding 80% sensitivity and 94% specificity. For the NCS, the SNAPs had the best diagnostic accuracy for DPN; each nerve had an extremely high AUC (median nerve, 0.971; ulnar nerve, 0.944; and sural nerve, 0.938; $P < 0.001$). These cutoffs also yielded very good sensitivity (93% - 94%) and specificity (80% to 92%). Some investigators have reported that sural nerve dysfunction is the most common indicator of peripheral nerve dysfunction, is the first to be affected, and correlates most closely with the neuropathological findings (Dyck et al., 1985; Dyck., 1988; Redmond et al., 1992). Dyck et al. (1985) found that the peroneal motor nerve had the highest degree of abnormality, followed by the sural, median sensory, and median motor nerves. Karsidag et al. (2005) also reported that the most affected nerves were the sural sensory, peroneal motor, posterior tibial motor, median motor, ulnar motor, median sensory, and ulnar sensory nerves. In our study, the sural nerve had a high AUG, as reported in previous reports. Furthermore, the CSA at TA showed the most effective parameter in the US examinations; it was suggested that the most useful and practical nerves for electrophysiological and sonographical studies in diabetic patients are the lower extremity nerves.

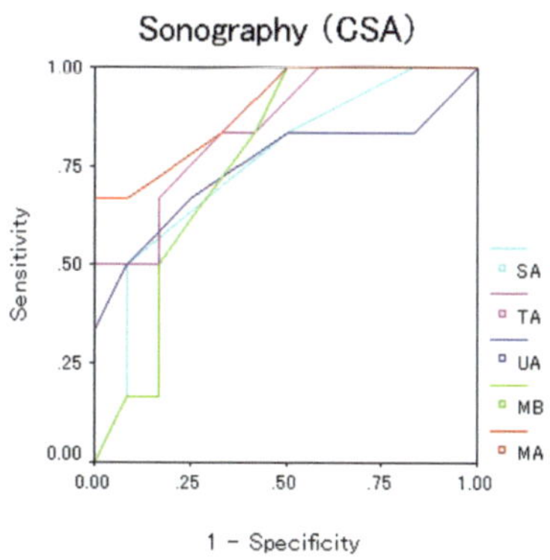

(a)

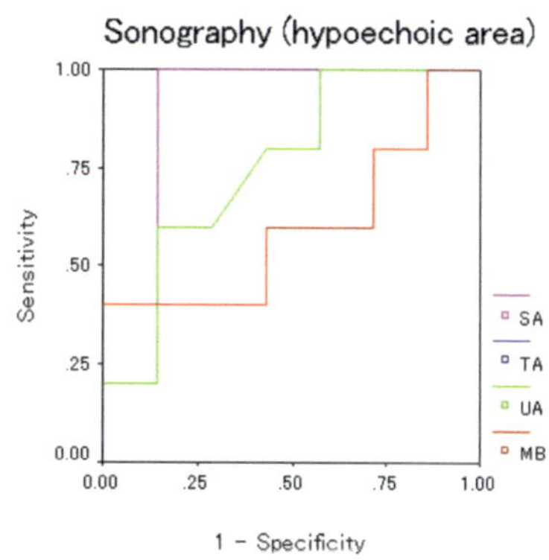

(b)

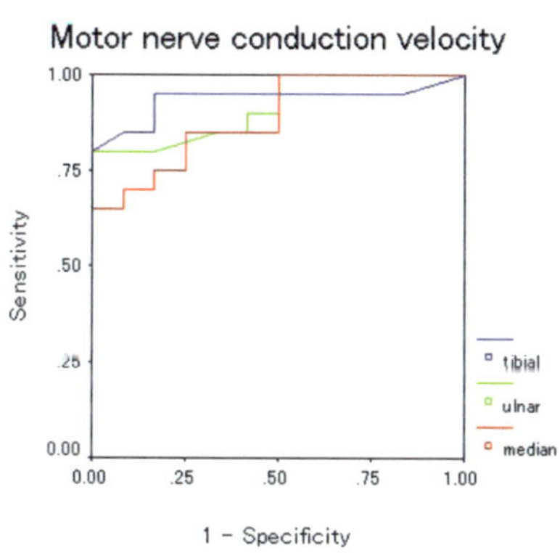

(c)

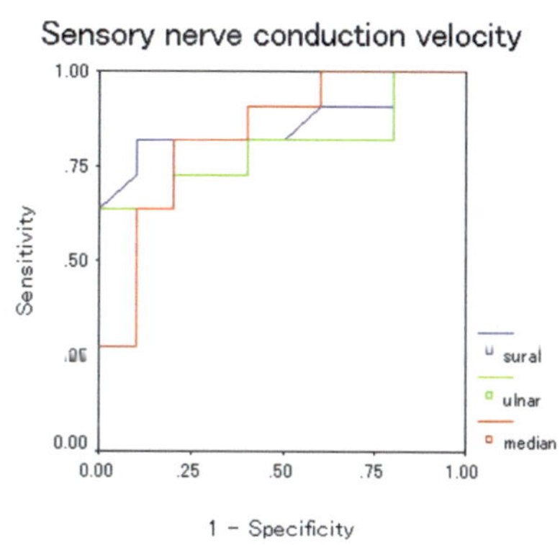

(d)

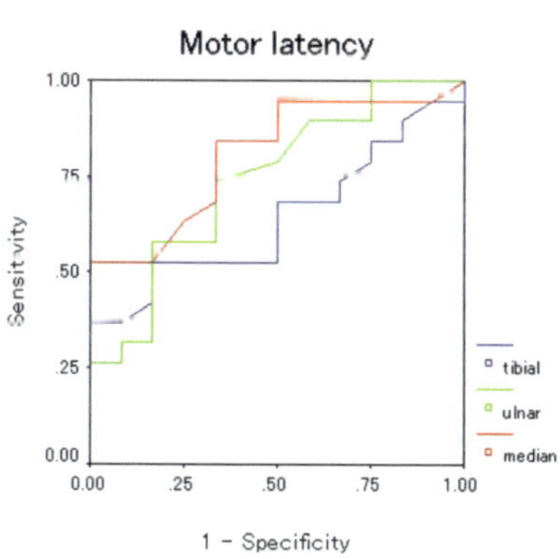

(e)

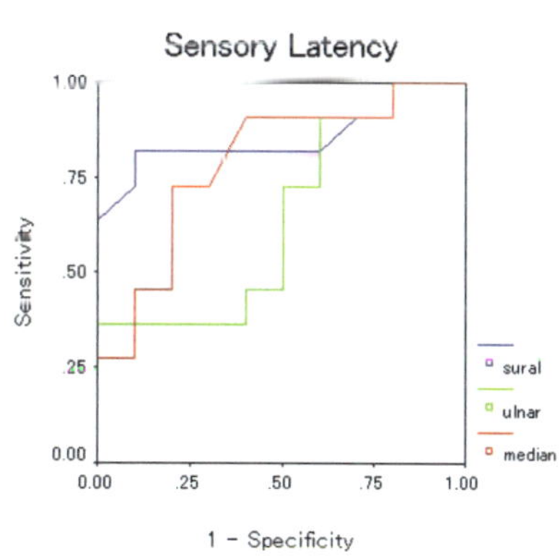

(f)

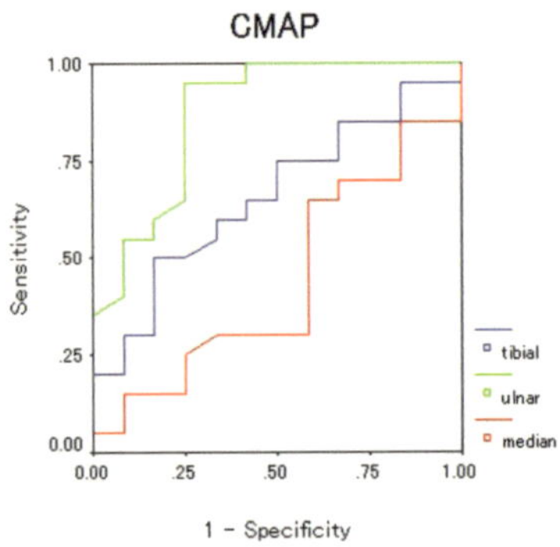

(g)

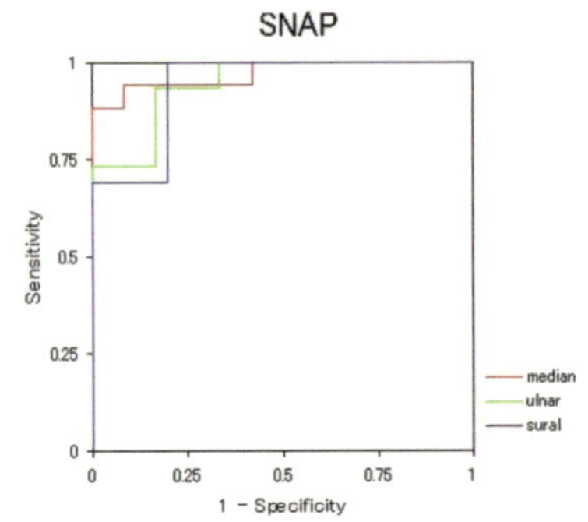

(h)

Fig. 7. Receiver operating characteristic curves fitted for difference modality. (a) When the ROC curve was fitted using CSA results of US, CSA at the TA was most effective. (b) When the ROC curve was fitted using hypoechoic area of US, SA at the sural nerve was most effective. (c) When the ROC curve was fitted using MCV results of NCS, MCV of the tibial nerve was most effective. (d) When the ROC curve was fitted using SCV results of NCS, SCV of the sural nerve was most effective. (e) When the ROC curve was fitted using motor DL results of NCS, latency of the median nerve was most effective. (f) When the ROC curve was fitted using sensory DL results of NCS, latency of the sural nerve was most effective. (g) When the ROC curve was fitted using CMAP results of NCS, CMAP of the ulnar nerve was most effective. (h) When the ROC curve was fitted using SNAP results of NCS, SNAP of the median nerve was most effective.

According to the ROC curve analysis, to investigate whether the use of US and NCS could accurately determine the presence of DPN, we compared the sensitivity and specificity of different parameters. Both sensitivity and specificity were higher in NCS than in US. These results were consistent with the current status that NCS is widely accepted as the more sensitive system of evaluation of polyneuropathy. Although sonographic measurements have insufficient sensitivity and specificity compared with those of the NCS, the ROC curves showed that AUCs were as high as 0.681 to 0.919, yielding 43% to 94% sensitivity and 50% to 94 % specificity. We promote the possibility of using sonography to diagnose DPN.

7. Conclusion

In this chapter, we have reviewed the current knowledge of neuropathy in type 2 DM and have introduced a sonographical examination for DPN. Based on our present data, it appears that both size and hypoechoic area of nerves were increased in patients with type 2 DM compared with controls. US is a noninvasive method that can be used to evaluate detailed nerve structures. The results from this preliminary study indicate that US might be considered as a valuable tool for the evaluation of DPN. In this work, we focused on the development of an objective method of quantitative analysis of echogenicity changes in peripheral nerves over a clarification of the mechanism. Some limitations of our study should be mentioned. First, a relatively small number of participants were studied and no adjustments were made for age differences. Second, our study was an ultrasonographic examination only; therefore, exactly what causes an increased hypoechoic area or CSA remains unknown. Furthermore, we must describe the property of sound waves. The property depends on both the object and the matrix in which it occurs, in that it relates to changes in acoustic impedance between 2 abutting structures. It is generally known that most nerves, including the median nerve, are surrounded by hyperechoic structures such as the tendons and that these hyperechoic structures may affect their appearance. Further investigation is required to clarify these findings in larger groups of diabetic patients using other modalities, such as magnetic resonance imaging.

Finally, there is little doubt that NCS are widely accepted as more sensitive than US in the evaluation of peripheral nerve disorders. However, US is able to directly show morphological changes in the peripheral nerves. Compared with NUS, US caused less discomfort to patients and was less time-consuming in our study. For these reasons, we promote the possibility of using this technique for the diagnosis of DPN.

8. Acknowledgements

The support of the clinical laboratory staff at the Gifu University Hospital is gratefully acknowledged. Authors also gratefully thank Dr. D. Fukuoka for helpful analysis of the echogenisity in the nerve.

9. References

Abe, M. (2004). Ultrasound measurement of the median nerve for carpal tunnel syndrome of the non-handicapped and the handicapped. J Phys Ther Sci, Vol. 16, No. 2, pp. 107-114, ISSN: 0915-5287.

Albers, JW.; Brown, MB.; Sima, AA.; Greene, DA. (1996). Nerve conduction measures in mild diabetic neuropathy in the Early Diabetes Intervention Trial: the effects of age, sex, type of diabetes, disease duration, and anthropometric factors. Tolrestat Study Group for the Early Diabetes Intervention Trial. Neurology, Vol. 46, No. 1, pp. 85-91, ISSN: 0028-3878.

Alemán, L.; Berná, JD.; Reus, M.; Martínez, F.; Doménech-Ratto, G.; Campos, M. (2008). Reproducibility of sonographic measurements of the median nerve. J Ultrasound Med, Vol. 27, No. 2, pp. 193-197, ISSN: 0278-4297.

Attarian, S.; Azulay, JP.; Boicraut, J.; Escande, N.; Pouget, J. (2001). Terminal latency index and modified F ratio in distinction of chronic demyelinating neuropathies. Clin Neurophysiol, Vol. 112, No. 3, pp. 457-463, ISSN: 1388-2457.

Cameron, NE.; Eaton, SE.; Cotter, MA.; Tesfaye, S. (2001). Vascular factors and metabolic interactions in the pathogenesis of diabetic neuropathy. Diabetologia, Vol. 44, No. 11, pp. 1973-1988, ISSN: 0012-186X.

Cartwright, MS.; Chloros, GD.; Walker, FO.; Wiesler, ER.; Cambell, WW. (2007). Diagnostic ultrasound for nerve transection. Muscle Nerve, Vol. 35, No. 6, pp. 796-799, ISSN: 0148-639X.

Chudzik, W.; Kaczorowska, B.; Przybyła, M.; Chudzik, B.; Całka, M. (2007). Diabetic neuropathy. Pol Merkur Lekarski, Vol. 22, No. 127, pp. 66-69, ISSN: 1426-9686.

Colak, A.; Kutlay, M.; Pekkafali, Z.; Saraçoglu, M.; Demircan, N.; Simşek, H.; Akin, ON.; Kibici, K. (2007). Use of sonography in carpal tunnel syndrome surgery: a prospective study. Neurol Med Chir, Vol. 47, No. 3, pp. 109-115, ISSN: 1349-8029.

Cornblath, DR.; Chaudhry, V.; Carter, K.; Lee, D.; Seysedadr, M.; Miernicki, M.; Joh, T. (1999). Total neuropathy score: validation and reliability study. Neurology, Vol. 53, No. 8, pp. 1660-1664, ISSN: 0028-3878.

Diabetes Control and Complications Trial (DCCT) Research Group. (1995). Effect of intensive diabetes treatment on nerve conduction in the Diabetes Control and Complications Trial. Ann Neurol, Vol. 38, No. 6, pp. 869-880, ISSN: 034-5134.

Duncan, I.; Sullivan, P.; Lomas, F. (1999). Sonography in the diagnosis of carpal tunnel syndrome. AJR Am J Roentgenol, Vol. 173, No. 3, pp. 681-684, ISSN: 0361-803X.

Dyck, PJ.; Karnes, JL.; Daube, J.; O'Brien, P.; Service, FJ. (1985). Clinical and neuropathological criteria for the diagnosis and staging of diabetic polyneuropathy. Brain, Vol. 108, No. 4, pp. 861-880, ISSN: 0006-8950.

Dyck, PJ. (1988). Detection, characterization, and staging of polyneuropathy: assessed in diabetics. Muscle Nerve, Vol. 11, No. 1, pp. 21-32, ISSN: 0148-639X.

Dyck, PJ.; Kratz, KM.; Lehman, KA.; Karnes, JL.; Melton, LJ 3rd.; O'Brien, PC.; Litchy, WJ.; Windebank, AJ.; Smith, BE.; Low, PA, et al. (1991). The Rochester Diabetic Neuropathy Study: design, criteria for types of neuropathy, selection bias, and reproducibility of neuropathic tests. Neurology, Vol. 41, No. 6, pp. 799-807, ISSN: 0028-3878.

Feldman, EL.; Stevens, MJ.; Thomas, PK.; Brown, MB.; Canal, N.; Greene, DA. (1994). A practical two-step quanttative clinical and electrophysiological assessment for the diagnosis and staging of diabetic neuropathy. Diabetes Care, Vol. 17, No. 11, pp. 1281-1289, ISSN: 0149-5992.

Fornage, BD. (1993). Sonography of peripheral nerves of the extremities. Radiol Med, Vol. 85, No. 5, pp. 162-167, ISSN: 0033-8362.

Greene, DA.; Lattimer, SA.; Sima, AAF. (1987). Sorbitol, phosphoinositides, and sodium-potassium–ATPase in the pathogenesis of diabetic complications. N Engl J Med, Vol. 316, No. 10, pp. 599-606. ISSN: 0028-4793.

Jayaraman, S.; Naidich, TP. (2004). The carpal tunnel: ultrasound display of normal imaging anatomy and pathology. Neuroimaging Clin N Am, Vol. 14, No. 1, pp. 103-113, ISSN: 1052-5149.

Kaplan, P.; Sahgal, V. (1978). Residual latency: new applications of an old technique. Arch Phys Med Rehabil, Vol. 59, No. 1, pp. 24-27, ISSN: 0003-9993.

Karsidag, S.; Morali, S.; Sargin, M.; Salman, S.; Karsidag, K.; Us, O. (2005). The electrophysiological findings of subclinical neuropathy in patients with recently diagnosed type 1 diabetes mellitus. Diabetes Res Clin Pract, Vol. 67, No. 3, pp. 211-219, ISSN: 0168-8227.

Khoury, V.; Cardinal, E.; Bureau, NJ. (2007). Musculoskeletal sonography: a dynamic tool for usual and unusual disorders. AJR Am J Roentgenol, Vol. 188, No. 1, pp. 63-73, ISSN: 0361-803X.

Lee, CH.; Choi, JW.; Kim, KA.; Seo, TS.; Lee, JM.; Park, CM. (2006). Usefulness of standard deviation on the histogram of ultrasound as a quantitative value for hepatic parenchymal echo texture; preliminary study. Ultrasound Med Biol, Vol. 32, No. 12, pp. 1817-1826, ISSN: 0301-5629.

Lee, D.; van Holsbeeck, MT.; Janevski, PK.; Ganos, DL.; Ditmars, DM.; Darian, VB. (1999). Diagnosis of carpal tunnel syndrome, Ultrasound versus electromyography. Radiol Clin North Am, Vol. 37, No. 4, pp. 859-872, ISSN: 0033-8389.

Oates, PJ. (2002). Polyol pathway and diabetic peripheral neuropaathy. Int Rev Neurobiol, Vol. 50, pp. 325-392, ISSN: 0074-7742.

Ogawa, K.; Sasaki, H.; Yamasaki, H.; Okamoto, K.; Matsuno, S.; Shono, T.; Doi, T.; Arimoto, K.; Furuta, H.; Nishi, M.; Nakao, T.; Nanjo, K. (2006). Peripheral nerve functions may deteriorate parallel to the progression of microangiopathy in diabetic patients. Nutr Metab Cardiovasc Dis, Vol. 16, No. 5, pp. 313-321, ISSN: 0939-4753.

Okamoto, M.; Abe, M.; Shirai, H.; Ueda, N. (2000). Diagnostic ultrasonography of the ulnar nerve in cubitial tunnel syndrome. J Hand Surg Br, Vol. 25, No. 5, pp. 499-502, ISSN: 0266-7681.

Osawa, H.; Mori, Y. (1996). Sonographic diagnosis of fatty liver using a histogram technique that compares liver and renal cortical echo amplitudes. J Clin Ultrasound, Vol. 24, No. 1, pp. 25-29, ISSN: 0091-2751.

Otsu, N. (1979). A threshold selection method from gray-level histogram. IEEE Trans. Systems Man Cybern, Vol. 9, No. 1, pp. 62-66, ISSN: 1083-4419.

Peer, S.; Bodner, G.; Meirer, R.; Willeit, J.; Piza-Katzer, H. (2001). Examination of postoperative peripheral nerve lesions with high-resolution sonography. Am J Roentgenol, Vol. 177, No. 2, pp. 415-419, ISSN: 0002-9580.

Perkins, BA.; Bril, V. (2003). Diabetic neuropathy: a review emphasizing diagnostic methods. Clin Neurophysiol, Vol. 114, No. 7, pp. 1167-1175. ISSN: 1388-2457.

Perkins, BA.; Olaleye, D.; Zinman, B.; Bril, V. (2001). Simple screening tests for peripheral neuropathy in the diabetes clinic. Diabetes Care, Vol. 24. No. 2, pp. 250-256, ISSN: 0149-5992.

Radziwill, AJ.; Steck, AJ.; Renaud, S.; Fuhr, P. (2003). Distal motor latency and residual latency as sensitive markers of anti-MAG polyneuropathy. J Neurol, Vol. 250, No. 8 , pp. 962-966, ISSN: 1121-8428.

Redmond, JM.; McKenna, MJ.; Feingold, M.; Ahmad, BK. (1992). Sensory testing versus nerve conduction velocity in diabetic polyneuropathy. Muscle Nerve, Vol. 15, No. 12, pp. 1334-1339, ISSN: 0148-639X.

Said, G. (2007). Diabetic neuropathy: a review. Nat Clin Pract Neurol, Vol. 3, No. 6, pp. 331-340, ISSN: 1745-8358.

Sernik, RA.; Abicalaf, CA.; Pimentel, BF.; Braga-Baiak, A.; Braga, L.; Cerri, GG. (2008). Ultrasound features of carpal tunnel syndrome: a prospective case-control study. Skeletal Radiol, Vol. 37, No. 1, pp. 49-53, ISSN: 0278-4297.

Silvestri, E.; Martinoli, C.; Derchi, LE., Bertolotto, M.; Chiaramondia, M.; Rosenberg, I. (1995). Echotexture of peripheral nerves: correlation between US and histologic findings and criteria to differentiate tendons. Radiology, Vol. 197, No. 1, pp. 291-296, ISSN: 0033-8419.

Solbiati, L.; De Pra, L.; Ierace, T.; Bellotti, E.; Derchi, LE. (1985). High-resolution sonography of the recurrent laryngeal nerve: anatomic and pathologic considerations. AJR Am J Roentgenol, Vol. 145, No. 5, pp. 989-993, ISSN: 0361 803X.

Stokvis, A., Van Neck, JW.; Van, Dijke, CF.; Van Wamel, A.; Coert, JH. (2009). High-resolution ultrasonography of the cutaneous nerve branches in the hand and wrist. J Hand Surg Eur, Vol. 34, No. 6, pp. 766-771, ISSN: 2043-6289.

Suzuki, E.; Yasuda, K.; Yasuda, K.; Miyazaki, S.; Takeda, N.; Inouye, H.; Omawari, N.; Miura, K. (1994). 1H-NMR analysis of nerve edema in the streptozotocin-induced diabetic rat. J Lab Clin Med, Vol. 124, No. 5, pp. 627-637, ISSN: 0022-2143.

Thomas, PK. (1997). Classfication, differentiatial diagnosis, and staging of diabetic peripheral neuropathy. Diabetes, Vol.46, No.2, pp. 54-57, ISSN: 0149-5992.

Vincent, AM.; Brownlee, M.; Russell, JW. (2002). Oxidative stress and programmed cell death in diabetic neuropathy. Ann N Y Acad Sci, Vol. 959, pp. 368-383. ISSN: 0077-8923.

Vinik, AI. (1999). Diabetic neuropathy: pathogenesis and therapy. Am J Med, Vol. 107, No. 2, pp. 17S-26S. ISSN: 0002-9343.

Watanabe, T.; Ito, H.; Morita, A.; Uno, Y.; Nishimura, T.; Kato, Y.; Takeda, J.; Seishima, M.; Matsuoka, T. (2009). Sonographic evaluation of the median nerve in diabetic patients: comparison with nerve conduction studies. J Ultrasound Med, Vol. 28, No. 6, pp. 727-734, ISSN: 0278-4297.

Watanabe, T.; Ito, H.; Sekine, A.; Katano, Y.; Nishimura, T.; Kawase, H.; Kato, Y.; Matsuoka, T.; Takeda, J.; Seishima, M. (2010). Sonographic evaluation of the peripheral nerve in diabetic patients: the relationship between nerve conduction studies, echo intensity, and cross-sectional area. J Ultrasound Med, Vol. 29, No. 5, pp 697-708, ISSN: 0278-4297.

Wiesler, ER.; Chloros, GD.; Cartwright, MS.; Smith, BP.; Rushing, J.;Walker, FO. (2006a). The use of diagnostic ultrasound in carpal tunnel syndrome. J Hand Surg Am, Vol. 31, No. 5, pp. 726-732, ISSN: 0363-5023.

Wiesler, ER.; Chloros, GD.; Cartwright, MS.; Shin, HW.; Walker, FO. (2006b). Ultrasound in the diagnosis of ulnar neuropathy at the cubital tunnel. J Hand Surg Am, Vol. 31, No. 5, pp. 1088-1093, ISSN: 0363-5023.

Wild, S.; Roglic, G.; Green, A.; Sicree, R.; King, H. (2004). Global prevalence of diabetes: estimates for the year 2000 and projections for 2030. Diabetes Care, Vol. 27, No. 5, pp. 1047-1053, ISSN: 1047-1053.

Yagihashi, S.; Yamagishi, S.; Wada, R. (2007). Pathology and pathogenetic mechanism of diabetic neuropathy: correlation with clinical signs and symptoms. Diabetes Res Clin Pract, Vol. 77, No. 1, pp. 184-189, ISSN: 1872-8227.

3

Diabetic Neuropathy – Nerve Morphology in the Upper Extremity

Niels Thomsen, Anders Bjorkman and Lars B. Dahlin
Department of Hand Surgery, Skåne University Hospital
Lund University
Sweden

1. Introduction

Diabetic neuropathy is the most common long-term complication of Type 1 and Type 2 diabetes, affecting approximately 10% within a year of diagnosis to 50% of subjects with diabetes for more than 25 years. Prevalence rates depend on diagnostic technique and the population under study (Dahlin et al., 2011; Rubino et al., 2007). Diabetic neuropathy associated with Type 1 diabetes tend to be more frequent, and develop more rapidly than in Type 2 diabetes. Gender differences seem to exist with males being more affected by neuropathy than females (Booya et al., 2005; Aaberg et al., 2008). Diabetes mellitus imposes a considerable burden on the nervous system and is the most common cause of peripheral nerve damage associated with a vast spectrum of neuropathy syndromes. The primary risk factor for the development of diabetic neuropathy is related to duration and severity of hyperglycaemia. Other independent risk factors for diabetic neuropathy include hypertension, hypercholesterolemia, smoking, increased body mass index and the presence of other complications of diabetes such as retinopathy and nephropathy (Adler et al., 1997). Diabetic neuropathy affects somatic as well as autonomic neurons of the peripheral nervous system with resultant morbidity and mortality for the patients and economic cost for the society and health care system. Interactions of pathogenic metabolic and vascular factors are responsible for the development of diabetic neuropathy. These complex mechanisms, which are not fully understood, need further clarification in order to develop new treatment strategies. The aim of this chapter is to describe methods and result in the evaluation of small and large nerve fibre pathology on the upper extremity.

2. Small nerve fibre morphology

Epidermal nerve fibres are predominantly unmyelinated C-fibres, which originate from the dorsal root ganglion, and are responsible for conveying thermal and nociceptive painful sensation. Small nerve fibres are believed to degenerate early in the course of diabetic neuropathy, and may even be affected in patients with impaired glucose tolerance (Loseth et al., 2008; Nebuchennykh et al., 2008).

An accepted method to evaluate small nerve fibre pathology is quantification of intraepidermal nerve fibre density (IENFD) using immunostaining with the cytoplasmatic neuronal marker protein gene product 9.5. In accordance with recommendations from the European Federation of Neurological Societies, the majority of studies report on results from the lower extremity (Lauria et al., 2005). It is generally believed that IENFD decreases with age, while the influence of gender seems controversial (Goransson et al., 2004). In healthy subjects, as well as in asymptomatic diabetic patients, a length dependent reduction of IENFD has been demonstrated (Umapathi et al., 2007). Using IENFD quantification at the ankle, the diagnosis of diabetic peripheral neuropathy was reported to have a sensitivity and specificity of about 75%. Skin biopsy has been reported to be the most sensitive measure for pre-diabetic neuropathy compared to nerve conduction studies, quantitative sensory testing, and a neuropathy score system (Smith et al., 2006).

A reduction in unmyelinated nerve fibre density has been established from skin biopsies on the lower leg as well as from sural nerve biopsy of patients with diabetes. Sorensen et al. (2006) demonstrated a significantly lower IENFD in a group of patients with diabetes having painful neuropathy in the lower extremity compared to a group of patients without pain. Likewise, other reports from studies on the lower leg have indicated that a reduction in IENFD among patients with diabetes may primarily be related to those suffering from painful small fibre neuropathy (Quattrini et al., 2007). On the other hand, complete denervation of the epidermis can be seen in patients with genetic insensitivity to pain, questioning whether loss of IENF is related to pain, or should be judged only as an indicator of neuropathy (Nolano et al., 2000).

Studies of IENFD in the upper extremity are sparse and have shown divergent results. Based on skin biopsies from the distal forearm a considerably reduced IENFD was demonstrated in patients with neuropathy compared to a healthy control group (Chien et al., 2001). However, aetiologies behind the neuropathy patient group were mixed with only 14% of the cases being due to diabetes. Another study compared skin biopsies of the forearm and the lower extremity in patients with diabetes, patients without diabetes suffering from neuropathy of different origin, and in a healthy control group (Pittenger et al., 2004). They demonstrated a significant difference in IENFD in the distal leg, but not in the forearm comparing patients with healthy controls subjects.

Normative range of IENFD in the wrist area has been investigated in two studies. Using immunofluorescence and light microscopy on 15µm thick sections from skin biopsies of various areas of the hand an IENFD of 10.3±8.3/mm (mean±SD) in glabrous skin of the proximal palm was reported. It was noted that inter-individual variability was high and that no specific pattern of distribution was found from fingertips to the palm (Kelly et al., 2005). A study on hairy skin from the distal forearm, using bright-field immunohistochemistry on 50µm thick sections reported a higher IENFD of 17.3±6.2/mm (Pan et al., 2001). Whether the difference in these results are caused by the study population, quantification technique or morphology in the hairy and glabrous skin remains unanswered as no comparative study on IENFD at the same anatomical level was performed.

In a recent study with matched patient groups, skin biopsies taken from hairy and glabrous skin at wrist level, demonstrated no difference in IENFD between patient with and without diabetes (Thomsen et al., 2009b). Furthermore, no differences were found between patients with Type 1 or Type 2 diabetes, or between subgroups of patients with diabetes with or without peripheral neuropathy. In addition, for both patients with and without diabetes,

IENFD was significantly higher in females compared to males and in hairy compared to glabrous skin. This is interesting, with the reported higher frequency of diabetic neuropathy in males than in females, suggesting that subjects with lower nerve fibre density would be more prone to develop neuropathy (Aaberg et al., 2008). Glabrous skin has been reported to have a higher heat pain threshold than hairy skin. Neurophysiological studies on monkeys provided a possible explanation for this phenomenal. The Aδ fibres consisted of both high threshold heat nociceptors and low threshold heat nociceptors, with glabrous skin being sparsely, if at all, innervated with low threshold Aδ fibres (Treede at al., 1995). Performing contact heat evoked potential stimulation others have confirmed these findings, that the glabrous surface of the hand is paucity innervated by low threshold nociceptors. These results on different nociceptive thresholds and receptors in glabrous versus hairy skin together with reported difference in thermal pain thresholds between male and female could explain these differences in the IENFD (Meh & Denislic, 1994). Furthermore, in order to functionally balance important inputs to the exploring surface of the glabrous skin, it seems reasonable that density of intraepidermal nociceptive nerve fibres is lower compared to the hairy skin.

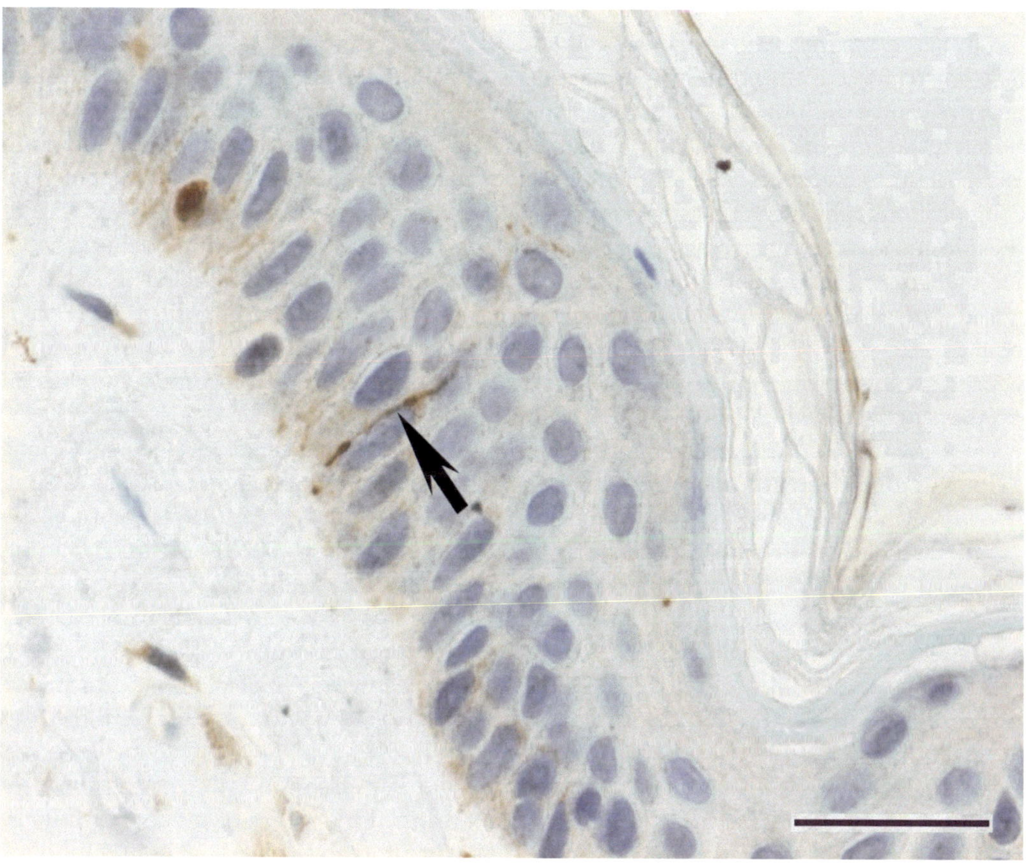

Fig. 1. Intraepidermal nerve fibre (arrow) from the dorsum of the wrist. Immunostained with protein gene product 9.5. Bar = 25 µm.

Small nerve fibres can also be assessed from a sural nerve biopsy. However, the biopsy procedure may cause long-term discomfort for the patient (Dahlin et al., 1997) and evaluation requires access to electron microscopy. A study, where patients underwent skin as well as sural nerve biopsy, concluded that IENFD measurement in the skin was more sensitive than evaluation of sural nerve biopsy to identify small fibre neuropathy (Herrmann et al., 1999).

As a non-invasive method for assessment of neuropathy, corneal confocal microscopy allows in vivo visualization of small nerve fibres in the cornea without taking a biopsy (Quattrini et al., 2007). The extent of corneal nerve damage and repair can be accurately defined. Reduction in corneal nerve density has been demonstrated to correlate with the severity of somatic neuropathy defined by intraepidermal nerve fibre loss. Abnormalities have been detected in minimal and mild neuropathy. Furthermore, nerve regeneration and its response to therapy may be quantified by detecting changes in corneal nerve branch density and tortuosity.

3. Large nerve fibre morphology

Sural nerve biopsy has been the method of choice to undertake neuropathological assessment for the diagnosis of peripheral neuropathies of unknown cause. Biochemical analysis can be performed, such as assessment of sorbitol, fructose and myo-inositol levels, which relates to clinical neuropathy (Sundkvist et al., 2000). Furthermore, it has been used to gain insight to the underlying pathology of nerve damage in diabetes. Due to the potential complication following sural nerve biopsy (wound infection, persistent pain, dysaesthesia of the affected skin, sensory loss and patient dissatisfaction with the procedure), demonstrated for both type 1 and type 2 diabetes, such procedures should be restricted to carefully selected cases and performed at surgical centres with a special interest in this field (Dahlin et al., 1997). Nerve biopsies require careful managing and evaluation by an experienced neuropathologist. For obvious reasons, most of our insight into nerve pathology relies on experimental studies.

From evaluation of sural nerve biopsies, it is known that the principal pathological lesions in human diabetic neuropathy are axonal degeneration and regeneration with loss of large myelinated nerve fibres, and segmental demyelination (Veves et al., 1991; Malik et al., 2005). Endoneurial microangiopathy has been demonstrated in such biopsies including basement membrane thickening, pericyte degeneration, endothelial cell hyperplasia, and luminal narrowing. Myelinated nerve fibre density has proven a reliable indicator of neuropathy in diabetic patients, correlating with clinical findings as well as to nerve conduction studies (Malik et al., 2001). Furthermore, a low myelinated fibre density may predict future nerve fibre loss and progression of neuropathy with time (Thrainsdottir et al., 2009).

With progression of disease, diabetic neuropathy may also affect the upper limb, in particular the mononeuropathies. Owing to the described morbidity of a nerve biopsy, as well as the length-dependent nature of diabetic neuropathy, only a few publications describe morphology of nerves in the upper limb. Due to limitations in acquiring a biopsy, which fulfils the criteria for nerve biopsy in the upper limb, results have so far have been provided from post-mortem subjects or amputated limbs (Reske-Nielsen & Lundbaek,

1968). Furthermore, the number of included cases are small, predominantly paraffin sections with limited detailed quantification.

In a post-mortem study of subclinical entrapment of the median and ulnar nerves a thickening of the perineurium and epineurium were observed. Furthermore, teased fibre analysis revealed thinning and retraction of the myelin as well as intercalated segments, suggestive of previous demyelination (Neary et al., 1975). The limited amount of human nerve tissue available for analysis, make us reliant on experimental models in order to understand the pathological features of nerve compression. It is clear that animal models with application of compression clamps or silicon tubes around a nerve, however valuable, are not an authentic reflection of chronic nerve compression in humans. However, acute and chronic compression models may serve as prototypes for analysis of intracellular signalling in Schwann cells and neurons during and after nerve compression (Dahlin et al., 2008). Acute nerve compression differs from chronic nerve compression involving mechanisms such as inflammation, and stretching and tethering of the nerve during joint movements. Schwann cells are believed to be one of the primary mediators of demyelination seen in nerve compression, possibly initiated by mechanical stimulus (Gupta & Steward, 2003).

Recently, a low morbidity procedure was presented, to assess large fibre pathology of the upper extremity (Thomsen et al., 2009a). The posterior interosseous nerve (PIN) biopsy is performed on the distal part of the dorsal forearm. The PIN is located on the interosseous membrane in the bottom of the fourth extensor compartment (Fig.2). A 3-4 cm long nerve biopsy can be harvested. Morphologic assessment of the PIN biopsies demonstrated a reduced myelinated nerve fibre density in patients with Type 2 diabetes compared to autopsy control subjects (Fig.2). It was argued that the PIN biopsy procedure fulfils the criteria for nerve biopsy described by Dyck (1968) as it has a constant location, is easy accessible, leaves no sensory or motor deficit and it is seldom subjected to trauma or entrapment. Furthermore, if a corroborative functional assessment is desirable, nerve conduction studies can be performed on the superficial sensory branch of the same nerve and at the same distal level as the nerve biopsy. The posterior interosseous nerve biopsy, performed under local anaesthesia and well tolerated by the patients, enables for the first time a larger scale human evaluation of nerve morphology in diabetes.

The posterior interosseous nerve biopsy performed on patients with carpal tunnel syndrome, demonstrated a significant reduction in myelinated nerve fibre and endoneurial capillary densities in patients with diabetes compared to patients without diabetes (Thomsen et al., 2009c). Surprisingly, these parameters were reduced for both patients with and without diabetes having carpal tunnel syndrome, compared to healthy control subjects without carpal tunnel syndrome. The finding suggests that distinct nerve pathology may exist even in patients without diabetes with idiopathic carpal tunnel syndrome. A reduction in endoneurial capillary density, which ultimately will lead to reduced endoneurial oxygenation, provides the first mechanistic foundation for axonal nerve damage through a hypoxic endoneural environment. A reduced number of nerve fibres may therefore represent an inborn impaired reserve capacity for the peripheral nervous system. Although not quantified, microangiopathy with reduplication of the basement membrane and thickening of the endothelium was observed in some of the diabetic patients. Gender differences need further investigation as a resent study on large nerve fibre function, represented by vibrotactile sense and electrophysiology demonstrated impaired function in males compared to females (Dahlin et al., 2011).

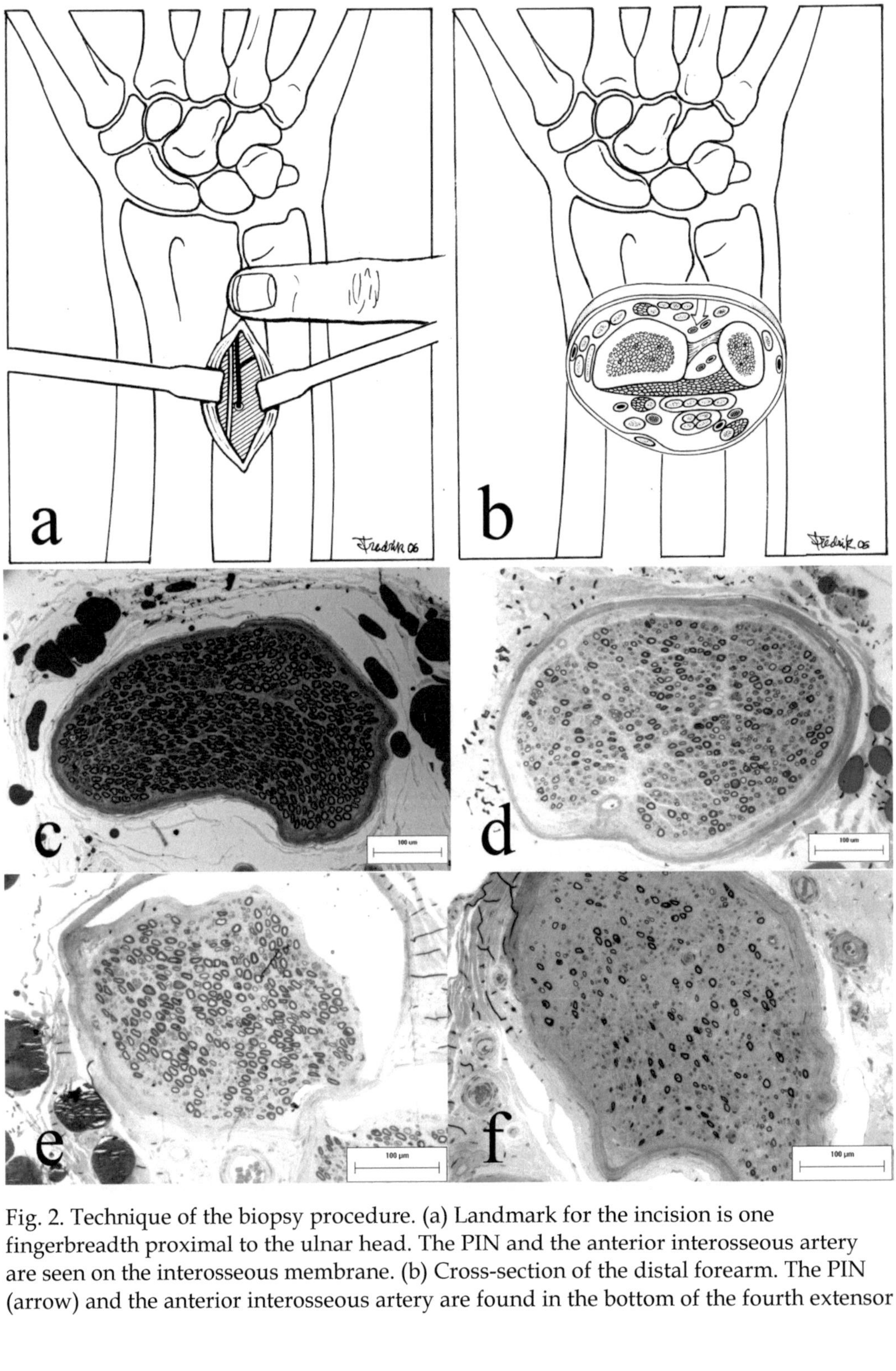

Fig. 2. Technique of the biopsy procedure. (a) Landmark for the incision is one fingerbreadth proximal to the ulnar head. The PIN and the anterior interosseous artery are seen on the interosseous membrane. (b) Cross-section of the distal forearm. The PIN (arrow) and the anterior interosseous artery are found in the bottom of the fourth extensor

compartment lying on the interosseous membrane.Light microscopic image of a PIN fascicle from (c) an autopsy control subject and (d) a diabetic subject. Note the lower myelinated fibre density in the diabetic patient compared to the autopsy control. From another patient (e) a PIN fascicle and (f) a sural nerve fascicle. Observe the lower myelinated fibre density in the sural nerve fascicle compared to the PIN fascicle. Reproduced with the courtesy of Wiley-Blackwell.

3. Conclusion

When evaluating small nerve fibre pathology in the upper extremity it is important to consider that the intraepidermal nerve fibre density is higher in female than in males and higher in hair than in glabrous skin. Differences between patients with and without diabetes needs further attention.

Studies on nerve morphology in the upper extremity can provide useful insight into the pathophysiology of diabetic neuropathies. Patients with diabetes demonstrate significant reduction in myelinated nerve fibre and endoneurial capillary densities in the upper extremity compared to patients without diabetes. These factors may predispose patients with diabetes to compression neuropathy, which is found with increased prevalence compared to patients without diabetes.

4. Acknowledgement

The studies on diabetic neuropathy from our group was supported by the Swedish Research Council (Medicine), Crafoord's Fund for Medical Research, Svenska Diabetesförbundet, Diabetesföreningen Malmö, Konsul Thure Carlsson Fund for Medical Research, Stiftelsen Sigurd och Elsa Goljes Minne, Region Skåne and Funds from the University Hospital Malmö, Sweden.

5. References

Aaberg ML, Burch DM, Hud ZR, Zacharias MP (2008) Gender differences in the onset of diabetic neuropathy. Journal of Diabetes & Its Complications 22:83-87

Adler AI, Boyko EJ, Ahroni JH, Stensel V, Forsberg RC, Smith DG (1997) Risk factors for diabetic peripheral sensory neuropathy. Results of the Seattle Prospective Diabetic Foot Study. Diabetes Care 20:1162-1167

Booya F, Bandarian F, Larijani B, Pajouhi M, Nooraei et al. (2005) Potential risk factors for diabetic neuropathy: a case control study. BMC Neurology 5:24.

Dahlin LB, Shyu BC, Danielsen N, Andersson SA (1989) Effects of nerve compression or ischaemia on conduction properties of myelinated and non-myelinated nerve fibres. An experimental study in the rabbit common peroneal nerve. Acta Physiol Scand 136:97-105

Dahlin LB, Eriksson KF, Sundkvist G (1997) Persistent postoperative complaints after whole sural nerve biopsies in diabetic and non-diabetic subjects. Diabet Med 14:353-356

Dahlin LB, Stenberg L, Luthman H, Thomsen NO (2008) Nerve compression induces activating transcription factor 3 in neurons and Schwann cells in diabetic rats. Neuroreport 19:987-990

Dahlin LB, Granberg V, Rolandsson I, Rosen I, Dahlin E et al. (2011) Disturbed vibrotactile sense in finger pulps in patients with type 1 diabetes - correlations with glycaemic level, clinical examination and electrophysiology. Diabet Med. In press

Chien HF, Tseng TJ, Lin WM, Yang CC, Chang YC, Chen RC, Hsieh ST (2001) Quantitative pathology of cutaneous nerve terminal degeneration in the human skin. Acta Neuropathol (Berl) 102:455-461

Dyck PJ, Lofgren EP (1968) Nerve biopsy. Choice of nerve, method, symptoms, and usefulness. Med Clin North Am 52:885-893

Dyck PJ, Kratz KM, Karnes JL et al. (1993) The prevalence by staged severity of various types of diabetic neuropathy, retinopathy, and nephropathy in a population-based cohort: the Rochester Diabetic Neuropathy Study. Neurology 43:817-824

Goransson LG, Mellgren SI, Lindal S, Omdal R (2004) The effect of age and gender on epidermal nerve fiber density. Neurology 62:774-777

Granovsky Y, Matre D, Sokolik A, Lorenz J, Casey KL (2005) Thermoreceptive innervation of human glabrous and hairy skin: a contact heat evoked potential analysis. Pain 115:238-247

Gupta R, Steward O (2003) Chronic nerve compression induces concurrent apoptosis and proliferation of Schwann cells. J Comp Neurol 461:174-186

Herrmann DN, Griffin JW, Hauer P, Cornblath DR, McArthur JC (1999) Epidermal nerve fiber density and sural nerve morphometry in peripheral neuropathies. Neurology 53:1634-1640

Kelly EJ, Terenghi G, Hazari A, Wiberg M (2005) Nerve fibre and sensory end organ density in the epidermis and papillary dermis of the human hand. Br J Plast Surg 58:774-779

Lauria G, Cornblath DR, Johansson O et al. (2005) EFNS guidelines on the use of skin biopsy in the diagnosis of peripheral neuropathy. Eur J Neurol 12:747-758

Loseth S, Stalberg E, Jorde R, Mellgren SI (2008) Early diabetic neuropathy: thermal thresholds and intraepidermal nerve fibre density in patients with normal nerve conduction studies. J Neurol 255:1197-1202

Malik RA, Veves A, Walker D et al. (2001) Sural nerve fibre pathology in diabetic patients with mild neuropathy: relationship to pain, quantitative sensory testing and peripheral nerve electrophysiology. Acta Neuropathol 101:367-374

Malik RA, Tesfaye S, Newrick PG et al. (2005) Sural nerve pathology in diabetic patients with minimal but progressive neuropathy. Diabetologia 48:578-585

Meh D, Denislic M (1994) Quantitative assessment of thermal and pain sensitivity. J Neurol Sci 127:164-169

Neary D, Ochoa J, Gilliatt RW (1975) Sub-clinical entrapment neuropathy in man. J Neurol Sci 24:283-298

Nebuchennykh M, Loseth S, Jorde R, Mellgren SI (2008) Idiopathic polyneuropathy and impaired glucose metabolism in a Norwegian patient series. Eur J Neurol 15:810-816

Nolano M, Crisci C, Santoro L et al. (2000) Absent innervation of skin and sweat glands in congenital insensitivity to pain with anhidrosis. Clin Neurophysiol 111:1596-1601

Nolano M, Provitera V, Crisci C et al. (2003) Quantification of myelinated endings and mechanoreceptors in human digital skin. Ann Neurol 54:197-205

Pan CL, Lin YH, Lin WM, Tai TY, Hsieh ST (2001) Degeneration of nociceptive nerve terminals in human peripheral neuropathy. Neuroreport 12:787-792

Pittenger GL, Ray M, Burcus NI, McNulty P, Basta B, Vinik AI (2004) Intraepidermal nerve fibers are indicators of small-fiber neuropathy in both diabetic and nondiabetic patients. Diabetes Care 27:1974-1979

Quattrini C, Tavakoli M, Jeziorska M et al. (2007) Surrogate markers of small fiber damage in human diabetic neuropathy. Diabetes 56:2148-2154

Reske-Nielsen E, Lundbaek K (1968) Pathological changes in the central and peripheral nervous system of young long-term diabetics. II. The spinal cord and peripheral nerves. Diabetologia 4:34-43

Rubino A, Rousculp MD, Davis K, Wang J, Bastyr EJ et al. (2007) Diagnosis of diabetic peripheral neuropathy among patients with type 1 and type 2 diabetes in France, Italy, Spain and the United Kingdom. Prim Care Diabetes 1:129-134

Smith AG, Russell J, Feldman EL et al. (2006) Lifestyle intervention for pre-diabetic neuropathy. Diabetes Care 29:1294-1299

Sorensen L, Molyneaux L, Yue DK (2006) The relationship among pain, sensory loss, and small nerve fibers in diabetes. Diabetes Care 29:883-887

Sundkvist G, Dahlin LB, Nilsson H et al. (2000) Sorbitol and myo-inositol levels and morphology of sural nerve in relation to peripheral nerve function and clinical neuropathy in men with diabetic, impaired, and normal glucose tolerance. Diabet Med 17:259-268

Thomsen NO, Mojaddidi M, Malik RA, Dahlin LB (2009a) Biopsy of the posterior interosseous nerve: a low morbidity method for assessment of peripheral nerve disorders. Diabet Med 26:100–104

Thomsen, NO, Englund E, Thrainsdottir S, Rosen I, Dahlin LB (2009b) Intraepidermal nerve fibre density at wrist level in diabetic and non-diabetic patients Diabet Med 26: 1120-6

Thomsen NO, Mojaddidi M, Malik RA, Dahlin LB (2009c) Reduced myelinated nerve fibre and endoneurial capillary densities in the forearm of diabetic and non-diabetic patients with carpal tunnel syndrome. Acta Neuropathol 118:785-791

Thrainsdottir S, Malik RA, Rosen I et al. (2009) Sural nerve biopsy may predict future nerve dysfunction. Acta Neurol Scand 120:38-46

Treede RD, Meyer RA, Raja SN, Campbell JN (1995) Evidence for two different heat transduction mechanisms in nociceptive primary afferents innervating monkey skin. J Physiol 483 (Pt 3):747-758

Umapathi T, Tan WL, Loke SC, Soon PC, Tavintharan S, Chan YH (2007) Intraepidermal nerve fiber density as a marker of early diabetic neuropathy. Muscle Nerve 35:591-598

Veves A, Malik RA, Lye RH et al. (1991) The relationship between sural nerve morphometric findings and measures of peripheral nerve function in mild diabetic neuropathy. Diabet Med 8:917-921

Part 2

Diabetes and Cardiovascular Disease

Residual Vascular Risk in T2DM: The Next Frontier

Michel P. Hermans[1], Sylvie A. Ahn[2] and Michel F. Rousseau[2]
[1]*Endocrinology & Nutrition, Cliniques universitaires St-Luc, Brussels*
[2]*Cardiology Division, Cliniques universitaires St-Luc, Brussels*
Belgium

1. Introduction

In T2DM, macro- and microvascular complications represent the major cause for morbi-/mortality, decreased quality of life and healthcare costs. Current guidelines for standards of care in T2DM emphasize the significance of multifactorial intervention on standard modifiable variables, in order to achieve recommended levels of blood glucose, LDL-C and blood pressure. T2DM patients achieving such targets represent a minority. Many of those not meeting those targets are exposed to high residual vascular risk (RVR) to develop incident micro- and macrovascular events and/or to suffer from progression of existing complications. Determining RVR in T2DM patients is of major relevance, as a substantial fraction of it is modifiable, including a lipid-related fraction, associated with both LDL and non-LDL lipids and lipoproteins. Atherogenic dyslipidemia (AD) is characterized by raised fasting triglycerides and low HDL-C. AD contributes to RVR of micro- and macrovascular disease in T2DM, even when LDL-C and/or hyperglycemia are controlled. The presence of a metabolic syndrome, or its score, is an additional means to capture modifiable components of RVR for micro- and macroangiopathy. AD is best prevented and addressed by therapeutic lifestyle changes, fibrates, or nicotinic acid. In the ACCORD Lipid trial, RVR of macrovascular events was high despite background simvastatin, and was substantially decreased in patients with AD following bitherapy with fenofibrate plus simvastatin. In FIELD and/or ACCORD trials, fenofibrate also decreased RVR of retinopathy progression, irrespective of baseline lipids, reduced albuminuria incidence and risk of diabetes-related lower-limb amputations. These data suggest a wider role for fenofibrate in the management of multisite microvessel RVR in T2DM. As regards other anti-dyslipidaemic drugs, ongoing trials will establish whether targeting low HDL-C with niacin reduces RVR in high-risk T2DM patients.

2. Standards of care in T2DM and target attainments

In type 2 diabetes mellitus (T2DM), vascular complications represent the major cause for morbi-/mortality, decreased quality of life and healthcare costs. These chronic, long-term complications arise in the setting of elevated residual vascular risk (RVR) factors. These factors may not only damage *macrovessels*, leading to premature-onset coronary artery disease (CAD), cerebrovascular disease (transient ischemic attack (TIA) and/or stroke), or peripheral arterial disease (PAD), but also affect *microvessels* leading to "diabetic complications", i.e. diabetes-specific long-term complications of chronic hyperglycemia: retinopathy, nephropathy or neuropathy. Certain vascular diabetic complications such as PAD, TIA/stroke, nephropathy or erectile dysfunction may arise from a combination of macro- and microangiopathies [1-6].

Low-density lipoprotein cholesterol (LDL-C)

Due to the overall efficacy of statins, and the relatively low baseline level of LDL-C in T2DM, LDL-C may be considered as the easiest-modifiable single parameter in diabetic patients [4,5,7-15]. However, in the recent *Centralized Pan-European survey on the under-treatment of hypercholesterolaemia* (CEPHEUS), a primary care survey from 8 European countries, under-treatment of hypercholesterolaemia was highly prevalent, with low total and LDL-C target attainment observed across countries [16,17]. In CEPHEUS, patients with the highest CV risk were T2DM patients with established cardiovascular disease (CVD) (i.e. patients in true secondary CV prevention). Yet, these highest-risk patients achieved the lowest level of LDL-C target attainment, with only 27% attaining the <70 mg/dL target. Moreover, only 58% of T2DM patients without CVD achieved LDL-C target <100 mg/dL. Eight modifiable variables were associated with LDL-C target attainment in CEPHEUS [17]:

1. normal body mass index;
2. being a non-smoker;
3. not having a metabolic syndrome (MetS) phenotype;
4. current treatment with a statin;
5. belonging to a medium-high CVD risk category;
6. good treatment adherence;
7. high patient's awareness of his/her current LDL-C level; and/or
8. frequency of cholesterol reviews.

Six non-modifiable factors were also associated with LDL-C target attainment:

1. age >70 years;
2. male gender;
3. history of diabetes;
4. history of hypertension;
5. absence of PAD; and/or
6. receiving LLD for secondary prevention.

Blood pressure (BP)

Controlling BP values in T2DM is of paramount importance, as it improves both macro- and microvascular outcomes. Such control is nevertheless challenging, as in the common form of T2DM, associated with the MetS and insulin resistance (IR), hypertension is not only highly prevalent, but also responds poorly to BP-lowering monotherapy intervention, and often requires multiple BP-lowering therapies on top of therapeutic lifestyle changes (TLC). In a recent study, only 16% of hypertensive T2DM treated with BP-lowering drug(s) in a tertiary-care setting achieved target BP <130<80 mmHg (<125<75 mmHg in case of proteinuria) [18].

Glycemic control and glycated haemoglobin (HbA_{1c})

Maintaining HbA_{1c} at target is an additional and constant challenge in T2DM, due to relentless loss of β-cell function over time and perpetual requirement for progressive stepping-up of glucose-lowering therapies [3,19,20]. Despite a large choice of oral and parenteral therapies to lower blood glucose, target attainment as regards glucose control, or that of its surrogate HbA_{1c}, remains suboptimal. Among U.S. adults with diabetes in 1999–2002, only 49.8% had an HbA_{1c} <7.0% [19], a proportion similar to that found 10 years later in the *OPtimal Type 2 dIabetes Management Including Benchmarking and Standard trEatment* (OPTIMISE) trial [21].

Multifactorial intervention

Current guidelines for standards of care in T2DM emphasize the significance of multifactorial intervention on major modifiable RFs to achieve recommended levels of glucose, LDL-C and BP [12-15]. In the Steno study, a multifactorial intervention aimed at achieving recommended levels of critical indicators, including HbA_{1c} as surrogate for contemporary glucose exposure, LDL-C and systolic BP (SBP), was highly effective in reducing (micro)vascular complications [22-24].

As each of these three major modifiable targets have distinct determinants, natural histories and responses to TLC or pharmacotherapy, it comes to no surprise that only a fraction of T2DM patients will reach all three targets in synchrony in real-life conditions, leaving a majority of T2DM patients exposed to incident micro-/macrovascular events over time, or to progression of existing complications [18,21].

Many factors associated with failure to meet critical targets (HbA_{1c}, LDL-C. SBP) in T2DM represent previously identified barriers to chronic diseases management:

- age;
- disease duration;
- ethnicity;
- hyperglycaemia, hypertension and dyslipidaemia are mostly asymptomatic conditions, both in primary or secondary prevention;
- chronic disease misrepresentation;
- faulty perception of risk related to metabolic diseases is frequently observed among many T2DM patients, especially from ethnic minorities;
- patients are often poorly compliant to TLC;
- impractical, conflicting, or competing guidelines;
- many patients are poorly adherent to prescribed treatment regimens and/or to self-monitoring of blood glucose;
- fear of hypoglycaemia;
- concerns about weight gain;
- fear, misperception of the natural history of T2DM and of the risk/benefit ratio of adding exogenous insulin;
- delaying tactics at the time when lifelong insulin supplementation is deemed necessary (insulinophobia);
- reluctance to resort to subcutaneous injections or to perform capillary blood glucose self-testing;
- variations among patients in pharmacological response to antidiabetic, lipid-lowering and/or BP-lowering drugs;
- reluctance of physicians and patients to increasing drug dosage or to switching drugs within classes, or to resorting to combined therapies;
- complex treatment schemes and side-effects;
- wrong perception of potential side-effects;

- insufficient counseling;
- physicians and healthcare providers inertia delaying diagnosis or stepping-up of successive interventions;
- insufficient or unfrequent laboratory follow-up;
- competing T2DM-related co-morbidities and complications: obstructive sleep apnoea syndrome, chronic kidney disease or left ventricular dysfunction;
- lack of patient empowerment and responsibility for self-care;
- social pressures and discrimination related to aspects of diabetes management;
- low socioeconomic or educational status;
- unsupportive/overstretched healthcare systems.

3. Residual vascular risk in T2DM

RVR in T2DM is best defined as "the residual risk of incident vascular events or progression of established vascular damage persisting in patients treated with current evidence-based recommended care, including risk from established risk factors, such as dyslipidemia, high blood pressure, hyperglycemia, inflammation and unhealthy lifestyles, and risk related to emerging or newer risk factors" [4,5].

Determining macro- and micro- RVR in T2DM patients after implementation of standards of care is especially relevant when dealing with a chronic condition in which a substantial fraction of risk remains addressable, eg. by further lowering of exposure levels to standards RFs for micro- and macroangiopathy. Besides those modifiable components to RVR, one should also consider in risk assessment non-gender, non-modifiable components of RVR in T2DM, such as ethnicity, certain polymorphisms, and familial histories for (*i*) premature-onset CVD; (*ii*) obesity; and/or (*iii*) impaired glucose homeostasis or diabetes.

For macrovascular RVR, the usual approach involves single-variable assessment (HbA_{1c}, SBP and LDL-C) and targeting with TLC and/or pharmacotherapy. Due to an overwhelmingly glucocentric approach to T2DM management, the hierarchy of priorities follows a sequence in which hyperglycemia control ranks first, followed on a par with BP control and LDL-C lowering with statin as preferred agent, and then with a needs assessment for aspirin therapy as antiplatelet agent in high-risk patients [12-15].

Combined assessment of the harmful effects of multiple coexisting modifiable variables on RVR is rarely done for an individual T2DM patient, even though multifactorial intervention was demonstrated to be highly-effective in reducing micro- and macrovascular RVR [22-24]. Various calculators were proposed to estimate absolute risk in nondiabetic and diabetic patients [25-31]. At present, the best means to predict macrovascular residual risk of CAD (nonlethal or lethal) and stroke (nonlethal or lethal) in patients in primary macrovascular prevention is the T2DM-specific calculator *United Kingdom Prospective Diabetes Study* (UKPDS) *Risk Engine* [25,27,28]. It computes risk from the following variables: (*i*) known T2DM duration, (*ii*) age, (*iii*) gender, (*iv*) ethnicity, (*v*) smoking status, (*vi*) atrial fibrillation, (*vii*) current HbA_{1c} level, (*viii*) SBP, (*ix*) total cholesterol and (*x*) high-density lipoprotein cholesterol (HDL-C).

In a diabetic RVR perspective, such calculations of absolute predicted risk should ideally be performed prior to, and following implementations of standards of care to control hyperglycemia, high BP and hypercholesterolemia, with updated levels as input for estimating the magnitude of risk reduction. Such an approach will yield relevant figures regarding (*i*) absolute vascular risk for CAD (nonlethal or lethal) and stroke (nonlethal or lethal), (*ii*) RVR for CAD (nonlethal or lethal) and stroke (nonlethal or lethal), together with (*iii*) absolute and (*iv*) relative decreases in CAD (nonlethal or lethal) and stroke (nonlethal or lethal) risks [25,27,28].

In order to illustrate RVR in T2DM from real-life conditions, we systematically assessed *UKPDS Risk* in 429 consecutive T2DM outpatients in primary macrovascular prevention. Eighty percent were White Caucasians, with a male-to-female ratio of 59:41. Mean age (1 standard deviation [SD]) was 62 (12) years, and known diabetes duration 12 (8) years. Sixteen percent were current smokers. Major modifiable variables in this cohort receiving standards of care in an academic setting were: total cholesterol: 173 (39) mg/dL; HDL-C: 48 (14) mg/dL; SBP: 137 (18) mmHg; and HbA_{1c}: 7.6 (1.47)%. The 10-year *UKPDS Risk Engine* estimated RVR values are illustrated in **Figure 1**. For the entire cohort, 10-year risk of CAD was high (almost 20%), a level in accordance with the status of *secondary-prevention equivalent* proposed for T2DM in primary macrovascular prevention [1,2]. According to gender, male T2DM patients had a 62% higher absolute risk for CAD than female patients, although the difference between genders was less marked for fatal CAD or stroke, and abolished for fatal stroke, illustrating the loss of protective effects afforded by the female gender in T2DM. Despite their primary CVD prevention status, those 429 patients had a high prevalence of microangiopathies: 46% (any microangiopathy); 21% (retinopathy); 23% (peripheral neuropathy); and 36% (albuminuria). These figures highlight the complexity of defining RVR in diabetic patients, who may at any time belong to different risk categories according to (*i*) the micro- *vs.* macrovascular level of dichotomy, and (*ii*) which target organs are under scrutiny.

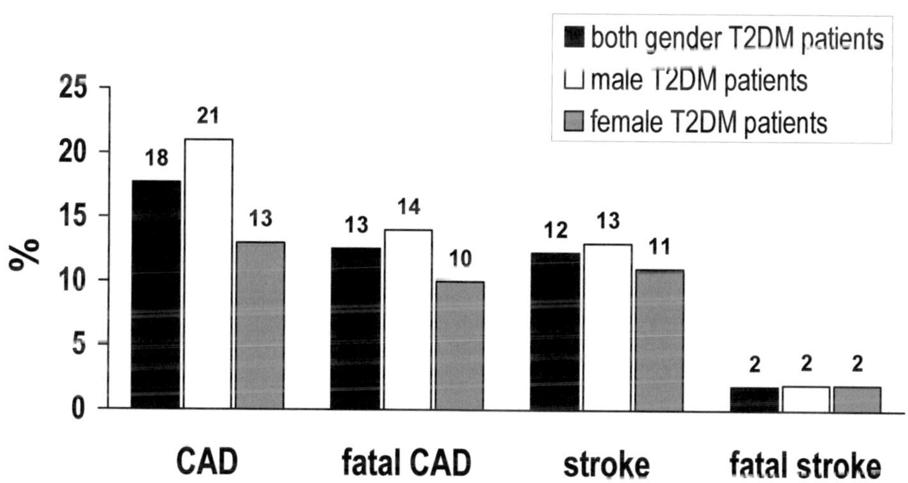

Fig. 1. *UKPDS Risk Engine*'s 10-year prediction estimates for developing non-fatal and fatal coronary artery disease (CAD), fatal CAD, non-fatal and fatal stroke in T2DM patients of both gender (n=429; solid bars), both groups in primary cardiovascular prevention.The UKPDS Risk Engine computes the following variables, i.e. (1) known T2DM duration, (2) age, (3) gender, (4) ethnicity, (5) smoking status, (6) atrial fibrillation, (7) HbA1c level, (8) systolic BP, (9) total cholesterol (C) and (10) HDL-C.

With respect to microangiopathy, individual RVR assessment is limited to an "educated guess" relating *hyperglycemia exposure time* (with known diabetes duration as surrogate) to *hyperglycemia severity* (with current HbA_{1c} as surrogate). Unfortunately, there exists no assigned microvascular calculator available for estimating 10-year absolute risk in major target organs, such as retina, kidney or peripheral nerves destined to diabetic patients or to prediabetic patients with rapid loss of β-cell function and as such at very high risk for new-onset T2DM. Such a limitation in microangiopathic RVR represents a truly unmet need for T2DM management. Such is also the case when it comes to estimating absolute RVR in end-organs at risk for combined micro- and macroangiopathies, such as PAD in lower limbs, cerebrovascular disease, certain subtypes of nephropathy, or erectile dysfunction. Other limitations of current risk calculators for T2DM patients include: (*i*) the complexity of the underlying pathophysiological processes; (*ii*) the poor predictive value of (micro)albuminuria as surrogate to diabetes-related nephropathy; (*iii*) the lack of effective clinical surrogate for early-neuropahy; and (*iv*) the exclusion of familial histories for diabetes, early-onset CVD, obesity and/or IR and of their mutual metabolic/vascular impacts [25-32].

4. Atherogenic dyslipidemia

A major component of modifiable RVR is lipid-related, both associated with LDL and non-LDL, including atherogenic dyslipidemia (AD). Epidemiological studies and landmark intervention trials clearly established that AD contributes to RVR for macrovascular disease in T2DM, even when LDL-C and/or hyperglycemia are controlled at baseline. The hallmark of AD is raised fasting TG and low HDL-C levels, two routinely available markers of a series of complex and deleterious metabolic abnormalities which affect, in a proatherogenic way, LDL and non-LDL lipoproteins composition and numbers. These abnormalities also diminish, in an antiatherogenic way, the dynamics and magnitude of reverse cholesterol transport [33-45].

The underlying process driving AD in T2DM or nondiabetic patients consists of (*i*) overproduction by the liver of TG-rich, apolipoprotein B_{100}(apoB)-carrying lipoproteins of the very-low density lipoprotein (VLDL) class, as a direct result of (*ii*) whole body IR and compensatory hyperinsulinemia, leading to (*iii*) raised portal insulin levels, which affect (*iv*) VLDL assembly and export by the hepatocyte, as a consequence of preserved insulin sensitivity of select pathways for lipogenesis and TG-rich lipoproteins synthesis [33,34,36,37,41,45].

Screening for AD provides a clinically-relevant and easy means to capture RVR associated with low HDL-C, high TG and their determinants. Such screening is not routinely performed due eg. to lack of general agreement on criteria or cut-offs based on current *vs.* baseline HDL-C and TG values. One way to diagnose AD consists of establishing the combined occurrence of high TG levels and low HDL-C. This seemingly easy estimation is rarely performed as such, due to (*i*) lack of consensual cut-off values across gender, race/ethnicities or underlying conditions; (*ii*) the requirement for baseline lipid values (prior to lipid-lowering drugs (LLD)); and (*iii*) the limiting fact that a *sine qua non* co-occurrence definition does not take into account the linearity of these non-LDL abnormalities, since both HDL-C and TG are continuous CVD risk variables [35,38,39,40,42,44,45]. Such an approach based on co-occurrence may also underestimate AD prevalence and severity in T2DM subpopulations with spontaneously low (Afro-

Americans, sub-Saharan Africans) or elevated TG levels [46-48]. A more rationale approach would be to use ratios between TG and HDL-C in order to incorporate each component's information as continuous variable while increasing the epidemiological potency by having the atherogenic TG variable as *numerator* together with the anti-atherogenic HDL-C as *denominator* [35,38,39,40,45]. We showed that *log*(TG)/HDL-C is a simple means to estimate AD and the residual CV risk it confers to T2DM patients. Thus, this AD surrogate ratio was associated with major cardiometabolic and glucose homeostasis determinants, as well as with poorer metabolic control, and related to macroangiopathy prevalence and estimated *UKPDS* CAD risk [44].

5. Metabolic syndrome

Low HDL-C and high TG are part of the MetS definition, either as individual AD component or in combination. The presence of a MetS phenotype or its score (from 0/5 to 5/5) is another simple means to capture RVR. Identifying a MetS phenotype may be used as a dichotomic state (presence *vs.* absence). In addition, score ranking within MetS syndrome categories, besides providing a stepwise surrogate for IR/hyperinsulinemia, also provides a simple means to determine increasing CV risk categories (from 1/5 to 5/5 for T2DM patients). While the MetS is not an absolute risk calculator, its presence hints to heightened relative RVR, as a result of exposure to standard CV RFs (underlying the current definition, such as hypertension and hyperglycemia) or due to the presence of AD. MetS ranking is also associated with lesser target achievement for key variables, such as HbA_{1c}, SBP or LDL-C. In addition, the MetS also associates with microangiopathy prevalence in major target organs [18,49-55].

6. New and emerging risk markers and factors

Many candidates RFs were proposed in the last decades to improve CVD risk assessment or RVR appraisal, although few, if any, are globally acknowledged in guidelines as part of standards of care and follow-up. These candidate RFs include eg. biological markers of low-grade subclinical systemic inflammation, markers of plaque instability, of endothelial dysfunction, or of proatherothrombotic conditions. None of these emerging markers/RFs are at present used as input variables in CVD risk calculators. Other emerging RFs for risk assessment in T2DM include potentially modifiable variables contributing to, or associated with RVR, such as the MetS phenotype, IR /hyperinsulinemia, adverse lifestyle habits (excessive caloric intake, Westernized diets, smoking, high ethanol intake, sedentarity), high-cardiometabolic risk anthropometrics (abnormal distribution/expansion of fat tissue, sarcopenia), or other comorbidites increasingly described as associated with the common form of T2DM (sleep-related breathing disorders, chronic kidney disease, left ventricular systolic/diastolic dysfunction, or non-alcoholic fatty liver disease) [56-74].

Table 1 enumerates a non-exhaustive series of non-modifiable and modifiable markers/RFs for micro-/macroangiopathy which may be at play in accruing RVR in T2DM patients, including inflammatory, behavioural/environnemental, and proatherothrombotic, whereas **Table 2** lists markers/RFs related to lipids and lipoproteins or to cardiometabolic factors involved in T2DM-related RVR [45,56-74].

Non-modifiable	Coagulation - haemostasis - platelets
age	platelet activity
male gender	platelet agregation
ethnicity	platelet size / volume
family history:	aspirin resistance
early-onset CVD	lipoprotein(a)
overweight / obesity	fibrinogen
IFG / IGT / T2DM	factor V, VII, and VIII
former tobacco smoking	fibrinopetide A
small size at birth for gestational age	PAI-1
right handedness	prothrombin fragments 1 + 2
genes / loci and polymorphisms associated with:	tissue-plasminogen activator
CVD	von Willebrand factor antigen
β-cell function loss	D-dimer
overweight / obesity	
	Varia
Inflammatory	cystatin-C
high-sensitivity C-reactive protein	asymmetric dimethylarginine
leucocyte count	nongenetic causes of iron overload
interleukin-6	hemochromatosis
matrix metalloproteinase 9	elevated ferritinaemia
serum amyloid A	Nt-proANP and Nt-proBNP
soluble CD_{40} ligand	endothelin-1
vascular / cellular adhesion molecules	urotensin II
lipoprotein-associated phospholipase A(2)	*Cytomegalovirus, Herpes simplex* virus
periodontal disease	*Helicobacter pylori*
	Chlamydia pneumoniae
Behavioural / environnemental	collagen vascular disease
current tobacco smoking	non-specific ST-segment ECG changes
air pollution (including airborne fine particles)	coronary artery calcifications
sedentary lifestyle (*surrogate* : TV viewing)	left ventricular dysfunction
physical inactivity	obstructive sleep apnoea / hypopnoea syndrome
quantitative / qualitative sarcopenia	psoriasis
psychosocial stress	rheumatoid arthritis
low socioeducative status	systemic lupus erythematosis
low income	HIV infection on highly-active antiretroviral therapy
decreased fruit and vegetable consumption	hypoglycemia unawareness

**: see Table 2 for lipid and cardiometabolic risk factors. ANP: Atrial natriuretic peptide; BNP: brain natriuretic peptide; CVD: cardiovascular disease; ECG: electrocardiogram; eGFR: estimated glomerular filtration rate; HIV: human immunodeficiency virus; IFG: impaired fasting glucose; IGT: impaired glucose tolerance; NAFLD: nonalcoholic fatty liver disease; PAI-1: plasminogen activator inhibitor type 1; T2DM type 2 diabetes mellitus; TV: television.*

Table 1. Micro or macrovascular disease risk factors/markers in T2DM patients: standard, emerging and candidate

7. Reducing residual vascular risk in T2DM

a. Targets attainment.

Reducing RVR must be part of a *continuum* in managing individual patients. RVR assessment is the next logical step after implementation of good clinical practices. Despite RFs identification and standards of care provision, all major modifiable RFs rarely attain all recommended targets for a given individual in real-life conditions [12-17,21-24]. This supports a more global approach to further reduce RVR [4-6,75-84]:

Lipids and lipoproteins	Cardiometabolic
total cholesterol	overweight - obesity (*surrogate* : increased BMI)
LDL-C	central fat distribution (*surrogate* : enlarged waist)
apolipoprotein B_{100}	hypertension
non-HDL-C	metabolic syndrome (presence *vs* . absence)
LDL particles number	metabolic syndrome (*score* : 3/5 - 4/5 - 5/5)
hypo-HDL-cholesterolaemia	insulin resistance / hyperinsulinaemia
decreased apolipoprotein A-I	dysadipokinemia (adiponectin, resistin, *etc* ...)
HDL subtypes distribution	non-alcoholic fatty liver / steatohepatitis / NAFLD
fasting hypertriglyceridemia	chronic hyperglycaemia (*surrogate* : elevated HbA_{1c})
postprandial hypertriglyceridemia	endothelial dysfunction
TG-rich lipoprotein remnants	erectile dysfunction
apolipoprotein CIII(+)-carrying apoB lipoproteins	(micro)albuminuria
oxidized LDL	glomerular hyperfiltration
antibodies to oxidized LDL	CKD - eGFR <60 ml/min/1.73 m^2
small-dense LDL	end-stage renal failure / dialysis
lipoprotein(a)	hyperuricemia
lipoproteins glycation	hyperhomocysteinemia
lipoprotein receptors glycation	vitamin D deficiency
lipid metabolism enzymes glycation	sympathetic nervous system hyperactivity

Apo: apolipoprotein; BMI: body mass index; C: cholesterol; CKD: chronic kidney disease; CVD: cardiovascular disease; eGFR: estimated glomerular filtration rate; HbA1c: glycated haemoglobin; HDL: high-density lipoprotein; LDL: low-density lipoprotein; NAFLD: nonalcoholic fatty liver disease; T2DM type 2 diabetes mellitus; TG: triclycerides (triacylglycerols).

Table 2. Lipid, lipoproteins and cardiomatabolic micro- and macrovascular disease risk factors/markers in TD2M patients: standard, emerging and candidate

1. continuous strive towards conventional target attainment, including reinforcement of TLC, higher drug dosages, drug switches or combination therapies;
2. addressing identified barriers to chronic diseases management using an individualized patient-based approach;
3. force-driving major modifiable RFs below recommended thresholds or physiological ranges ("*the lower is better*" paradigm);
4. impacting upon emerging risk factors, but this often means venturing beyond guidelines, or using off-label medications, or resorting to newer therapies not always supported by evidence from randomized clinical trials.

b. Non-LDL dyslipidemia and macroangiopathic RVR

As regards non-LDL dyslipidemia, AD can be improved by TLC, fibrates, or nicotinic acid [45,85-93] In T2DM, data from the recent *Action to Control Cardiovascular Risk in Diabetes* (ACCORD) Lipid trial reinforce the residual risk hypothesis for macroangiopathy, since despite achieving a mean LDL-C of 80 mg/dl, patients in the pre-specified subgroup with AD (defined as having both baseline TG >204 mg/dl and baseline HDL-C ≤34 mg/dl; numbering 17% of the ACCORD cohort) experienced a 70% higher relative rate (7% higher absolute rate) of incident major CV events (composite of CVD death, nonfatal myocardial infarction and nonfatal stroke) over a mean 4.7 year follow-up when compared to patients without AD [94,95].

In ACCORD Lipid, although in the whole T2DM cohort the main macrovascular outcome was negative, a prespecified subgroup of T2DM patients with AD treated with combination LLD therapy [simvastatin *plus* fenofibrate] had a 31% reduction in major CV events, compared to those treated with simvastatin alone (12.4% incidence [simvastatin *plus* fenofibrate] *vs.* 17.3% [simvastatin monotherapy]), amounting to a 5% absolute RVR reduction. The number-needed-to-treat was low, calculated at 20 T2DM patients with AD receiving LLD biotherapy over 5 years to prevent one major CV event. This number compares very favourably with those from landmark intervention trials with LLD in diabetic or nondiabetic populations. When primary outcome in the whole cohort was analyzed according to gender, another prespecified analysis, data for men showed a strong indication that they benefited from combination therapy (11.2% [fenofibrate] *vs.* 13.3% events [placebo]), while data for women were not as conclusive. Thus, whereas the *P* value for interaction related to gender was significant (0.0106), the confidence interval of the effect in females (9.1% [fenofibrate] *vs.* 6.6% events [placebo]) was not only wide, but also encroached the line of unity.

In ACCORD, AD was present in only one-sixth of the population under study, a subgroup which however markedly benefited in terms of macrovascular RVR reduction from combined therapy [94,95]. Whether in real-life conditions a higher proportion of T2DM patients might benefit from combination therapy [simvastatin *plus* fenofibrate] as a result of having AD as a comorbidity, is a tentative hypothesis. In ACCORD Lipid, the low recorded AD prevalence was a result not only of inclusion criteria, sequential exclusion of tertiles, intrinsic characteristics of the study population, and a relatively high proportion of volunteers of Afro-American ethnicity, who often have naturally low-to-normal triglycerides levels and less prone to suffer from AD [46-48].

We sought to investigate whether AD prevalence was akin to that observed in the ACCORD Lipid trial in an unselected, mostly Caucasian T2DM patients sample (*n*=974), consecutively attending our academic diabetes clinic. As ACCORD Lipid cutoffs, based on study-specific tertiles are unapplicable to other T2DM populations, we selected another approach to define AD, based on the co-occurrence of low HDL-C and high TG, with cutoffs derived from the harmonized definition of the MetS [51,53,55]. We also checked patient's file in order to retrieve pre-LLD HDL-C and TG values in patients on lipid-lowering drug(s), in order to establish the true, unbiased presence of AD (**Table 3**).

With such criteria and stringent use of baseline lipids values, we observed a higher prevalence of AD (35%), similar in both genders. In our survey, mean pre-LLD triglycerides were 203 mg/dl *vs.* 167 mg/dl for current values, representing an average difference of 36 mg/dl (18%), a difference sufficient to otherwise underestimate AD prevalence unless pre-LLD TG values are available. Such a confounding effect of LLD was not observed as regards HDL-C. In this analysis, the expected differences in the general population between genders were observed for HDL-C and apolipoprotein A-I level. Female patients also had significantly higher total cholesterol and significantly lower AD ratio [*log*(TG)/HDL-C] levels (**Table 3**).

Whatever AD prevalence data, notwithstanding the beneficial effects of fenofibrate on microvascular residual risk, a substantial proportion of unselected T2DM patients may potentially benefit from combination therapy to substantially decrease a modifiable component of AD-related RVR [94,95]. Such a likely assumption needs however to be confirmed from both epidemiological sources documenting the real-life prevalence of AD, and also from prospective randomised controlled trials, in which only fenofibrate-naïve patients with untreated AD would be included, with AD defined by consensual criteria, such as MetS thresholds for non-LDL dyslipidemia or trial-dependent AD cutoffs derived *a posteriori* on tertiles of non-LDL lipids at study entry such as in ACCORD Lipid [45]. Future trial should also investigate whether triple therapy (simvastatin *plus* fenofibrate *plus* nicotinic acid), aimed at further correction of most aspects of hypercholesterolemia and AD, will provide proportionate benefit for RVR in T2DM.

		both genders	males	females	*p*
n		*974*	*637*	*337*	
atherogenic dyslipidemia *	%	**35**	**35**	**35**	*NS*
pre-LLD total cholesterol	$mg.dl^{-1}$	**230** (43)	**225** (42)	**240** (43)	*<0.0001*
pre-LLD LDL-C	$mg.dl^{-1}$	**145** (35)	**143** (35)	**150** (35)	*0.0170*
pre-LLD HDL-C	$mg.dl^{-1}$	**47** (13)	**45** (12)	**52** (15)	*<0.0001*
pre-LLD TG	$mg.dl^{-1}$	**203** (167)	**201** (155)	**208** (193)	*NS*
anti-dyslipidemic drug(s)	%	**65**	**66**	**63**	*NS*
statin - fenofibrate - ezetimibe	%	**53 - 21 - 3**	**55 - 22 - 3**	**51 - 18 - 3**	*NS*
total cholesterol	$mg.dl^{-1}$	**179** (43)	**175** (42)	**186** (44)	*0.0001*
non-HDL-C	$mg.dl^{-1}$	**132** (42)	**130** (41)	**135** (42)	*NS*
apolipoprotein B_{100}	$mg.dl^{-1}$	**90** (27)	**89** (27)	**92** (27)	*NS*
LDL-C	$mg.dl^{-1}$	**99** (35)	**98** (35)	**102** (36)	*NS*
HDL-C	$mg.dl^{-1}$	**47** (14)	**44** (13)	**52** (15)	*<0.0001*
apolipoprotein A-I	$mg.dl^{-1}$	**149** (30)	**143** (28)	**163** (31)	*<0.0001*
triglycerides	$mg.dl^{-1}$	**167** (120)	**171** (128)	**161** (105)	*NS*
***log* (TG).$HDL\text{-}C^{-1}$**		**0.051** (0.025)	**0.054** (0.026)	**0.046** (0.021)	*<0.0001*

*Mean (1 SD) values; * : atherogenic dyslipidemia was defined as the concurrence of low HDL-C (<40 mg/dl in males; <50 mg/dl in females) and elevated fasting triglycerides (>150 mg/dl in both genders) as defined by the NCEP-ATP III cutoffs used to define the discrete lipid components of the metabolic syndrome score. Lipid values used to define AD were baseline (pre-LLD) lipids levels in patients treated with LLD(s). HDL-C: high-density lipoprotein cholesterol; LDL-C: low-density lipoprotein cholesterol; LLD: lipid lowering drug(s); T2DM: type 2 diabetes mellitus; TG: triglycerides. p: statistical value from Student's t test; NS: not significant (p value = or > 0.05).*

Table 3. Atherogenic dyslipidemia prevalence, lipid-lowering drug(s) therapy, and baseline vs. current lipids and lipoproteins values in unselected T2DM patients

c. Microangiopathic residual vascular risk

Diabetic eye disease includes diabetic retinopathy (DRP) and non-vessel comorbidities, such as cataract or glaucoma [96]. DRP is a microangiopathy affecting the retinal blood vessels resulting predominantly from poor metabolic control, which produces microvascular occlusion and leakage, leading to progressive retinal damage which may end in complete visual loss as a result of maculopathy or ischemic/proliferative retinopathy [96-100]. Few modifiable risk factors are identified with respect to DRP: poor metabolic (i.e. glycemic) control; hypertension, especially if poorly-controlled; LDL and non-LDL dyslipidemia; anemia and possibly, tobacco smoking. The recently published ACCORD Eye substudy highlighted the limits of conventional approaches based on near-normalization of two key modifiable variables (HbA_{1c} and high blood pressure). In ACCORD, DRP outcomes were defined as a ≥3-steps DRP progression on the EDTRS scale, or development of DRP requiring laser therapy or vitrectomy [101-103].

While glycemic control intensification significantly reduced the rate of progression of DRP (by a relative 33% and an absolute 3.1%, respectively), it was associated with serious safety concerns, as higher all-cause mortality was observed in the intensive glycemic control group [104]. This led to premature termination of the glycemic arm of the ACCORD trial. Another source of disappointment from the ACCORD trial for microvascular RVR reduction was the lack of efficacy of BP normalization to improve primary DRP outcomes [105]. These findings highlights the current pitfalls of current approaches to DRP management based on a "*the lower the better*" paradigm for the two major standard modifiable risk factors, i.e. HbA_{1c} and BP [104].

As regards lipids, landmark statin trials in T2DM or in subgroups with T2DM failed to identify a beneficial effect of LDL- lowering on any type on diabetic microangiopathies. On the other hand, epidemiological evidence links AD with RVR for diabetic retinopathy and/or nephropathy in T2DM [4-6,100,104]. The *REsiduAl risk, Lipids and Standard Therapies* (REALIST) studies are two *Residual Risk Reduction Initiative*-initiated worldwide epidemiological retrospective case-control surveys designed to assess AD-related macro- and microvascular residual risk. These are performed in non-diabetic and T2DM patients (REALIST MICRO) receiving current standards of care, with LDL-C levels at or near goal, treated or not with a statin. Pilot results from REALIST MICRO show a highly-significant and strong association between AD and microangiopathy incidence, even when LDL-C is controlled [107,108].

In the ACCORD Eye substudy, fenofibrate decreased RVR of DRP progression, assessed using the validated EDTRS scale, and irrespective of baseline lipids. The efficacy of fenofibrate was most obvious in patients with DRP at baseline, i.e. those in secondary DRP prevention [101-104]. Such a beneficial effect confirms the previously documented benefits of fenofibrate on DRP. This, in the *Fenofibrate Intervention and Event Lowering in Diabetes* (FIELD) study, a previous other large randomised controlled trial, a decreased requirement for DRP-related laser therapy was observed in T2DM treated with fenofibrate (*vs.* placebo). Such decreased requirement was however neither a primary outcome endpoint nor a "hard endpoint" for DRP progression assessment [88,104,106].

Results from ACCORD Eye therefore markedly raise the level of clinical evidence for a beneficial effect of this PPAR-α agonist on DRP. The FIELD study also showed that fenofibrate decreased new-onset albuminuria and diabetes-related non-traumatic amputations in T2DM patients [109]. In a recent assessment of fenofibrate's renal effects (FIELD washout sub-study), decreased albuminuria and reduced estimated glomerular filtration rate (eGFR) loss over 5 years were observed in patients allocated to the fenofibrate arm [110]. These observations confirm that fenofibrate not only reduces albuminuria or delay its onset, but also diminishes the natural history of progressive eGFR impairment in T2DM, despite an early and reversible increase in plasma creatinine [104,110-114]. As regards other LLD, future trials will establish whether targeting low HDL-C with nicotinic acid, alone or on top of background statin, reduces RVR of macroangiopathy in high-risk T2DM patients [90-93,115]. Safe and effective combination of LLDs (bi- or tritherapies) targeting most aspects of dyslipidemia are likely to become standards of care in high-risk populations such as patients with T2DM [45,75,91,104,115-118].

8. Benchmarking

Innovative approaches are needed to improve individual and overall target achievement with the aim of reducing RVR. Benchmarking targeting physicians is one of those newer approaches. The goal of the non-interventional randomised OPTIMISE trial was to investigate in 6 European countries the effect of physician's benchmarking on quality of care, assessed according to the percentage of T2DM patients achieving pre-set targets for three key modifiable variables (HbA_{1c}, LDL-C and SBP), as recommended by international guidelines. At baseline, the percentage of patients achieving targets was highly unsatisfactory: 51% (HbA_{1c}); 27% (SBP); and 35% (LDL-C), with a mere 5% reaching all three targets at study entry. Physicians were randomly assigned to receive either benchmarked feedback or non-benchmarked feedback on their patients' modifiable outcome indicators (HbA_{1c}, fasting glycaemia, total cholesterol, HDL-C, LDL-C and TG). At study end, the percentage of patients achieving all targets almost doubled, suggesting that benchmarking may be an innovative approach to improve target attainment of modifiable variables affecting RVR in T2DM patients [21,119,120].

9. References

Haffner SM, Lehto S, Rönnemaa T, Pyörälä K, Laakso M. Mortality from coronary heart disease in subjects with type 2 diabetes and in nondiabetic subjects with and without prior myocardial infarction. N Engl J Med 1998;339:229-34

Juutilainen A, Lehto S, Rönnemaa T, Pyörälä K, Laakso M Type 2 diabetes as a 'coronary heart disease equivalent'. An 18-year prospective population-based study in Finnish subjects. Diabetes Care 2005;28:2901-7

Hermans MP. Diabetic macro- and microvascular disease in type 2 diabetes. Diabetes Vasc Dis Res 2007;4:S7-11.

Fruchart J-C, Sacks F, Hermans MP, Assmann G, Brown V, Ceska R, Chapman J, Dodson PM, Fioretto P, Ginsberg HN, Kadowaki T, Lablanche J-M, Marx N, Plutzky J, Reiner Z, Rosenson RS, Staels B, Stock JK, Sy R, Wanner C, Zambon A, Zimmet P. Executive statement: the Residual Risk Reduction Initiative: a call to action to reduce residual vascular risk in dyslipidemic patients. A condensed position paper by the Residual Risk Reduction Initiative (R3i). Diab Vasc Dis Res 2008;5:319-35.

Fruchart J-C, Sacks F, Hermans MP, Assmann G, Brown WV, Ceska R, Chapman MJ, Dodson PM, Fioretto P, Ginsberg HN, Kadowaki T, Lablanche J-M, Marx N, Plutzky J, Reiner Z, Rosenson RS, Staels B, Stock JK, Sy R, Wanner C, Zambon A, Zimmet P for the Residual Risk Reduction Initiative. The Residual Risk Reduction Initiative: a call to action to reduce residual vascular risk in patients with dyslipidemia. Am J Cardiol 2008; 102(suppl): 1-34.

Fioretto P, Dodson PM, Ziegler D, Rosenson RS. Residual microvascular risk in diabetes: unmet needs and future directions. Nat Rev Endocrinol. 2010;6:19-25.

Brown G, Albers JJ, Fisher LD, Schaefer SM, Lin JT, Kaplan C, Zhao XQ, Bisson BD, Fitzpatrick VF, Dodge HT. Regression of coronary artery disease as a result of intensive lipid-lowering therapy in men with high levels of apolipoprotein B. N Engl J Med 1990;323:1289-98.

LaRosa JC, Grundy SM, Waters DD, Shear C, Barter P, Fruchart JC, Gotto AM, Greten H, Kastelein JJ, Shepherd J, Wenger NK. Intensive lipid lowering with atorvastatin in patients with stable coronary disease. N Engl J Med 2005;352:1425-35.

Alsheikh-Ali AA, Lin JL, Abourjaily P, Ahearn D, Kuvin JT, Karas RH. Prevalence of low high-density lipoprotein cholesterol in patients with documented coronary heart disease or risk equivalent and controlled low-density lipoprotein cholesterol. Am J Cardiol 2007;100:1499-1501.

Brunzell JD, Davidson M, Furberg CD, Goldberg RB, Howard BV, Stein JH, Witztum JL. Lipoprotein management in patients with cardiometabolic risk: consensus conference report from the American Diabetes Association and the American College of Cardiology Foundation. J Am Coll Cardiol 2008;51:1512-24.

Forrester JS. Redefining normal low-density lipoprotein cholesterol: a strategy to unseat coronary disease as the nation's leading killer. J Am Coll Cardiol 2010;56:630-6.

Graham I, Atar D, Borch-Johnsen K, Boysen G, Burell G, Cifkova R, Dallongeville J, De Backer G, Ebrahim S, Gjelsvik B, Herrmann-Lingen C, Hoes A, Humphries S, Knapton M, Perk J, Priori SG, Pyorala K, Reiner Z, Ruilope L, Sans-Menendez S, Scholte op Reimer W, Weissberg P, Wood D, Yarnell J, Zamorano JL; Other experts who contributed to parts of the guidelines:, Walma E, Fitzgerald T, Cooney MT, Dudina A; European Society of Cardiology (ESC) Committee for Practice Guidelines (CPG), Vahanian A, Camm J, De Caterina R, Dean V, Dickstein K, Funck-Brentano C, Filippatos G, Hellemans I, Kristensen SD, McGregor K, Sechtem U, Silber S, Tendera M, Widimsky P, Zamorano JL, Hellemans I, Altiner A, Bonora E, Durrington PN, Fagard R, Giampaoli S, Hemingway H, Hakansson J, Kjeldsen SE, Larsen ML, Mancia G, Manolis AJ, Orth-Gomer K, Pedersen T, Rayner M, Ryden L, Sammut M, Schneiderman N, Stalenhoef AF, Tokgözoglu L, Wiklund O, Zampelas A. European guidelines on cardiovascular disease prevention in clinical practice. Fourth Joint Task Force of the European Society of Cardiology and other Societies on Cardiovascular Disease Prevention in Clinical Practice. Executive summary. Eur Heart J 2007;28:2375-414.

Ryden L, Standl E, Bartnik M, Van den Berghe G, Betteridge J, de Boer MJ, Cosentino F, Jonsson B, Laakso M, Malmberg K, Priori S, Ostergren J, Tuomilehto J, Thrainsdottir I, Vanhorebeek I, Stramba-Badiale M, Lindgren P, Qiao Q, Priori SG, Blanc JJ, Budaj A, Camm J, Dean V, Deckers J, Dickstein K, Lekakis J, McGregor K, Metra M, Morais J, Osterspey A, Tamargo J, Zamorano JL, Deckers JW, Bertrand M, Charbonnel B, Erdmann E, Ferrannini E, Flyvbjerg A, Gohlke H, Juanatey JR, Graham I, Monteiro PF, Parhofer K, Pyorala K, Raz I, Schernthaner G, Volpe M, Wood D. Guidelines on diabetes, pre-diabetes, and cardiovascular diseases: executive summary. The Task Force on Diabetes and Cardiovascular Diseases of the European Society of Cardiology (ESC) and of the European Association for the Study of Diabetes (EASD). Eur Heart J 2007;28:88-136.

Genest J, McPherson R, Frohlich J, Anderson T, Campbell N, Carpentier A, Couture P, Dufour R, Fodor G, Francis GA, Grover S, Gupta M, Hegele RA, Lau DC, Leiter L, Lewis GF, Lonn E, Mancini GB, Ng D, Pearson GJ, Sniderman A, Stone JA, Ur E. 2009 Canadian Cardiovascular Society/Canadian guidelines for the diagnosis and treatment of dyslipidemia and prevention of cardiovascular disease in the adult - 2009 recommendations. Can J Cardiol 2009;25:567-79.

American Diabetes Association. Clinical practice recommendations 2010. Diabetes Care 2010;33:S1-100.

Ferrieres J, Tocque-Le Gousse E, Fabry C, Hermans MP on behalf of the French CEPHEUS investigators. Assessment of lipid-lowering treatment in France. Arch Cardiovasc Dis 2008; 101:557-63.

Hermans MP, Castro Cabezas M, Strandberg T, Ferrieres J, Feely J, Elisaff M, Michel G, Sansoy V. Centralized Pan-European survey on the under-treatment of hypercholesterolaemia (CEPHEUS): overall findings from eight countries. Curr Med Res Opin 2010;26:445-54.

Hermans MP, Amoussou-Guenou KD, Ahn SA, Rousseau MF, Everaert L, Aerts A. The elusive type 2 diabetes individual achieving tight blood pressure target: A phenotypic study. Diab Metab Syndr 2010;4:215-9.

Resnick HE, Foster GL, Bardsley J, Ratner RE : Achievement of American Diabetes Association clinical practice recommendations among U.S. adults with diabetes, 1999–2002: the National Health and Nutrition Examination Survey. Diabetes Care 2006;29:531-7.

Munoko Th, Hermans MP. Phenotypic characterization of first generation Maghrebian migrants with type 2 diabetes: a gender-based comparison with a reference North-Caucasian Belgian cohort. Diab Met Syndr 2008;2:115-24.

Hermans MP, Muls E, Michel G, Elisaf M, Brotons C, Matthys A. Optimal type 2 diabetes management including benchmarking and standard treatment. Baseline European results. Atherosclerosis Supplements 2010;11:44.

Gaede P, Vedel P, Larsen N, Jensen GV, Parving HH, Pedersen O. Multifactorial intervention and cardiovascular disease in patients with type 2 diabetes. N Engl J Med 2003;348:383-93.

Stratton IM, Cull CA, Adler AI, Matthews DR, Neil HA, Holman RR. Additive effects of glycaemia and blood pressure exposure on risk of complications in type 2 diabetes: a prospective observational study (UKPDS 75). Diabetologia 2006;49:1761-9.

Gaede P, Lund-Andersen H, Parving HH, Pedersen O. Effect of a multifactorial intervention on mortality in type 2 diabetes. N Engl J Med 2008;358:580-91.

Stevens RJ, Kothari V, Adler AI, Stratton IM; United Kingdom Prospective Diabetes Study (UKPDS) Group. The UKPDS Risk Engine: a model for the risk of coronary heart disease in type 2 diabetes. Clin Science 2001;101:671-9.

Assmann G, Cullen P, Schulte H. Simple scoring scheme for calculating the risk of acute coronary events based on the 10-year follow-up of the prospective cardiovascular Münster (PROCAM) study. Circulation 2002;105:310-5.

Kothari V, Stevens RJ, Adler AI, Stratton IM, Manley SE, Neil HA, Holman RR. UKPDS 60: risk of stroke in type 2 diabetes estimated by the UK Prospective Diabetes Study risk engine. Stroke 2002;33:1776-81.

Stevens RJ, Coleman RL, Adler AI, Stratton IM, Matthews DR, Holman RR. UKPDS 66: risk factors for myocardial infarction case fatality and stroke case fatality in type 2 diabetes. Diabetes Care 2004;27:201-7.

Coleman RL, Stevens RJ, Retnakaran R, Holman RR. Framingham, SCORE and DECODE do not provide reliable cardiovascular risk estimates in type 2 diabetes. Diabetes Care 2007;30:1292-3.

Eichler K, Puhan MA, Steurer J, Bachmann LM. Prediction of first coronary events with the Framingham score: a systematic review. Am Heart J 2007;153:722-31.

Wilson PW. Risk scores for prediction of coronary heart disease: an update. Endocrinol Metab Clin North Am 2009;38:33-44.

Ragé M, Van Acker N, Knaapen MW, Timmers M, Streffer J, Hermans MP, Sindic C, Meert T, Plaghki L. Asymptomatic small fiber neuropathy in diabetes mellitus: investigations with intraepidermal nerve fiber density, quantitative sensory testing and laser-evoked potentials. J Neurol. 2011 Apr 7. [Epub ahead of print]

Davis RA. Cell and molecular biology of the assembly and secretion of apolipoprotein B-containing lipoproteins by the liver. Biochim Biophys Acta 1999;1440:1-31.

Brites FD, Bonavita CD, De Geitere C, Cloës M, Delfly B, Yael MJ, Fruchart J, Wikinski RW, Castro GR. Alterations in the main steps of reverse cholesterol transport in male patients with primary hypertriglyceridemia and low HDL-cholesterol levels. Atherosclerosis 2000;152:181-92.

Dobiásová M, Frohlich J. The plasma parameter log (TG/HDL-C) as an atherogenic index: correlation with lipoprotein particle size and esterification rate in apoB-lipoprotein-depleted plasma (FERHDL). Clin Biochem 2001;34:583-8.

Blasiole DA, Davis RA, Attie AD. The physiological and molecular regulation of lipoprotein assembly and secretion. Mol Biosyst 2007;3:608-19.

Adiels M, Olofsson S-O, Taskinen M-R, Borén J. Overproduction of very low–density lipoproteins is the hallmark of the dyslipidemia in the metabolic syndrome. Arterioscler Thromb Vasc Biol 2008;28:1225-36.

da Luz PL, Favarato D, Faria-Neto JR Jr, Lemos P, Chagas AC. High ratio of triglycerides to HDL-cholesterol predicts extensive coronary disease. Clinics (Sao Paulo) 2008;63:427-32.

Bittner V, Johnson BD, Zineh I, Rogers WJ, Vido D, Marroquin OC, Bairey-Merz CN, Sopko G. The triglyceride/high-density lipoprotein cholesterol ratio predicts all-cause mortality in women with suspected myocardial ischemia: a report from the Women's Ischemia Syndrome Evaluation (WISE). Am Heart J 2009;157:548-55.

Cordero A, Andrés E, Ordoñez B, León M, Laclaustra M, Grima A, Luengo E, Moreno J, Bes M, Pascual I, Civeira F, Pocoví M, Alegría E, Casasnovas JA and MESYAS (MEtabolic Syndrome Active Subjects) Study Investigators. Usefulness of triglycerides-to-high-density lipoprotein cholesterol ratio for predicting the first coronary event in men. Am J Cardiol 2009;104:1393-7.

Watts GF, Ooi EMM, Chan DC. Therapeutic regulation of apoB100 metabolism in insulin resistance in vivo. Pharmacology & Therapeutics 2009;123:281-91.

Assmann G, Cullen P, Schulte H. Non-LDL-related dyslipidemia and coronary risk: a case-control study. Diab Vasc Dis Res 2010;7:204-12.

Costet P. Molecular pathways and agents for lowering LDL-cholesterol in addition to statins. Pharmacol Ther 2010;126:263-78.

Hermans MP, Ahn SA, Rousseau MF. log(TG)/HDL-C is related to both residual cardiometabolic risk and β-cell function loss in type 2 diabetes males. Cardiovasc Diabetol. 2010;9:88.

Hermans MP, Fruchart JC. Reducing residual vascular risk in patients with atherogenic dyslipidaemia: where do we go from here? Clinical Lipidology 2010;5:811-26.

Sumner AE, Vega GL, Genovese DJ, Finley KB, Bergman RN, Boston RC. Normal triglyceride levels despite insulin resistance in African Americans: role of lipoprotein lipase. Metabolism 2005;54:902-9.

Dehout F, Haumont S, Gaham N, Amoussou-Guenou KD, Hermans MP. Metabolic syndrome in Bantu subjects with type 2 diabetes from sub-Saharan extraction: prevalence, gender differences and HOMA-hyperbolic product. Diab Metab Syndr 2008;2:5-11.

Paramsothy P, Knopp R, Bertoni AG, Tsai MY, Rue T, Heckbert SR. Combined hyperlipidemia in relation to race/ethnicity, obesity, and insulin resistance in the Multi-Ethnic Study of Atherosclerosis (MESA). Metabolism 2009;58:212-9.

Bonora E, Targher G, Formentini G, Calcaterra F, Lombardi S, Marini F, Zenari L, Saggiani F, Poli M, Perbellini S, Raffaelli A, Gemma L, Santi L, Bonadonna RC, Muggeo M. The metabolic syndrome is an independent predictor of cardiovascular disease in Type 2 diabetic subjects. Prospective data from the Verona Diabetes Complications Study. Diabet Med 2004;21:52-8.

Bruno G, Merletti F, Biggeri A, Bargero G, Ferrero S, Runzo C, Prina Cerai S, Pagano G, Cavallo-Perin P; Casale Monferrato Study. Metabolic syndrome as a predictor of all-cause and cardiovascular mortality in Type 2 diabetes: the Casale Monferrato Study. Diabetes Care 2004;27:2689-94.

Grundy SM, Cleeman JI, Daniels SR, Donato KA, Eckel RH, Franklin BA, Gordon DJ, Krauss RM, Savage PJ, Smith SC Jr, Spertus JA, Costa F; American Heart Association; National Heart, Lung, and Blood Institute. Diagnosis and management of the metabolic syndrome: an American Heart Association/National Heart, Lung, and Blood Institute Scientific Statement. Circulation 2005;112:2735-52.

Metascreen Writing Committee. The metabolic syndrome is a risk indicator of microvascular and macrovascular complications in diabetes. Results from Metascreen, a multicenter diabetes clinic-based survey. Diabetes Care 2006;29:2701-7.

Alberti KG, Eckel RH, Grundy SM, Zimmet PZ, Cleeman JI, Donato KA, Fruchart JC, James WP, Loria CM, Smith SC Jr; International Diabetes Federation Task Force on Epidemiology and Prevention; National Heart, Lung, and Blood Institute; American Heart Association; World Heart Federation; International Atherosclerosis Society; International Association for the Study of Obesity. Harmonizing the metabolic syndrome: a joint interim statement of the International Diabetes Federation Task Force on Epidemiology and Prevention; National Heart, Lung, and Blood Institute; American Heart Association; World Heart Federation; International Atherosclerosis Society; and International Association for the Study of Obesity. Circulation. 2009;120:1640-5.

Hermans MP, Ahn SA, Amoussou-Guenou KD, Rousseau MF. Impact of metabolic syndrome on microvascular complications in type 2 diabetes. Diab Metab Syndr 2010;4:150-4.

Sadikot S, Hermans MP. Here we go again ... The metabolic syndrome revisited! Diab Metab Syndr 2010;4:111-20.

Davignon J, Cohn JS. Triglycerides: a risk factor for coronary heart disease. Atherosclerosis 1996;124(Suppl):S57-64.

Fruchart JC, Duriez P. HDL and triglyceride as therapeutic targets. Curr Opin Lipidol 2002;13:605-16.

Lu W, Resnick HE, Jablonski KA, Jones KL, Jain AK, Howard WJ, Robbins DC, Howard BV. Non-HDL cholesterol as a predictor of cardiovascular disease in type 2 diabetes : The Strong Heart Study. Diab. Care 2003;26.16-23.

Fruchart JC, Nierman MC, Stroes ES, Kastelein JJ, Duriez P. New risk factors for atherosclerosis and patient risk assessment. Circulation 2004;109(23 Suppl 1):III15-9.

Yusuf S, Hawken S, Ôunpuu S, Dans T, Avezum A, Lanas F et al. on behalf of the INTERHEART investigators, Effect of potentially modifiable risk factors associated with myocardial infarction in 52 countries (the INTERHEART study): case-control study. Lancet 2004;364:937-52.

Assmann G, Cullen P, Fruchart JC, Greten H, Naruszewicz M, Olsson A, Paoletti R, Riesen W, Stoll M, Tikkanen M, von Eckardstein A; International Task Force for Prevention of Coronary Heart Disease. Implications of emerging risk factors for therapeutic intervention. Nutr Metab Cardiovasc Dis 2005;15:373-81.

Walldius G, Jungner I. The apoB/apoA-I ratio: a strong, new risk factor for cardiovascular disease and a target for lipid-lowering therapy--a review of the evidence. J Intern Med 2006;259:493-519.

Assmann G, Schulte H, Cullen P, Seedorf U. Assessing risk of myocardial infarction and stroke: new data from the Prospective Cardiovascular Münster (PROCAM) study. Eur J Clin Invest 2007;37:925-32.

Bansal S, Buring JE, Rifai N, Mora S, Sacks FM, Ridker PM. Fasting compared with nonfasting triglycerides and risk of cardiovascular events in women. JAMA 2007;298:309-16.

Hermans MP, Ahn SA, Rousseau MF. The non-HDL-C/HDL-C ratio provides cardiovascular risk stratification similar to the ApoB/ApoA1 ratio in diabetics: Comparison with reference lipid markers. Diab Metab Syndr 2007;1:23-8.

Assmann G, Schulte H, Seedorf U. Cardiovascular risk assessment in the metabolic syndrome: results from the Prospective Cardiovascular Munster (PROCAM) Study. Int J Obes (Lond) 2008;32(Suppl 2):S11-6.

Kawakami A, Osaka M, Tani M, Azuma H, Sacks FM, Shimokado K, Yoshida M. Apolipoprotein CIII links hyperlipidemia with vascular endothelial cell dysfunction. Circulation 2008;118:731-42.

Ridker PM, Danielson E, Fonseca FA, Genest J, Gotto AM Jr, Kastelein JJ, Koenig W, Libby P, Lorenzatti AJ, MacFadyen JG, Nordestgaard BG, Shepherd J, Willerson JT, Glynn RJ; JUPITER Study Group. Rosuvastatin to prevent vascular events in men and women with elevated C-reative protein. N Engl J Med 2008;359:2195-207.

Hermans MP, Ahn SA, Rousseau MF. Cardiometabolic phenotype and UKPDS risk in male type 2 diabetic patients with obstructive sleep apnoea syndrome. Diabetes Metab Syndr 2009;3:50-4.

Hermans MP, Ahn SA, Rousseau MF. Erectile dysfunction, microangiopathy and UKPDS risk in type 2 diabetes. Diabetes Metab 2009;35:484-9.

Mendivil CO, Zheng C, Furtado J, Lel J, Sacks FM. Metabolism of very-low-density lipoprotein and low-density lipoprotein containing apolipoprotein C-III and not other small apolipoproteins. Arterioscler Thromb Vasc Biol 2010;30:239-45.

Sarwar N, Sandhu MS, Ricketts SL, Butterworth AS, Di Angelantonio E, Boekholdt SM, Ouwehand W, Watkins H, Samani NJ, Saleheen D, Lawlor D, Reilly MP, Hingorani AD, Talmud PJ, Danesh J. Triglyceride Coronary Disease Genetics Consortium and Emerging Risk Factors Collaboration. Triglyceride-mediated pathways and coronary disease: collaborative analysis of 101 studies. Lancet 2010;375:1634-9.

Zheng C, Khoo C, Furtado J, Sacks FM. Apolipoprotein C-III and the metabolic basis for hypertriglyceridemia and the dense low-density lipoprotein phenotype. Circulation 2010;121:1722-34.

Hermans MP, Sacks FM, Ahn SA, Rousseau MF. Non-HDL-cholesterol as valid surrogate to apolipoprotein B100 measurement in diabetes: discriminant ratio and unbiased equivalence. Cardiovasc Diabetol. 2011;10:20.

Davidson MH. Reducing residual risk for patients on statin therapy: the potential role of combination therapy. Am J Cardiol 2005;96(9A):3K-13K.

Libby PL. The forgotten majority. Unfinished business in cardiovascular risk reduction. J Am Coll Cardiol 2005;46:1225-8.

Shepherd J, Barter P, Carmena R, Deedwania P, Fruchart JC, Haffner S, Hsia J, Breazna A, LaRosa J, Grundy S, Waters D for the Treating to New Targets Investigators. Effect of lowering LDL cholesterol substantially below currently recommended levels in patients with coronary heart disease and diabetes: The Treating to New Targets (TNT) study. Diabetes Care 2006;29:1220-6

Barter P, Gotto AM, LaRosa JC, Maroni J, Szarek M, Grundy SM, Kastelein JJ, Bittner V, Fruchart JC. Treating to New Targets Investigators. HDL cholesterol, very low levels of LDL cholesterol, and cardiovascular events. N Engl J Med 2007;357:1301-10.

Friedewald VE Jr, Ballantyne CM, Davidson MH, Guyton JR, Roberts WC. The editor's roundtable: lipid management beyond statins - reducing residual cardiovascular risk. Am J Cardiol 2008;102:559-67.

Jones PH. Expert perspective: reducing cardiovascular risk in metabolic syndrome and type 2 diabetes mellitus beyond low-density lipoprotein cholesterol lowering. Am J Cardiol 2008;102:41L-7L.

Miller M, Cannon CP, Murphy SA, Qin J, Ray KK, Braunwald E; PROVE-IT TIMI 22 Investigators. Impact of triglyceride levels beyond low-density lipoprotein cholesterol after acute coronary syndrome in the PROVE-IT TIMI 22 trial. J Am Coll Cardiol 2008;51:724-30

Schramm TK, Gislason GH, Køber L, Rasmussen S, Rasmussen JN, Abildstrøm SZ, Hansen ML, Folke F, Buch P, Madsen M, Vaag A, Torp-Pedersen C. Diabetes patients requiring glucose-lowering therapy and nondiabetics with a prior myocardial infarction carry the same cardiovascular risk: a population study of 3.3 million people. Circulation 2008;117:1945-54

Sulkes D, Brown BG, Krauss RM, Segrest JP, Sniderman AD, Roberts WC. The editor's roundtable: expanded versus standard lipid panels in assessing and managing cardiovascular risk. Am J Cardiol 2008;101:828-42.

Ridker PM, Genest J, Boekholdt SM, Libby P, Gotto AM, Nordestgaard BG, Mora S, MacFadyen JG, Glynn RJ, Kastelein JJ; JUPITER Trial Study Group. HDL cholesterol and residual risk of first cardiovascular events after treatment with potent statin therapy: an analysis from the JUPITER trial. Lancet 2010;376:333-9.

Volek JS, Fernandez ML, Feinman RD, Phinney SD. Dietary carbohydrate restriction induces a unique metabolic state positively affecting atherogenic dyslipidemia, fatty acid partitioning, and metabolic syndrome. Prog Lipid Res 2008;47:307-18.

Katcher HI, Hill AM, Lanford JL, Yoo JS, Kris-Etherton PM. Lifestyle approaches and dietary strategies to lower LDL-cholesterol and triglycerides and raise HDL-cholesterol. Endocrinol Metab Clin North Am 2009;38:45-78.

Fruchart JC. Peroxisome proliferator-activated receptor-α (PPARα): at the crossroads of obesity, diabetes and cardiovascular disease. Atherosclerosis 2009;205:1-8.

Vergès B. Role for fibrate therapy in diabetes: evidence before FIELD. Curr Opin Lipidol 2005;16:648-51.

Jun M, Foote C, Lv J, Neal B, Patel A, Nicholls SJ, Grobbee DE, Cass A, Chalmers J, Perkovic V. Effects of fibrates on cardiovascular outcomes: a systematic review and meta-analysis. Lancet 2010;375:1875-84.

Taylor AJ, Villines TC, Stanek E, Devine PJ, Griffen L, Miller M, Weissman NJ, Turco M. Extended-release niacin or ezetimibe and carotid intima-media thickness. New Engl J Med 2009;361: 2113-22.

Chapman MJ, Redfern JS, McGovern ME, Giral P. Niacin and fibrates in atherogenic dyslipidemia: pharmacotherapy to reduce cardiovascular risk. Pharmacol Ther 2010;126:314-45.

AIM HIGH: Niacin plus statin to prevent vascular events. ClinicalTrials.gov identifier: NCT00120289.

HPS2-THRIVE. Treatment of HDL to reduce the incidence of vascular events. ClinicalTrials.gov Identifier: NCT00461630.

ACCORD Study Group, Ginsberg HN, Elam MB, Lovato LC, Crouse JR 3rd, Leiter LA, Linz P, Friedewald WT, Buse JB, Gerstein HC, Probstfield J, Grimm RH, Ismail-Beigi F, Bigger JT, Goff DC Jr, Cushman WC, Simons-Morton DG, Byington RP. Effects of combination lipid therapy in type 2 diabetes mellitus. N Engl J Med 2010;362:1563-74.

Fruchart J-C, Sacks FM, Hermans MP. Implications of the ACCORD lipid study : perspective from the Residual Risk Reduction Initiative (R3i). Curr Med Res Opin 2010;26:1793-7.

Hermans MP, Ahn SA, Rousseau MF. Statin therapy and cataract in Type 2 diabetes. Diabetes Metab 2011;37:139-43.

UK Prospective Diabetes Study Group. Tight blood pressure control and risk of macrovascular and microvascular complications in type 2 diabetes. UKPDS 38. BMJ 1998;317:703-13.

Misra A, Kumar S, Kishore Vikram A, Kumar A. The role of lipids in the development of diabetic microvascular complications: implications for therapy. Am J Cardiovasc Drugs 2003;3:325-338.

Dodson PM. Medical treatment for diabetic retinopathy: do the FIELD microvascular study results support a role for lipid lowering? Practical Diabetes International 2008;25:76-79.

Dodson PM. Diabetes and the Eye. In: Diabetic Retinopathy, Dodson PM (ed). Oxford University Press, Oxford, pp 33-44, 2009.

Chew EY, Ambrosius WT, Howard LT, Greven CM, Johnson S, Danis RP, Davis MD, Genuth S, Domanski M; ACCORD Study Group. Rationale, design, and methods of the Action to Control Cardiovascular Risk in Diabetes Eye Study (ACCORD-EYE). Am J Cardiol 2007;99(12A):103i-11i.

ACCORD Study Group; ACCORD Eye Study Group, Chew EY, Ambrosius WT, Davis MD, Danis RP, Gangaputra S, Greven CM, Hubbard L, Esser BA, Lovato JF, Perdue LH, Goff DC Jr, Cushman WC, Ginsberg HN, Elam MB, Genuth S, Gerstein HC, Schubart U, Fine LJ. Effects of medical therapies on retinopathy progression in type 2 diabetes. N Engl J Med 2010;363;233-44.

Matthews DR. Fenofibrate and statin therapy, compared with placebo and statin, slows the development of retinopathy in type 2 diabetes patients of 10 years duration: the ACCORD study. Evid Based Med 2011 Apr;16(2):45-6.

Hermans MP. Prevention of microvascular diabetic complications by fenofibrate: lessons from FIELD and ACCORD. Diabetes Vasc Dis Res 2011 (*in press*).

Cushman WC, Grimm RH, Cutler JA for the ACCORD study group. Rationale and Design for the Blood Pressure Intervention of the Action to Control Cardiovascular Risk in Diabetes (ACCORD) Trial. Am J Cardiol 2007;99(suppl):44i-55i.

Hermans MP. Impact of fenofibrate on type 2 diabetes patients with features of the metabolic syndrome: subgroup analysis from FIELD. Curr Cardiol Rev 2010;6:112-8.

Carey VJ, Bishop L, Laranjo N, Harschfield BJ, Kwiat C, Sacks FM. Contribution of high plasma triglycerides and low high-density lipoprotein cholesterol to residual risk of coronary heart disease after establishment of low-density lipoprotein cholesterol control. Am J Cardiol 2010;106:757-63.

Rajamani K, Colman PG, Li LP, Best JD, Voysey M, D'Emden MC, Laakso M, Baker JR, Keech AC; FIELD study investigators. Effect of fenofibrate on amputation events in people with type 2 diabetes mellitus (FIELD study): a prespecified analysis of a randomised controlled trial. Lancet 2009;373:1780-8.

Millán Núñez-Cortés J, Montoya JP, Salas XP, Hernández Mijares A, Carey VJ, Hermans MP, Sacks FM, Fruchart JC. The REALIST (REsiduAl risk, LIpids and Standard Therapies) study: an analysis of residual risk attributable to lipid profile in acute coronary syndrome. Endocrinol Nutr 2011;58:38-47.

Davis TM, Ting R, Best JD, Donoghoe MW, Drury PL, Sullivan DR, Jenkins AJ, O'Connell RL, Whiting MJ, Glasziou PP, Simes RJ, Kesäniemi YA, Gebski VJ, Scott RS, Keech AC; Fenofibrate Intervention and Event Lowering in Diabetes Study investigators. Effects of fenofibrate on renal function in patients with type 2 diabetes mellitus: the Fenofibrate Intervention and Event Lowering in Diabetes (FIELD) Study. Diabetologia 2011;54:280-90.

Keech A, Simes RJ, Barter P, Best J, Scott R, Taskinen MR, Forder P, Pillai A, Davis T, Glasziou P, Drury P, Kesaniemi YA, Sullivan D, Hunt D, Colman P, d'Emden M, Whiting M, Ehnholm C, Laakso M. Effects of long-term fenofibrate therapy on cardiovascular events in 9795 people with type 2 diabetes mellitus (the FIELD study): randomised controlled trial. Lancet 2005;366:1849-61.

Scott R, O'Brien R, Fulcher G, Pardy C, D'Emden M, Tse D, Taskinen MR, Ehnholm C, Keech A; Fenofibrate Intervention and Event Lowering in Diabetes (FIELD) Study Investigators. The effects of fenofibrate treatment on cardiovascular disease risk in 9795 people with type 2 diabetes and various components of the metabolic syndrome: the FIELD study. Diabetes Care 2009,32:493-8.

Effect of fenofibrate on progression of coronary-artery disease in type 2 diabetes: the Diabetes Atherosclerosis Intervention Study, a randomised study. Lancet 2001;357:905 10.

Ansquer JC, Foucher C, Rattier S, Taskinen MR, Steiner G; DAIS Investigators. Fenofibrate reduces progression to microalbuminuria over 3 years in a placebo-controlled study in type 2 diabetes: results from the Diabetes Atherosclerosis Intervention Study (DAIS). Am J Kidney Dis 2005;45:485-93.

Polonsky TS, Davidson MH. Reducing the residual risk of 3-hydroxy-3-methylglutaryl coenzyme A reductase inhibitor therapy with combination therapy. Am J Cardiol 2008;101(8A):27B-35B.

Rosenson RS. Management of non-high-density lipoprotein abnormalities. Atherosclerosis 2009;207:328-35.

Rosenson RS, Davidson MH, Pourfarzib R. Underappreciated opportunities for low-density lipoprotein management in patients with cardiometabolic residual risk. Atherosclerosis 2010;213/1-7.

Sacks FM, Carey VJ, Fruchart JC. Combination lipid therapy in type 2 diabetes. N Engl J Med 2010;363:692-4.

Hermans MP, Muls E, Nobels F, Krzentowski G, Claes N, Debacker N, Matthys A. Evaluating benchmarking to optimize management of type 2 diabetes patients: the Belgian data from the OPTIMISE study. Acta Cardiol 2011;66:124-5.

Brotons C, Elisaf M, Hermans MP, Michel G, Muls E, Matthys A. Evaluating benchmarking to optimize management of type 2 diabetic patients: HbA_{1c} control in the European OPTIMISE study. Diabetes 2011 (*in press*).

5

Type 2 Diabetes and Fibrinolysis

Ján Staško, Peter Chudý, Daniela Kotuličová,
Peter Galajda, Marián Mokáň and Peter Kubisz
Comenius University in Bratislava, Jessenius Faculty of Medicine in Martin
Slovakia

1. Introduction

Type 2 diabetes (DM2) is associated with complex hemostasis disorders characterised with enhanced coagulation, platelet dysfunction and hypofibrinolysis. These pathological conditions predispose type 2 diabetics towards increased morbidity and mortality due to thrombotic complications. In fact, DM2 is considered the most frequent acquired thrombophilic state. Under physiological conditions, fibrinolytic system is responsible for the lysis of fibrin clot, thus maintaining the blood fluidity. It was first described by Astrup in 1956. The most important molecule in fibrinolytic system is plasmin, which cleaves fibrin clot. It is released in its inactive form called plasminogen from the liver to the blood stream and gets activated by tissue plasminogen activator (t-PA), urokinase plasminogen activator (u-PA), clotting factor XII (FXII) and kallikrein. Plasmin deactivation occurs via several molecules. The best known and most important is α2-plasmin inhibitor (α-2PI). Another one, which was described in early nineteen nineties, is called thrombin-activatable fibrinolysis inhibitor (TAFI). Plasminogen activation and thus plasmin formation is inhibited by plasminogen activator inhibitor type 1 (PAI-1), PAI-2 and PAI-3. Fibrinolysis disorder due to disequilibrium between plasminogen activators and its inhibitors is the most characteristic feature of prothrombotic state associated with diabetes. The fibrinolytic activity in DM2 is influenced by numerous factors, the most crucial ones are glycaemic control, insulinaemia, blood lipid profile, blood pressure, genetic factors and different sorts of medication (Brummel-Ziedins et al., 2009, Alzahrani & Ajjan, 2010a).

2. Fibrinolysis

2.1 Plasminogen and its activation

Under physiological conditions, fibrinolytic system is responsible for the lysis of fibrin clot, thus maintaining the blood fluidity. The central protein in whole fibrinolytic system is plasmin, a serin protease, which cleaves fibrin clot. Plasminogen, the single-chain proenzyme of plasmin, is a protein of 791 amino acids, m.w. 92 000 synthesized primarily in the liver (Raum et al., 1980). The lysine-binding domains of plasminogen mediate its specific interactions with fibrin, cell surface receptors and other proteins, including its circulating inhibitor α2-plasmin inhibitor (α2-PI), which is also known as α2-antiplasmin (Hajjar et al., 1986; Plow et al., 1991). Activation of plasminogen, by cleavage of a single Arg-Val peptide bond at position 560–561 (Holvoet et al., 1985), gives rise to the active serine protease, plasmin.

Plasminogen can be converted to plasmin by both t-PA and u-PA. t-PA is a molecule of m.w. 72 000 which consists of 527 amino acids (Pennica et al., 1983). Cleavage of the Arg275-Ile276 peptide bond by plasmin converts t-PA to a disulphide-linked, two-chain form (Pennica et al., 1983). While single-chain t-PA is less active than two-chain t-PA in the fluid phase, both forms demonstrate equivalent activity when fibrin bound. The t-PA is synthesized and secreted primarily by endothelial cells. u-PA is the second endogenous plasminogen activator. Single-chain u-PA or prourokinase, is a glycoprotein of m.w. 54 000, consisting of 411 amino acids. Cleavage of the Lys158-Ile159 peptide bond by plasmin or kallikrein converts single-chain u-PA to a disulphide-linked two-chain derivative. The u-PA has much lower affinity for fibrin than t-PA, and is an effective plasminogen activator in both the presence and the absence of fibrin (Gurewich et al., 1984). Fibrin, the major plasmin substrate, regulates its own degradation by binding both plasminogen and t-PA on its surface, thereby localizing and enhancing plasmin generation. The affinity between t-PA and plasminogen is low in the absence of fibrin, but increases significantly in its presence. Once formed, plasmin cleaves fibrin, generating soluble degradation products, and exposing carboxy-terminal lysine (Lys) residues. 'Kringles' 2 of t-PA, and 1 and 4 of plasminogen contain lysine-binding sites, which mediate further binding to fibrin, leading to enhanced plasmin generation and fibrin removal (Plow et al., 1991).

This binding can be blocked by the recently discovered thrombin-activatable fibrinolysis inhibitor (TAFI). When activated by thrombin-thrombomodulin complex, TAFI removes carboxy-terminal Lys residues, thereby attenuating plasmin generation, stabilizing fibrin thrombi, and establishing a regulatory connection between coagulation and fibrinolysis. Fibrin dissolution is also regulated by inhibitors of plasminogen activation, such as PAI-1, and by inhibitors of plasmin itself, such as α2-PI. In addition, plasmin bound to fibrin is protected from α2-PI, due to occupancy of its lysine-binding sites. TAFI, on the other hand, decreases this protection by deleting plasmin-binding Lys residues on fibrin. Moreover, diverse cell types promote plasmin generation through their expression of cell surface receptors (Cesarman-Maus & Hajjar, 2005). Endothelial cells, monocytes, macrophages, neutrophils and some tumour cells, all bind plasminogen, as well as t-PA and/or u-PA. Their receptors localize cell surface fibrinolytic activity, serve as cofactors in acute or ongoing plasmin generation, and provide specialized environments that are protected from circulating inhibitors. Under certain conditions, proteases that are traditionally classified within the intrinsic arm of the coagulation cascade have been shown to activate plasminogen directly. These include kallikrein, factor XIa and factor XIIa, but normally account for no more than 15% of total plasmin-generating activity in plasma (Cesarman-Maus & Hajjar, 2005). In addition, the membrane type 1 matrix metalloproteinase (MT1-MMP) appears to exert fibrinolytic activity in the absence of plasminogen. Factor VII-activating protease has also been reported to serve as an in vitro activator of single-chain PLG activators, but its role *in vivo* remains to be determined (Römisch et al., 1999). Plasminogen together with its activators t-PA and u-PA, urokinase receptor (uPAR), plasminogen activator inhibitors PAI-1, PAI-2, PAI-3 (which is identical to the protein C inhibitor) and protease nexin forms the plasminogen activator system (PAS). (Brummel-Ziedins et al., 2009; Schmitt et al., 1997).

2.2 Inhibition of fibrinolysis

The major plasmin inhibitor is α2-PI. It is a single-chain glycoprotein of m.w. 70 000. α2-PI is also a constituent of platelet α granules (Plow & Collen, 1981). Thus, plasmin released into

flowing blood or in the vicinity of a platelet-rich thrombus, is immediately neutralized by α2-PI. α2-PI is cleaved at its Arg364-Met365 peptide bond, and then forms a lysine-binding site-dependent α2-PI–plasmin complex, which is cleared in the liver (Plow et al., 1991).
The PAI-1 is the most important and most rapidly acting physiological inhibitor of both tPA and uPA. This single chain glycoprotein of m.w. 52 000 is released by endothelial cells, monocytes, macrophages, hepatocytes, adipocytes and platelets (Ny et al, 1986). Release of PAI-1 is stimulated by many cytokines, growth factors and lipoproteins common to the global inflammatory response. After the release, PAI-1 quickly converts to an inactive form and circulates in plasma. Activation occurs by conformational change through binging to negatively charged phospholipids. It builds up a 1:1 complex binding with t-PA, thus inactivating it. This process is catalyzed by fibrin, which binds PAI-1 and enhances the t-PA plasma clearance. The complex dissociates from fibrin and is removed from circulation by liver (Cesarman-Maus & Hajjar, 2005).
PAI-2, the less important inhibitor of plasmin activation, is a 393 amino acid member of the serpin family. It was originally purified from human placenta. Functionally, PAI-2 inhibits both two-chain t-PA and two-chain u-PA with comparable efficiency, but it is less effective towards single-chain t-PA, and does not inhibit prourokinase. Significant levels of PAI-2 are found in human plasma only during pregnancy (Ye et al, 1987).

2.3 Plasminogen activator inhibitor type 1

2.3.1 Regulation of plasminogen activator inhibitor type 1 levels

PAI-1 is synthesized after stimulation. Its gene is localized on chromosome 7. In the circulation PAI-1 is rapidly converted (half-life 5 min.) to a latent inactive form which represents the major form of PAI-1 in plasma. Vitronectin stabilizes the active form of PAI-1 in plasma and prolonges its half-life 2 to 4-fold. The vitronectin levels are increased in relation to the cytokine dependent synthesis in the liver and hence the PAI-1 active form circulates in plasma during inflammation at high concentration. PAI-1 is removed from the circulation in the liver, in particular through binding at low density lipoprotein receptor-related protein (LRP), with the half-life of 10 min. (Lijnen, 2004; Loskutoff & Mimuro, 1991; Schleef & Loskutoff, 1988; Wiman, 1995).
According to multicompartmental and multifactorial model, the regulation of the PAI-1 plasma levels is complex and depends on multiple sites of PAI-1 synthesis and various stimuli, including hormones involved in the lipid and glucose metabolism. PAI-1 is synthesized in vascular (endothelium, vascular smooth muscles, platelets storage pool) and extravascular, i.e. metabolic (adipocytes, hepatocytes) compartments. These two PAI-1 compartments are regulated in a different way with various effect of insulin on PAI-1 synthesis. Factors regulating the PAI-1 production include stimulating effects of insulin, proinsulin, very low density lipoproteins (VLDL), inflammatory cytokines and oxidative stress (Galajda et al., 1997b, 1998a, 1998e, 1999; Galajda & Mokáň, 2001).

2.3.1.1 PAI-1 metabolic compartment

PAI-1 metabolic compartment is formed by visceral adipocytes, stromal fat cells (in particular macrophages) and hepatocytes. These cells regulate the postprandial changes of fibrinolysis in splanchnic system. The principle site of PAI-1 production in mice is adipose tissue. The cultures of visceral adipocytes are more important source of PAI-1 *in vitro* than hepatocytes. Experimental studies of PAI-1 *in vivo* found that PAI-1 production in obese mice is 7-fold increased in adipocytes whilst it is only 2-fold higher in hepatocytes compared to lean mice. In human adipose tissue, PAI-1 production is localized mainly in the stromal fat cells and macrophages. Adipose tissue can be the principal source of PAI-1. Visceral adipose tissue produces 5-fold higher amount of PAI-1 compared to subcutaneous adipose tissue and levels of PAI-1 in obese subjects are related rather to the amount of visceral than subcutaneous fat. Thus PAI-1 levels are better correlated with indices of the central obesity (waist-to-hip ratio - WHR). Insulin stimulates PAI-1 production in adipose tissue with synergistic effect of VLDL and free fat acids (FFAs). Therefore the adipose tissue is the most important source of PAI-1 related to insulin. Moreover, experimental studies in mice proved that the insulin application increases the expression of PAI-1 mRNA much more in adipose tissue than in the liver. Locally formed corticoids, inflammatory cytokines (TNF) and growth factors (TGF-β) can also stimulate the PAI-1 production in visceral adipose tissue. Under certain circumstances, hepatocytes can be an important source of PAI-1, especially in fatty liver disease. Insulin, proinsulin (PI) including des-31,32-split form and insulin like growth factor (IGF-1) stimulate production of PAI-1 in the liver. The most potent form among them is des-31,32-split PI, whilst PI and insulin stimulate the production of PAI-1 in liver with lower effect. The PAI-1 production is also stimulated by hyperlipidemia. VLDL act relatively rapidly and in synergy with insulin (Alessi et al., 1988, 1997, 2006; Hamsten & Eriksson, 1994; Juhan-Vague et al., 1991; Juhan-Vague & Alessi, 1997; Lijnen, 2004; Lijnen et al., 2005; Loskutoff & Mimuro, 1991; Loskutoff & Samad, 1998; Schneider & Sobel, 1996; Samad & Loskutoff, 1997).

2.3.1.2 PAI-1 vascular compartment

PAI-1 vascular compartment includes endothelium, subendothelial pool (vascular smooth muscles, fibroblasts, macrophages) and a rapid release pool (platelets). PAI-1 is released to circulation mainly from the endothelium. Vascular smooth muscles can participate in regulation of PAI-1 levels under certain conditions. The platelets are the only cells in human body which store PAI-1. The total amount of PAI-1 is 4-fold higher in platelets compared to plasma, but they do not significantly impact on the PAI-1 plasma levels. The platelet PAI-1 plays a role in the local accumulation and action of the inhibitor. In our DM2 patients, hyperinsulinemic (HI) non-diabetics and healthy controls the PAI-1 levels did not correlate with platelet factor 4 (PF_4) - the marker of platelet activation. This finding supports the hypothesis about more significant effect of the endothelium on PAI-1 plasma levels than the release of PAI-1 from platelet α granules (Galajda et al., 1997a; Galajda & Mokáň, 2001). Regulation of PAI-1 production in the endothelium has some specifics and differs from its regulation in metabolic compartment. The inflammatory cytokines as tumor necrosis factor (TNF), interleukin 1 (IL-1), transforming growth factor β (TGF-β), thrombin and angiotensin II and metabolic factors as proinsulin, hyperglycaemia, oxidative stress and lipids including VLDL and FFAs represent important stimulators of PAI-1 synthesis in the endothelium. On the contrary insulin inhibits synthesis of PAI-1 in the endothelium induced by TGF-β, probably due to activated cGMP and cAMP systems. Insulin along with leptin also stimulates the PAI-1 production in vascular smooth muscles (Eriksson et al., 1998; Hamsten & Eriksson, 1994; Kawai et al., 1996; Kim et al., 1997; Li et al., 1997; Peiretti et al., 1997; Vaughan, 1997, 2005; Yamauchi et al., 1997).

2.3.2 The control of PAI-1 levels in circulation

PAI-1 levels depend on the PAI-1 expression and release from various tissues which are induced by the stimulatory effects of different factors. Adipose tissue, liver and vascular endothelium are considered to be the most important sources of PAI-1 production.

2.3.2.1 Genetic factors

Up to 100-fold individual variability of PAI-1 levels has been described in the general population. Genetic factors take part in this variability in only as much as 3-5%. Increased PAI-1 levels are associated with several known PAI-1 gene polymorphisms. One of them is the PAI-1 promotor region gene polymorphism **-844** G/A (Xho I) which represents a potential binding site for Ets transcription factor. Another one is the polymorphism **-675 4G/5G** which affects the binding of nuclear proteins involved in the regulation of PAI-1 gene transcription. The PAI-1 5G allele leads to binding of a repressor protein thereby decreasing gene transcription. Consequently, higher plasma PAI-1 concentrations have been found among homozygotes for the 4G- allele compared to heterozygotes and homozygotes for the 5G-allele (Burzotta et al, 2003; Dawson et al., 1993; Eriksson et al, 1995). Majority of the europoid population are heterozygous carriers of the 4G/5G allele with a frequency of approximately 50%. Total frequency of 4G allele associated with a higher PAI-1 production is 52-54% in europoid, 30-46% in mongoloid and 24% in negroid population. Another polymorphism **Hind III** in the 3´-end of PAI-1 gene is associated with different regulation of PAI-1 by metabolic factors. Allele 2/2 is linked with more potent stimulatory effect of VLDL on PAI-1 production in the endothelial cell culture while a less frequent allele 1/1 (present in 20% of general population), is characterized by the stimulatory effect of insulin on PAI-1 production in endothelial cells *in vitro*. Recently identified **G12078A dimorphism** in 3´-end of PAI-1 can influence the PAI-1 levels by modifying of post-transcription mechanisms (Green, 1996; Lijnen, 2004; Mansfield et al., 1997; McCormack et al., 1996).

2.3.2.2 Insulin, proinsulin and insulin resistance

The grade of insulin resistance (IR) is responsible for 49% interindividual variability of the PAI-1 levels in europoid men and 29% variability in women. It is a principle factor associated with PAI-1 levels but it includes various stimulatory mechanisms. Insulin is considered to be one of the main physiologic regulators of PAI-1 levels, it is responsible for a linkage of PLG system with human metabolic activity. The effect of insulin is different in various compartments of the PAI-1 production. Adipose tissue is the most important source of circulating PAI-1, its *in vivo* production is insulin dependent. Insulin stimulates the PAI-1 synthesis in synergy with VLDL and FFAs. Insulin also enhances the PAI-1 production in the liver. The effect of insulin on PAI-1 production in the endothelium is rather more complex. Insulin impacts neither PAI-1 basal production in the culture of human endothelial cells *in vitro* nor PAI-1 production in the vessels of mice splanchnic system after insulin application *in vivo*. On the contrary, insulin can inhibit PAI-1 production in the culture of endothelial cells induced by TGFβ *in vitro*. The inhibitory effect of insulin on the PAI-1 endothelial production can be mediated by cGMP and cAMP. Insulin increases the activity of cGMP by stimulation of NO production, it also increases the amount of cAMP by subsequent cGMP dependent inhibition of specific phosphodiesterase (PDE_3). The decrease of PAI-1 during postprandial HI can be explained by inhibitory effect of insulin on the PAI-1 production in endothelium *in vivo*. Similarly, we confirmed the significantly decreased PAI-1 levels which were independent from other metabolic parameters in our DM2 patients with endothelial dysfunction on long-term insulin treatment compared to those treated with oral antidiabetics **(Table 1 and 2)** (Galajda & Mokáň, 2001). These findings verify the inhibitory effect of insulin on PAI-1 production in the endothelial cells. On the other hand some studies found locally increased PAI-1 levels in human antebrachial vessels which were induced by the insulin application. This finding can be explained either by the release of PAI-1 from the vascular smooth muscles, as insulin stimulates PAI-1 release from the muscles *in vitro* or by heterogeneity of insulin effect on different types of endothelium. Another explanation can be found in the interindividual differences in human endothelial response to insulin as it was proved in Hind III polymorphism of PAI-1 gene. In this polymorphism a less frequent allele 1/1 is associated with stimulatory effect of insulin on PAI-1 production in the culture of human umbilical vein endothelial cells (HUVEC). **Proinsulin (PI)** including its incomplete split forms (des-31,32; des-61,62) stimulates the PAI-1 synthesis in liver and endothelial cells. The des-31,32 split PI form has the most potent stimulatory effect on PAI-1 production in hepatocytes whereas PI stimulates PAI-1 production with the same effect as insulin. **Insulin-like growth factor 1 (IGF-1)** stimulates, similarly to insulin, the PAI-1 production in the liver but not in the endothelium. **C-peptide,** which possesses certain hormonal activity of insulin, does not influence the PAI-1 production (Alessi et al., 1988, 1997, 2007; Alessi & Juhan-Vague, 2006; Grant et al., 1990; Gray et al., 1997; Juhan-Vague et al., 1991; Lijnen 2004; Nagi et al., 1990; Nordt et al., 1994; Panahloo et al., 1996; Pandolfi et al., 1996; Yamauchi, et al., 1997).

2.3.2.3 Free fat acids and lipoproteins with very low density

VLDL are important molecules stimulating PAI-1 synthesis. From among them, the bigger $VLDL_1$ stimulate PAI-1 production more than the smaller $VLDL_2$. Unsaturated FFAs are proper stimulators of PAI-1 released from the VLDL, which intracellularly activate specific VLDL/FA - inducible transcription factor. This factor binds at -672 to -657 site of the PAI-1 gene promotor region marked as VLDL/FA-RE. This site has 67% homology with binding sites of so called peroxisome proliferator-activated receptors (PPARs) and is situated next to -675G promotor which is responsible for the binding of PAI-1 transcription repressor (factor B). Binding of VLDL/FA - inducible transcription factor at VLDL/FA-RE decreases the binding of transcription repressor (factor B) resulting in the increased PAI-1 production. VLDL increase synthesis of PAI-1 in the endothelium by this mechanism whilst in hepatocytes VLDL stimulate the PAI-1 synthesis synergistically with insulin by stabilization of mRNA. The monounsaturated, ω-3 and ω-6 polyunsaturated FFAs have a stimulatory effect on PAI-1 production in hepatocytes and endothelium *in vitro* while saturated FFAs do not influence PAI-1 production. Regulation of PAI-1 by PPARs has different mechanisms. Binding of PPARγ to corresponding bond sites (PPRE) on PAI-1 gene promotor can be associated with the increased basal mRNA expression for PAI-1 but the main effect is inhibition of PAI-1 production induced by inflammatory cytokines TNF and IL-1. Also the application of glitazones for patients with DM2 is associated with decreased PAI-1 independently on metabolic control and in correlation with decreased insulin and FFAs. Activation of PPARα by fibrates do not influence basal production of PAI-1 in the endothelium *in vitro,* but significantly decreases PAI-1 production mediated by TGFβ. The fibrates decrease PAI-1 production stimulated by insulin in hepatocytes *in vitro.* (Alessi & Juhan-Vague, 2006; Alessi et al., 2007; Asplund-Carlson et al., 1993; Eriksson et al., 1998; Li et al., 1997; Nilsson et al., 1998; Schneider & Sobel, 1996; Stiko-Rahm et al., 1990).

2.3.2.4 Inflammatory cytokines, growth factors, leptin

Inflammatory cytokines TNF, IL-1, IL-6 stimulate very effectively PAI-1 synthesis. TNF induces PAI-1 production in endothelium and adipose tissue more than in hepatocytes. IL-1 is an important stimulator of PAI-1 production in endothelium. Inflammatory cytokines have an increased effect on the 4G/5G promotor region PAI-1 gene polymorphism. The 5G allele has a bond site for inhibitory transcription factor and therefore the 4G insertion causes dramatic response to IL-1 with the increased PAI-1 levels. IL-6 also increases PAI-1 production in hepatocytes. Leptin, hormon of adipocytes, stimulates PAI-1 production in vascular smooth muscles. Adiponectin inhibits PAI-1 production in adipose tissue. TGFβ stimulates the endothelial PAI-1 production while growth factors related to the receptor protein tyrosine kinase (PTK) like insulin and IGF-1, do not act on PAI-1 synthesis in the endothelium but stimulate PAI-1 production in hepatocytes. This regulation is connected with indirect inhibitory effect of PAI-1 on the endothelial proliferation that needs proteolytic phenotype mediated by plasmin. Mentioned growth factors related to the receptor PTK induce endothelial proliferation. On the contrary, TGFß inhibits their growth effect, directly blocks the endothelial proliferation and increases PAI-1 endothelial production with an indirect antiproliferative effect. TGFß increases PAI-1 production in adipocytes and its effect is several times higher compared to insulin (Alessi & Juhan-Vague, 2006; Kawai et al., 1996; Loskutoff & Samad, 1998; Peiretti et al., 1997; Samad & Loskutoff, 1997; Vaughan, 2005).

2.4 Tissue plasminogen activator

t-PA is a serine protease which cleaves plasminogen to plasmin. t-PA has a structure of glycoprotein with two polypeptide chains (m.w.70 kDa) and disulphide-linked bond. Fibrin acts as a main cofactor of t-PA activity in the activation of fibrinolysis. tPA is synthesized particulary in the endothelium. After its synthesis by gene localized at 8th chromosome the t-PA is either stored in reserved compartment of the endothelium which is different from Weibel-Palade bodies or released to the circulation. t-PA is bound in circulation on the surface proteoglycan layer of endothelium or minority of t-PA circulates in plasma bound in complexes with its inhibitor PAI 1. Release of t-PA from the endothelium differs according to the types of vessels and takes part on heterogeneity of the fibrinolytic potential of vessels. The most of t-PA is localized on the surface of veins, especially in the upper part of body (release of t-PA in the veins of arms is 10 times higher than in the veins of legs), less of t-PA is produced in microvascular circulation and in aorta, and at least is localized in the endothelium of arteries. The highest release of t-PA was found in splanchnic system and coronary arteries. Liver is the site of t-PA uptake with a half-life of 5 min. (Hinsgbergh, 1988; Jern et al., 1997b).

2.4.1 The effects on t-PA levels

The t-PA antigen and activity levels depend on various factors.

2.4.1.1 Release of t-PA from stories in granules

The t-PA is stored in reserved granules of the endothelium which are different from Weibel-Palade bodies for vWF and small vesicules for protein S. Rapid degranulation and the t-PA release to plasma appears after the Ca_i-dependent stimulus. Factors activating receptors of phosphoinositol system by G-protein signaling pathway such as thrombin, acetylcholine, bradykinin, histamin, platelet activating factor (PAF) and endothelin stimulate the t-PA release by this way. Hormones like catecholamines activating cAMP system via β-receptors and vasopressin via V_2-receptor also increase the t-PA release to plasma. Physical or mental stress is associated with the activation of fibrinolysis and increased t-PA but without changes in PAI-1 levels. The t-PA released by stress is dependent on the intensity and duration of the stressor action. Strong or long-acting stressor against decreases the release of t-PA and increases PAI-1 production (Chandler et al., 1995; Kooistra et al., 1994; Teger-Nilsson et al., 1991).

2.4.1.2 Formation of complexes with PAI-1

The most of circulating t-PA antigen is coupled in complex with PAI-1 and only 5% of total t-PA circulates in free form. Measurement of the total t-PA by enzyme immunosorbent assay (EIA) does not distinguish the amount of free and bound t-PA. Close correlation between t-PA and PAI-1 can be explained especially by the increased level of t-PA/PAI-1 complexes because the PAI-1 level is fundamental for t-PA level. But only a small amount of circulating t-PA is in active form and therefore the t-PA activity does not correlate with t-PA antigen (Loo et al., 1995; Wiman, 1991).

2.4.1.3 Endothelial damage

t-PA is bound on the surface proteoglycan layer of endothelium and can be released to plasma after the endothelial damage. The increased t-PA levels correlate with vWF a TM in patients with coronary or peripheral atherosclerosis supporting the role of t-PA as a marker of endothelial damage. The t-PA levels are also an independent predictive marker for the risk of acute coronary events. So, the increased t-PA levels reflect severity of the endothelial dysfunction and are associated with a deterioration of fibrinolytic activity in plasma (Blann et al., 1995; Galajda et al., 1998d; Galajda & Mokáň, 2001).

2.5 Thrombin activatable fibrinolysis inhibitor

Thrombin-activatable fibrinolysis inhibitor (TAFI) is a procarboxypeptidase and member of the family called metallocarboxypeptidases. Activation of TAFI occurs by trypsin, plasmin, thrombin and meizothrombin. The catalytic efficiency of thrombin to activate TAFI is increased about three orders of magnitude in the presence of thrombomodulin. Thus, the thrombin-thrombomodulin complex is most likely the physiologic activator of TAFI. TAFI removes C-terminal lysine residues from partially degraded fibrin, thus inhibiting further plasminogen activation. It could be stated that TAFI acts as an important link between coagulation and fibrinolysis (Bajzar et al., 1996; Staško et al., 2004).

3. Fibrinolysis in diabetes mellitus type 2

Fibrinolysis disorder due to excessive PAI-1 production is the most characteristic feature of the prothrombotic state associated with DM2. Of all the various haemostatic measures, PAI-1 has been most consistently associated with insulin resistance (IR) and is generally accepted as being an important part of the risk cluster.

3.1 PAI-1 in patients with diabetes mellitus type 2

PAI-1 levels are strongly correlated with components of the IR syndrome such as body mass index (BMI), blood pressure, plasma triglycerides (TG) and insulin in healthy subjects with IR, DM2 patients, and patients with known coronary heart disease (CHD). Elevated PAI-1 levels were an independent risk factor for the development of DM2 in healthy subjects in the Insulin Resistance Atherosclerosis Study (IRAS), suggesting that they may be a very early risk marker for the development of the metabolic syndrome and DM2. This view was supported by subsequent serial analysis of PAI-1 in the IRAS in which baseline and follow-up PAI-1 levels were higher in subjects who subsequently converted to DM2. This link is strengthened by interventional studies, in which PAI-1 levels fell following improved insulin sensitivity (weight loss, exercise, metformin therapy). Festa et al. suggested that a fall in PAI-1 may in itself be associated with a reduction in conversion to DM2. However, the observation that elevated PAI-1 precedes the development of DM2 and is, in the presence of IR, independent of glycaemia (Natali et al., 2006) provides compelling evidence that abnormalities in fibrinolysis occur very early in the course of these disorders. (Juhan-Vague et al., 1987, 1989, 1993; Mansfield et al., 1997; Grant, 2007; Sakkinen et al., 2000; Vague et al., 1986; Landin et al., 1990a, 1990b; Hamsten et al., 1987; Sundell et al., 1989; Asplund-Carlson et al., 1993; Meigs et al., 2000; Festa et al., 1999, 2002, 2006; Natali et al., 2006). Our work also proved PAI-1 to be increased in early stages of diabetes (Kubisz et al., 2010).

3.1.1 PAI-1 as a predictive factor of cardiovascular risk

The role of PAI-1 as a predictive factor of cardiovascular risk is different compared to parameters of subclinical inflammation (CRP, fibrinogen) and endothelial dysfunction (von Willebrand factor - vWF) that are the independent cardiovascular risk factors but their predictive role for the risk of DM2 development is dependent on presence of obesity. PAI-1 was supposed as a risk factor for development of coronary heart disease (CHD) due to the results of Northwick Park Heart Study that found an independent relation of decreased fibrinolytic activity to the risk of future CHD. However, metaanalysis of the studies showed that PAI-1 levels have not independent effect as a predictor of the CHD risk. Paradoxically the increased levels of t-PA can be predictive for development of CHD. The IRAS study confirmed that increased PAI-1 levels have strong effect as a predictor of DM2 risk that is independent from obesity (Alessi & Juhan-Vague, 2006; Festa et al., 2002; Lowe et al., 2004; Lowe, 2005; Meade et al. 1993).

3.1.2 Heterogeneity of the insulin effects on PAI-1 levels in diabetes mellitus type 2

It was considered in previous model that the overproduction of PAI in IR states is a result of direct stimulatory effect of the portal hyperinsulinaemia (HI). This was confirmed by a stimulatory effect of insulin in the culture of hepatocytes *in vitro*, by the increased PAI-1 levels during oral glucose tolerance test (OGTT) and clinically proved by the correlation of PAI-1 levels to insulinaemia. The endothelial production of PAI-1 was considered as independent on insulin. This model was modified by a discovery that the principal source of PAI-1 which is dependent on insulin is adipose tissue but there are some controversies. The effect of insulin is different in adipose tissue, liver and vascular system, dependent on duration and character of concurrent factors and influenced by clearence of PAI-1 in liver and endothelial cells (Jokl et al., 1994; Juhan-Vague et al., 1991; Potter van Loon et al., 1993; Galajda & Mokáň, 2001).

3.1.2.1 Dependence on compartment

Insulin stimulates production of PAI-1 in visceral adipose tissue and liver. On the contrary insulin in the endothelial cells inhibits production of PAI-1 induced by cytokines. However, insulin has a stimulatory effect on PAI-1 synthesis in the subendothelial compartment, which is probably responsible for a local release of PAI-1 in the vascular stream of forearm muscles during infusion of insulin. The increased PAI-1 levels in subjects with IR can be a result of either the stimulatory effect of HI on adipose tissue mass in obesity or the missing inhibitory effect of insulin on endothelium in IR (Jern et al., 1997a; Juhan-Vague et al., 1991; Negri et al., 1997; Yamauchi et al., 1997).

3.1.2.2 Dependence on duration of insulin action

Decreased PAI-1 levels were found after a short-term insulin infusion or HI clamp. The same PAI-1 decrease was showed also in the control group with an administration of physiological solution without HI induction. These results confirmed that short-term application of insulin does not influence the PAI-1 levels and that PAI-1 decrease is a result of the PAI-1 diurnal rhytm variability. The PAI-1 levels after a long-term application of insulin in DM2 subjects were found decreased independently on other metabolic parameters. This effect can be caused by the stimulatory action of proinsulin during insulin treatment. We proved the inhibitory effect of insulin especially in DM2 subjects with endothelial dysfunction. This result supports, in accordance with an evidence of the inhibitory effect of PAI-1 on endothelium *in vitro,* the possibility of a direct inhibitory action of insulin during its long-term application (Galajda et al., 1998a, 1998b; Galajda & Mokáň, 2001; Nordt et al., 1993; Panahloo & Yudkin, 1996).

3.1.2.3 Dependence on concurrent factors

Short-term infusion of insulin, lipids or glucose does not influence PAI-1 levels but their mixed application leads to the increased PAI-1 levels. Synergistical effect of insulin and lipids on PAI-1 levels was confirmed also in the culture of hepatocytes. Insulin supports the stimulatory effect of glucose on PAI-1 synthesis in the endothelial cells but it inhibits the PAI-1 production in the endothelium mediated by cytokines (Calles-Escandon et al., 1998; Panahloo & Yudkin, 1996; Schneider & Sobel, 1996; Yamauchi et al., 1997).

3.1.2.4 Dependence on PAI-1 clearence.

PAI-1 synthesized by a visceral adipose tissue under the stimulation by insulin forms complexes with the increased t-PA produced in splanchnic system. Liver is a site of the rapid and effective uptake of these complexes. Rapid uptake of PAI-1/t-PA complexes can be responsible for the postprandial PAI-1 decrease. Intravenous application of glucose leads to the rapid PAI-1 decrease accelerated by sulodexid. This result supports the endothelial uptake of PAI-1. The similar finding was confirmed in subjects with diabetes mellitus type 1 (DM1) and it supposes the idea that postprandial PAI-1 levels variability can be independent on insulin (Ceriello et al., 1993; Jern et al., 1997b).

3.1.3 The effect of insulin treatment on PAI-1 levels in subjects with DM2

Insulin treatment in DM2 is associated with a decrease of PAI-1 levels. This is opposite to the confirmed stimulatory effect of insulin on PAI-1 levels in adipose tissue and liver. Although insulin has not the effect on basal PAI-1 production in endothelial culture *in vitro,* it inhibits the PAI-1 production induced by cytokines. This effect can exist also *in vivo.* In our clinical study we examined two groups of subjects with DM2 treated by sulphonylurea derivates (DM2-SU) and those treated 2-3 months by insulin (DM2-INS) (**table 1, table 2**).

	DM2 - SU (n=17)	**DM2 - INS** (n=11)	p
PAI-1 (ng/ml)	48,1 (14-108)	27,9 (2-53)	<0,05
t-PA (ng/ml)	8,1 (4,4-11,8)	8,8 (4,6-14,0)	n.s.
vWF (IU/ml)	1,0 (0,7-1,4)	1,0 (0,8-1,3)	n.s.
TFPI(ng/ml)	60,1 (33,2-84,3)	69,1 (29.1-86,7)	n.s.
TM (ng/ml)	27,8 (10-45)	31,0 (11-50)	n.s.
PF$_4$ (ng/ml)	52,1 (1-172)	50,8 (6-106)	n.s.
CP (ng/ml)	1,5 (0,5-5,9)	1,7 (0,4-3,8)	n.s.
TG (mM/l)	2,7 (0,9-6,8)	2,9 (0,4-7,4)	n.s.

DM2-SU (diabetics treated by sulphonylurea derivates), DM2-INS (diabetics treated by insulin), PAI-1 (plasminogen activator inhibitor type 1), t-PA (tissue plasminogen activator), vWF (von Willebrand factor), TFPI (tissue factor pathway inhibitor), TM (thrombomodulin), PF$_4$ (platelet factor 4), CP (C-peptid), TG (triglycerids)

Table 1. Subjects with diabetes mellitus type 2 without endothelial dysfunction

	DM2 - SU (n=17)	**DM2 - INS** (n=13)	p
PAI-1 (ng/ml)	80,7 (43-217)	16,7 (7-34)	<0,0001
t-PA (ng/ml)	13,7 (5,6-25,3)	7,1 (3,4-18,9)	<0,01
vWF (IU/ml)	1,9 (1,3-2,4)	1,8 (1,0-2,3)	n.s.
TFPI(ng/ml)	81,4 (50,2-107,1)	89,0 (47,3-112,8)	n.s.
TM (ng/ml)	54,7 (2-104)	46,9 (13-179)	n.s.
PF$_4$ (ng/ml)	70,1 (3-126)	68,3 (6-146)	n.s.
CP (ng/ml)	1,8 (0,6-7,9)	1,7 (0,9-5,6)	n.s.
TG (mM/l)	2,3 (0,9-8,2)	2,3 (0,9-6,1)	n.s.

DM2-SU (diabetics treated by sulphonylurea derivates), DM2-INS (diabetics treated by insulin), PAI-1 (plasminogen activator inhibitor type 1), t-PA (tissue plasminogen activator), vWF (von Willebrand factor), TFPI (tissue factor pathway inhibitor), TM (thrombomodulin), PF$_4$ (platelet factor 4), CP (C-peptid), TG (triglycerids)

Table 2. Subjects with diabetes mellitus type 2 with endothelial dysfunction

These two groups did not differ by metabolic parameters (glycaemia, glycosylated HbA1c, triglycerides, BMI), endothelial and platelet parameters (vWF, thrombomodulin-TM, PF$_4$). We found the significantly decreased PAI-1 levels in the insulin treated subjects compared to those with sulphonylurea derivates. These results can admit the inhibitory effect of insulin on PAI-1 levels independently to metabolic parameters. We evaluated also the influence of endothelial dysfunction measured by the endothelial markers. We found the significantly increased PAI-1 levels in subjects treated with sulphonylurea in subgroup with the increased vWF levels. Our results supported the idea that presence of the endothelial dysfunction was associated with the increased PAI-1 levels and this relation was not influenced by treatment with sulphonylurea derivates. There were confirmed decreased PAI-1 levels in subjects treated with insulin especially in those with the endothelial dysfunction when compared groups of subjects treated with insulin and sulphonylurea derivates. In accordance with the confirmed inhibitory insulin effect on PAI-1 production mediated by cytokines in the endothelium *in vitro* our results suppose the possibility of direct inhibitory action of insulin *in vivo* (Galajda et al., 1998b, 1998c; Galajda & Mokáň, 2001).

3.1.4 The effect of microalbuminuria on PAI-1 levels

Several studies found high PAI-1 levels in DM2 subjects with normo- and microalbuminuria. These results are in agreement with our results. We suggest decreased fibrinolysis in DM2 subjects presenting with increased levels of PAI-1 in both normoalbuminuric (NAU) and microalbuminuric (MAU) diabetics. We found a positive correlation between PAI-1 levels and BMI in the MAU group and between PAI-1 and triglycerids in our NAU subjects, which proves that obesity, dyslipidemia and hypofibrinolysis are closely linked together (Chudý et al., 2011; Soares et al., 2007; Umpaichitra et al., 2005; Sobel et al., 2005).

3.2 t-PA in subjects with diabetes mellitus type 2

The t-PA levels were described to be increased in DM2 in an early phase of disease while t-PA levels in DM1 are increased later in presence of vascular complications. There is a correlation between t-PA and PAI-1 levels in subjects with DM2 and the principle cause of the t-PA increase is formation of the t-PA/PAI-1 complexes. Therefore it seems that the relation between t-PA and some parameters of IR as HI, BMI and arterial hypertension (AH) is mediated by correlation of IR parameters with PAI-1. The t-PA/PAI-1 complexes are increased in diabetics of both types with AH, microangiopathy (nephropathy including microalbuminuria) and macroangiopathy, however t-PA levels are increased in the early phase in DM2 subjects and also dependence between t-PA levels and PAI-1 and IR is higher in the phase of complications than dependence between t-PA and presence of complications in DM2. (Cho et al., 1994; Collier et al., 1992; Kvasnička et al., 1997).

t-PA was considered to be a marker of endothelial dysfunction because the circulating t-PA is of endothelial origin. However, EIA does not distinguish between a free t-PA and circulating t-PA bound in t-PA/PAI-1 complexes. Due to this problem with interpretation of t-PA results it is necessary to evaluate t-PA levels together with PAI-1 levels in relation to the type of disease. In our study we verified the relation between t-PA and PAI-1 levels in subjects with DM1 and DM2, treated by insulin (DM2-INS) or oral antidiabetics (DM2-AD), subjects with IR and HI and healthy controls (**table 3**). Since the PAI-1 levels are increased due to the extravascular production in adipose tissue it is evident that t-PA levels in complex with PAI-1 could not reflect a severity of the endothelial dysfunction in DM2 subjects. In accordance with other studies we confirmed the correlation between t-PA and PAI-1 in DM2 subjects treated with oral antidiabetics (DM2-AD) and subjects with IR. This correlation was even more significant in control healthy group (**table 3**). In subjects with DM2 and IR there is the increase of PAI-1 levels with the determinant effect on t-PA antigen levels. It was proved by the increased t-PA/PAI-1 complexes levels and inverse correlation between t-PA antigen and t-PA activity. Since the circulating PAI-1 is of combined vascular and extravascular origin with a close relation to parameters of IR there is not possible to consider the t-PA levels as a marker of endothelial dysfunction in DM2 and IR. But it can be of benefit to measure t-PA levels as a marker of endothelial dysfunction e.g. in subjects with DM1 and normal PAI-1 levels. The t-PA plasma levels increase in the period of vascular complications and correlate with endothelial markers in subjects with DM1. Predictive value of the increased t-PA levels for worse disease prognosis was confirmed in subjects with atherosclerosis. The levels of t-PA and PAI-1 antigen in our subjects with DM1 did not correlate and the PAI-1 levels were in most of them normal. Thus the t-PA increase can reflect its release from the endothelium and measurement of t-PA in this case can be considered as a marker of endothelial dysfunction. We did not prove the correlation between t-PA and PAI-1 levels in DM2 subjects treated with insulin (DM2-INS). Insulin can inhibit the endothelial production of PAI-1 with the following decrease of tPA/PAI-1 complexes levels but insulin does not influence the t-PA release from endothelium and t-PA plasma levels. This can be explanation of the absent correlation between t-PA and PAI-1 levels in our DM2 subjects treated with insulin (Galajda & Mokáň, 2001).

	t-PA (ng/ml)	**PAI-1 (ng/ml)**	**Correlation t-PA/PAI-1 p**
DM1 (n=19)	4 (1-13)	7 (4-99)	n.s.
DM2-INS (n=27)	8 (1-17)	28 (2-270)	n.s.
DM2-AD (n=39)	11 (2-26)	58 (14-217)	p<0,05
NDIAB (n=22)	7 (2-15)	35 (6-217)	p<0,01
NORMAL (n=22)	3 (2-13)	9 (16-50)	p<0,01

DM1 (subjects with diabetes mellitus type 1), DM2 (subjects with diabetes mellitus type 2, treated by insulin - INS, oral antidiabetics - AD), NDIAB (hyperinsulinemic nondiabeticics), NORMAL (healthy controls), t-PA (tissue plasminogen activator) and plasminogen activator inhibitor type 1 (PAI-1)

Table 3. Correlations between tPA and PAI-1 levels

3.3 Thrombin activatable fibrinolysis inhibitor in subjects with diabetes mellitus type 2

Hori et al. found TAFI antigen levels and activity to be significantly higher in plasma of DM2 subjects compared to healthy controls. The plasma levels of TAFI antigen and D-dimers were inversely and significantly correlated in all DM2 subjects. These observations support the role of TAFI in the mechanism of diabetes-associated hypofibrinolysis (Hori et al., 2002).

Yano at al. found that the plasma levels of TAFI were significantly increased in DM2 subjects with microalbuminuria (MAU) compared to those in DM2 subjects with normoalbuminuria (NAU) and in normal subjects (Yano et al., 2003). Yener et al. observed in normotensive DM2 subjects without diabetes-related complications that PAI-1 level was significantly elevated, but level of TAFI antigen did not differ from healthy controls (Yener et al., 2009).

Our results in DM2 subjects (Chudý et al., 2011) showed that TAFI was significantly increased only in the MAU group compared to the controls (**table 4**). Neither the difference in TAFI levels between NAU and controls, nor the difference between diabetic subgroups MAU and NAU were statistically significant. These results indicate that the disease progression in DM2 subjects leads to more profound TAFI mediated inhibition of fibrinolysis (Chudý et al., 2011).

	NAU (n=42)	**MAU** (n=42)	**controls** (n=42)
TAFI (μg/mL)	63.5 (48-88)	72 (59-122)**	47 (36-55)
PAI-1 (ng/mL)	71.95 (57-90.9)**	102 (63.4-124.4)**	27.9 (10.2-47.7)
t-PA (ng/mL)	10.6 (8.7-12.9)	11.4 (7.9-15.6)*	8.15 (4.9-11.7)
F1+2 (nmol/L)	2.05 (1.7-5.3)**	2.9 (1.5-9.2)**	0.8 (0.5-1.4)**

* $0.05<p<0.1$, ** $p<0.01$ compared to the control group.

TAFI: thrombin-activable fibrinolysis inhibitor, PAI-1: plasminogen activator inibitor type 1, t-PA: tissue plasminogen activator, F1+2: prothrombin fragments 1+2, NAU: normoalbuminuric group, MAU: microalbuminuric group

Table 4. Levels of TAFI, PAI-1, t-PA and F1+2 in subjects with DM2 based on albuminuria and in controls

Recent results are concordant with those of previous studies (Hori et al., 2002; Yano et al., 2003; Yener et al., 2009). We found no significant correlation between TAFI and PAI-1 in either group of subjects. This suggests that TAFI mediated inhibition of fibrinolysis in DM2 might be regulated independently from PAI-1. While PAI-1 is up-regulated mainly in obesity and in endothelial dysfunction, TAFI is activated in conditions of enhanced coagulation activation, which was also proved by positive correlation between TAFI and F1+2 in our MAU group as well as TAFI and fibrinogen in the NAU group. TAFI may be up-regulated by arterial hypertension, which is supported by the significantly positive correlation found between TAFI and systolic blood pressure in our MAU subjects, while dyslipidemia defined by elevated total cholesterol seems to down-regulate TAFI, which is supported by significant inverse correlation between TAFI and total cholesterol in our MAU subjects (Chudý et al., 2011). This finding is in agreement with previous study in subjects with essential hypertension where diastolic blood pressure significantly correlated with TAFI concentrations in untreated subjects, and in beta-blocker-treated subjects (Malyszko & Tymcio, 2008).

Our work also suggests fibrinolysis inhibition mediated by TAFI in early stages of diabetes defined by microalbuminuria in type 2 diabetic subjects without macrovascular complications (Chudý et al., 2011).

3.4 Modulation of hypofibrinolysis in subjects with diabetes mellitus type 2

In subject with DM2 there is hemostatic balance tipped towards a hypofibrinolytic phenotype which, coupled with atheromatous vascular changes and platelet hyperreactivity, predisposes to increased cardiovascular ischemic events (Alzahrani & Ajjan, 2010a). In the next section various agents used in diabetes are discussed.

3.4.1 Hypoglycaemic agents

3.4.1.1 Metformin

This agent is usually used in DM2 subjects. Metformin lowers PAI-1 levels *in vivo*. This beneficial effect of metformin on fibrinolysis (and on clot structure) may, in part, explain findings from the UK prospective Diabetes Study (UKPDS), which demonstrated reduced CHD risk in metformin users compared with other hypoglycaemic agents (UKPDS Group, 1998). Metformin therapy was associated with enhanced fibrinolytic potential of the clot in 850 DM2 subjects, further providing mechanistic explanation for the cardioprotective properties of this agent (Alzahrani et al., 2010b).

3.4.1.2 Sulphonylureas

Gliclazide has been shown to reduce clot permeability, creating a prothrombotic clot structure that is resistant to fibrinolysis (Dhall & Nair, 1994). Improving glycemic control with glipizide is associated with a fall in PAI-1 levels thereby enhancing fibrinolysis (Cefalu et al, 2002).

3.4.1.3 Thiazolidinediones

Thiazolidinediones are peroxisome proliferator-activated receptor (PPAR) - γ stimulators and possess antithrombotic properties. These agents lower PAI-1 levels which improves fibrinolysis (Haffner et al., 2002; Buckingham, 2005; Chen et al., 2010; Perriello et al., 2007). Clinical studies have shown that glitazones can delay progression of atherothrombotic lessions although the pioglitazone as well as rosiglitazone have failed to show a reduction in cardiovascular events in DM2 subjects (Dormandy et al., 2005; Nissen & Wolski, 2007; Home et al., 2009).

3.4.1.4 Gliptins and GPL-1 agonists

Number of clinical outcome studies are currently underway to clarify the role of these relatively new agents used in DM2 subjects in prevention of cardiovascular complications (De Caterina et al., 2010). Both native GLP-1 and the GLP-1 analogue liraglutide attenuate glucose-stimulated PAI-1 expression in human vascular endothelial cells (Liu et al., 2009).

3.4.1.5 Insulin

Insulin-treated DM2 subjects are at greater risk of cardiovascular events compared with non-insulin-treated subjects, which may be a reflection of longer disease duration increasing the risk of complications (Margolis et al., 2008). Hyperinsulinemia increases PAI-1 levels, which explains elevated levels of this protein in insulin-resistant states (Alessi & Juhan-Vague, 2008). In healthy individuals, insulin has antithrombotic effects. But according to the results of some recent studies the insulin treatment is associated with prothrombotic changes in the presence of IR and diabetes, as it increases fibrinogen and PAI-1 levels (Alzahrani & Ajjan, 2010a).

3.4.2 Anti-platelet agents

3.4.2.1 Aspirin

Aspirin has been shown to acetylate fibrinogen, resulting in a less compact clot structure that is easier to lyse (Ajjan et al., 2009b). Ajjan et al. have shown in DM1 subjects that addition of aspirin to plasma samples *ex vivo* resulted in either no effect or a paradoxical increase in clot lysis time in the presence of poor glycemic control, and this was reversed once glycemic control improved (Ajjan et al., 2009a).

3.4.2.2 Thienopyridines

Ticlopidine, clopidogrel´s precursor, has been associated with a reduction in plasma fibrinogen levels in a meta-analysis (Mazoyer et al., 1994). However, this was not confirmed in a randomized multi-centre study, which showed no difference in fibrinogen levels comparing subjects treated with cloppidogrel or aspirin following acute myocardial infarction (Woodward et al., 2004).

3.4.3 Lipid-lowering agents

3.4.3.1 Statins

Statins affect the fibrinolytic system through upregulation of thrombomodulin expression and reduction in plasma PAI-1 levels. Indirect effects on the coagulation system are related to lowering cholesterol levels which may be associated with reduced PAI and improved tPA release (Tekin et al., 2004; Masamura et al., 2003; Ludwig et al., 2005).

3.4.3.2 Fibrates

Fibrates are PPARα activators and are mainly used in subjects with raised triglyceride levels or in those intolerant to a statin. Fibrinogen and PAI-I levels are reduced in hyperlipidemic subjects following fibrate treatment (Okopien et al., 2001). Clinical study failed to show a reduction in cardiovascular events in diabetes subjects on fibrate treatment, but this may be related to a study design that has been repeatedly criticised (Keech et al., 2005).

3.4.3.3 Ezetimibe

Recent animal work has shown that PAI-1 expression in aortic and adipose tissue is reduced following ezetimibe administration (Yamamoto et al., 2009). The exact mechanism is unknown but may be related to decreased levels of oxidised low-density lipoprotein.

3.4.4 Angiotensin-converting enzyme inhibitor and angiotensin receptor blocker

The renin–angiotensin system has a role in hypofibrinolysis by stimulating PAI-1 synthesis. Both angiotensin-converting enzyme inhibitor (ACEI) and angiotensin receptor blocker (ARB) reduce fibrinogen levels (Makris et al., 2004) thereby reducing the risk of cardiovascular events. ACEI can also modulate PAI-1 levels in diabetes subjects, whereas ARB has a less consistent effect (Fogari et al., 2002; Sola et al, 2005).

4. Conclusion

Diabetes mellitus is a metabolic disorder associated with increased vascular risk. Fibrinolysis disorders characterized with increased PAI-1 and t-PA antigens are considered a risk factor for future development of diabetes. This prothrombotic state is in diabetics further enhanced by decrease in t-PA activity and increase in TAFI antigen and activity. Consistant antidiabetics therapy may improve diabetes related hypofibrinolytic condition.

5. Acknowledgement

This work was supported by project "Center of Excellence for Perinatology Research" (CEPV I, ITMS 26220120016 and CEPV II, ITMS 26220120036), project "Support of human resources development using the most modern methods and forms of education at JLF UK in Martin" (ITMS 26110230031) and Vega 1/0018/10.

6. References

Ajjan, R.A.; Standeven, K.F.; Khanbhai, M., et al. (2009a). Effects of aspirin on clot structure and fibrinolysis using a novel in vitro cellular system. *Arterioscler. Thromb. Vasc. Biol.*, Vol.29, pp. 712–717.

Ajjan, R.A.; Standeven, K.F.; Mughal, S., et al. (2009b). An interaction between glycation and acetylation may be one mechanism for the reduced clinical efficacy of aspirin in individuals with diabetes. *Eur. J. Cardiol.*, Vol.30: p. 885.

Alessi, M.C.; Juhan-Vague, I.; Kooistra, T., et al. (1988). Insulin stimulates the synthesis of plasminogen activator inhibitor 1 by hepatocellular cell line HepG2. *Thromb. Haemost*, Vol.60, pp. 491-494.

Alessi, M.C.; Peiretti, F.; Morange, P., et al. (1997). Production of plasminogen activator inhibitor 1 by human adipose tissue. Possible link between visceral fat accumulation and vascular disease. *Diabetes* , Vol.46, pp. 860 -867.

Alessi, M.C. & Juhan-Vague, I. (2006). PAI-1 and metabolic syndrome. Links, causes and consequences. *Arterioscler. Thromb. Vasc. Biol., Vol.*26, pp. 2200-2207.

Alessi, M.C.; Poggi, M. & Juhan-Vague, I. (2007). Plasminogen activator inhibitor, adipose tissue and insulin resistance. *Curr. Opin. Lipidol.*, Vol.18, pp. 240-245.

Alessi, M.C. & Juhan-Vague I. (2008). Metabolic syndrome, haemostasis and thrombosis. *Thromb. Haemost.*, Vol.99, pp. 995–1000.

Alzahrani, S.H. & Ajjan, RA. (2010a). Coagulation and fibrinolysis in diabetes. *Diabetes & Vascular Disease Research*, Vol.7, No.4, pp. 260-273.

Alzahrani, S.H.; Hess, K.; Baxter, P.D., et al. (2010b). Fibrin clot structure/fibrinolysis and relationship with cardiac ischaemia and inflammatory markers in older individuals with type 2 diabetes. *Diabetes*; 70th Scientific Session, p. 817P.

Asplund-Carlson, A.; Hamsten, A.; Wiman, B., et al. (1993). Relationship between plasma plasminogen activator inhibitor-1 activity and VLDL triglyceride concentration, insulin level and insulin sensitivity: studies in randomly selected norms and hypertriglyceridaemic men. *Diabetologia*, Vol.36, pp. 817-825.

Bajzar, L.; Morser, J. & Nesheim M. (1996). TAFI, or Plasma Procarboxypeptidase B, Couples the Coagulation and Fibrinolytic Cascades through the Thrombin-Thrombomodulin Complex. *J. Biol. Chem.*, Vol.271, pp. 16603-8.

Blann, A.D.; Dobrotova, M.; Kubisz, P., et al. (1995). Von Willebrand factor, soluble P-selectin, tissue plasminogen activator and plasminogen activator inhibitor in atherosclerosis. *Thromb. Haemost.*, Vol.74, No.2, pp. 626-630.

Brummel-Ziedins, K.; Orfeo, T.; Swords J.N., et al. (2009). Blood coagulation and fibrinolysis. In: Greer JP, Foerster J, Rodgers JM, editors. *Wintrobe´s Clinical Hematology*, 12th edition. Lippincott Wiliams & Wilkins, Baltimore, pp. 528-619.

Buckingham, R.E. (2005). Thiazolidinediones: Pleiotropic drugs with potent anti-inflammatory properties for tissue protection. *Hepatol. Res.*, Vol.33, pp. 167-170.

Burzotta, F.; Iacoviello, L.; Di Castelnuovo, A., et al. (2003) 4G/5G PAI-1 promoter polymorphism and acute-phase levels of PAI-1 following coronary bypass surgery: a prospective study. *J Thromb Thrombolysis*, Vol.16, pp. 149-54.

Calles-Escandon, J.; Mirza, S.A.; Sobel, B.E., et al. (1998). Induction of hyperinsulinemia combined with hyperglycemia and hypertriglyceridemia increases plasminogen activator inhibitor 1 in normal human subjects. *Diabetes*, Vol.47, pp. 290-293.

Cefalu, W.T.; Schneider, D.J.; Carlson, H.E., et al. (2002). Effect of combination glipizide GITS/metformin on fibrinolytic and metabolic parameters in poorly controlled type 2 diabetic subjects. *Diabetes Care*, Vol.25, pp. 2123-2128.

Ceriello, A.; Quatraro, A.; Marchi, E., et al. (1993). Impaired fibrinolytic response to increased thrombin activation in type 1 diabetes mellitus: Effect of the glycosaminoglycan sulodexide. *Diabetes Metabolism*, Vol.19, pp. 225-229.

Cesarman-Maus, G. & Hajjar, K.A. (2005). Molecular mechanisms of fibrinolysis. *Br. J. Haematol.*, Vol.129, No.3, pp. 307-21.

Collier, A.; Rumley, A.; Rumley, A.G., et al. (1992). Free radical activity and hemostatic factors in NIDDM patients with and without microalbuminuria. *Diabetes*, Vol.41, pp. 909-913.

Dawson, S.J.; Wiman, B.; Hamsten, A., et al. (1993) The two allele sequences of a common polymorphism in the promoter of the plasminogen activator inhibitor-1 (PAI-1) gene respond differently to interleukin-1 in HepG2 cells. *J Biol Chem*, Vol.268, pp. 10739-45.

De Caterina, R; Madonna, R.; Sourij, H. et al. (2010). Glycaemic control in acute coronary syndromes: prognostic value and therapeutic options. *Eur. Heart J.*, Vol.31, pp. 1557–1564.

Dhall, D.P. & Nair, C.H. (1994). Effects of gliclazide on fibrin network. *J. Diabetes Complications*, Vol.8, pp. 231-234.

Dormandy, J.A.; Charbonnel, B.; Eckland, D.J. et al. (2005). Secondary prevention of macrovascular events in patients with type 2 diabetes in the PROactive Study (PROspective pioglitAzone Clinical Trial In macroVascular Events): a randomised controlled trial. *Lancet*, Vol.366, pp. 1279–1289.

Eriksson, P.; Kallin, B.; van 't Hooft, F.M., et al. (1995) Allele-specific increase in basal transcription of the plasminogen-activator inhibitor 1 gene is associated with myocardial infarction. *Proc Natl Acad Sci USA*, Vol.92, pp. 1851-5.

Eriksson, P.; Nilsson, L.; Karpe, F., et al. (1998). Very low density lipoprotein response element in the promoter region of the human plasminogen activator inhibitor-1 gene implicated in the impaired fibrinolysis of hypertriglyceridemia. *Arterioscler. Thromb. Vasc. Biol.*, Vol.18, pp. 20-26.

Festa, A.; D'Agostino, R.; Mykkanen, L., et al. (1999). Relative contribution of insulin and its precursors to fibrinogen and PAI-1 in a large population with different states of glucose tolerance. The Insulin Resistance Atherosclerosis Study (IRAS). *Arterioscler. Thromb. Vasc. Biol.*, Vol.19, pp. 562–568.

Festa, A.; D'Agostino, R.; Tracy, R.P., et al. (2002). Elevated levels of acute phase proteins and plasminogen activator inhibitor - 1 predict the development of type 2 diabetes: the Insulin Resistance Atherosclerosis Study. *Diabetes*, Vol.51, pp. 1131 - 1137.

Festa, A.; Williams, K.; Tracy, R., et al. (2006). Progression of plasminogen activator inhibitor-1 and fibrinogen levels in relation to incident type 2 diabetes. *Circulation*, Vol.113, pp. 1753–1759.

Fogari, R.; Mugellini, A.; Zoppi, A., et al. (2002). Losartan and perindopril effects on plasma plasminogen activator inhibitor-1 and fibrinogen in hypertensive type 2 diabetic patients. *Am. J. Hypertens.*, Vol.15, pp. 316–320.

Galajda, P.; Martinka, E.; Baláž, D., et al. (1997a). Plasminogen activator inhibitor (PAI-1) and markers of endothelial dysfunction in patients with diabetes mellitus. *Vnitřní Lék.*, Vol.43, pp. 744-747.

Galajda, P.; Šutarík, Ľ.; Vladár, Ľ., et al. (1997b). Plasminogen activator inhibitor (PAI-1) and diabetes mellitus. I. Regulation of PAI-1 levels. *Vnitřní Lék.*, Vol.43, pp. 804-808.

Galajda, P.; Šutarík, Ľ.; Vladár, Ľ., et al. (1998a). Plasminogen activator inhibitor (PAI-1) and diabetes mellitus. II. PAI-1 in the insulin resistance states. *Vnitřní Lék.*, Vol.44, pp. 111-114.

Galajda, P.; Martinka, E.; Staško, J., et al. (1998b). Plasminogen activator inhibitor type-1 (PAI-1) levels are decreased in NIDDM patients treated by insulin. *Clin. Appl. Thromb. Hemost.*, Vol.4, pp. 138-139.

Galajda, P.; Baláž, D.; Martinka, E., et al. (1998c). Insulin treatment inhibites PAI-1 production in NIDDM patients with endothelial dysfunction. *Clin. Appl. Thromb. Hemost.*, Vol.4, pp. 250-252.

Galajda, P.; Martinka, E.; Kubisz, P., et al. (1998d). Tissue plasminogen activator (tPA) in patients with diabetes mellitus. *Vnitřní Lék.*, 44, , s. 661-664.

Galajda, P.; Kubisz, P. & Mokáň, M. (1998e). Multicompartmental and multifactorial model of PAI-1 production I. Experimental studies. *Vnitřní Lék.*, Vol.44, pp. 718-721.

Galajda, P.; Kubisz, P. & Mokáň, M. (1999). Multicompartmental and multifactorial model of PAI-1 production. II. Clinical studies. *Vnitřní Lék.*, Vol.45, pp. 62-66.

Galajda, P. & Mokáň, M. (2001). Disorders of hemostasis in diabetes mellitus. *JLF UK and Prokonzult Martin*, 255 p.

Grant, P.J.; Kruithof, E.K.O.; Felley, C.P., et al. (1990). Short-term infusions of insulin, triacylglycerols and glucose do not cause acute increases in plasminogen activator inhibitor 1 concentrations in man. *Clin. Sci.*, Vol.79, pp. 513-516.

Grant, P.J. (2007). Diabetes mellitus as a prothrombotic condition. *J. Intern. Med.*, Vol.262, No.2, pp. 157-72.

Gray, R.P.; Panahloo, A.; Mohamed-Ali, V., et al. (1997). Proinsulin-like molecules and plasminogen activator inhibitor type 1 (PAI-1) activity in diabetic and non-diabetic subjects with and without myocardial infarction. *Atherosclerosis*, Vol.130, pp. 171-178.

Green, F.R. (1996). Genetic and enviromental determinants of factor VII, fibrinogen and PAI-1. *Fibrinolysis*, Vol.10, No.S2, pp. 7-8.

Gurewich, V.; Pannell, R.; Louie, S., et al. (1984). Effective and fibrin-specific clot lysis by a zymogen precursor from urokinase (pro-urokinase). A study in vitro and in two animal species. *J. Clin. Invest.*, Vol.73, No.6, 1731-1739.

Haffner, S.M.; Greenberg, A.S.; Weston, W.M., et al. (2002). Effect of rosiglitazone treatment on nontraditional markers of cardiovascular disease in patients with type 2 diabetes mellitus. *Circulation*, Vol.106, pp. 679–684.

Hajjar, K.A.; Harpel, P.C.; Jaffe, E.A., et al. (1986). Binding of plasminogen to cultured human endothelial cells. *J. Biol. Chem.*, Vol.261, No.25, pp. 11656-11662.

Hamsten, A.; Defaire, U.; Wallidus, G., et al. (1987). Plasminogen activator inhibitor in plasma: a risk factor for recurrent myocardial infarction. *Lancet*, ii, 3–9.

Hamsten, A. & Eriksson, P. (1994). Fibrinolysis and atherosclerosis: an Update. *Fibrinolysis*, Vol.8, No.S1, pp. 253-262.

Holvoet, P.; Lijnen, H.R. & Collen D. (1985). A monoclonal antibody specific for Lys-plasminogen. Application to the study of the activation pathways of plasminogen in vivo. *J. Biol. Chem.*, Vol.260, No.22, pp. 12106-12111.

Home, P.D.; Pocock, S.J.; Beck-Nielsen, H., et al. (2009). Rosiglitazone evaluated for cardiovascular outcomes in oral agent combination therapy for type 2 diabetes (RECORD): a multicentre, randomised, open-label trial. *Lancet*, Vol.373, pp. 2125–2135.

Hori, Y.; Gabazza, E.C.; Yano, Y., et al. (2002). Insulin resistance is associated with increased circulating level of thrombin-activatable fibrinolysis inhibitor in type 2 diabetic patients. *J. Clin. Endocrinol. Metab.*, Vol.87, No.2, pp. 660-665.

Chandler, W.L.; Levy, W.C. & Stratton, J.R. (1995). The circulatory regulation of tPA and uPA secretion, clearence, isoproterenol and phenylephrine. *Circulation*, Vol.92, pp. 2984-2994.

Chen, I.C.; Chao, T.H.; Tsai, W.C., et al. (2010). Rosiglitazone reduces plasma levels of inflammatory and hemostatic biomarkers and improves global endothelial function in habitual heavy smokers without diabetes mellitus or metabolic syndrome. *J. Formos. Med. Assoc.*, Vol.109, pp. 113–119.

Cho, Y.W.; Yang, D.H.; Oh, D.Y., et al. (1994). Plasma tPA and PAI-1 antigen concentration in non-insulin dependent diabetic patients - implication for diabetic retinopathy. *Diab Res Clin. Pract*, Vol.22, pp. 123-128.

Chudý, P.; Kotuličová, D.; Staško, J., et al. (2011). The relationship among TAFI, t-PA, PAI-1 and F1+2 in type 2 diabetic patients with normoalbuminuria and microalbuminuria. *Blood Coagul. Fibrinolysis*, doi: 10.1097/MBC.0b013e328346f8ca

Jern, C.; Selin, E.; Tengborn, L., et al. (1997a). Sympathoadrenal activation and muscarin receptor stimulation induce acute release of tissue-type plasminogen activator but not von Willebrand factor across the human foream. *Thromb. Haemost.*, Vol.78, pp. 887-891.

Jern, C.; Seeman-Lodding, H.; Biber, B., et al. (1997b). An experimental multiple-organ model for the study of regional net release/uptake rates of tissue-type plasminogen activator in the intact pig. *Thromb. Haemost.*, Vol.78, pp. 1150-1156.

Jokl, R.; Lazarchick, J.; Johnston, P.S., et al. (1994). Postprandial activation of fibrinolysis with type 2 diabetes mellitus. *Abstracts of 15th International Diabetes Federation Congres*, Kobe, p. 301.

Juhan-Vague, I.; Vague, P.; Alessi, M., et al. (1987). Relationships between plasma insulin, triglyceride, body mass index and plasminogen activator inhibitor 1. *Diab. Metab.*,Vol.13, pp. 331–336.

Juhan-Vague, I.; Roul, C.; Alessi, M, et al. (1989). Increased plasminogen activator inhibitor activity in non insulin dependent diabetic patients. Relationship with plasma insulin. *Thromb. Haemost.*, Vol.61, pp. 370–373.

Juhan-Vague, I., Alessi, M.C. & Vague, P. (1991). Increased plasminogen activator inhibitor 1 levels. A possible link between insulin resistance and atherothrombosis. *Diabetologia*, Vol.34, pp. 457- 462.

Juhan-Vague, I.; Thompson, S. & Jespersen, J. (1993). Involvement of the hemostatic system in the insulin resistance syndrome: a study of 1500 patients with angina pectoris. *Arterioscler. Thromb.*, Vol.13, pp. 1865–1873.

Juhan-Vague, I. & Alessi, M.C. (1997). PAI-1, obesity, insulin resistance and risk of cardiovascular events. *Thromb. Haemost.*, Vol.78, pp. 656-660.

Kawai, Y.; Matsumoto, Y. & Watanabe, K. (1996). Hemodynamic forces modulates effects of cytokines on fibrinolytic activity of endothelial cells. *Blood*, Vol.87, pp. 2314-2321.

Keech, A.; Simes, R.J.; Barter, P., et al. (2005). Effects of long-term fenofibrate therapy on cardiovascular events in 9795 people with type 2 diabetes mellitus (the FIELD study): randomised controlled trial. *Lancet*, Vol.366, pp. 1849–1861.

Kim, D.K.; Kim, J.W. & Kim, S. (1997). Polymorphism of angiotensin converting enzyme gene is associated with circulating levels of plasminogen activator inhibitor-1. *Arterioscler. Thromb. Vasc. Biol.*, Vol.17, pp. 3242-3247.

Kooistra, T.; Schrauwen, Y.; Arts, J., et al. (1994). Regulation of endothelial cell t-PA synthesis and release. *Int. J. Hematol.*, Vol.59, pp. 233-255.

Kubisz, P.; Chudý, P.; Staško, J., et al. (2010). Circulating vascular endothelial growth factor in the normo- and/or microalbuminuric patients with type 2 diabetes mellitus. *Acta Diabetol.*, Vol.47, No.2, pp. 119-124.

Kvasnička, J.; Škrha, J.; Perušičová, J., et al. (1997). The occurrence of the cardiovascular risk factors - fibrinogen, t-PA, PAI-1 and inflammation in insulin-dependent diabetes mellitus (IDDM) and in non-insulin dependent diabetes mellitus (NIDDM). *Cor Vasa*, Vol.39, pp. 146-150.

Landin, K.; Stigendal, L.; Eriksson, E., et al. (1990a). Abdominal obesity is associated with impaired fibrinolytic activity and elevated plasminogen activator inhibitor-1. *Metabolism*, Vol.39, pp. 1044–1048.

Landin, K.; Tengborn, L. & Smith, U. (1990b). Elevated fibrinogen and plasminogen activator inhibitor (PAI-1) in hypertension are related to metabolic risk factors for cardiovascular disease. *J. Intern. Med.*, Vol.227, pp. 273–278.

Li, X.N.; Grenett, H.E.; Benza, R.L., et al. (1997). Genotype-specific transcriptional regulation of PAI-1 expression by hypertriglyceridemic VLDL and Lp(a) in cultured human endothelial cells. *Arterioscler. Thromb. Vasc. Biol.*, Vol.17, pp. 3215-3223.

Lijnen, H.R. (2004). Pleiotropic functions of plasminogen activator inhibitor-1. *J. Thromb. Haemost.*, Vol.3, pp. 35-45.

Lijnen, H.R.; Alessi, M.C.; Van Hoef, B., et al. (2005). On the role of plasminogen activator inhibitor -1 in adipose tissue development and insulin resistance in mice. *J. Thromb. Haemost.*, Vol.3, pp. 1174 - 1179.

Liu, H.; Dear, A.E.; Knudsen, L.B., et al. (2009). A long-acting glucagon-like peptide-1 analogue attenuates inductionof plasminogen activator inhibitor type-1 and vascular adhesion molecules. *J. Endocrinol.*, Vol.201, pp. 59–66.

Loo, J.C.W.; Haverkate, F. & Thomson, S.G. (1995). Hemostatic factors and the risk of myocardial infarction. *N. Engl. J. Med.*, Vol.333, pp. 389-390.

Loskutoff, D.J. & Mimuro, J. (1991). Type 1 plasminogen activator inhibitor. In: Haber, E. & Braunwald, E., editors. *Thrombolysis, Basic Contributions and Clinical Progress*, Mosby Year Book, St.Louis, pp. 93-104.

Loskutoff, D.J. & Samad, F. (1998). The adipocyte and hemostatic balance in obesity. Studies of PAI-1. *Arterioscler. Thromb. Vasc. Biol.*, Vol.18, pp. 1-6.

Lowe, G.D.O.; Danesh, J.; Lewington, S., et al. (2004). Tissue plasminogen activator antigen and coronary heart disease. Prospective study and meta-analysis. *Eur. Heart J.*, Vol.25, pp. 252-259.

Lowe G. D. O. (2005). Circulating inflammatory markers and risk of cardiovascular and non-cardiovascular disease. *J. Thromb. Haemost.*, Vol.3, pp. 1618 - 1627.

Ludwig, S.; Dharmalingam, S.; Erickson-Nesmith, S., et al. (2005). Impact of simvastatin on hemostatic and fibrinolytic regulators in Type 2 diabetes mellitus. *Diabetes Res. Clin. Pract.*, Vol.70, pp. 110–118.

Makris, T.K.; Stavroulakis, G.; Papadopoulos, D.P., et al. (2004). Eprosartan effect onfibrinolytic/hemostatic variables in arterial hypertension: a comparative study to losartan. *Drugs Exp. Clin. Res.*, Vol.30, pp. 125–132.

Małyszko, J. & Tymcio, J. (2008). Thrombin activatable fibrinolysis inhibitor and other hemostatic parameters in patients with essential arterial hypertension. *Pol. Arch. Med. Wewn.*, Vol.118, pp. 36-41.

Mansfield, M.W.; Stickland, M.H. & Grant, P.J. (1997). PAI-1 concentrations in first-degree relatives of patients with non-insulin-dependent diabetes: metabolic and genetic associations. *Thromb. Haemost.*, Vol.77, pp. 357-361.

Margolis, D.J.; Hoffstad, O. & Strom, B.L. (2008). Association between serious ischemic cardiac outcomes and medications used to treat diabetes. *Pharmacoepidemiol. Drug Saf.*; Vol.17, pp. 753–759.

Masamura, K.; Oida, K.; Kanehara, H., et al. (2003). Pitavastatin-induced thrombomodulin expression by endothelial cells acts via inhibition of small G proteins of the Rho family. *Arterioscler. Thromb. Vasc. Biol.*, Vol.23, pp. 512–517.

Mazoyer, E.; Ripoll, L.; Boisseau, M.R. et al. (1994). How does ticlopidine treatment lower plasma fibrinogen? *Thromb. Res.*, Vol.75, pp. 361–370.

McCormack, L.J.; Nagi, D.K. & Stickland, M.H. (1996). Promoter (4G/5G) plasminogen activator inhibitor-1 genotype in Pima Indians: Relationship to plasminogen activator inhibitor-1 levels and features of the insulin resistance syndrome. *Diabetologia*, Vol.39, pp. 1512 -1518.

Meade, T.W.; Ruddock, V.; Stirling, Y., et al. (1993). Fibrinolytic activity, clotting factors an long-term incidence of ischaemic heart disease in Northwick Park Heart Study. *Lancet*, Vol.342, pp. 1076 - 1079.

Meigs, J.; Mittleman, M., Nathan, D. et al. (2000). Hyperinsulinaemia, hyperglycaemia and impaired hemostasis. the Framingham Offspring Study. *JAMA*, Vol.283, pp. 221–228.

Nagi, D.K.; Hendra, T.J.; Ryle, A.J., et al. (1990). The relationships of concetration of insulin, intact proinsulin and 32-33 split proinsulin with cardiovascular risk factor in type 2 (non-insulin dependent) diabetic subjects. *Diabetologia*, Vol.33, pp. 632-640.

Natali, A.; Toschi, E.; Baldeweg, X., et al. (2006). Clustering of insulin resistance with vascular dysfunction and low grade inflammation in type 2 diabetes. *Diabetes*, Vol.55, pp. 133–140.

Negri, F.; Morale, M.; Ferrini, L., et al. (1997). Role of insulin in the physiological regulation of PAI-1 expression by endothelial cells. *Thromb. Haemost.*, Vol.77, p. 749.

Nilsson, L.; Banfi, C.; Diczfalusy, U., et al. (1998). Unsaturated fatty acids increase plasminogen activator inhibitor-1 expression in endothelial cells. *Arterioscler. Thromb. Vasc. Biol.*, Vol.18, pp. 1679-1685.

Nissen, S.E. & Wolski, K. (2007). Effect of rosiglitazone on the risk of myocardial infarction and death from cardiovascular causes. *N. Engl. J. Med.*; Vol.356, pp. 2457–2471.

Nordt, T.K.; Klassen, K.J.; Schneider, D.J., et al. (1993). Augmentation of synthesis of plasminogen activator inhibitor type-1 in arterial endothelial cells by glucose and its implications for local fibrinolysis. *Arterioscler. Thromb.*, Vol.13, pp. 1822-1828.

Nordt, T.K.; Schneider, D.J. & Sobel, B.E. (1994). Augmentation of the synthesis of plasminogen activator inhibitor type-1 by precursors of insulin. A potential risk factor for vascular disease. *Circulation*, Vol.89, pp. 321-330.

Ny, T.; Sawdey, M.; Lawrence, D., et al. (1986). Cloning and sequence of a cDNA coding for the human beta-migrating endothelial-cell-type plasminogen activator inhibitor. *Proc. Natl. Acad. Sci. U S A.*, Vol.83, No.18, pp. 6776-6780.

Okopien, B.; Cwalina, L.; Lebek, M., et al. (2001). Effects of fibrates on plasma prothrombotic activity in patients with type IIb dyslipidemia. *Int. J. Clin. Pharmacol. Ther.*, Vol.39, pp. 551–557.

Panahloo, A. & Yudkin, J.S. (1996). Diminished fibrinolysis in diabetes mellitus and its implication for diabetic vascular disease. *Coronary Artery Disease*, Vol.7, pp. 723-731.

Pandolfi, A.; Giaccari, A.; Morviducci, L., et al. (1996). Acute hyperinsulinemia decreases plasma fibrinolytic activity in the rat. *Diabetologia*, Vol.39, No.S1, p. A279.

Peiretti, F.; Alessi, M.C.; Henry, M., et al. (1997). Intracellular calcium mobilisation suppresses the TNFa stimulated synthesis of PAI-1 in human endothelial cells. *Arterioscler. Thromb. Vasc. Biol.*, Vol.17, pp. 1550-1560.

Pennica, D.; Holmes, W.E.; Kohr, W.J., et al. (1983). Cloning and expression of human tissue-type plasminogen activator cDNA in E. coli. *Nature*, Vol.301 (5897), pp. 214-221.

Perriello, G.; Pampanelli, S.; Brunetti, P., et al. (2007). Long-term effects of pioglitazone versus gliclazide on hepatic and humoral coagulation factors in patients with type 2 diabetes. *Diabetes & Vascular Disease Research*, Vol.4, pp. 226–230.

Plow, E.F. & Collen, D. (1981). The presence and release of alpha-2-antiplasmin from human platelets. *Blood.*,Vol.58, No.6, pp. 1069-1074.

Plow, E.F.; Felez, J. & Miles, L.A. (1991). Cellular regulation of fibrinolysis. *Thromb. Haemost.*, Vol.66, No.1, pp. 32-36.

Potter van Loon, B.J.; Kluft, C.; Radder, J.K., et al. (1993). The cardiovascular risk factor plasminogen activator inhibitor type 1 is related to insulin resistance. *Metabolism*, Vol.42, pp. 945-949.

Raum, D.; Marcus, D.; Alper, C.A., et al. (1980). Synthesis of human plasminogen by the liver. *Science.*, Vol.208 (4447), pp. 1036-1037.

Römisch, J.; Vermöhlen, S.; Feussner, A., et al. (1999). The FVII activating protease cleaves single-chain plasminogen activators. *Haemostasis.*, Vol.29, No.5, pp. 292-299.

Sakkinen, P.; Wahl, P.; Cushman, M., et al. (2000). Clustering of procoagulation, inflammation, and fibrinolysis variables with metabolic factors in insulin resistance syndrome. *Am. J. Epidemiol.*, Vol.152, pp. 897–907.

Samad, F. & Loskutoff, D.J. (1997). The fat mouse: a powerful genetic model to study elevated plasminogen activator inhibitor 1 in obesity/NIDDM. *Thromb. Haemost.*, Vol.78, pp. 652-655.

Schleef, R.R. & Loskutoff, D.J. (1988). Fibrinolytic system of vascular endothelial cells. Role of plasminogen activator inhibitors. *Haemostasis*, Vol.18, pp. 328-341.

Schmitt, M.; Harbeck, M.; Thomssen C, et al. (1997). Clinical impact of the plasminogen activation system in tumor invasion and metastasis: Prognostic relevance and target therapy. *Thromb. Haemost.*, Vol.78, pp. 285-296.

Schneider, D.J. & Sobel, B.E. (1996). Synergistic augmentation of expression of plasminogen activator inhibitor type-1 induced by insulin, very low density lipoproteins and fatty acids. *Coronary Artery Disease*, Vol.7, pp. 813-817.

Soares, A.L.; Sousa Mde, O.; Dusse, L.M., et al. (2007). Type 2 diabetes: assessment of endothelial lesion and fibrinolytic system markers. *Blood Coagul. Fibrinolysis*, Vol.18, pp. 395-399.

Sobel, B.E.; Tilton, L.; Neimane, D., et al. (2005). Increased tissue-type plasminogen activator: a facade in the fibrinolytic system in type 2 diabetes. *Coronary Artery Disease*, Vol.16, pp. 31-35.

Sola, S.; Mir, M.Q.; Cheema, F.A., et al. (2005). Irbesartan and lipoic acid improve endothelial function and reduce markers of inflammation in the metabolic syndrome: results of the Irbesartan and Lipoic Acid in Endothelial Dysfunction (ISLAND) study. *Circulation*, Vol.111, pp. 343–348.

Staško, J., Hudeček, J. & Kubisz, P. (2004). Thrombin activatable fibrinolysis inhibitor (TAFI) and its role in regulation of fibrinolysis. *Vnitřní Lék.*, Vol.50, No.1, pp. 36-44.

Stiko-Rahm, A.; Wiman, I.; Hamsten, A., et al. (1990). Secretion of plasminogen activator inhibitor 1 from cultured human umbilical vein endothelial cells is induced by very low density lipoprotein. *Arteriosclerosis*, Vol.10, pp. 1067-1073.

Sundell, I.; Nilsson, T.; Hallmans, G., et al. (1989). Interrelationships between plasma levels of plasminogen activator inhibitor, tissue plasminogen activator, lipoprotein (a), and established cardiovascular risk factors in a North Swedish Population. *Atherosclerosis*, Vol.80, pp. 9–16.

Teger-Nilsson, A.-C.; Larsson, T.; Hjemdahl, P., et al. (1991). Fibrinogen and plasminogen activator inhibitor-1 levels in hypertension and coronary heart disease. Potential effects of beta blockade. *Circulation*, Vol.84, pp. 72-77.

Tekin, A.; Tekin, G.; Guzelsoy, D., et al. (2004). Effects of atorvastatin (10 mg) on hemostatic and inflammatory parameters in hyperlipidemic patients with angiographically proven coronary artery disease. *Am. J. Cardiol.*, Vol.94, pp. 206–209.

Umpaichitra, V.; Hussain, M.M. & Castells, S. (2005). Plasminogen activator inhibitor-1 and tissue plasminogen activator in minority adolescents with type 2 diabetes and obesity. *Pediatr. Res.*, Vol.58, pp. 483-487.

Vague, P.; Juhan-Vague, I.; Aillaud, M., et al. (1986). Correlation between blood fibrinolytic activity, plasminogen activator inhibitor level, plasma insulin level, and relative body weight in normal and obese subjects. *Metabolism*, Vol.35, pp. 250–253.

Vaughan, D.E. (1997). The renin-angiotensin system and fibrinolysis. *Am. J. Cardiol.*, Vol.79, S5A, pp. 12-16.

Vaughan, D.E. (2005). PAI-1 and atherothrombosis. *J. Thromb. Haemost.*, Vol.3, pp. 1879-1883.

Wiman, B. & Hamsten, A. (1991). Impaired fibrinolytic function in thrombotic disease. In: Haber, E., Braunwald, E., editors. *Thrombolysis, Basic Contribution and Clinical Progress*. Mosby Year Book, St.Louis, pp. 123-132.

Wiman, B. (1995). Plasminogen activator inhibitor 1 (PAI-1) in plasma: its role in thrombotic disease. *Thromb. Haemostas.*, Vol.74, pp. 71-76.

Woodward, M.; Lowe, G.D.; Francis, L.M., et al. (2004). A randomized comparison of the effects of aspirin and clopidogrel on thrombotic risk factors and C-reactive protein following myocardial infarction: the CADET trial. *J. Thromb. Haemost.*, Vol.2, pp. 1934–1940.

Yamamoto, K.; Shibayama, S.; Takeshita, K., et al. (2009). A novel cholesterol absorption inhibitor, ezetimibe, decreases adipose-derived and vascular PAI-1 expression in vivo. *Thromb. Res.*, Vol.124, pp. 644–645.

Yamauchi, K.; Shigematsu, S.; Nakajima, K., et al. (1997). Insulin differentially modified TGFβ action in blood vessel cells. *Diabetes*, Vol.46, No.S1, p. 388A.

Yano, Y.; Kitagawa, N.; Gabazza, E.C., et al. (2003). Increased plasma thrombin-activatable fibrinolysis inhibitor levels in normotensive type 2 diabetic patients with microalbuminuria. *J. Clin. Endocrinol. Metab.*, Vol.88, No.2, pp. 736-741.

Ye, R.D.; Wun, T.C. & Sadler, J.E. (1987). cDNA cloning and expression in Escherichia coli of a plasminogen activator inhibitor from human placenta. *J. Biol. Chem.*, Vol.262, No.8, pp. 3718-3725.

Yener, S.; Comlekci, A.; Akinci B, et al. (2009). Soluble CD40 ligand, plasminogen activator inhibitor-1 and thrombin-activatable fibrinolysis inhibitor-1- antigen in normotensive type 2 diabetic subjects without diabetic complications. Effects of metformin and rosiglitazone. *Med. Princ. Pract.*, Vol.18, pp. 266-271.

6

Diabetes and Aspirin Resistance

Subhashini Yaturu and Shaker Mousa
Stratton VA Medical Center/Albany Medical College; Pharmacy Research Institute
Albany College of Pharmacy and Health Sciences
Albany, NY
USA

1. Introduction

Cardiovascular disease (CVD) is the leading cause of morbidity and mortality in patients with diabetes mellitus (DM). DM is considered as a coronary artery disease equivalent for future risk of vascular events. There are 3 different classes of platelet-inhibiting drugs: cyclooxygenase-1 (COX-1) inhibitors (aspirin), ADP $P2Y_{12}$ receptor antagonists (thienopyridines), and platelet glycoprotein (GP) IIb/IIIa inhibitors, and these platelet inhibitors are mostly used for the prevention and treatment of atherothrombotic disorders.
Aspirin inhibits the COX-1 enzyme and therefore blocks platelet thromboxane A_2 synthesis. In 2007, the American Diabetes Association (ADA) and the American Heart Association (AHA) jointly recommended primary prevention strategy in those with diabetes, and that was modified by The U.S. Preventive Services Task Force recently; they did not differentiate their recommendations based on the presence or absence of diabetes. ADA recommends the use of low-dose aspirin (75–162 mg/day) for secondary prevention of cerebrovascular and cardiovascular events in all diabetic patients. In this chapter we discuss the cardiovascular risk in diabetes, what aspirin resistance means, the mechanism of aspirin resistance in diabetes including platelet activity, methods that are useful to identify aspirin resistance, and methods and management of aspirin resistance.

2. Diabetes and cardiovascular risk

Prevalence of diabetes is increasing rapidly worldwide. Diabetes is projected to affect 300 million people around the world by 2025. Type 2 diabetes is the most common form of diabetes. The prevalence of type 2 diabetes increases with age. Type 2 DM creates a prothrombotic state that is related to endothelial dysfunction, impaired fibrinolysis, increased levels of coagulation factors, and high platelet reactivity.(Carr 2001) Diabetes is considered as a coronary artery disease equivalent for future risk of vascular events http://www.nhlbi.nih.gov/guidelines/cholesterol/atglance.pdf. Despite a decline in mortality from CVD over the past decade, DM remains a key risk factor for CVD. Individuals with diabetes are at a 2- to 4-fold increased risk of cardiovascular events compared with age- and sex-matched individuals without diabetes. In diabetic patients over the age of 65 years, 68% of deaths are from coronary heart disease (CHD) and 16% are from stroke.(Pignone, Alberts et al. 2010) National Health and Nutrition Examination Survey data suggest that declines in all-cause mortality have occurred among men with DM but not women. Mortality rates among individuals with DM remain approximately 2-fold higher compared to individuals without DM.(Preis, Hwang et al. 2009) Mechanisms leading to prothrombotic state are shown in the Figure 1.

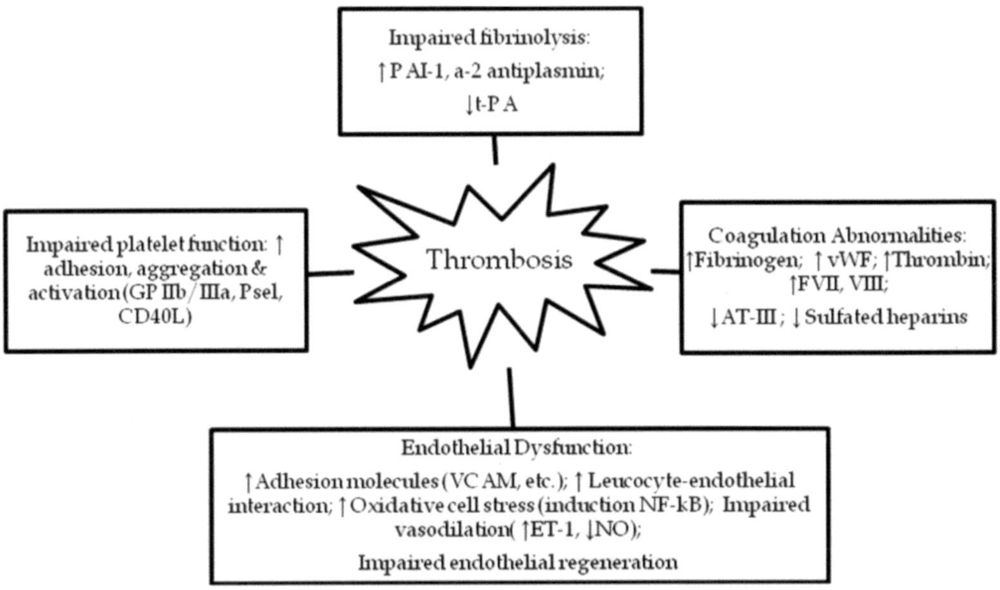

Fig. 1. Mechanisms leading to prothrombotic states in type 2 diabetes

3. Aspirin

Aspirin is one of the most important therapeutic agents used in the prevention of CVD (both primary and secondary) in patients with diabetes. Long-term aspirin administration in patients at high risk of occlusive vascular events reduced up to 34% of nonfatal myocardial infarction (MI), 25% of nonfatal stroke, and 18% of all-cause mortality. Low-dose aspirin (as low as 81 mg/day) irreversibly inhibits the COX-1 enzyme, by acetylating the serine residue at position 529, consequently impairing the transformation of arachidonic acid to prostaglandin (G2/H2), and TX A2, which is a potent mediator of platelet aggregation and activation. Aspirin's effect on COX-2 is minimal in doses <1200 mg per day.(Bucchi, Bodzenta et al. 1986; Frolich 1997) Equivalent doses of the enteric-coated aspirin are said to be as effective as plain aspirin.(Cox, Maree et al. 2006) Lower bioavailability of these preparations and poor absorption from the higher pH environment of the small intestine may result in inadequate platelet inhibition, particularly in heavier patients.(Cox, Maree et al. 2006)

3.1 Aspirin as a primary prevention strategy in diabetes mellitus

The Japanese Primary Prevention of Atherosclerosis With Aspirin for Diabetes (JPAD) trial (Ogawa, Nakayama et al. 2008) was the first prospectively designed trial to evaluate the use of aspirin (81 mg or 100 mg) in the primary prevention of cardiovascular events in patients with type 2 diabetes (n = 2,539) aged 30–85 years in Japan, and reported that aspirin use was associated with a 32% reduction in the risk of the primary end point at 4.7 years of follow up. The ongoing trials that will provide insights into the appropriateness of aspirin usage in diabetic patients include the Aspirin and Simvastatin Combination for Cardiovascular Events Prevention Trial in Diabetes (ACCEPT-D).(De Berardis, Sacco et al. 2007) Results of the Prevention Of Progression of Arterial Disease And Diabetes (POPADAD) trial have been reported, with no benefit with aspirin or antioxidants in primary prevention of cardiovascular events.(Belch, MacCuish et al. 2008) ADA recommends enteric-coated aspirin at a dosage of 81–325 mg to be used as a preventive strategy in high-risk diabetic individuals.(Pignone, Alberts et al. 2010) An important consideration is that patients may acquire additional risk factors over time, which would necessitate a reassessment of their overall risk profile. Several meta-analyses have explored the benefit of aspirin therapy in the primary prevention of major adverse cardiovascular events (MACE) among patients with diabetes.(Baigent, Blackwell et al. 2009; Calvin, Aggarwal et al. 2009; De Berardis, Sacco et al. 2009; Pignone, Alberts et al. 2010; Younis, Williams et al. 2010; Zhang, Sun et al. 2010) There are several tools to calculate the risk. Tools that can be used in patients with diabetes are available from several sources, for example: UKPDS Risk Engine: http://www.dtu.ox.ac.uk/riskengine/index.php; ARIC CHD Risk Calculator: http://www.aricnews.net/riskcalc/html/RC1.html; American Diabetes Association Risk Assessment Tool, Diabetes PHD: http://www.diabetes.org/phd. The AHA has issued similar guidelines and recommends 75–160 mg/day of aspirin as a primary prevention strategy in high-risk individuals, defined as those with a 10-year risk of coronary artery disease (CAD) over 10%.

3.2 Aspirin as a secondary prevention strategy in diabetes mellitus

Two large meta-analyses of major secondary prevention trials by the Antithrombotic Trialists' Collaboration (ATC) showed oral aspirin to be protective in patients at high risk for CVD, including those with diabetes (1994; 2002). The meta-analyses included 287 secondary prevention trials involving 212,000 high-risk patients with acute or prior vascular disease or another condition that increased their risk of vascular disease. Of note, a low dose of aspirin (75–150 mg/day) was found to be at least as effective as higher daily doses. In more than 4,500 diabetic patients studied in the ATC, the incidence of vascular events was also reduced from 23.5% in the control group to 19.3% in the group treated with antiplatelet therapy ($P <$ 0.01) and from 17.2% to 13.7% in the ~42,000 nondiabetic patients ($P < 0.00001$). The ADA recommends the use of aspirin (81–325 mg/day) as a secondary prevention measure in diabetic patients with atherosclerotic disease. (Pignone, Alberts et al. 2010)

3.3 Aspirin resistance

Aspirin resistance, defined as failure of suppression of thromboxane generation, increases the risk of cardiovascular events in a high-risk population.(Eikelboom, Hirsh et al. 2002) Causes of aspirin resistance include concurrent use of nonsteroidal anti-inflammatory drugs such as ibuprofen that may compete with aspirin at the COX-1 receptor site,(Catella-Lawson, Reilly et al. 2001) polymorphisms in the *COX-1* gene,(Eikelboom, Hirsh et al. 2002; Halushka and Halushka 2002) poor glucose control, body weight, and conditions associated with a high platelet turnover.(Zimmermann, Wenk et al. 2003; Zimmermann, Kurt et al. 2005; Guthikonda, Lev et al. 2007; Modica, Karlsson et al. 2007)

3.4 Terminology (Ben-Dor, Kleiman et al. 2009)

The lack of agreement on a standardized definition for "aspirin resistance" has contributed to the disparity in reports of its incidence among different studies. Whereas some use the term "aspirin treatment failure," others like to call it "aspirin non responsiveness." The term *aspirin resistance* has been used to describe the occurrence of cardiovascular events despite regular aspirin intake at recommended doses.

3.5 Diabetes and aspirin resistance

The benefit of aspirin in diabetic patients has been consistently documented in several trials. Aspirin is recommended for primary and secondary prevention in DM. Yet, in the meta-analysis of the ATC, the event rate of DM patients on treatment was similar to that of non-DM patients off treatment.(2002) In the Primary Prevention Project Trial, aspirin treatment reduced cardiovascular events and deaths in high-risk non-diabetic patients, but not in patients with type 2 DM (T2DM). Furthermore, in the recent Japanese Primary Prevention of Atherosclerosis with Aspirin for Diabetes Study,(Ogawa, Nakayama et al. 2008) a low dose of aspirin in primary prevention did not reduce the risk of cardiovascular events at 4 years in diabetic patients. Other studies in secondary prevention similarly suggested that aspirin might be less effective in T2DM, especially in patients with poor metabolic control, than in non-DM patients, the underlying mechanism being still debated. Since platelets play a key role in the development of atherothrombotic events, the dysfunctional status of platelets in DM patients may contribute to the enhanced atherothrombotic risk of these patients. It has been proposed that reduced sensitivity to aspirin in diabetic patients might be owing to accelerated thrombopoiesis,(DiMinno, Silver et al. 1986) or to reduced platelet permeability to aspirin caused by membrane glycosylation.(Winocour, Watala et al. 1992)

The mechanisms that lead to increased platelet reactivity observed in patients with DM can be grouped together into the following aetiopathogenic categories: a) hyperglycaemia, b) insulin deficiency and resistance, c) associated metabolic conditions, and d) other cellular abnormalities (as shown in Figure 2). Poor glucose control and body weight are also proposed to contribute to aspirin resistance. (Watala, Golanski et al. 2004; Singla, Antonino et al. 2009) Poorly controlled patients with diabetes have the greatest platelet reactivity. High platelet reactivity was defined as >46% for 5 micromol/L ADP-induced and >59% for 20 micromol/L ADP-induced platelet activity and may require alternative antiplatelet strategies, and further clinical investigations are warranted.(Singla, Antonino et al. 2009)

Platelets: Platelets play a key role in the development of atherothrombotic events. Platelets are essential for primary hemostasis and repair of the endothelium, but they also play a key role in the development of acute coronary syndromes and contribute to cerebrovascular events. Platelet adhesion is an essential function in response to vascular injury and is generally viewed as the first step during which single platelets bind through specific membrane receptors to cellular and extracellular matrix constituents of the vessel wall and tissues. Beyond acute activation as a consequence of vascular injury, circulating platelets are actively involved in all phases of the atherogenetic process, from atherosclerotic plaque formation to plaque inflammation and rupture. (Davi and Patrono 2007; Ruggeri and Mendolicchio 2007; Langer and Gawaz 2008)

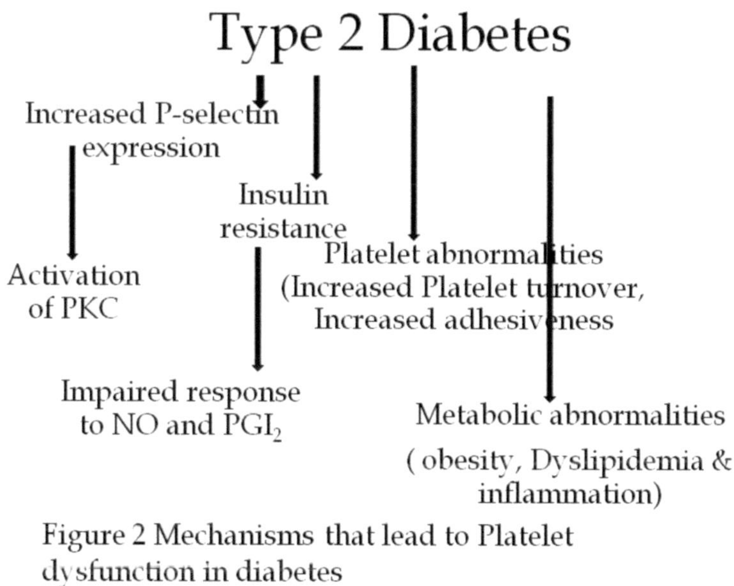

Fig. 2. Mechanisms that lead to Platelet dysfunction in diabetes

Mechanism of aspirin resistance in diabetes: Increased platelet reactivity observed in patients with DM may be secondary to several factors. Acute hyperglycemia as well as poor control of diabetes is associated with increased platelet reactivity. Comparative studies of patients with good glycemic control show they have better response to aspirin compared to the patients with poor glycemic control. Although this might implicate that better glucose control leads to less incidence of aspirin non-responsiveness, the clinical significance of such findings should be carefully inspected, since in 2 of the largest trials assessing the role of aspirin on primary prevention of cardiovascular events in patients with type 2 diabetes, low-dose aspirin did not decrease the risk of cardiovascular events when compared to placebo. Insulin resistance, TNF-alfa and IL-6 are shown to affect platelet reactivity. The clinical determinants that help identify aspirin resistance in diabetes are suggested to be CVD, microalbuminuria, poor diabetes control, and increased waist circumference.(Yassine, Davis-Gorman et al. 2010)

Platelet abnormalities in Type 2 diabetes: The abnormalities described in patients with diabetes are listed here.

1. Increased production of thromboxane A2 from arachidonic acid. (Halushka, Mayfield et al. 1981; Halushka, Rogers et al. 1981)
2. Increase in platelet-dependent thrombin generation.
3. Increased expression of platelet surface adhesion molecules such as CD31, CD49b, CD62P, and CD63, leading to increased platelet activation.
4. Increased platelet surface receptors such as P-selectin, GP Ib, and GP IIb/IIIa. (Gresele, Guglielmini et al. 2003)
5. Reduced vascular synthesis of the anti-aggregants PGI2 and NO, shifting balance towards aggregation and vasoconstriction.
6. Disordered calcium homeostasis that affects platelet shape change, secretion, aggregation, and thromboxane formation (Halushka, Mayfield et al. 1981; Halushka, Rogers et al. 1981).

7. Decreased platelet insulin receptor number and affinity and failure to reduce platelet responses to the agonists ADP, collagen, thrombin, arachidonate, and PAF.
8. Glycation of circulating LDL rendering platelets hypersensitive. Glycated LDL causes an increase in intracellular calcium concentration and platelet NO production, as well as inhibition of the platelet membrane Na+/K+-ATPase activity.

Key: GP = glycoprotein; PGI2 = prostacyclin; NO = nitric oxide; ADP = adenosine diphosphate; PAF = platelet-activating factor; LDL= low-density lipoprotein; Na+/K+-ATPase = Na+/K+-adenosine triphosphatase

An accelerated platelet turnover represented by the presence of a higher number of reticulated platelets has been observed in patients with DM.(Guthikonda, Alviar et al. 2008) The dysfunctional status of platelets in patients with DM may contribute to the enhanced atherothrombotic risk of these patients. Platelets obtained from diabetic patients show increased adhesiveness, hyperfunction both spontaneous as well as in response to agonists. These observed hyperfunctions are attributed to increased expression, activation or abundance of surface membrane receptors for agonists as well as cell matrix components, increased binding of fibrinogen, altered membrane fluidity, changes in activation mechanisms and signaling pathways. Changes in platelets in diabetes include enhanced GP receptor binding of agonists and adhesive proteins; decreased membrane fluidity; enhanced activation of the arachidonic acid pathway resulting in increased TxA_2 formation; altered PI turnover leading to changes in diacylglycerol and inositol triphosphate production, calcium mobilization, and protein phosphorylation; impaired responses to antiaggregants resulting in decreased PGI_2 receptor binding, cyclic nucleotide production and cyclic nucleotide-dependent protein phosphorylation; and reduced sensitivity to the inhibitory actions of insulin. These changes translate to impaired PGI_2 stimulation of cAMP and blindness to the inhibitory actions of both PGI_2 and NO. Platelet dysfunction coupled with decreased endothelial production of these antiaggregatory agents conspire to amplify the risk of CVD in patients with type 2 diabetes.(Vinik, Erbas et al. 2001)

Metabolic control and platelet reactivity

In the early 1960s Bridges *et al* showed that both *in vitro* as well as *in vivo* administration of glucose increased platelet stickiness.(Bridges, Dalby et al. 1965) Combined hyperinsulinemia and hyperglycemia in healthy volunteers increased circulating tissue factor, plasma thrombin generation, and coagulation factors VII and VIII activities, suggesting that the coagulation system had been activated.(Boden and Rao 2007) Chronic hyperglycemia has been identified as a causal factor for *in vivo* platelet activation and platelet hyperreactivity in DM patients as evidenced by enhanced TXA2 biosynthesis.(Davi, Gresele et al. 1997; Davi, Ciabattoni et al. 1999) Of note, T2DM platelets are characterized by enhanced thromboxane biosynthesis and tight metabolic control, shown to lead to a reduction of thromboxane levels.(Davi, Catalano et al. 1990) Acute, short-term hyperglycemia induces an increased activation of platelets exposed to high shear stress conditions *in vitro* (filtration method) or *in vivo* (bleeding time). *In vivo* platelet activation is reflected by an increased urinary excretion of 11-dehydro-TxB (2).(Gresele, Guglielmini et al. 2003) This acute hyperglycemia-induced enhancement of platelet activation is resistant to aspirin: an NO -donating agent suppresses it.(Gresele, Marzotti et al. 2010) LDL, a circulating complex of lipids and proteins that is increased in hypercholesterolemia, enhances platelet function and sensitizes platelets via binding of apoB-100 to a receptor on the platelet membrane and via transfer of lipids to the platelet membrane.(Relou, Hackeng et al. 2003) Hyperglycemia also induces an increase in nonenzymatic glycation of LDL (glycLDL), which renders them more susceptible to oxidative stress.(Angiolillo 2007)

Insulin and platelet reactivity

The T2DM patients had platelet aggregation and shear-induced platelet function significantly increased compared to nondiabetic patients using all assays. Platelet aggregation was increased in ITDM (n = 68) compared with NITDM (n = 133) patients after P2Y12-specific stimuli. Insulin treatment was the strongest predictor of ADP-induced aggregation. Platelet function profiles were similar between ITDM and NITDM using assays non-specific to the P2Y12 pathway. Platelet dysfunction was independent of glycemic control and inflammatory status.(Angiolillo, Bernardo et al. 2006)

NF-kB is a transcription factor that stimulates numerous genes and activates inflammatory responses related to insulin resistance. Salicylates inhibit NFkB activation. This inhibition was shown to be associated with a significant decrease in IL-6 and TNF-α release, mediated through inhibition of IKKβ activity.

Platelet activity measures

A major urinary metabolite of thromboxane A2 synthesized from extra renal sources is 11-dehydro thromboxane B2. A major portion of this metabolite is believed to come from the platelet, but there are additional cellular sources. In the Heart Outcomes Prevention Evaluation (HOPE) trial, patients whose urinary 11-dehydro thromboxane B2 levels were in the highest quartile had an odds ratio of 2 for having a myocardial infarction and an odds ratio of 3.5 for a risk of having a cardiovascular-related death compared to those patients in the lowest quartile. Serum aspirin esterase (AE) activity may account for part of aspirin pharmacokinetics and has been proposed as one source of variation in aspirin effectiveness.(Adebayo, Williams et al. 2007) Elevated MPV values are associated with a shortened bleeding time and increased thromboxane B2 plasma levels. Thus, MPV could be considered an indicator of platelet function.(Vizioli, Muscari et al. 2009) Diabetic patients with coronary heart disease have significantly higher MPV values compared to control patients.(Tavil, Sen et al. 2010)

Methods that directly measure the capacity of platelets to synthesize TxA_2 are certainly preferable. Of these, the urinary levels of the TxB_2 metabolite, 11-dehydrothromboxane B_2, represent a time-integrated index of TxA_2 biosynthesis *in vivo*.(Patrono, Ciabattoni et al. 1986) 11-dehydro-TxB_2 is the most abundant urinary metabolite of TxB_2. Detection in the urine of this metabolite, which is not formed in the kidney, reflects systemic TxA_2 formation, which largely, albeit not exclusively, occurs in the platelets. It has been calculated that about 30% of the urinary metabolite derives from extra-platelet sources, as in inflammatory diseases, the contribution of extra-platelet sources may increase in atherosclerosis and inflammatory conditions.(Catella and FitzGerald 1987) Test measures consider the end products of the TxA_2pathway such as serum TxB_2, or urine 11-dehydro-TxB_2, for assessing aspirin activity.(Eikelboom, Hirsh et al. 2002) In fact, these 2 tests may better reflect the amount of TxA_2 derived from sources other than platelets such as macrophages and monocytes, and on the COX-2 linked pathway of arachidonic acid, which is blocked by aspirin at very high doses (1200 mg/ day) only.(Bucchi, Bodzenta et al. 1986) Urinary 11-dehydro- TxB_2 concentration is affected by renal production of this substance. However, measurement of this metabolite is still commonly used in trials assessing aspirin resistance, due to its low cost and ease of measurement.(Eikelboom, Hirsh et al. 2002)

In aspirin-treated patients, elevated urinary 11-dehydro thromboxane B_2 levels identify patients who are relatively resistant to aspirin and who may benefit from additional antiplatelet therapies or treatments that more effectively block in vivo thromboxane production or activity.(Eikelboom, Hirsh et al. 2002)

Clinical implications

The clinical implication of aspirin resistance as measured *in vitro* by the inability of aspirin to reduce platelet activation and aggregation by failure to suppress the platelet production of TXA has not yet been elucidated via prospective trials that have controlled for confounders, such as hypertension, and dyslipidemia. Large meta-analyses have found low-dose aspirin to be as effective as high-dose aspirin in preventing vascular events, making a dose-dependent improvement in laboratory response clinically irrelevant. Causes of aspirin resistance include poor compliance, inadequate dose, drug interactions, genetic polymorphisms of cyclooxygenase-1, increased platelet turnover, and upregulation of nonplatelet pathways of thromboxane production. At present, there is no standardized approach to the diagnosis and no proven effective treatment for aspirin resistance. Further research exploring the mechanisms of aspirin resistance is needed in order to better define aspirin resistance, as well as to develop a standardized laboratory test that is specific and reliable, and can correlate with the clinical risk of vascular events.

Management

Factors that need to be considered in the approach to patients with suspected treatment failure include: compliance with aspirin use, ensure the optimal dose and drug form (avoid use of enteric-coated aspirin formulations), evaluate concomitant infections or inflammatory conditions, and assess possible drug–drug interactions. Several approaches have been evaluated for treatment failure and some of these approaches are based on laboratory testing for evidence of resistance. The role of testing in directing management is still controversial. Management strategies are currently limited to dosing alteration and introduction of other anti platelet agents. However, these measures have not met the expected efficacy or safety.

Increased aspirin doses: The idea of increasing aspirin dose has been assayed in many studies, as there is some evidence that response to aspirin may be dose dependent.(ten Berg, Gerritsen et al. 2002) Because patients with diabetes exhibit a higher prevalence of aspirin resistance on standard aspirin doses (81 mg/day) and have significantly higher ADP- and collagen-induced platelet aggregation, 11-dehydro- TxB_2 levels and the aspirin resistance may be partially overcome by higher aspirin doses.(DiChiara, Bliden et al. 2007) Laboratory and genetic inconsistency, as well as dose dependence, is seen when agonists other than arachidonic acid (the most specific in assessing aspirin resistance), such as ADP, collagen, and epinephrine, are used for *in vitro* assessment of platelet inhibition by aspirin.(McCabe, Harrison et al. 2005; Assadian, Lax et al. 2007; Gurbel, Bliden et al. 2007). The Clopidogrel vs Aspirin in Patients at Risk of Ischaemic Events (CAPRIE) trial compared the efficacy for secondary prevention of clopidogrel (75 mg daily) versus aspirin (325 mg daily) in a high-risk population (n = 19,185) consisting of patients with a history of recent MI, recent ischaemic stroke, or established peripheral artery disease.(Diener, Bogousslavsky et al. 2004) The benefit of clopidogrel therapy was higher (15.6% vs. 17.7%; $P = 0.042$) in DM patients, despite the increased incidence of ischaemic outcomes in this subgroup. The absolute reduction in events was highest among diabetic patients requiring insulin therapy.(Diener,

Bogousslavsky et al. 2004) In large, well-designed multicentre trials, such as CURE, COMMIT, and CLARITY-TIMI 28, the addition of clopidogrel to aspirin therapy improved outcomes in patients with acute coronary syndromes.(Plosker and Lyseng-Williamson 2007) *Addition of other antiplatelet agents*: Dual antiplatelet therapy using acetylsalicylic acid and clopidogrel is of great importance following coronary stenting. Clopidogrel, a thienopyridine, works by irreversibly inhibiting ADP binding to the P2Y12 receptors on the platelet surface, and ultimately interfering with platelet-fibrinogen binding. The PLATO (PLATelet Inhibition and Patient Outcomes) study has shown that ticagrelor, an agent with a similar mechanism of action to clopidogrel and still in phase III trials, showed a significant reduction of a combined endpoint of cardiovascular death, myocardial infarction, or stroke as compared with clopidogrel (hazard ratio 0.84; 95%CI 0.75, 0.94; P = 0.0025).(Cannon, Harrington et al. 2010) In the subgroup of patients undergoing coronary artery bypass graft (CABG) within 7 days after the last study drug intake, ticagrelor compared with clopidogrel was associated with a substantial reduction in total and cardiovascular mortality without excess risk of CABG-related bleeding.(Held, Asenblad et al. 2011) Addition of dipyridamole to aspirin can lead to significant platelet inhibition in aspirin-resistant patients. The addition of dipyridamole to aspirin appears to be more effective than aspirin alone in the prevention of secondary vascular events in stroke patients and does not cause an increase in haemorrhagic events compared to aspirin alone in an identical dose.(Diener, Darius et al. 2001; Diener, Darius et al. 2001) There is also a suggestion that dipyridamole may partially compensate for aspirin resistance in patients with ischaemic stroke via an alternative antithrombotic mechanism.(Serebruany, Malinin et al. 2005; Serebruany, Malinin et al. 2006) In a study to determine whether treatment with dipyridamole or clopidogrel, in addition to aspirin, is more effective at reducing embolization and transient ischemic attacks, King and associates have shown that both dipyridamole and clopidogrel reduced embolization to a similar extent.(King, Bath et al. 2011) Other antiplatelet agents that may be more potent via alternative pathways are under investigation.

Statins to improve aspirin resistance: There is evidence that statins may be useful in treating aspirin resistance. Tirnaksiz and associates reported that in a study of patients with stable coronary artery disease, 11.2% were found to be aspirin resistant as measured by PFA-100, with a closure time of <186 seconds with collagen/adrenaline cartridges.(Tirnaksiz, Pamukcu et al. 2009) After 3 months of statin therapy (atorvastatin 10 mg/day), 65% of the aspirin-resistant patients became aspirin sensitive by PFA-100 measurements (P < 0.0001).(Tirnaksiz, Pamukcu et al. 2009) Tekten and his colleagues have shown that statins reduced platelet aggregation.(Tekten, Ceyhan et al. 2004)

Another recommendation is that because saturated fat ingestion increases *in vivo* thromboxane production despite aspirin therapy, diabetic patients on ASA therapy should have low dietary saturated fat intake and aggressive lipid management.**(Yassine, Davis-Gorman et al. 2010)**

4. Conclusion

Aspirin is recommended for primary prevention and secondary prevention of CVD in patients with type 2 diabetes. Aspirin resistance is common in patients with type 2 diabetes. Further studies are required to answer the question, will improving glycemic control in patients with poor glycemic control cause a change in responsiveness to aspirin? The relationship of the adipokines TNF-alfa and IL-6 to aspirin non-responsiveness needs further evaluation. Prospective randomized trials are needed to prove the clinical benefits of adapting the dosing of clopidogrel or switching to alternative compounds in high-risk patients with impaired antiplatelet effectiveness according to the result of platelet function assays.

5. References

(1994). "Collaborative overview of randomised trials of antiplatelet therapy--I: Prevention of death, myocardial infarction, and stroke by prolonged antiplatelet therapy in various categories of patients. Antiplatelet Trialists' Collaboration." BMJ 308(6921): 81-106.

(2002). "Collaborative meta-analysis of randomised trials of antiplatelet therapy for prevention of death, myocardial infarction, and stroke in high risk patients." BMJ 324(7329): 71-86.

Adebayo, G. I., J. Williams, et al. (2007). "Aspirin esterase activity - Evidence for skewed distribution in healthy volunteers." Eur J Intern Med 18(4): 299-303.

Angiolillo, D. J. (2007). "Antiplatelet therapy in type 2 diabetes mellitus." Curr Opin Endocrinol Diabetes Obes 14(2): 124-131.

Angiolillo, D. J., E. Bernardo, et al. (2006). "Insulin therapy is associated with platelet dysfunction in patients with type 2 diabetes mellitus on dual oral antiplatelet treatment." J Am Coll Cardiol 48(2): 298-304.

Assadian, A., J. Lax, et al. (2007). "Aspirin resistance among long-term aspirin users after carotid endarterectomy and controls: flow cytometric measurement of aspirin-induced platelet inhibition." J Vasc Surg 45(6): 1142-1147; discussion 1147.

Baigent, C., L. Blackwell, et al. (2009). "Aspirin in the primary and secondary prevention of vascular disease: collaborative meta-analysis of individual participant data from randomised trials." Lancet 373(9678): 1849-1860.

Belch, J., A. MacCuish, et al. (2008). "The prevention of progression of arterial disease and diabetes (POPADAD) trial: factorial randomised placebo controlled trial of aspirin and antioxidants in patients with diabetes and asymptomatic peripheral arterial disease." BMJ 337: a1840.

Ben-Dor, I., N. S. Kleiman, et al. (2009). "Assessment, mechanisms, and clinical implication of variability in platelet response to aspirin and clopidogrel therapy." Am J Cardiol 104(2): 227-233.

Boden, G. and A. K. Rao (2007). "Effects of hyperglycemia and hyperinsulinemia on the tissue factor pathway of blood coagulation." Curr Diab Rep 7(3): 223-227.

Bridges, J. M., A. M. Dalby, et al. (1965). "An Effect of D-Glucose on Platelet Stickiness." Lancet 1(7376): 75-77.

Bucchi, F., A. Bodzenta, et al. (1986). "Effects of 1 gram oral or intravenous aspirin on urinary excretion of thromboxane B2 and 6-keto-PGF1 alpha in healthy subjects." Prostaglandins 32(5): 691-701.

Calvin, A. D., N. R. Aggarwal, et al. (2009). "Aspirin for the primary prevention of cardiovascular events: a systematic review and meta-analysis comparing patients with and without diabetes." Diabetes Care 32(12): 2300-2306.

Cannon, C. P., R. A. Harrington, et al. (2010). "Comparison of ticagrelor with clopidogrel in patients with a planned invasive strategy for acute coronary syndromes (PLATO): a randomised double-blind study." Lancet 375(9711): 283-293.

Carr, M. E. (2001). "Diabetes mellitus: a hypercoagulable state." J Diabetes Complications 15(1): 44-54.

Catella-Lawson, F., M. P. Reilly, et al. (2001). "Cyclooxygenase inhibitors and the antiplatelet effects of aspirin." N Engl J Med 345(25): 1809-1817.

Catella, F. and G. A. FitzGerald (1987). "Paired analysis of urinary thromboxane B2 metabolites in humans." Thromb Res 47(6): 647-656.

Cox, D., A. O. Maree, et al. (2006). "Effect of enteric coating on antiplatelet activity of low-dose aspirin in healthy volunteers." Stroke 37(8): 2153-2158.

Davi, G., I. Catalano, et al. (1990). "Thromboxane biosynthesis and platelet function in type II diabetes mellitus." N Engl J Med 322(25): 1769-1774.

Davi, G., G. Ciabattoni, et al. (1999). "In vivo formation of 8-iso-prostaglandin f2alpha and platelet activation in diabetes mellitus: effects of improved metabolic control and vitamin E supplementation." Circulation 99(2): 224-229.

Davi, G., P. Gresele, et al. (1997). "Diabetes mellitus, hypercholesterolemia, and hypertension but not vascular disease per se are associated with persistent platelet activation in vivo. Evidence derived from the study of peripheral arterial disease." Circulation 96(1): 69-75.

Davi, G. and C. Patrono (2007). "Platelet activation and atherothrombosis." N Engl J Med 357(24): 2482-2494.

De Berardis, G., M. Sacco, et al. (2007). "Aspirin and Simvastatin Combination for Cardiovascular Events Prevention Trial in Diabetes (ACCEPT-D): design of a randomized study of the efficacy of low-dose aspirin in the prevention of cardiovascular events in subjects with diabetes mellitus treated with statins." Trials 8: 21.

De Berardis, G., M. Sacco, et al. (2009). "Aspirin for primary prevention of cardiovascular events in people with diabetes: meta-analysis of randomised controlled trials." BMJ 339: b4531.

DiChiara, J., K. P. Bliden, et al. (2007). "The effect of aspirin dosing on platelet function in diabetic and nondiabetic patients: an analysis from the aspirin-induced platelet effect (ASPECT) study." Diabetes 56(12): 3014-3019.

Diener, H. C., J. Bogousslavsky, et al. (2004). "Aspirin and clopidogrel compared with clopidogrel alone after recent ischaemic stroke or transient ischaemic attack in high-risk patients (MATCH): randomised, double-blind, placebo-controlled trial." Lancet 364(9431): 331-337.

Diener, H. C., H. Darius, et al. (2001). "Cardiac safety in the European Stroke Prevention Study 2 (ESPS2)." Int J Clin Pract 55(3): 162-163.

Diener, H. C., H. Darius, et al. (2001). "[Does early high dosage dipyridamole in prevention of secondary stroke induce cardiac events?]." Z Kardiol 90(5): 348-351.

DiMinno, G., M. J. Silver, et al. (1986). "Trial of repeated low-dose aspirin in diabetic angiopathy." Blood 68(4): 886-891.

Eikelboom, J. W., J. Hirsh, et al. (2002). "Aspirin-resistant thromboxane biosynthesis and the risk of myocardial infarction, stroke, or cardiovascular death in patients at high risk for cardiovascular events." Circulation 105(14): 1650-1655.

Frolich, J. C. (1997). "A classification of NSAIDs according to the relative inhibition of cyclooxygenase isoenzymes." Trends Pharmacol Sci 18(1): 30-34.

Gresele, P., G. Guglielmini, et al. (2003). "Acute, short-term hyperglycemia enhances shear stress-induced platelet activation in patients with type II diabetes mellitus." J Am Coll Cardiol 41(6): 1013-1020.

Gresele, P., S. Marzotti, et al. (2010). "Hyperglycemia-induced platelet activation in type 2 diabetes is resistant to aspirin but not to a nitric oxide-donating agent." Diabetes Care 33(6): 1262-1268.

Gurbel, P. A., K. P. Bliden, et al. (2007). "Evaluation of dose-related effects of aspirin on platelet function: results from the Aspirin-Induced Platelet Effect (ASPECT) study." Circulation 115(25): 3156-3164.

Guthikonda, S., C. L. Alviar, et al. (2008). "Role of reticulated platelets and platelet size heterogeneity on platelet activity after dual antiplatelet therapy with aspirin and clopidogrel in patients with stable coronary artery disease." J Am Coll Cardiol 52(9): 743-749.

Guthikonda, S., E. I. Lev, et al. (2007). "Reticulated platelets and uninhibited COX-1 and COX-2 decrease the antiplatelet effects of aspirin." J Thromb Haemost 5(3): 490-496.

Halushka, M. K. and P. V. Halushka (2002). "Why are some individuals resistant to the cardioprotective effects of aspirin? Could it be thromboxane A2?" Circulation 105(14): 1620-1622.

Halushka, P. V., R. Mayfield, et al. (1981). "Increased platelet arachidonic acid metabolism in diabetes mellitus." Diabetes 30(Suppl 2): 44-48.

Halushka, P. V., R. C. Rogers, et al. (1981). "Increased platelet thromboxane synthesis in diabetes mellitus." J Lab Clin Med 97(1): 87-96.

Held, C., N. Asenblad, et al. (2011). "Ticagrelor versus clopidogrel in patients with acute coronary syndromes undergoing coronary artery bypass surgery: results from the PLATO (Platelet Inhibition and Patient Outcomes) trial." J Am Coll Cardiol 57(6): 672-684.

King, A., P. M. Bath, et al. (2011). "Clopidogrel versus dipyridamole in addition to aspirin in reducing embolization detected with ambulatory transcranial Doppler: a randomized trial." Stroke 42(3): 650-655.

Langer, H. F. and M. Gawaz (2008). "Platelet-vessel wall interactions in atherosclerotic disease." Thromb Haemost 99(3): 480-486.

McCabe, D. J., P. Harrison, et al. (2005). "Assessment of the antiplatelet effects of low to medium dose aspirin in the early and late phases after ischaemic stroke and TIA." Platelets 16(5): 269-280.

Modica, A., F. Karlsson, et al. (2007). "Platelet aggregation and aspirin non-responsiveness increase when an acute coronary syndrome is complicated by an infection." J Thromb Haemost 5(3): 507-511.

Ogawa, H., M. Nakayama, et al. (2008). "Low-dose aspirin for primary prevention of atherosclerotic events in patients with type 2 diabetes: a randomized controlled trial." JAMA 300(18): 2134-2141.

Patrono, C., G. Ciabattoni, et al. (1986). "Estimated rate of thromboxane secretion into the circulation of normal humans." J Clin Invest 77(2): 590-594.

Pignone, M., M. J. Alberts, et al. (2010). "Aspirin for primary prevention of cardiovascular events in people with diabetes: a position statement of the American Diabetes Association, a scientific statement of the American Heart Association, and an expert

consensus document of the American College of Cardiology Foundation." Diabetes Care 33(6): 1395-1402.
Plosker, G. L. and K. A. Lyseng-Williamson (2007). "Clopidogrel: a review of its use in the prevention of thrombosis." Drugs 67(4): 613-646.
Preis, S. R., S. J. Hwang, et al. (2009). "Trends in all-cause and cardiovascular disease mortality among women and men with and without diabetes mellitus in the Framingham Heart Study, 1950 to 2005." Circulation 119(13): 1728-1735.
Relou, I. A., C. M. Hackeng, et al. (2003). "Low-density lipoprotein and its effect on human blood platelets." Cell Mol Life Sci 60(5): 961-971.
Ruggeri, Z. M. and G. L. Mendolicchio (2007). "Adhesion mechanisms in platelet function." Circ Res 100(12): 1673-1685.
Serebruany, V., A. Malinin, et al. (2006). "Dipyridamole decreases protease-activated receptor and annexin-v binding on platelets of post stroke patients with aspirin nonresponsiveness." Cerebrovasc Dis 21(1-2): 98-105.
Serebruany, V. L., A. I. Malinin, et al. (2005). "Effects of clopidogrel and aspirin in combination versus aspirin alone on platelet activation and major receptor expression in patients after recent ischemic stroke: for the Plavix Use for Treatment of Stroke (PLUTO-Stroke) trial." Stroke 36(10): 2289-2292.
Singla, A., M. J. Antonino, et al. (2009). "The relation between platelet reactivity and glycemic control in diabetic patients with cardiovascular disease on maintenance aspirin and clopidogrel therapy." Am Heart J 158(5): 784 e781-786.
Tavil, Y., N. Sen, et al. (2010). "Coronary heart disease is associated with mean platelet volume in type 2 diabetic patients." Platelets 21(5): 368-372.
Tekten, T., C. Ceyhan, et al. (2004). "The effect of atorvastatin on platelet function in patients with coronary artery disease." Acta Cardiol 59(3): 311-315.
ten Berg, J. M., W. B. Gerritsen, et al. (2002). "High-dose aspirin in addition to daily low-dose aspirin decreases platelet activation in patients before and after percutaneous coronary intervention." Thromb Res 105(5): 385-390.
Tirnaksiz, E., B. Pamukcu, et al. (2009). "Effect of high dose statin therapy on platelet function; statins reduce aspirin-resistant platelet aggregation in patients with coronary heart disease." J Thromb Thrombolysis 27(1): 24-28.
Vinik, A. I., T. Erbas, et al. (2001). "Platelet dysfunction in type 2 diabetes." Diabetes Care 24(8): 1476-1485.
Vizioli, L., S. Muscari, et al. (2009). "The relationship of mean platelet volume with the risk and prognosis of cardiovascular diseases." Int J Clin Pract 63(10): 1509-1515.
Watala, C., J. Golanski, et al. (2004). "Reduced sensitivity of platelets from type 2 diabetic patients to acetylsalicylic acid (aspirin)-its relation to metabolic control." Thromb Res 113(2): 101-113.
Winocour, P. D., C. Watala, et al. (1992). "Decreased platelet membrane fluidity due to glycation or acetylation of membrane proteins." Thromb Haemost 68(5): 577-582.
Yassine, H. N., G. Davis-Gorman, et al. (2010). "Clinical determinants of aspirin resistance in diabetes." Diabetes Res Clin Pract 90(1): e19-21.
Yassine, H. N., G. Davis-Gorman, et al. (2010). "Effect of glucose or fat challenge on aspirin resistance in diabetes." Int J Endocrinol 2010: 820876.

Younis, N., S. Williams, et al. (2010). "Role of aspirin in the primary prevention of cardiovascular disease in diabetes mellitus: a meta-analysis." Expert Opin Pharmacother 11(9): 1459-1466.

Zhang, C., A. Sun, et al. (2010). "Aspirin for primary prevention of cardiovascular events in patients with diabetes: A meta-analysis." Diabetes Res Clin Pract 87(2): 211-218.

Zimmermann, N., M. Kurt, et al. (2005). "Is cardiopulmonary bypass a reason for aspirin resistance after coronary artery bypass grafting?" Eur J Cardiothorac Surg 27(4): 606-610.

Zimmermann, N., A. Wenk, et al. (2003). "Functional and biochemical evaluation of platelet aspirin resistance after coronary artery bypass surgery." Circulation 108(5): 542-547.

7

Diabetic Cardiomyopathy

Dike Bevis Ojji
Cardiovacular Medicine, Internal Medicine,
University Of Abuja Teaching Hospital, Gwagwalada, Abuja
Nigeria

1. Introduction

Diabetes Mellitus is a syndrome characterized by hyperglycaemia and disturbances of carbohydrate, fat and protein metabolism associated with absolute or relative deficiencies in insulin secretion and, or insulin action.[1] It is a genetically and clinically heterogeneous group of disorders that share glucose intolerance in common.[2] It is the most common endocrine metabolic disorder world wide affecting people of all races and of different social conditions[2]. It is estimated that approximately 120 million people have diabetes mellitus worldwide and this number is expected to double in the next 25 year.[4] The major part of the increase in the prevalence of diabetes mellitus is expected in the developing countries.[5] In most African populations, it is said that the high prevalence of impaired glucose tolerance (IGT) suggests that public health impact of diabetes could increase in these communities in the future.[6]

Diabetes mellitus is characterized by acute and long term complications and these result in increased morbidity and mortality in diabetics especially in developing countries due to inadequate facilities for treatment and the inability of patients to afford the cost of care.[7] The cardiovascular, renal, retinal and neuropathic long-term complications lead to premature disability and death.[7]

Heart disease has been singled out as a major cause of death in patients with diabetes mellitus,[8,9] and the risk of atherosclerotic coronary artery disease is substantially increased in patients with both overt diabetes and asymptomatic hyperglycaemia.[10] Several studies have suggested that diabetes may be associated with left ventricular (LV) structural and functional abnormalities in addition to, and independent of atherosclerosis.[11,12] In the Framingham Cohort, diabetes was associated with higher LV mass in women but not men[13]. High blood pressure (BP), obesity and abnormal lipid profile, which often co-exist with diabetes, tend to be associated with preclinical cardiovascular abnormalities,[14] and may contribute to the association of diabetes mellitus with cardiovascular events.

However, there is increasing evidence that diabetics have abnormalities of left ventricular function in the absence of clinical heart disease[15,16] which is an entity called diabetic cardiomyopathy.

Diastolic left ventricular abnormalities have been disclosed in the past by cardiac catheterisation[17] and abnormal systolic time interval using phonocardiograms,[18,19] and presently by abnormal left ventricular filling using standard and digitised echocardiography,[20,21] radionuclide studies[22] and subsequently by Doppler echocardiography.[22,23]. Non-invasive methods of assessing left function have confirmed that it is frequently impaired in young asymptomatic diabetics,[24,25] in maturity onset diabetics [26] and in those with retinopathy and nephropathy.[27,28] In diabetes, the left ventricle is not usually dilated or hypertrophied[29] and abnormalities of function are predominantly in diastole, with delayed opening of the mitral valve. Reduced ejection and abnormal systolic function is probably a late event.[19,20]

Possible mechanisms for diabetic cardiomyopathy include excessive myocardial fibrosis,[30] interstitial accumulation of glycoproteins and slow sarcoplasmic calcium reuptake[31] or altered release from a dysfunctional coronary endothelium of mediators such as nitric oxide and endothelin which exert paracrine myocardial effects on diastolic properties [32,34].

2. Diastolic dysfunction

2.1 What is diastolic dysfunction?

Diastolic dysfunction can be defined as a condition in which myocardial relaxation and filling are impaired and incomplete.[34] In its most severe form, diastolic dysfunction results in overt symptoms of congestive heart failure.[35] In modest cases, symptoms of dyspnoea and fatigue occur only during stress or activity such as exercise when heart rate and/or end diastolic volume increase[36]. In its mildest forms, diastolic dysfunction can be manifested as slow or delayed pattern of relaxation and filling with little or no elevation in diastolic pressure and no cardiac symptoms.[37] Some factors that have been implicated in left ventricular diastolic dysfunction include: diabetes mellitus, coronary artery disease, hypertensive heart disease, hypertrophic cardiomyopathy, valvular heart disease, cardiac transplantation, cardiac amyloidosis [38] and aging.[39]

2.2 Prevalence of diastolic dysfunction

The prevalence of asymptomatic diastolic dysfunction was estimated at 27% in an epidemilogic study, and was found to increase with age [40]. Results of early studies suggested that as many as 40% of patients with heart failure symptoms have diastolic heart failure. More recent studies showed that of patients hospitalised for heart failure, 35% to 40% present with diastolic heart failure.[41,42] In the community setting, this number was found to be between 45%and 55%.[43,44] Two recent studies found the prevalence of diastolic heart failure in women to be 1.5-to 2-fold greater than in men.[45,46]. In a study of 86 normotensive type 2 diabetic patients (43% of whom were women, mean age of 43 years and mean glycosylated haemoglobin of 6.5g/dl), greater than 40% had diastolic dysfunction on Doppler echocardiography.[47] In 1989, Shapiro et al reported a prevalence of 40% amongst a mixed patient population of both type1 and type2 diabetics.[48]

In a study of one-hundred and twenty Nigerian normotensive type 2 diabetic subjects, only 29% of the diabetic subjects had normal filling function compared to 58% of the normal controls.[49]

2.3 Clinical evidences for diabetic cardiomyopathy

The Framingham study was the first to demonstrate an increased risk of heart failure in patients with diabetes mellitus.[50] When the incidence of heart failure in men and women with diabetes mellitus was compared with that of non diabetic men and women, the incidence in individuals with diabetes was found to be 2- and 5-fold greater respectively.[51] Since then, additional trials like Studies of Left Ventricular Dysfunction (SOLVD),[52] the Heart Outcomes Prevention Evaluation (HOPE) study[53] and the Cardiovascular Health Study (CHS)[54] have identified diabetes mellitus as a major risk factor for the development of heart failure. It has been found that close to 30% of patients with diastolic heart failure have diabetes mellitus.[55]

Left ventricular diastolic dysfunction is proposed to be the first stage of diabetic cardiomyopathy.[27,56] In the Strong Heart Study[57] which enrolled 2,411 Native Americans, individuals with diabetes mellitus had evidence of impaired left ventricular relaxation on Doppler echocardiography. In that study, the association between diabetes mellitus and abnormal left ventricular relaxation was independent of age, blood pressure, LV mass and LV systolic function. The abnormalities were more severe in the diabetes-hypertension group, showing the additive deleterious effects on active LV relaxation when both of these conditions are present. Poirier et al[58] reported that patients with well-controlled diabetes and without overt coronary artery disease, hypertension or heart failure have lower levels of exercise performance on maximal treadmill testing than do age-matched controls. This exercise limitation correlated with the severity of diastolic dysfunction as assessed by Doppler echocardiography.

Several workers have studied the correlation between left ventricular diastolic function and factors such as duration of diabetes mellitus, glycaemic control, microangiopathy, microalbuminuria and systemic hypertension. In the study of thirty patients with type 2 diabetes mellitus, Fiorini et al[59] found no correlation between duration of diabetes mellitus and diastolic dysfunction. Also, in the study of one hundred and twenty-five (125) type I diabetics, some workers[60] found no correlation between duration of diabetes and diastolic dysfunction. Also, other workers[61] in the study of twelve (12) type I diabetic patients found that diastolic abnormalities are not related to the duration of the disease. However, Bertoni et al[62] in the study of twenty-six (26) young subjects with type 1 diabetes mellitus of at least three years duration, found that there is a correlation between diastolic dysfunction and duration of diabetes mellitus.

In the Veterans Affairs Co-operative Study in type 2 Diabetes Mellitus (VACSDM)[63], it was found that two years of intensive glycaemic control did not affect the left ventricular systolic or diastolic functions in patients with type 2 diabetes. Also in the study of twenty normotensive patients with a new diagnosis of type 2 diabetes mellitus, some workers[64] found that diastolic function was impaired at diagnosis and was not affected by an improvement in the glycaemic control.However,Felicio et al[65] in the study of fifty-six hypertensive patients with type 2 diabetes mellitus concluded that even though there was no correlation between diastolic dysfunction and glycaemic control, improvement in glycaemic control may contribute to LVH regression in hypertensive patients with type 2 diabetes mellitus.

Cecchi et al[66] in the study of forty recently diagnosed type 1 diabetics (with and without microangiopathy) showed that slight preclinical diastolic dysfunction is present in young recently diagnosed type 1 diabetic without microangiopathy. But it was found that more severe dysfunction is present when there is also microangiopathy. Some other workers[56] confirmed this in the study of 26 young subjects with type 1 diabetes mellitus. They showed that there is an often sub-clinical cardiac abnormality in young diabetics resulting in impairment of diastolic function that is correlate with the presence of clinical complications such as nephropathy and retinopathy.

Liu et al in the strong Heart study[57] showed that albuminuria is independently associated with LV systolic and diastolic dysfunction in type 2 diabetics. Some other workers[67] in the study of forty-two patients with mild-to-moderate essential hypertension and type 2 diabetes mellitus found that an elevated urinary albumin excretion is associated with an increased left ventricular mass index. They also found that urinary albumin excretion is associated with a higher prevalence of concentric left ventricular hypertrophy pattern, a depressed midwall systolic performance and a markedly impaired diastolic function. Also Mori et al[68] in the study of twenty-one type 2 diabetics found that left ventricular diastolic function may be related to both hypertension and proteinuria.

In the study of ten age-controlled type 2 diabetes, it was found by Poirier et al[69] that left ventricular diastolic dysfunction and cardiac autonomic neuropathy are associated in patients with otherwise uncomplicated well-controlled type 2 diabetes mellitus.

3. Pathogeesis of diabetic cardiomyopathy

The pathogenesis of diabetic cardiomyopathy has been illustrated in figure1.The morphologic changes in the diabetic heart include myocyte hypertrophy, increased matrix collagen, interstitial fibrosis, and intra-myocardial microangiopathy.[70] These changes are probably consequences of altered myocardial glucose and fatty acid metabolism due to diabetes.[50] Chronic hyperglycaemia leads to nonenzymatic glycation of vascular and membrane proteins, producing advanced glycation end products (AGEs) and reactive oxygen species.[67] Once AGEs develop in the arterial wall and myocardium, they form stable and irreversible crosslinks with adjacent collagen polymers thereby decreasing the compliance of the blood vessels and myocardium.[67] The AGEs and reactive oxygen species will also affect ion channel, calcium homeostasis, and mitochondrial function, as well as initiating apoptosis, leading to contractile dysfunction-glucotoxicity.[67]

Diabetes is also characterised by an increased turnover of free fatty acids. The increased free fatty acid turnover leads to increased myocardial oxygen consumption and enhances the intracellular accumulation of intermediates, leading to deleterious effects-lipotoxicity.[67] These effects include interference with ATP-dependent ion pumps and mobilisation of intracellular calcium, thereby creating calcium overload and relaxation abnormalities. Impaired glucose oxidation also leads to lactic acid accumulation that further promotes the degradation of free fatty acids.[68]

Other myocardial changes in diabetes include impairment of beta-receptor signal transudation and induction of fetal gene pattern.[70,71] The fetal gene pattern leads to upregulation of beta-myosin heavy chain and downregulation of alpha-myosin heavy chain gene which is the fast –contracting isoform of myosin heavy chain that contains much greater ATPase activity than does beta-myosin heavy chain.[72] In addition, there is downregulation of the SERCA gene,[73] leading to impaired myocardial calcium handling.[74] These changes in gene expression are closely associated with abnormalities in diastolic function.[75]

To support the theory that abnormalities in high-energy phosphate metabolism may cause diastolic dysfunction in diabetes, magnetic resonance imaging study demonstrated LV diastolic dysfunction in 12 asymptomatic, normotensive, nonobese patients with well-controlled diabetes when compared with control subjects matched for age, sex, body mass index, and blood pressure.[76] These findings were associated with a significantly lower ratio of myocardial phosphocreatine to ATP in-patients with diabetes compared with controls.[91]

Results of previous studies in non-diabetic individuals with LV hypertrophy suggested that the lower phosphocreatine content and the switch in substrate preference from glucose to fatty acids may lead to lower levels of ATP in the sarcomeres that cannot be overcome by increased mitochondrial ATP production[77]. Lower cytosolic ATP concentrations are associated with impaired calcium sequestration by the sarcoplasmic reticulum and impaired relaxation of cardiomyocytes[76].

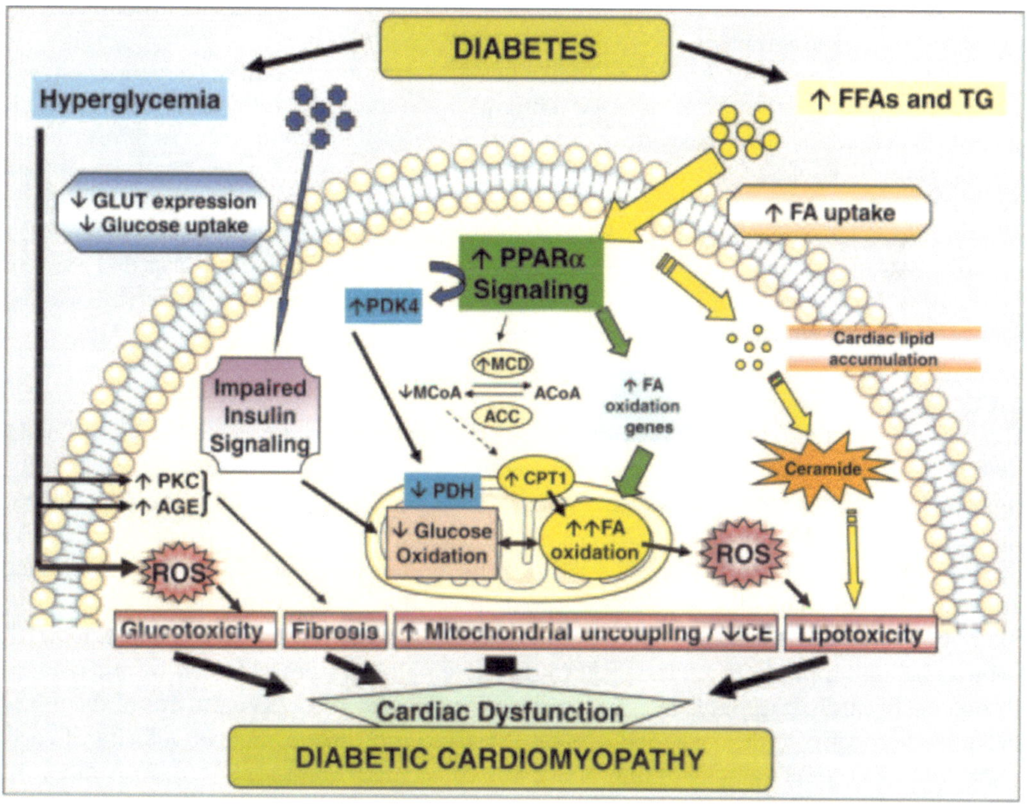

Increased free FA (FFA) activates PPAR- signaling, leading to the increased transcription of many genes involved in FA oxidation. Increased FA oxidation leads to the generation of ROS at the level of the electron transport chain. ROS, which also can be generated by extramitochondrial mechanisms such as NADPH oxidase, plays a critical role in several pathways involved in the pathogenesis of diabetic cardiomyopathy, including lipotoxicity, cell death, and tissue damage, as well as mitochondrial uncoupling and reduced cardiac efficiency. TG= triglycerides; GLUTs= glucose transporters; PDK4=pyruvate dehydrogenase kinase 4; MCD=malonyl-coenzyme A decarboxylase;MCoA= malonyl-coenzyme A; ACoA=acetyl-coenzyme A; ACC= acetyl coenzyme A carboxylase; CPT1= carnitine palmitoyl-transferase 1; PDH= pyruvate dehydrogenase; CE= cardiac efficiency; PKC= protein kinase C; and AGE= glycation end products

4. Diagnosing diastolic dysfunction

Differentiating between diastolic and systolic dysfunction on clinical grounds is very difficult, although clues may be given by the patient's past history, clinical presentation, physical examination, radiographic and electrocardiographic findings.[78] Exertional dyspnoea because of pulmonary congestion is frequently an early event in diastolic dysfunction.[78]
More commonly, estimates of left ventricular size and systolic function are needed in order to determine whether congestive heart failure is caused by systolic or diastolic dysfunction. These measurements can be made using echocardiography, radionuclide ventriculography, or contrast ventriculography.[79]
Precisely, the definite diagnosis of diastolic dysfunction or failure depends on the observation of an appropriate upward shift of the (end-) diastolic pressure - volume relation.[80] Therefore, objective evidence of ventricular diastolic dysfunction requires cardiac catheterisation with volume determinations using frame-by-frame analysis of left ventricular contrast angiograms or impedance measurements and high - fidelity measurements of ventricular pressure with a micromanometer.[81] However, due to the invasive nature, high cost, and limited availability of haemodynamic studies, this remains impractical for widespread use or for serial follow-up examinations[82] thereby leaving echocardiography as the gold standard.

4.1 Echocardiography

Doppler echocardiography has become the most widely used and accepted method for the diagnosis and follow-up of patients with diastolic dysfunction. Its reliability, reproducibility, ease of performance, and advances in applications over the past decade makes it the ideal tool for the assessment of "diastology"[83]. The basis of the Doppler echocardiographic assessment of diastolic function relies on a careful, integrated approach.[84,85] The main stay of this approach involves the recording of flow velocities across the mitral valve and within the pulmonary veins to assess filling patterns and estimate left ventricular filling pressure indirectly.[85] Mitral flow velocities are obtained by pulse-wave Doppler echocardiography placing the sample volume located between the tips of the mitral valve leaflet during ventricular diastole (as shown in figure 2). The peak velocity of early rapid filling (E), peak velocity of late filling caused by atrial contraction (A), E/A ratio, the interval from the peak of E velocity to its extrapolation to baseline or the deceleration time (DT) and the interval from aortic valve closure to mitral valve opening or isovolumic relaxation time (IVRT) is measured.[86]
Pulmonary venous flow is measured using pulse-wave Doppler echocardiography with sample volume located 1-2cm into a pulmonary vein, proximal to its insertion into the left atrium(as shown in figure 3). The systolic peak velocity which is biphasic in 30% of cases (S), diastolic peak velocity (D), the S/D ratio, atrial systolic reversal velocity (A) are measured.[87]
Based on Doppler echocardiographic studies, diastolic filling is classified into:[86] normal, impaired relaxation or mild diastolic dysfunction, moderate diastolic dysfunction or pseudo normal filling and severe diastolic dysfunction or restrictive filling.

4.2 Normal filling

The determinants of LV filling, ventricular relaxation and effective chamber compliance change with increasing age. This leads to different diastolic filling patterns for different groups.[88] In normal young individuals aged (20s - 30s), LV relaxation is rapid, the majority of filling (85-95%) occurring in early diastole and only a small proportion (5-15%) occurring with atrial contraction. This results in mitral inflow parameters of E/A between 1-2 (mean1.8), and relatively short deceleration time (mean 182msec) and isovolumetric relaxation time (mean 71msec). Pulmonary venous inflow usually shows a slight systolic predominance (S>D) with a mean pulmonary 'A' of 0.19m/sec.[89]

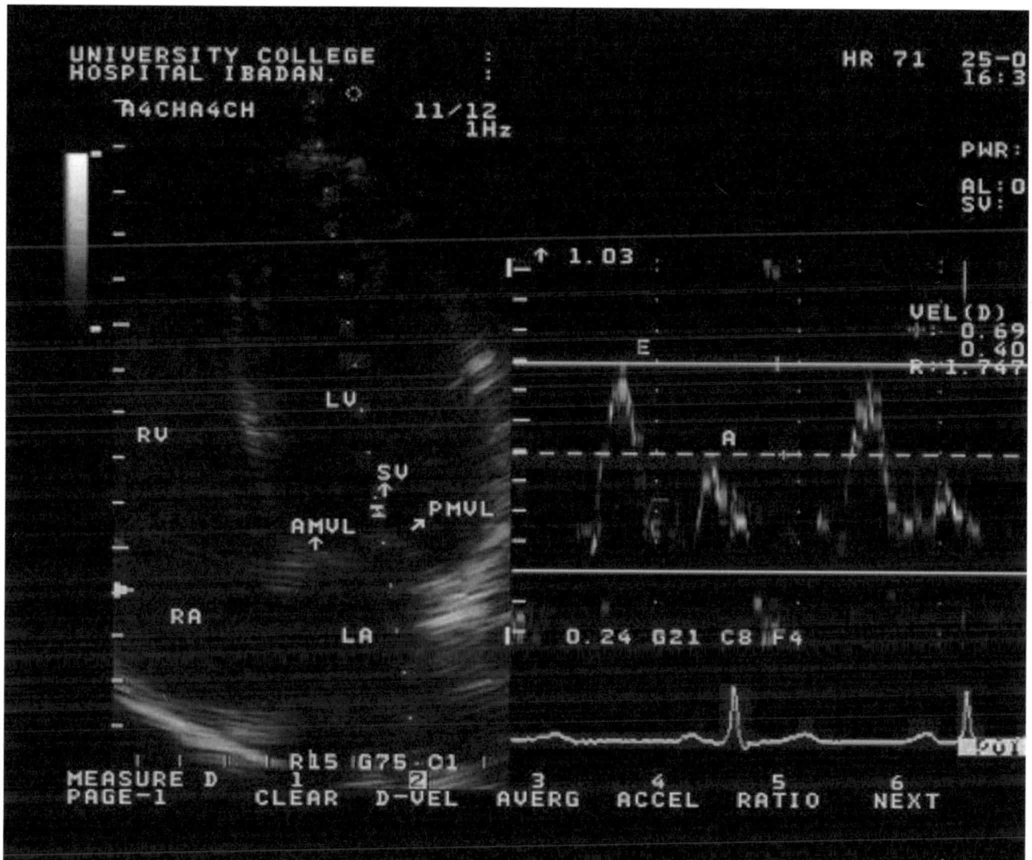

RV =Right Ventricle
LV=Left Ventricle
RA=Right Atrium
LA =Left Atrium
SV=Sample Volume
AMVL=Anterior Mitral Valve Leaflet
PMVL=Posterior Mitral Valve Leaflet
E=Mitral E wave
A=Mitral A wave

Fig. 2.Echocardiogram showing measurement of Transmitral Flow Velocity Profile ('E' and 'A' Waves)

With aging, the rate of LV relaxation decreases with slower and less filling in early diastole and an increased contribution to LV filling by atrial contraction. This leads to a prolongation of the IVRT and DT, a reduction in E velocity, and an increase in A velocity with a subsequent reduction in E/A ratio. Individuals >65 years have the following average parameters: E/A ratio of less than 1, a mean DT greater than 214msec, and IVRT greater than of 94msec. As pulmonary D parallels the pulmonary S velocity, the pulmonary venous flow now shows diastolic predominance (D>S). As well, the A increases slightly, but does not exceed the upper limit of normal (0.35m/sec).[90]

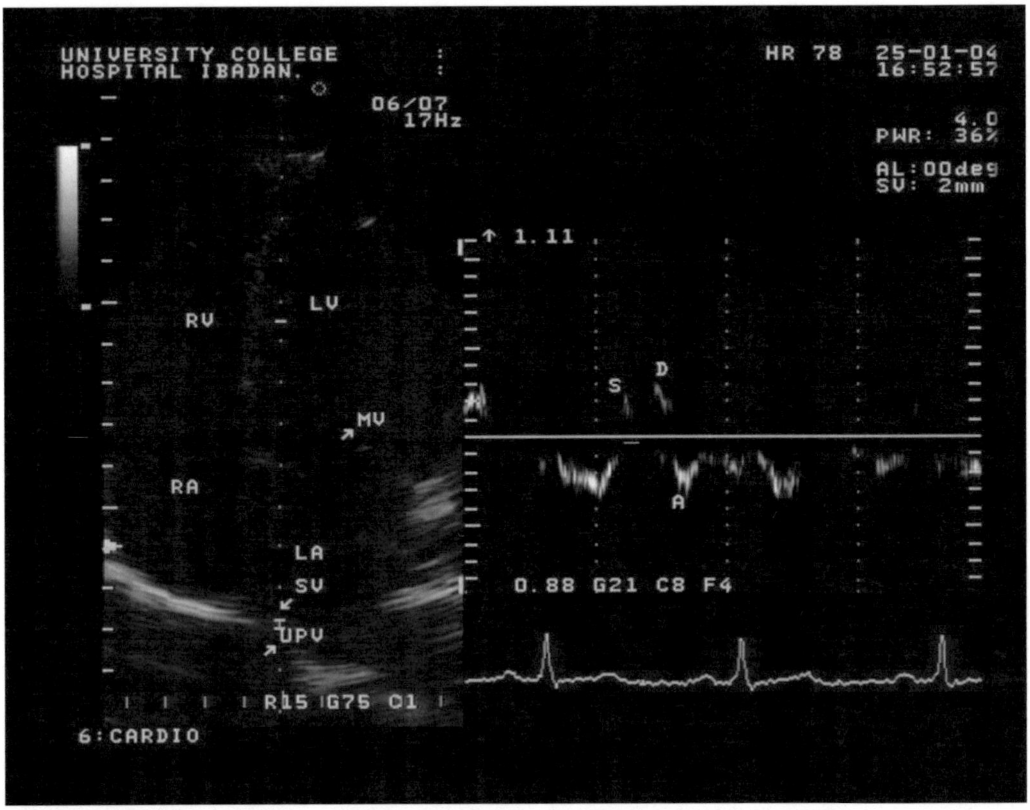

LV=Left Ventricle,
RV =Right Ventricle,
RA=Right Atrium,
A =Left Atrium,
SV=Sample Volume,
UPV= Upper Pulmonary Vein (Right),
S=Pulmonary Vein Systolic Velocity,
D=Pulmonary Vein Diastolic velocity,
A=Pulmonary Reverse flow Velocity

Fig. 3. Echocardiogram showing measurement of Pulmonary Flow Velocity Profile

4.3 Mild diastolic dysfunction

This represents the earliest stage of diastolic dysfunction. There is impaired LV relaxation with initially normal LV filling pressures, leading to decreased early filling and increased filling with atrial contraction. Mitral inflow patterns show an E/A less than 1 which is abnormal for the age. The IVRT is prolonged (>100msec), with prolongation of the DT (>200msec). Pulmonary venous inflow normally remains normal with systolic predominance (S>D), and with pulmonary 'A'<0.35m/sec.[90]

4.4 Moderate diastolic dysfunction

As diastolic dysfunction progresses, LV relaxation becomes further impaired and LV stiffness increases.[90] In an attempt to maintain LV filling and cardiac output, the filling pressure, specifically left atrial (LA) pressure becomes elevated. This increased transmitral pressure gradient leads to increased early filling with the E/A ratio 'normalizing' to a value >1, with prolongation of IVRT and DT to high values. This mitral pattern is similar to the pattern in normal individuals, leading to the term 'pseudonormal'. The differentiation from normal is done on the basis of an abnormal response to the valsalva manoeuvre or as abnormal pulmonary venous flow pattern.[90]

4.5 Severe diastolic dysfunction

As diastolic dysfunction progresses further, LV relaxation continues to be impaired, however, it is marked by rising LV filling pressures and a markedly reduced LV compliance. This mimics the physiology of restrictive cardiomyopathy.[90] The increased LA pressure causes an early mitral valve opening and rapid early filling (increased E velocity). As early rapid filling occur into a noncompliant LV, there is rapid equalization of LV and LA pressured leading to a shortened DT.[90] Atrial contraction into a noncompliant LV with high diastolic pressure leads to a reduced A velocity. Therefore, the E/A ratio is >2, and occasionally >4 to 5. Pulmonary venous inflow shows a marked blunting of systolic inflow (PS<<PD) corresponding to the markedly elevated LA pressure and reduced LA compliance.[87]

5. Conclusion

Abnormal left ventricular relaxation seen in diabetics, independent of other factors has been shown to contribute to the incidence of congestive heart failure despite normal left ventricular ejection fraction.[55] It is therefore another cause of clinical cardiovascular morbidity. In addition, reduced or increased mitral E/A ratio has been shown to be independently associated with increased all cause mortality as well as cardiovascular mortality.[91]

It is therefore necessary to detect early, diabetic patients with left ventricular diastolic dysfunction and commence treatment modalities such as use of selective β - blockers and ACE inhibitor.[131] However, there have not been prospective intervention studies to determine the reversibility and effectiveness of such treatments.

6. References

Bennett PH. Diabetes - Definition and Pathogenesis. In: Kahn CR, Weir GC. (Eds). Joslin's Diabetes Mellitus. Thirteenth edition. Lea and Febiger (Publishers), Philadelphia. 1994: 193-200.

National Diabetes Data Group. Classification and diagnosis of Diabetes Mellitus and other categories of glucose intolerance. Diabetes 1979; 28: 1039-1057.

Famuyiwa OO. Important considerations in the care of diabetic patients in Nigeria. International diabetes Digest 1993; 4: 48-51.

King H, Rewers M.WHO Ad Hoc Diabetes Reporting Group. Global estimates for prevalence of diabetes and impaired glucose tolerance in adults. Diabetes care 1993; 16:157-177.

King H. Diabetes Mellitus: a growing international health care problem. International Diabetes Monitor 1997; 9:1-6.

King H, Rewers M.WHO Ad Hoc Diabetes Reporting Group. Global estimates for prevalence of diabetes and impaired glucose tolerance in adults. Diabetes care 1993; 16:157-177.

World Health Organisation. Prevention of Diabetes Mellitus: report of a WHO study group. WHO Technical report series 1994; 844.

Rubler S, Sajadi RM, Araoye MA, Holford FD. Non invasive estimation of myocardial performance in patients with diabetes. Effect of alcohol administration. Diabetes 1978; 27: 127-34.

D'Elia JA, Weinrauch LA, Healy RW, Libertino JA, Bradley R, Leland OS. Myocardial dysfunction without coronary artery disease in diabetic renal failure. Am J cardiol 1979; 43: 193-19.

Shapiro LM, Howat AP, Calter MM. Left ventricular function in diabetes mellitus. 1. Methodology and prevalence and spectrum of abnormalities. Br Heart J 1981; 45: 122-128.

Shapiro LM, Leatherdale BA, Mackinnon J, Fletcher RF. Left Ventricular Function in diabetes mellitus. II. Relation between clinical features and left ventricular function. Br Heart J 1981; 45: 129-132.

Sanderson JE, Brown DJ, Rivellese A, Kohner E. Diabetic Cardiomyopathy? An echocardiographic study of young diabetes. Br Med J 1978; 1: 404-407.

Galderisi M, Anderson KM, Wilsion PWF, et al. Echocardiogrephic evidence for the existence of a distinct diabetic Cardiomoyopathy (the Framingham study} Am J Cardiol.1991; 68; 85-89.

Devereux RB, Alderman MH. Role of preclinical cardiovascular disease in the evolution from risk factor exposure to development of morbid events. Circulation 1993, 88; 1444-1455.

Ahmed SS, Jaferi GA, Narany RM, et al. Preclinical abnormality of left ventricular function in diabetes mellitus. Am Heart J.1975; 89:153-158.

Grossman E, Shemesh J, Shamiss A, et al. Left Ventricular mass in diabetes- hypertension. Arch Intern Med. 1992; 152:1001-1004.

Regan TJ, Lyons MM, Ahmed SS, et al. Evidence for cardiomyopathy in familial diabetes mellitus. J Clin Invest 1977; 60: 885-899.

Shapiro LM, Howat AP, Calter MM. Left ventricular function in diabetes mellitus. 1. Methodology and prevalence and spectrum of abnormalities. Br Heart J 1981; 45: 122-128.

Shapiro LM, Leatherdale BA, Mackinnon J, Fletcher RF. Left Ventricular Function in diabetes mellitus. II. Relation between clinical features and left ventricular function. Br Heart J 1981; 45: 129-132.

Sanderson JE, Brown DJ, Rivellese A, Kohner E. Diabetic cardiomyopathy? An echocardiographic study of young diabetics. Br. Med J 1978; i: 404-7.

Danielsen R, Nordrehaug JE, Lien E, Vik-Mo H. Subclinical left ventricular abnormalities in young subjects with long-term type 1 diabetes mellitus detected by digitized M-mode echocardiography. Am J Cardiol 1987; 60: 143-146.

Takenaka K, Sakamoto T, Amano K, Oku J, Murakami T, Toda I, Kawakubo K, Sugimoto T. Left Ventricular filling determined by Doppler echocardiography in diabetes mellitus. Am J Cardiol 1988; 61: 1140-1143.

Zarich SW, Arbuckle BE, Cohen LR, Roberts H, Nesto RW. Diastolic abnormalities in young asymptomatic diabetic patients assessed by Pulsed Doppler echocardiography. JACC 1988; 12: 114-130.

Rynkiewicz A, Semetkowska-Jurkiewicz E,Wyrzkowski B. systolic time. Intervals in young diabetics. Br Heart J 1980; 44:280-3.

Ahmed SS, Jaferi GA, Narang RM, Regan TJ; Preclinical abnormality of left ventricular function in diabetes mellitus. Am Heart J 1975; 89: 153-8.

Shapiro LM, Leatherdale BA, Loyne ME, Fletcher RF, Mackinnon J.Prospective study of heart disease in untreated maturity onset diabetes. Br Heart J 1980;44:342-8.

Seneviratine BIB. Diabetic cardiomyopathy: the preclinical phase Br Med J 1977; i : 1444-6.

Sanderson JE, Brown DJ, Rivellese A, Kohner E. Diabetic Cardiomyopathy; An echocardiographic study of young diabetics Br Med J 1978; i: 404-7.

Shapiro LM, Leatherdale Ba, Mackinnon J, Fletcher RF. Left ventricular function in diabetes mellitus. II: Relation between clinical features and left ventricular function.Br Heart J 1981; 45:129-32.

Hoeven KH, Factor SM. A comparison of the pathological Spectrum of hypertensive, diabetic and hypertensive-diabetic heart disease. Circulation 1990:82:848-55.

Goetzche O. Myocardial cell dysfunction in diabetes mellitus.A review of clinical and experimental studies.Diabetes1986;35:1158-62.

Paulus WJ. Paracrine coronary endothelial modulation of diastolic left ventricular function in man: implications for diastolic heart failure. J Cardiac Failure 1996;2:S155-164.

Shah AM. Paracrine modulation of heart cell function by endothelial cells. Cardiovasc Res 1996;31:847-67.

Gaasch WH, Schick EC, Zile MR. Management of left ventricular diastolic dysfunction. In: Smith TW (ed). Cardiovascular therapeutics. A companion to Braunmwald's Heart Disease, Philadelphia: W.B. Sanders company, 1996;237-242.

Lorell BH. Significance of diastolic dysfunction of the heart. Am.Rev. Med 1991; 42:411-436.

Bonow RO, Udelson JE. Left ventricular diastolic dysfunction as a cause of congestive heart failure: mechanisms and management. Ann Intern Med 1992; 117:502-510.

Zile MR. Diastolic dysfunction and heart failure in hypertrophied hearts. CHF 1998; 4:32-42.

Catherine Paillole, Micheal Dahan, Frederic Paycha et al. Am J cardiol 1989; 64:1010-1016.

Zile MR, Brusaert DL. New concepts in diastolic dysfunction and diastolicheart failure.1.Diagnosis, prognosis and measurements of diastolic function. Circulation 2002; 105:1387-1393.

Redfield MM, Jacobsen SJ, Burnett JC Jr et al. Burden of systolic and diastolic ventricular dysfunction in the community: appreciating the scope of the heart failure epidemic. JAMA>2003;289:194-202.

Vasan RS, Benjamin EJ, Levy D.Prevalence, clinical features and prognosis of diastolic heart failure: an epidemiological perspective's Am Coll Cardiol.1995; 26:1565-1574.

Smith GL, Masoudi FA,Vaccarino V, et al. Outcomes in heart failure patients with preserved ejection fraction: mortality, readmission, and functional decline. J Am Coll Cardiol.2003;41:1510-1518.

EF, Rocco TA, Lindenmuth NW, et al. Systolic versus diastolic heart failure in community practice: clinical features, outcomes, and the use of angiotensin-converting enzyme inhibitors. Am J Med.2000;109:605-613.

Pernenki R, Vinson JM, Shah AS, et al. Course and prognosis in patients Greater than 70years of age with congestive heart failure and normal Versus abnormal left ventricular ejection fraction. AM J Cardiol.1997;79:216-219.

Vasan RS, Larson MG, Benjamin EJ, et al. Congestive heart failure in Subjects with normal versus reduced left ventricular ejection fraction: Prevalence and mortality in population based cohort. J AM Coll Cardiol.1999;33:1948-1955.

Senni M, Triboulloy CM, Rodeheffer RJ, et al. Congestive heart failure in the community: a study of all incident cases in Olmsted county, Minnesota, in 1991.Circulation 1998;98:2282-2289.

Kitzman DW, Gardin JM, Gottdiener JS, et al., for Cardiovascular Health Study Research Group. Importance of heart failure with preserved systolic function in patients greater than 65years of age. Am J Cardiol.2001;87:413-419.

Lindenfeld J, Krause-Steinrauf H, Salenro J. Where are all the women with heart failure? J Am Coll Cardiol.1997; 30:1417-1419.

Ojji D, Parsonage W, Dooris M, Adebiyi A, Oladapo O, Adeleye J, Aje A, Ogah O, Adebayo A, Falase A, Atherton J. J Natl Med Assoc. 2008 Sep;100(9):1066-72

Jonathan P P, Liviu K, Mihai G, Robert O B. New Insights into Diastolic Heart Failure: Role of Diabetes Mellitus. Am J Med.2004; 116 (5A): 64S-75S.

Kannel WB, Hjortland M, Castelli W P. Role of diabetes in congestive Heart failure: the Framingham study. Am J Cardiol.1974; 34:29-34.

Parker AB, Yusuf S, Naylor CD. The relevance of sub-group-specific treatment effects: the studies of Left Ventricular Dysfunction (SOLVD) revisited. Am Heart J.2002; 144:941-947.

Arnold JM, Yusuf S, Young J, et al. Prevention of heart failure in patients in the Heart Outcomes Prevention Evaluation (HOPE Study. Circulation. 2003; 107:1284-1290.

Gottdiener JS, Arnold AM, Aurigemma GP, et al. Predictors of Congestive heart failure in the elderly: the Cardiovascular Health Study. J Am Coll Cardiol.2000; 35:1628-1637.

O'Connor CM, Gattis WA, Shaw L, et al. Clinical characteristics and long-term outcomes of patients with heart failure and preserved systolic function. Am J Cardiol.2000;86:863-867.

Raev DC. Which left ventricular function is impaired earlier in the evolution of diabetic cardiomyopathy? : an echocardiographic study of young type 1 diabetic patients. Diabetes Care.1994;17:633-639.

Liu JE, V,Robbins DC,Palmieri V,Bella JN,Roman MJ,et al.The impact of diabetes on left ventricular filling pattern in normotensive and hypertensive adults: the Strong Heart Study.J Am Coll Cardiol.2003; 41:2022-2028.

Poirier P, Bogaty P, Philippon F, Garneau C, Fortin C et al. Diastolic dysfunction in normotensive men with well-controlled type 2 diabetes:importance of manoeuvres in echocardiographic screening for preclinical diabetic cardiomyopathy. Diabetes Care.2001;24:5-10.

Fiorini G, Scotti LA, Parmigiani ML, Ferrari M, Pezzoli P et al. An echocardiographic study of left ventricular diastolic in patients with type2 diabetes mellitus. Cardiol 1995 Jan; 25(1):17-25.

Illan F, Valdes-Chavarri M, Tebar J, Garcia A, Pascual H et al. Anatomic and functional cardiac abnormalities. Clin Invest.1992 May;70(5):403-10.

Chiarella F, Viviani GL, Belloti P, Briata P, Domenicucci S et al. Left Ventricular Diastolic Function in Type1 Diabetes Mellitus.G Ital Cardiol 1986Jul; 16(7): 544.

Bertoni PD, Morandi G, Di Michele R, Canziani R et al. Altered diastolic function of the left ventricle in juvenile diabetes. G Ital Cardiol 1984 Nov; 14(11): 839-46.

Pitale SU, Abraira C, Emanuele NV, McCarren M, Hendreson WG et al. Two years intensive glycaemic control and left Ventricular function in the Veterans Affairs Co-operative study in type 2 diabetes mellitus. Diabetes Care 2000 Sep;23(9):1316-20.

Gough SC, Smyllie J,Barker M, Berkin KE, Rice PJ et al. Diastolic dysfunction is not related to changes in glycaemic control over 6 months in type 2 diabetes mellitus. A cross sectional study. Acta Diabetol 1995 Jun;32(2);110-5.

Felicio JS, Ferreira SR, Plavnik FL, Moises V, Kohlmann O et al. Effect of blood glucose on left ventricular mass in patients with hypertension and type2 diabetes mellitus. Hypertens 2000 Nov; 3(11): 1149-54.

Cecchi E, Pomari F, Brusasco G, Angelino P, Blatto A, et al. Preclinical left ventricular diastolic dysfunction in insulin dependent diabetes.G Ital Cardiol 1994 Jul;24(7):839-44.

Poirier P, Garneau C, Bogaty P, Nadeau A, Marois L et al. Preclinical diabetic cardiomyopathy: relation of Cardiovascular diastolic dysfunction to cardiac autonomic neuropathy in men with uncomplicated well-controlled type 2 diabetes. Metabolism 2003 Aug; 52(8): 1056-617.

Hardin N. The myocardial and vascular pathology of diabetic Cardiomyopathy. Coron. Artery Dis.1996; 7:99-108.

Young ME, McNulty P, Taegtmeyer H. Adaptation and mal-adaptation of the heart in diabetes. II. Potential mechanisms.Circulation.2002;105:1861-1870

Rodrigues B, Cam MC, McNeill JH. Metabolic disturbances in diabetic Cardiomyopathy. Mol Cell Biol Biochem.1998; 180:53-57

Rupp H, Elimban V, Dhalla NS. Modification of myosin isoenzymes and SR Ca (2+)-pump ATPase of the diabetic rat heart by lipid-lowering interventions. Mol Cell Biochem. 1994; 132:69-80.

Bristow MR. Why does the myocardium fail?:insights from basic Science.Lancet.1998; 352:S8 S14.

Depre C, Young ME, Ying J, et al. Streptozotocin-induced changes in Cardiac gene expression in the absence of severe contractile dysfunction. J Mol Cardiol.2000; 32;985-996.

Golfman L, Dixon IM, Takeda N, et al. Differential changes in cardiac Myofibrillar and sarcoplasmic reticular gene expression in alloxan-induced diabetes. Mol cell Biochem.1999; 200:15 25.

Flasheim CE, Grupp Il, Matlib MA. Mitochondrial dysfunction accompanies diastolic dysfunction in diabetic rat heart. Am J Physiol.1996; 271:H192-H202.

Bristow MR. Etomoxir: A new approach to treatment of chronic heart Failure. Lancet. 2000; 356:1621-1622.

Diamant M, Lamb HJ, Groeneveld Y, et al. Diastolic dysfunction is Associated with altered myocardial metabolism in asymptomatic normotensive patients with well-controlled type 2 diabetes mellitus. Am Coll Cardiol.2003; 42:328-335.

Bonito A. Doppler assessment of left ventricular systolic and diastolic function. In: Bonita A (ed).Echocardiography. The Normal Examination and Echocardiographic Measurements, Brisbane: Fergies, 2000;189-227

European Study Group on Diastolic Heart Failure.How to diagnose diastolic heart failure. Eur Heart J 1999;19:990-1003.

Zile MR. Diastolic heart failure: Diagnosis, mechanisms, and Treatment. Cardiology Rounds, 1999; 3(3): 1-6.

Mirsky I. Assessment of diastolic function: suggested methods and future considerations. Circulation 1984; 69:836-41.

Shah PM, Pai RM. Diastolic heart failure. Curr.Probl. Cardiol. 1992; 17:783-86.

Clarkson P, Wheeldon NM, Macdonald TM. Left ventricular diastolic dysfunction. QJM 1994; 87:143-148

Nishimura RA, Tajik AJ: Evaluation of diastolic filling of the left Ventricle in health and disease: Doppler echocardiography is the clinician's Rosetta stone. J Am Coll Cardiol 1997; 30:8-18.

Oh JL, Appleton CP, Hatle LK, Nishimura RA, Seward JB, Tajik AJ. The non-invasive assessment of left ventricular diastolic function with two-dimensional and Doppler echocardiography. J Am Soc echocard 1997; 10:246-270.

Appleton CP, Hatle LK, Popp RL. Relation of transmitral flow velocity Patterns to left ventricular diastolic function: new insights from a combined haemodynamic and Doppler echocardiography.J Am Coll Cardiol 1988;12:426-440.

Rakowski H, Appleton CP et al. Canadian Consensus Recommendation for the Measurement and Reporting of Diastolic Dysfunction by Echocardiography. J Am Soc Echocardiog.1996; 9:736-60.

Vasan RS, Levy D. Defining diastolic heart failure. A call for standardized diagnostic criteria. Circulation 2000;101:2118-2121

Packer M. Abnormalities of diastolic function as potential cause of exercise intolerance in chronic heart failure. Circulation 1990;81(111):78-86

Gilbert J, Glantz S. Determinants of left-ventricular filling and of the diastolic pressure-volume relation. Circ Res 1989; 64: 827-852

Bella JN, Palmieri V, Roman MJ. Prognostic significance of abnormal peak early to late diastolic filling ratio in middle-aged to elderly American Indians: The Strong Heart Study (abstr).JACC 2000;35:293A.

8

AF and Diabetes Prognosis and Predictors

Carlo Pappone, Francesca Zuffada and Vincenzo Santinelli
Department of Arrhythmology, Maria Cecilia Hospital, Cotignola, Ravenna, Italy

1. Introduction

Although approximately 10% of atrial fibrillation (AF) patients have no evident cardiac disorder (so-called "lone" AF), the arrhythmia usually occurs in patients with structural heart disease. Hypertension, coronary heart disease, valvular heart disease, dilated cardiomyopathy, and heart failure are the most frequent cardiovascular comorbidities associated with AF, but this arrhythmia is frequently found also in diabetic patients, with prevalence rates estimated to be at least double than among patients without diabetes (1). Comorbidities may induce atrial fibrosis and loss of myocardial tissue which have an apparent clear impact in facilitating AF by reducing the conduction velocity and possibly creating areas of conduction block. Fibrosis may be either a substrate for AF or a result of fibrillating atria and part of the so-called structural remodeling. Since atrial enlargement is often present in AF patients with or without comorbidities, it is difficult to establish if it represents the cause or the consequence of the arrhythmia. AF affects one in 25 adults aged 60 or over and nearly one in 10 adults aged 80 or over. Due to symptoms and the increased risk of ischemic stroke and death in elderly patients, AF is a source of considerable concern, and its impact is likely to increase as the number of individuals affected by AF rises nearly 2.5-fold during the next 50 years. The economic repercussions on national health systems around the world will be considerable. Like AF, diabetes mellitus is a global health problem with an estimated worldwide prevalence of 2.8% in 2000, which will increase to 4.4% in 2030 (2). At least 10.3 million Americans carry a diagnosis of diabetes mellitus. Another 5.4 million of people are estimated to have undiagnosed diabetes. Approximately 90% of patients with diabetes have the type 2 variety. The onset of type 2 diabetes usually precedes clinical diagnosis by several years. As a result, an increasing prevalence of type 2 diabetes cannot be divorced from the rising prevalence of atrial fibrillation in our society. Diabetic patients have at least twice the risk of vascular complications and cardiovascular death, compared with those without diabetes(3,4). Several epidemiological and pathological data have reported that diabetes is an independent predictor of cardiovascular disease (CVD) in both men and women. CVDs are considered as the cause of death in ≈65% of people with diabetes. To make matters worse, when patients with diabetes develop clinical CVD, they sustain a worse prognosis for survival than do CVD patients without diabetes. These observations suggest that it is imperative to promote coordinated efforts on behalf of cardiologistis, electrophysiologistis, neurologists, and primary-care providers to meet the increasing challenge of stroke and death prevention and rhythm management in the growing population of patients with atrial fibrillation and diabetes. Since among patients with AF type 2 diabetes is frequently associated with cardiovascular comorbidities including coronary artery disease, heart failure and hypertension (AF has been observed three times higher in patients with hypertension)(5) it is very difficult to evaluate its independent predictive value for arrhythmia progression, thromboembolic and cardiac adverse events including death (6,7). To assess whether diabetes further increases the already high risk among patients with AF and concomitant cardiovascular diseases, a prospective large number of patients with a long-term follow-up is required. We report here our long-term experience in a large and selected population of patients with paroxysmal AF in order to identify predictors of outcome, including AF progression, ischemic stroke and cardiovascular death.

2. Study population

Patients with history of documented paroxysmal AF with at least 2 or more episodes of symptomatic or asymptomatic AF lasting >1 hour were recruited for this 4-year prospective follow-up study. Exclusion and inclusion criteria are reported in Table 1. Patients with arrhythmia due to potentially reversible causes such as acute or recent (<6 months) myocardial infarction, recent cardiac surgery, New York Heart Association class III-IV heart failure, severe valvular heart disease requiring surgery, uncontrolled hypertension, acute pulmonary disease, WPW syndrome, a history of long-QT syndrome, Brugada syndrome, pericarditis, substance abuse, electrolyte imbalance, hyper or hypothyroidism were excluded. Patients with hepatic diseases, history of thromboembolism including stroke or TIA, contraindication to anticoagulation therapy, or any condition that would make survival for 1 year unlikely were also excluded. Patients scheduled to undergo catheter ablation or implantation of a pacemaker or defibrillator were also excluded. All participants had to have been on stable therapy for AF and any underlying cardiovascular disorders for at least 1 month before enrollment. Patients were allowed to continue all previously prescribed treatments for these conditions (including antiarrhythmic drugs, amiodarone, beta-blockers, and ACE inhibitors).

2.1 Follow-up

Serial control visits with ECG, 48-h Holter, echocardiography, and laboratory testing were scheduled at 1, 3, 6 months and thereafter once annually for 4 years. If a recurrence of AF was detected, the patient was asked to come in for an office visit to confirm the findings. Baseline evaluation included a past medical history of cardiovascular and endocrine disorders as well as a history of precipitating events. A complete blood count, urinalysis, thyroid-function tests, hepatic panel, lipid profile, and serum chemical measurements were obtained at baseline and at each control visit thereafter. Transesophageal echocardiography was performed at baseline to rule out atrial thrombi and annually. Recurrent episodes were pharmacologically managed by conventional ADT (propafenone, flecainide, and/or sotalol as first-line drugs in patients without structural heart disease or amiodarone as a single drug or in combination in patients with structural heart disease or in case of first-line drugs failure) according to AF management guidelines (8,9). Electrical cardioversion was performed if necessary or in patients with persistent AF refractory to ADT. Antithrombotic therapy with warfarin (INR between 2.0 and 3.0) was initially applied after stroke risk assessment according to the current AF guidelines recommendations (8,9). Patients with comorbidities or those with at least one moderate risk factor for thromboembolism regardless of AF clinical form were prescribed warfarin. Electrical cardioversion was performed for a maximum of 3 attempts. Patients with recurrent AF were followed monthly in an outpatient setting. The outcomes evaluated in this analysis were arrhythmia progression, cardiovascular mortality and major thromboembolic events.

Inclusion criteria:
Age between 18 and 85
Exclusion criteria:
Left ventricular ejection fraction <30%
NYHA functional class III-IV
Left atrial size >60mm
AF burden > 2 episodes/month
Uncorrected severe valvular heart disease
Contraindication to anticoagulation
Presence of left atrial thrombus
Patients scheduled to undergo catheter ablation or implantation of a pacemaker or defibrillator
Prior attempt at catheter or surgical ablation for atrial fibrillation
Recent (6 months) history of myocardial infarction
Cardiac surgery for congenital, valvular, aortic or coronary heart disease
History of cerebrovascular accidents
Pregnancy
Life expectancy less than 1 year
Significant comorbidities: cancer, end stage renal disease, severe obstructive lung disease, cirrhosis, etc
Inability or unwillingness to provide written informed consent

Table 1. Inclusion and Exclusion Criteria

2.2 Definitions

Paroxysmal AF was defined as recurrent AF that was self-terminating within 7 days. Persistent AF is defined as AF that was sustained beyond 7 days, or lasting less than 7 days but requiring pharmacologic or electrical cardioversion for termination. Ischemic stroke was defined as neurological deficit of sudden onset lasting >24 hours and caused by ischemia. Cardiovascular (CV) death was defined as death due to cardiovascular causes (myocardial infarction or heart failure).

3. Results

3.1 Study population

Among 5210 screened patients with paroxysmal AF, 1931 (mean age, 61.5 years, M, 47.2%) fulfilled inclusion and exclusion criteria and completed a 4-year follow-up period. Baseline clinical characteristics of the study population are shown in Table 1. Many patients had a history of hypertension with hypetensive heart disease (44.8%) or coronary artery disease (31.6%). A total of 9.5% of patients had recent heart failure and 8.8% had valvular heart disease often with mitral valve disease. Type 2 diabetes mellitus was present in 13.9% of patients and in many of them (85 patients) diabetes was of long duration (median duration 15 years) and poor controlled with oral antidiabetic therapy as assessed by glycosylated hemoglobin (median 8%)). AF burden was 2.05±0.2 (episodes/month). At the time of enrollment, 35% of the patients were receiving amiodarone alone or in combination, 25.2% were receiving beta-blockers or sotalol, 20% were receiving ACE inhibitors, and only 20% of them were receiving chronic anticoagulant therapy with warfarin. Class I antiarrhythmic agents were prescribed in 30% of patients. Adverse drug reactions occurred in 115 patients during class I antiarrhythmic drugs (75 patients), amiodarone alone (30 patients) or in combination (10 patients). No serious complications developed and long-term antiarrhythmic drug therapy was not permanently discontinued in any patient.

3.2 Atrial fibrillation progression

At 4 years, 1452 patients had had at least a recurrence of AF , 183 patients remained in stable sinus rhythm on antiarrhythic drug therapy and the remaining 276 patients had progressed to persistent AF despite conventional ADT alone or in combination. Intensive Holter recordings revealed that in 68/183 patients, of whom 50 with diabetes mellitus, AF progression was silent. The baseline characteristics of patients with and without AF progression were compared for demographics at study entry (Table 2). Patients who progressed were older and had more comorbidities including type 2 diabetes and higher baseline AF burden than those who did not. On the baseline echocardiogram, patients with AF progression had larger left atrial diameters. The median interval between the onset of recurrent paroxysmal and persistent AF was 33.5 months (range 5-38). Patients who progressed received more frequently drugs associated with heart failure (ACE inhibitors and/or diuretics) and many of them had oral anticoagultion therapy with warfarin. Electrical cardioversion was more frequently used before and after progression but the arrhythmia recurred 32±18 days after electrical cardioversion requiring multiple hospitalizations.

3.3 Complications

Cardiovascular events. During a median follow-up of 35 months, 84 patients died due to cardiovascular causes (Table 2) with a cumulative 4-year cardiovascular mortality rate of 4.3%. All patients were older than 65 years of age and all had comorbidities including heart failure, diabetes, coronary artery disease and hypertensive cardiomyopathy alone or in combination. Arrhythmia progression occurred in 49/84 (58.3%) before death which was commonly due to worsening of heart failure or acute heart failure (55 patients) secondary to inadequate control of the ventricular rate at the time of recurrent episodes of persistent arrhythmia at rapid ventricular rate (115 ±15 bpm) or hypertensive crises with pulmonary edema (29 patients). All patients at the time of death were on amiodarone therapy and warfarin. *Thromboembolic events.* During a median follow-up of 25 months, thromboembolism developed in 140 patients (Table 2) with a 4-year cumulative stroke rate of 7.3%. Arrhythmia progression occurred in 58/140 (41.4%) before thromboembolic events. All patients at the time of thromboembolism were on warfarin but subtherapeutic doses were found in many of them (40%).

Variables	All Patients (n=1931)	No AF Progression (n=1655)	AF Progression (n=276)	p-value
Male sex, n (%)	911(47.2)	1095(66.1)	165 (59.7)	0.024
Age, (years)	61.5±7.4	61.2±7.4	62.4±7.2	0.021
Hypertension, n (%)	865 (44.8)	718 (43.8)	147 (53.2)	0.001
Heart Failure, n (%)	184 (9.5)	119 (7.1)	65 (23.5)	<0.001
Diabetes mellitus, n (%)	270 (13.9)	188 (11.3)	82 (29.7)	<0.001
Valvular disease, n (%)	171 (8.8)	141 (8.5)	35 (12.6)	0.020
Coronary artery disease	611 (31.6)	514 (31)	93 (33.6)	0.382
LA diameter, (mm)	42±3.3	41.5±3.2	42.8±3.4	<0.001
LV EF, (%)	54±5.3	54±5.0	51±6.5	<0.001
AF burden, (episodes/month)	2.2 ±0.5	2.2±0.4	2.4 ±0.7	<0.001
AF duration, (months)	50.4±7.3	53±3.5	58±4.6	<0.001
Thromboembolism, n (%)	140 (7.2)	82 (4.9)	58 (21)	<0.001
CV Death, n (%)	84 (4.3)	36 (2.1)	48 (17.3)	<0.001

Table 2. Baseline characteristics of patients with paroxysmal AF

3.4 Risk factors of progression, thromboembolic events and death

Multivariate analysis demonstrated that many comorbidities including diabetes mellitus, heart failure, and coronary artery disease were common predictors of arrhythmia progression as well as of thromboembolic events and death (Tables 3-5). In addition, low ejection fraction, left atrial enlargment, female gender, and older age also predicted all adverse events. AF burden was a strong predictor of arrhythmia progression but did not predict thromboembolic events/death. Diabetes and heart failure were the strongest predictors of all events. (Tables 3-5).

Covariates	Regression Coefficient	p-value	Adjusted HR	95% CI	
AF burden	0.545	<0.001	1.724	1.449	2.051
Ejection fraction	-0.070	<0.001	0.933	0.912	0.954
Sex	0.335	0.031	1.398	1.032	1.894
Age	0.043	0.001	1.044	1.018	1.070
Coronary artery disease	0.328	0.015	1.388	1.067	1.806
Heart failure	0.674	<0.001	1.963	1.412	2.728
Diabetes mellitus	0.568	<0.001	1.765	1.301	2.396
Left atrial diameter	0.050	0.007	1.051	1.013	1.090
Valvular disease	0.537	0.004	1.712	1.191	2.460

Table 3. Multivariate Cox analysis for AF progression

4. Discussion

This is the largest prospective long-term study which provides additional data on predictors of arrhythmia progression and prognosis among a selected population with paroxysmal AF which represents the vast majority of patients with paroxysmal AF commonly seen in clinical practice. The long-term results while confirming the role of associated comorbidities to predict AF progression, clearly demonstrate that type 2 diabetes is one of the strongest predictor of both arrhythmia progression and prognosis. AF burden of at least 2 episodes/month was a strong predictor of arrhythmia progression but this arrhythmia burden, unlike diabetes and cardiovascular comorbidities did not predict stroke and death. AF progression was discrete and at 4 years occurred only in a minority of patients (14.3%), most of whom with advancing age and comorbidities.

Covariates	Regression Coefficient	p-value	Adjusted HR	95% CI	
Ejection fraction	-0.043	0.005	0.958	0.930	0.987
Sex	0.696	0.004	2.005	1.256	3.202
Age	0.120	<0.001	1.128	1.082	1.176
Coronary artery disease	1.345	<0.001	3.839	2.207	6.678
Heart failure	1.407	<0.001	4.085	2.533	6.587
Diabetes mellitus	1.705	<0.001	5.500	3.208	9.431
Left atrial diameter	0.102	<0.001	1.108	1.056	1.162

Table 4. Multivariate Cox analysis for thromboembolism

Covariates	Regression Coefficient	p-value	Adjusted HR	95% CI	
Ejection fraction	-0.066	<0.001	0.936	0.904	0.970
Sex	1.576	<0.001	4.836	2.017	11.594
Age	0.057	0.054	1.059	0.999	1.121
Coronary artery disease	0.741	0.051	2.097	0.996	4.417
Heart failure	2.557	<0.001	12.891	4.977	33.387
Diabetes mellitus	1.628	<0.001	5,092	2,233	11.615
Left atrial diameter	0.059	0.065	1.061	0.996	1.130

Table 5. Multivariate Cox analysis for cardiovascular death

4.1 Predictors of AF progression, ischemic stroke and death

Risk factors for the transition from paroxysmal to persistent forms of AF may be similar to those predisponing to incident AF, but there are very limited data on their identification for secondary prevention in order to reduce arrhythmia progression and associated complications such as thromboembolic events or death. Patients with AF have a substantial risk of stroke, which is modified by the presence or absence of several risk factors. These risk factors have been used to develop thromboembolic risk stratification schemes, which have arbitrarily divided the risk into low, intermediate, and high risk strata. Multivariate pooled analysis demonstrated that cardiovascular comorbidities and diabetes were independently predictive of arrhythmia progression as well as of stroke and CV death while baseline AF burden of 2 episodes/month was a strong predictor of arrhythmia progression, but at 4 years was not sufficient to predict serious adverse events and death. Our data also demonstrate that advancing age, female gender and the presence of coronary artery disease are independently predictive of adverse events including death. These findings suggest that in patients with paroxysmal AF thromboembolic risk stratification schemes using these risk factors are useful. Therefore, potential additional risk factors listed in the 2006 ACC/AHA/ESC guidelines (8) as "less validated or weaker risk factors" including female gender, age 65-74 years, and coronary artery disease should be instead considered as independent strong risk factors. Many of these variables have been expressed in the CHA2DS2-VASc (Congestive heart failure, Hypertension, Age>75 years, Diabetes mellitus, previous Stroke/transient ischemic attack, Vascular disease, Age 65-74 years, Sex category,) score, which has been proposed to complement the CHADS2 score.

4.2 Silent progression of AF

In the present study, AF progression from paroxysmal to persistent AF was silent in many patients as documented by the intensive Holter monitoring. Of note, about a half of patients with AF progression had diabetes mellitus. These findings are important in terms of pathophysiology and therapy suggesting that oral anticoagulation therapy with warfarin in patients at high risk should be frequently and constantly monitored to avoid subtherapeutic intensity (INR below 2.0) regardless of the presence of symptoms. In the absence of an accurate arrhythmia monitoring by intermittent ECG recordings, asymptomatic transition to more persistent forms, particularly in diabetic patients, may be undetected increasing the risk of theromboembolic and cardiovascular complications.

4.3 Comparison with previous studies

The results of the present study extend the results of previous studies on AF progression from paroxysmal to persistent AF (10-14). In the CARAF (Canadian Registry of Atrial Fibrillation Study) study, underlying heart disease and age were reported as independent factors of AF progression (10). Nieuwlaat et al reported univariate analysis of AF progression in the Euro Heart Survey (EHS), but independent risk factors were not analyzed (11). De Vos et al (12) have recently reported interesting data on the clinical correlates of AF progression and prognosis in the patients enrolled in the Euro Heart Survey of AF (13). In agreement with our data but during a much shorter follow-up period (only 1 year), progression to persistent AF occurred in 15% of Euro Heart Survey patients. Based on these data, the Authors have suggested a new risk stratification score (HATCH) to identify patients prone to arrhythmia progression. Recently, we have reported AF progression in 106 patients with first of whom 52 with comorbidities AF and diabetes was a strong predictor of arrhythmia progression (14). The present study reports additional data among a large patient population with paroxysmal AF. A predefined baseline AF burden before enrollment was purposively included to enhance the clinical applicability of the results and, unlike the study by de Vos et al (12), patients with AF who required pharmacological cardioversion for restoration of sinus rhythm were considered as persistent AF patients and then were excluded. The results at 4 years while confirming the independent role of many cardiovascular comorbidities as predictors of AF progression, for the first time show type 2 diabetes mellitus as a strong independent predictor of AF progression, thromboembolism and cardiovascular death. In the analysis of de Vos and colleagues (12), diabetes also occurred more frequently in patients who progressed as compared with those who did not (19% vs 14%), but no significant differences were found and this may be due to several reasons including a shorter follow-up, misclassification of paroxysmal AF in many patients and a less accurate rhythm monitoring. Analysis of AF progression and predictors of prognosis requires a well defined AF burden prior to enrollment which should not be based on the patients'reported history alone as it may be unreliable. Previous trials frequently have been based exclusively on electrocardiography performed at scheduled visits or on the patient's report of symptoms which may explain why different rates of progression and predictors have been reported. Recently, the results of the ADVANCE study suggested that AF in diabetic patients should be regarded as a marker of adverse outcome and prompt aggressive management of all risk factors (15). Although it seems to be conceivable that many comorbidities including type 2 diabetes should be independent predictors of stroke and mortality in patients with nonvalvular atrial fibrillation, available data do not provide strong support. The results of the present study demonstrate that type 2 diabetes as well as cardiovascular comorbidities are independently predictors of thromboembolism and cardiovascular death. We believe that patients with paroxysmal AF without prior stroke with at least one risk factor such as advancing age, underlying heart or metabolic disease and a well defined baseline arrhythmia burden, as those enrolled in the present study, indeed represent the vast majority of patients with AF commonly seen in real life clinical practice. Large clinical studies require years for completion, but they are required to determine the impact of several risk factors on mortality and other long-term outcomes. In our experience, older patients, particularly females with cardiovascular comorbidity and diabetes mellitus are at highest risk of adverse outcomes and require chronic anticoagulation therapy with warfarin.

5. Conclusions

Our experience provides new evidence on characteristics and outcome among a large cohort of selected patients with paroxysmal AF with a minimal use of anticoagulation treatment. These data, while confirming the role of many cardiovascular comorbidities in predicting adverse outcomes, demonstrate that diabetes mellitus is an independent strong predictor of AF progression, stroke and CV death. AF progression in diabetics may be frequently silent which may result in higher risk of adverse outcome.

6. References

[1] Movahed MR, Hashemzadeh M, Jamal MM. Diabetes mellitus is a strong, independent risk for atrial fibrillation and flutter in addition to other cardiovascular disease. Int J Cardiol 2005;105:315–318.

[2] Wild S, Roglic G, Green A, Sicree R, King H. Global prevalence of diabetes; estimates for year 2000 and projections for 2030. Diabetes Care 2004;21:1047–1053.

[3] Asia Pacific Cohort Studies Collaboration. The effects of diabetes on the risks of major cardiovascular diseases and death in the Asia-Pacific region. The Asia Pacific Cohort Studies Collaboration. Diabetes Care 2003;26:360–366.

[4] Huxley R, Barzi F, Woodward M. Excess risk of fatal coronary heart disease associated with diabetes in men and women: meta-analysis of 37 prospective cohort studies. BMJ 2006;332:73–78.

[5] Ostgren CJ, Merlo J, Ra°stam L, Lindblad U. Atrial fibrillation and its association with type 2 diabetes and hypertension in a Swedish community.Diabetes Obes Metab 2004;6:367–374.

[6] Kannel WB, Abbott RD, Savage DD, McNamara PM. Epidemiologic features of chronic atrial fibrillation: the Framingham study. N Engl J Med 1982;306: 1018–1022.

[7] Friberg J, Scharling H, Gadsbøll N, Truelsen T, Jensen GB, Copenhagen City Heart Study. Comparison of the impact of atrial fibrillation on the risk of stroke and cardiovascular death in women versus men (The Copenhagen City Heart Study). Am J Cardiol 2004;94:889–894

[8] Fuster V, Ryden LE, Cannom DS, et al. ACC/AHA/ESC 2006 guidelines for the management of patients with atrial fibrillation-executive summary: a report of the American College of Cardiology/American Heart Association Task Force on Practice Guidelines and the European Society of Cardiology Committee for Practice Guidelines (Writing Committee to Revise the 2001 Guidelines for the Management of Patients With Atrial Fibrillation). J Am Coll Cardiol 2006;48:854 –906.

[9] Fuster V, Rydén LE, Cannom DS, Crijns HJ, Curtis AB, Ellenbogen KA, Halperin JL, Kay GN, Le Huezey JY, Lowe JE, Olsson SB, Prystowsky EN, Tamargo JL, Wann LS. 2011 ACCF/AHA/HRS Focused Updates Incorporated Into the ACC/AHA/ESC 2006 Guidelines for the Management of Patients with Atrial Fibrillation: a report of the American College of Cardiology Foundation/American Heart Association Task Force on Practice Guidelines Developed in partnership with the European Society of Cardiology and in collaboration with the European Heart Rhythm Association and the Heart Rhythm Society. J Am Coll Cardiol. 2011;57:e101-98

[10] Kerr CR, Humphries KH, Talajic M, Klein GJ, Connolly SJ, Green M, Boone J, Sheldon R, Dorian P, Newman D. Progression to chronic atrial fibrillation after the initial diagnosis of paroxysmal atrial fibrillation: results from the Canadian Registry of Atrial Fibrillation. Am Heart J. 2005;149:489-96.

[11] Nieuwlaat R, Prins MH, Le Heuzey JY, Vardas PE, Aliot E, Santini M, Cobbe SM, Widdershoven JW, Baur LH, Lévy S, Crijns HJ. Prognosis, disease progression, and treatment of atrial fibrillation patients during 1 year: follow-up of the Euro Heart Survey on atrial fibrillation. Eur Heart J. 2008;29:1181-9.

[12] De Vos CB, Pisters R, Nieuwlaat R, Prins MH, Tieleman RG, Coelen RJ, van den Heijkant AC, Allessie MA, Crijns HJ. Progression from paroxysmal to persistent atrial fibrillation clinical correlates and prognosis. J Am Coll Cardiol. 2010;55:725-31.

[13] Nieuwlaat R, Capucci A, Camm AJ, Olsson SB, Andresen D, Davies DW, Cobbe S, Breithardt G, Le Heuzey JY, Prins MH, Lévy S, Crijns HJ; Atrial fibrillation management: a prospective survey in ESC member countries: the Euro Heart Survey on Atrial Fibrillation. Eur Heart J. 2005;26:2422-34.

[14] Pappone C, Radinovic A, Manguso F, Vicedomini G, Ciconte G, Sacchi S, Mazzone P, Paglino G, Gulletta S, Sala S, Santinelli V. Atrial fibrillation progression and management: A 5-year prospective follow-up study. Heart Rhythm 2008;5:1501-7.

[15] Du X, Ninomiya T, de Galan B, Abadir E, Chalmers J, Pillai A, Woodward M, Cooper M, Harrap S, Hamet P, Poulter N, Lip GY, Patel A. Risks of cardiovascular events and effects of routine blood pressure lowering among patients with type 2 diabetes and atrial fibrillation: results of the ADVANCE study. Eur Heart J. 2009;30:1128-35.

9

Detection of Silent Ischemia in Patients with Type 2 Diabetes

Babes Elena Emilia and Babes Victor Vlad
University Oradea, Faculty of Medicine and Pharmacy
Romania

1. Introduction

The prevalence of diabetes mellitus has reached epidemic proportions and constitutes a major public health problem. Diabetes mellitus affects an estimated 171 million people worldwide in 2000 and this number is projected to double to 366 million by 2030 (Wild et al., 2004). Silent myocardial ischemia is common in diabetic patients and may delay or mask the diagnosis of coronary artery disease, particularly in its early stages.

2. Diabetes, a coronary artery disease risk equivalent

Coronary artery disease is the leading cause of morbidity and mortality in individuals with type 2 diabetes mellitus. Coronary artery disease is more severe, more prevalent and occurs at younger age in patients with type 2 diabetes mellitus. Using a range of diagnostic methods, the overall prevalence of coronary artery disease is reported to be as high as 55% in patients with diabetes, compared with 2% to 4% in the general population (Hammoud et al., 2000). In an asymptomatic and uncomplicated cohort of type 2 diabetic patients, 46, 3% had evidence of coronary calcification indicative of coronary atherosclerosis (Anand et al., 2006). In an autopsy study of diabetic patients the prevalence of anatomic coronary artery disease was 50% to 81% (Goraya et al., 2002)
An estimated 80% of diabetic patients die from cardiovascular disease, 75% of which is attributed to coronary artery disease (American Diabetes Association, 1998). In general diabetic patients have more extensive atherosclerosis with a higher prevalence of multivessel coronary artery disease, frequent silent myocardial ischemia and infarction with a higher cardiac event rate when compared with non-diabetic patients (Goraya et. al, 2002; Nesto et al., 1998; Stamler et al., 1993). Patients with diabetes without previous myocardial infarction or cardiovascular disease have been shown to have a similar prognosis as persons without diabetes but with prior myocardial infarction or cardiovascular disease (Haffner et al., 1998). Based on these data, diabetes is considered a coronary artery disease risk-equivalent according to current Framingham Risk Score Adult Treatment Program III guidelines and secondary prevention of coronary artery disease is recommended for all adult diabetic patients
(http://www.nhlbi.nih.gov/giudelines/cholesterol/atp3_rpt.htm).

3. Silent ischemia - prevalence and prognosis in diabetic patients

Silent ischemia is a common, under-recognized condition that is associated with an adverse prognosis. It is a marker of a significant underlying coronary artery disease and therefore of future cardiovascular events. Myocardial ischemia is often asymptomatic in patients with diabetes mellitus and coronary artery disease is frequently in an advanced stage when it becomes clinically manifest.

A number of studies have confirmed the presence of silent ischemia in diabetic patients. The reported prevalence of myocardial ischemia varied between studies from 6% to 59% (MiSAD group, 1997; Miller et al, 2004; Rajagopalan et al., 2005; Zellweger et al., 2004; Wackers et al., 2004; Scognamiglio et al., 2006). This variation is probably related to differences in patient selection, stress methodology and imaging techniques. Autopsy studies have identified a high prevalence of coronary atherosclerosis in patients with diabetes, even among those without clinical coronary heart disease. Almost 75% of diabetic decedents without clinical coronary artery disease have high grade coronary atherosclerosis (Goraya et al., 2002).

The importance of identifying silent ischemia is highlighted by the poor outcomes associated with silent ischemia in patients with type 2 diabetes. Silent ischemia was significantly related to future coronary events in asymptomatic diabetic patients after 2, 8 years (risk ratio: 21) (Rutter et al., 1999). Similarly, 5-year follow-up of the MISAD (Milan Study on Atherosclerosis and Diabetes) cohort showed that abnormal baseline scintigraphy was associated with fivefold increase in fatal and nonfatal cardiac events (risk ratio: 5,47) (Faglia et al., 2002). Diabetic patients with inducible ischemia on stress myocardial perfusion imaging using single-photon emission computed tomography (SPECT) have a significantly higher annual cardiac death or myocardial infarction rate than nondiabetic patients with ischemia (10% vs. 8%)(Shaw & Iskandrian, 2004). In one study of female diabetic patients with high-risk stress SPECT perfusion scan characterized by a multivessel disease pattern only 60% survived without infarction in the next 3 years. For male diabetic patients with high-risk scan this value was 79% (Giri et al., 2002). Similarly diabetic patients with abnormal stress echocardiography have a worse prognosis that non-diabetic patients (Cortigiani et al., 2006). Diabetic patients with coronary atherosclerosis as determined by computed tomography calcium scanning have a worse outcome regarding cardiac death and nonfatal infarction that non-diabetic patients with the same coronary artery calcium score (Raggi et al., 2004). Compared with nondiabetic patients diabetic patients with zero coronary artery calcium score had a similar annual mortality rate of 0, 36%. It seems that 48% of diabetic patients had coronary artery calcium score compatible with significant coronary artery disease (Khaleeli et al., 2001).

The exact reason for the poor prognosis associate with silent ischemia is unclear. Silent ischemia confirms the presence of significant coronary artery disease and therefore this population is more at risk for future coronary events. Also repeat episodes of silent ischemia could lead to progressive fibrosis which can progress to left ventricular systolic dysfunction or life threatening arrhythmias. Myocardial biopsies from hypokinetic territories supplied by stenosed coronary arteries have shown areas of fibrosis and myocite death in the absence of infarction (Schaper, 1988).

4. Diagnostic of silent ischemia, which test should be used in which diabetic patient

There are numerous non-invasive test available for myocardial ischemia detection: exercise stress test, Holter ECG monitoring, stress myocardial perfusion imaging, stress echocardiography and other non-invasive techniques can detect the atherosclerotic disease: as carotid-intimae-media thickness evaluation via high resolution ultrasound or coronary artery calcium scoring via computed tomography or computed tomography coronary angiography. It is unclear if for screening the detection of early markers of coronary artery disease is preferred over the actual visualisation of myocardial ischemia.

4.1 Exercise stress test

Exercise stress test is the most widely available, inexpensive and commonly used test used to detect coronary artery disease. It has been well validated in the general population and it can be used as the first diagnostic test for patients with an intermediate risk of having coronary artery disease. Given the differences in presentation of coronary artery disease within the diabetic population and the high incidence of silent myocardial ischemia, various groups have attempted to evaluate whether exercise ECG has similar accuracy in a diabetic population. Few data exist regarding the relationship between exercise ECG test results and coronary artery disease risk in persons with type 2 diabetes mellitus and most studies have involved small samples.

In a prospective study (Blandine et al., 1999) 203 diabetic patients without angina and with normal resting ECG were screened with exercise ECG test (stress nuclear imaging was used if exercise ECG was contraindicate or inconclusive). Sixteen percent had abnormal stress test whereas 9% had silent coronary artery disease as defined by angiography. In a study (Bacci et al., 2002) which evaluated 206 higher risk asymptomatic type 2 diabetes patients with peripheral arterial disease and at least 2 cardiovascular risk factors, 19% had an abnormal test and the positive predictive accuracy of the exercise ECG was 79%. These studies collectively support the notion that among higher-risk cohorts of asymptomatic patients with type 2 diabetes nearly 1/3 may have unrecognized coronary artery disease and exercise ECG may be useful in identifying these patients. In an evaluation of the correlation between the ECG exercise stress test and coronary angiography in 59 diabetic patients the sensitivity and specificity were 75% and 77% (Paillole et al., 1995). The mean positive predictive value of exercise ECG for predicting angiographic coronary disease varies between 70 and 90% (Bacci et al., 2002; Blandine et al., 1999).

Regarding the prognostic value of exercise stress test a study on 68 asymptomatic male veterans (Rubler et al., 1987) with diabetes mellitus found that exercise ECG testing had 50% sensitivity and 83% specificity for predicting subsequent cardiac events over an average of 41 months of follow-up. In the Milan study on Atherosclerosis and Diabetes (Faglia et al., 2002) 735 asymptomatic diabetic patients were screened for coronary artery disease and followed-up for 5 years. In all patients exercise ECG was performed with a positive test prompting stress nuclear testing. Among the subjects with normal exercise ECG test the incidence of cardiac events was significantly lower compared to those with abnormal stress testing ($p<0, 0001$). These data suggest that asymptomatic patients with uncomplicated type 2 diabetes who have a negative exercise ECG test have a lower cardiac event rate and relatively favourable prognosis.

In diabetic patients the value of exercise ECG testing is limited because its low sensitivity requires a workload that is difficult to achieve owing to comorbidities such as peripheral neuropathy, peripheral arterial diseases, poor physical fitness and obesity. The specificity of exercise testing is limited and false positive results are common in patients without angina. Furthermore the specificity is lower in diabetes because of the presence of microvascular disease (Bacci et al., 2002). Exercise ECG has moderate sensitivity and specificity for detection of coronary artery disease. During intermediate follow up exercise ECG has been shown to have a good predictive value for coronary events. It can identify a subgroup of asymptomatic diabetic patients who have significant coronary artery disease as defined by angiography and in lower risk diabetic cohorts it may offer short term prognostic reassurance to those asymptomatic patients with negative test. Parameters including exercise capacity and heart rate recovery offer significant information particularly in diabetic patients who may not experience angina during exercise and who may have increased autonomic dysfunction (Albers et al., 2006). Application of exercise ECG as a screening tool in type 2 diabetes is limited as the test is often inconclusive (Djaberi et al., 2008).

4.2 Holter ECG monitoring

The prevalence of silent myocardial ischemia as assessed by Holter ECG monitoring varies between 35% and 58% (Chiariello et al., 1985; Aronow et al., 1992). Comparison between diabetic patients and nondiabetic individuals in Asymptomatic Cardiac Ischemia Pilot (ACIP) study showed that despite more extensive and diffuse coronary disease, diabetic ACIP patients tended to have less measurable ischemia during the 48-hour ambulatory ECG (Caracciolo et al, 1996). Comparing exercise ECG and ambulatory ECG for detection of silent ischemia in diabetes a study revealed that ambulatory ECG identified ischemia only in diabetics with three vessel disease but exercise ECG also revealed ischemia in one or two vessel disease (Ahluwalia et al., 1995). Regarding the prognostic value, in one study patients with silent ischemia detected on ambulatory ECG had a higher incidence of new coronary events (87%) than those without silent ischemia (51%) during 40 month follow-up period (Aronow et al., 1992). Further studies are necessary to evaluate the prognostic value of silent ischemia detected by ambulatory ECG.

In conclusion the diagnostic value of ambulatory ECG for coronary heart disease is poor. The predictive value of ischemia detected by ambulatory ECG has not been extensively evaluated (Djaberi et al., 2008).

4.3 Stress echocardiography

Stress echocardiography imaging provides improved sensitivity and specificity compared with exercise ECG testing. There are limited data regarding the utility of stress echocardiography in patients with diabetes particularly in those who are asymptomatic. In a study, 52 patients with diabetes were referred for cardiac assessment using dobutamine stress echocardiography (Hennessy et al., 1997). Sensitivity, specificity and positive and negative predictive values of dobutamine stress echocardiography for coronary artery disease detection were 82%, 54%, 84% and 50% respectively. Although the study was limited by the small size of the cohort it demonstrated similar diagnostic accuracy for dobutamine stress echocardiography in a diabetic population as in the general population. In another study on 55 diabetics who underwent dobutamine stress echocardiography and angiography the sensitivity and specificity of stress echocardiography were 81% and 85% (Elhendy et al., 1998). The efficacy of dobutamine stress echocardiography was compared to exercise ECG testing and SPECT nuclear perfusion imaging in 56 asymptomatic diabetic patients with three additional cardiovascular risk factors but normal resting ECG. Participants underwent all forms of noninvasive stress testing but coronary angiography was only performed if at least one test was abnormal (47%), which precluded the measurement of diagnostic sensitivity and specificity. Positive predictive value was 69% for dobutamine stress echocardiography, 60% for exercise ECG and 75% for thallium SPECT (Penfornis et al., 2001).

A study was performed on 1899 asymptomatic diabetic patients which underwent dipyridamole myocardial contrast echocardiography and in those with myocardial perfusion defects the anatomy of coronary vessels was analyzed by coronary angiography (Scognamiglio et al., 2006). Patients were divided in two groups according to the number of risk factors for coronary artery disease. In the two study groups the prevalence of abnormal myocardial contrast echocardiography (59 vs. 60%) and of significant coronary artery disease (64, 6% vs. 65, 5%) was similar irrespective of risk profile. The criteria of ≥ 2 risk factors did not help to identify asymptomatic patients with a higher prevalence of coronary artery disease and is only related to a more severe coronary artery disease with unfavourable coronary anatomy. The findings of this study suggest that a substantial number of asymptomatic diabetic patients have myocardial perfusion defects and significant coronary artery disease independent of risk factor profile. As a consequence a large number of asymptomatic diabetic patients with few risk factors might have occult coronary artery disease and might be missed on the basis of 1998 American diabetes association guidelines (ADA, 1998).

Several studies have evaluated the prognostic value of stress echocardiography among diabetic patients. In a prospective study stress echocardiography plus an exercise ECG were used to screen 71 diabetic patients with unknown asymptomatic cardiac disease and two or more cardiovascular risk factors. Those who obtained an abnormal result in one test underwent coronary angiography and if necessary revascularization. Compared with patients randomised to the control arm (n=70) coronary events were significantly reduced in the screening arm during follow-up (Faglia et al, 2005). The preclinical diagnosis of coronary artery disease by stress echocardiography may therefore be effective. However more studies are needed to determine the prognostic role of stress echocardiography in screening for cardiac disease in asymptomatic diabetic patients.

Stress echocardiographic imaging provides improved sensitivity and specificity compared with exercise ECG testing. Increasing data are available to support both its diagnostic accuracy and its prognostic role. The presence of resting left ventricular systolic dysfunction and stress induced wall motion abnormalities provides incremental prognostic information to clinical and exercise parameters in multiple studies. Patients referred for pharmacological stress echocardiography demonstrate a higher risk for cardiovascular events than those referred for exercise testing which likely reflects more severe underlying cardiovascular disease and comorbidities. Diabetic patients with normal stress echocardiography appear to have a greater risk for subsequent cardiovascular events than non-diabetic patients, particularly beyond 2 years. The sensitivity and specificity of stress echocardiography for diagnosing extensive coronary artery disease are satisfactory. However the predictive value of a positive test in type 2 diabetes needs to be further analysed (Djaberi et al., 2008).

4.4 Nuclear single photon emission computed tomography (SPECT) myocardial perfusion imaging

Nuclear SPECT myocardial perfusion imaging has been employed in several series to test the prevalence of silent ischemia or to analyse the prognostic impact of perfusion abnormalities in diabetes. It is known that perfusion abnormalities precede abnormalities in systolic function in the ischaemic cascade (Nesto & Kowalchuk, 1987). Accordingly comparisons between myocardial perfusion imaging and stress echocardiography have shown a higher sensitivity for myocardial perfusion imaging for the detection of multi-vessel and single-vessel coronary artery disease (Schinkel et al., 2003).

In asymptomatic diabetic patients the rate of silent myocardial ischemia diagnosed by stress myocardial perfusion imaging ranges from 6 to 59% (Zellweger et al., 2004; Faglia et al., 2002; , De Lorenzo et al., 2002; Wackers et al., 2004; Rajagapolan et al., 2005; Vanzetto et al., 1999; Cosson et al., 2004). This wide range in the prevalence of silent ischemia is related to differences in patient selection, stress methodology and imaging techniques. In retrospective data base analyses of patients with diabetes referred for stress testing a high prevalence (41-58%) of abnormal stress myocardial perfusion imaging and a high cardiac event rate were found (Giri et al., 2002; Kang et al., 1999; Rajagapolan et al., 2005). A retrospective analysis performed by on 1427 diabetic patients referred for myocardial perfusion imaging reported an abnormal in 58% and high risk scan in 18% of subjects (Rajagopalan et al., 2005). Sixty-one percent of patients with high risk results had angiographically high risk coronary artery disease. According to SPECT imaging scans patients were categorized as being at high, intermediate or low risk with significant difference regarding annual mortality rate($p<0,001$) between groups. It is likely that these patients were referred for stress testing because of typical or atypical symptoms and/or perceived clinical high risk.

The retrospective database analyses of known asymptomatic patients with diabetes referred for stress testing showed a lower prevalence of abnormal stress myocardial perfusion imaging and cardiac event rate (Zellweger et al., 2004; Miller et al., 2004; De Lorenzo et al., 2002, Prior et al., 2005). These patients may not be representative of asymptomatic patients with diabetes in the larger population because they were referred for stress myocardial perfusion imaging for example before noncardiac surgery. The mean prevalence of ischemia ranged from 26-39% although Miller et al. reported abnormal myocardial perfusion imaging in 59% asymptomatic patients. But in the study performed by Miller et al. higher risk population was studied including patients with antianginal medication and ECG abnormalities (Q waves, ST-T changes). Because of the retrospective nature of these two types of studies the true prevalence of silent ischemia is uncertain. In general a higher percentage of perfusion defects have been detected in retrospective studies.

Several prospective studies showed lower prevalence of silent coronary artery disease ranging from 6 to 22%. There were important differences in design and stress testing methodology. In the Milan study on Atherosclerosis and Diabetes (MiSAD) asymptomatic patients with diabetes were first screened with exercise stress test and only if this test was abnormal stress myocardial perfusion imaging was performed. It is possible that because the low sensitivity of exercise ECG the overall observed prevalence of silent coronary artery disease was low 6% (Faglia et al., 2002). In DIAD (Detection of Ischemia in Asymptomatic Diabetics) a large prospective study, 1124 type 2 diabetic asymptomatic patients were enrolled. Half of the patients were randomized to an adenosine Tc 99 m sestamibi myocardial perfusion imaging and half were not. In the imaging cohort 22% of the individuals showed abnormal myocardial perfusion imaging and 1 in every 18 subjects (5, 5%) showed moderate to severe perfusion defects indicative of a poor prognosis. Coronary artery disease would remain undetected in as many as 41% of type 2 diabetic patients if 1998 American Diabetes Association recommendations for coronary artery disease screening were strictly followed. Although the study could not demonstrate benefit from routine screening stress myocardial perfusion imaging allowed a good stratification of risk. The 12% participants with moderate or large perfusion defects had higher event rates (2, 4% per year) compared with participants with small or no defects that had low event rates (0, 4% per year) (Wackers et al., 2004). In a study, 510 asymptomatic patients with diabetes had pre-screening performed using electron-beam computed tomography. If the coronary artery calcification score was 100 Agatston units or greater stress myocardial perfusion imaging was performed (Anand et al., 2006). The prevalence of silent coronary artery disease in this study was 13% and established cardiovascular risk factors failed to predict silent ischemia. These two recent prospective studies indicated that the prevalence of silent coronary artery disease in asymptomatic patients is considerably lower than was suggested by retrospective database analyses. Regarding the prognostic role of myocardial perfusion imaging, in pooled studies including both diabetic and non-diabetic patients and symptomatic as well as asymptomatic patients a normal stress myocardial perfusion imaging has been associated with a cardiac event rate of < 1% per year (Iskander & Iskandrian, 1998). With abnormal stress myocardial perfusion imaging studies the extent and severity of myocardial ischemia strongly predicts short and long term risks of coronary events (Hachamovitch et al., 1998). A study was performed on 180 asymptomatic adult-onset diabetic patients referred to exercise myocardial perfusion imaging to detect asymptomatic obstructive coronary artery disease (De Lorenzo et al., 2002). In this study a short-term follow-up was conducted to correlate the imaging findings with patients outcome. A positive test result was reported in 26% of all subjects and clinical variables were not associated with the type of defect or subsequent events. During follow-up two percent of hard events and 5% of total events occurred in patients with normal SPECT. These numbers increased to 9% of hard events and 38% of total events in those with an abnormal SPECT. Male sex and perfusion abnormalities were independent predictors of cardiac events. The presence of an abnormal SPECT in asymptomatic patients seemed to provide added prognostic value over clinical predictors alone. In a multicenter cohort consisting of 370 asymptomatic patients with diabetes with at least two additional cardiovascular risk factors silent ischemia was identified in 35% of patients using stress SPECT imaging as well as ECG stress testing (Valensi et al., 2005). During follow-up there was a significant association between positive stress test results and subsequent cardiac events only in patients > 60 years.

Myocardial perfusion imaging showed good sensitivity but poor specificity (possibly because microvascular disease) for diagnosing coronary artery disease in diabetes. Intermediate follow-up has shown good predictive value of myocardial perfusion imaging for coronary events in type 2 diabetes (Djaberi et al., 2008).

4.5 Coronary artery calcium scores

The presence of coronary calcium is indicative of coronary atherosclerosis. Coronary calcification can be detected noninvasively be electron beam computed tomography and more recently multislice computed tomography. Diabetic patients without manifest coronary artery disease have a higher coronary artery calcium score that non-diabetic independent of classical risk factors (Hoff et al., 2003; Schurgin et al., 2001, Reaven & Sacks, 2005). Also coronary artery calcium scores show significantly more progression over time in patients with diabetes that in nondiabetics (Raggi et al., 2005).

A substantial body of evidence has established that coronary artery calcium measurement provides potent risk stratification for asymptomatic diabetics. In a cohort of 10.377 asymptomatic individuals which included 903 diabetics the mean coronary artery calcium score was significantly higher in subjects with diabetes than in those without diabetes and for every increase in coronary artery calcium score there was a greater increase in mortality for diabetic patients than for nondiabetic patients (Raggi et al., 2004).

In the presence of multiple cardiac risk factors, the prevalence of coronary artery calcium is increased. In asymptomatic patients with three or more cardiac risk factors the prevalence of coronary artery calcium was significantly increased (Moser et al., 2003). An Agatston score greater than 400 is a threshold for further testing with myocardial perfusion imaging (Moser et al., 2003). These data suggest that coronary artery calcium scoring may have value as an approach to enrich target population of asymptomatic patients with diabetes for screening.

Currently only limited data are available on the relative values of coronary artery calcium and myocardial perfusion imaging for detection silent coronary artery disease and prognostic evaluation. Wong et al. studied 1043 patients without known coronary artery disease (140 patients with diabetes) with coronary artery calcium scoring and stress myocardial perfusion imaging (Wong et al., 2005). A coronary artery calcium score lower than 100 was associated with absence of stress induced ischemia on myocardial perfusion imaging. The likelihood of stress-inducible ischemia increased in parallel with increasing coronary artery calcium score and was greater in diabetics. A recent study explored the combined use of coronary artery calcium assessment and myocardial perfusion imaging in asymptomatic patients with diabetes (Anand et al., 2006). The study evaluated 510 asymptomatic patients with type 2 diabetes using initially electron beam computed tomography to assess coronary artery calcium. If coronary artery calcium score was greater than 100 (25%) stress myocardial perfusion imaging was performed. For comparison, 53 randomly selected patients with a coronary artery calcium score of 100 or less also underwent stress myocardial perfusion imaging. Patients with coronary artery calcium score of 10 or less had no abnormalities on myocardial perfusion imaging. The prevalence of abnormal myocardial perfusion imaging studies increased at higher coronary artery calcium scores. From patients with a coronary artery calcium score between 101 and 400, 23% had abnormal myocardial perfusion imaging and this number increased to 71, 4% of patients with a coronary artery calcium score greater than 1000. Sequential use of electron beam computed tomography and myocardial perfusion imaging may optimize screening of asymptomatic diabetic patients. During a mean follow-up of 18±5 months, no events occurred in patients with coronary artery calcium score of 10 or less; as compared with 82% of events occurring in patients with a coronary artery calcium score greater than 400. The coronary artery calcium score and the extent of myocardial perfusion imaging abnormalities were the only predictors of future cardiac events (Anand et al., 2006). The calcium score was demonstrated to be superior to the established risk factors in predicting silent ischemia and cardiac events. Other studies (He et al., 2000; Berman et al., 2004) found also that the prevalence of stress-induced ischemia on myocardial perfusion was very low if the coronary artery calcium score was lower than 100 Agatston units and increased in parallel to the coronary artery calcium score. Of patients with coronary artery calcium score 400 or greater, 46% had demonstrable stress-induced myocardial ischemia on myocardial perfusion imaging (He et al., 2000). The decision to perform coronary artery calcium scoring should be based on clinical judgment, only if the results have the potential to change the management of the patient (Bax et al., 2007).

4.6 Multislice computed tomography coronary angiography

In type 2 diabetes multislice computed tomography angiography has demonstrated a higher percentage of noncalcified and calcified plaques and a relatively lower percentage of mixed plaques in diabetes (Pundziute et al., 2007) which can be explained by the rapid progression of atherosclerosis. The sensitivity and specificity is 81% and 82% respectively for detection of coronary stenosis (Schuijf et al., 2004). The diagnostic accuracy of multislice computed tomography angiography is similar in diabetic and nondiabetic individuals (Schuijf et al., 2005). Importantly negative predictive value of multislice computed tomography angiography in diabetes was to be found 98% - 100 %(Berman et al., 2004). The prevalence of coronary heart disease has been assessed by multislice computed tomography angiography in 70 asymptomatic patients with type 2 diabetes. The majority of the patients (80%) had atherosclerosis: obstructive coronary artery disease in 26% and nonobstructive coronary heart disease in 54% of patients (Wong et al., 2005).

Thus, results on the use of noninvasive multislice computed tomography angiography for coronary heart disease screening and as a prognostic indicator in the diabetic population appear promising but further studies in larger population groups are needed.

Multislice computed tomography angiography has good sensitivity, specificity and negative predictive value for identification of coronary heart disease in diabetic patients. However assessment of coronary heart disease by multislice computed tomography in asymptomatic type 2 diabetic patients should be limited to patients at high-risk because of exposure to high radiation and contrast as well as cost factors (Djaberi et al., 2008).

4.7 Carotid intimae-media thickness in type 2 diabetes

Mean common carotid intimae-media thickness in middle aged individuals is higher in diabetic patients versus controls. In diabetics without a history of myocardial infarction carotid intimae-media thickness is similar to that in non diabetic with a history of myocardial infarction (Lee et al., 2004). Progression of maximal carotid intimae-media thickness in the Insulin Resistance Atherosclerosis Study was twice as high in person with diabetes versus controls (Wagenknecht et al., 2003) but other studies report lower rates (van der Meer et al., 2003). In type 2 diabetes prevalent cardiovascular disease is associated with a higher carotid intimae-media thickness (Lee et al., 2004). Carotid intimae-media thickness was shown to be an independent predictor of cardiovascular events (Bernard et al., 2005). Folsom and colleagues analysed carotid intimae-media thickness in a large cohort that included 1500 diabetic participants and they found that carotid intimae-media thickness has predictive value for future coronary events only in combination with other novel risk factors (Folsom et al., 2003). Carotid intimae media thickness is increased in type 2 diabetic patients with cardiovascular disease and is an independent predictor of coronary events. However the magnitude of its predictive value when added to other risk factors is questionable (Djaberi et al., 2008).

4.8 Arterial stiffness in type 2 diabetes

Diabetic patients have increased arterial stiffness (Weber et al., 2004, Cruickshank et al., 2002). Compromised carotid distensibility and pulse wave velocity have been demonstrated even before the onset of diabetes, in patients with impaired glucose tolerance. Arterial stiffness in diabetes is related to prevalent cardiovascular disease (Fukui et al., 2003) and has shown to be an independent predictor of coronary heart disease (Hatsuda et al., 2006). Pulse wave velocity does seem to have a reasonable value for mortality prediction in patients with impaired glucose tolerance and type 2 diabetes (Cruickshank et al., 2002). Vascular stiffness is increased in type 2 diabetic patients with cardiovascular disease and has been shown to predict cardiovascular mortality (Djaberi et al., 2008)

4.9 Flow mediated dilation in type 2 diabetes

Type 2 diabetes is associated with endothelial dysfunction. Insulin-mediated dilation being at least in part nitric-oxid dependent, insulin resistance may cause endothelial dysfunction. Clustering of risk factors such as dyslipidemia, hypertension and obesity in the metabolic syndrome play an additional role. The predictive value of endothelial dysfunction in epicardial coronary arteries of diabetic patients has been established for long-term coronary events (Nitenberg et al., 2005). Flow mediated dilation is a marker of endothelial dysfunction. The potential of flow mediated dilation for the identification of type 2 diabetic patients at risk for cardiovascular disease is unknown.

Surrogate markers of atherosclerosis: carotid intimae media thickness, arterial stiffness and flow mediated dilation are abnormal long time before the onset of diabetes. These measurements can be useful for the identification of at risk patients during early stages of atherosclerosis. Further studies are necessary to evaluate whether these measurements will provide any additional prognostic value in combination with risk scores (Djaberi et al., 2008).

4.10 Coronary angiography

Coronarography is an invasive diagnostic tool, the gold standard for identifying obstructive lesions and will be considered in the presence of ischemia revealed by noninvasive screening tests.

4.11 Cardiovascular magnetic resonance imaging

Cardiovascular magnetic resonance imaging studies can provide information regarding coronary stenoses and flow, evaluation of myocardial perfusion and metabolism, wall motion during stress and evidence of infarction. There are limited data to support the use of cardiovascular magnetic resonance in asymptomatic patients.

4.12 Biomarkers

A simple, inexpensive blood test for B type natriuretic peptide (BNP) or N terminal prohormone B type natriuretic peptide (NT-proBNP) is a candidate for screening tool of silent myocardial ischemia. BNP is of value in predicting silent ischemia at exercise testing in type 2 diabetic patients (Rana et al., 2006). Hamano et al. showed in a recent study that NT-proBNP has a very high negative predictive value which enables to focus on patients with silent ischemia independent of microalbuminuria (Hamano et al., 2010). Cosson et al. conclude that NT-proBNP helps to better define diabetic patients with silent ischemia independently of cardiac structure and function (Cosson et al., 2009).

5. Deciding who to investigate? Which are the patients with diabetes at high risk that should be screened?

Population screening is not feasible but diabetic patients with high risk of silent ischemia should be identified and investigated further. It still remains under debate what would be the best strategy for proper patient selection to screening and if screening will alter patient outcome when added to primary preventive measures. Several studies of asymptomatic patients with type 2 diabetes have specifically examined whether risk factor burden is predictive of silent ischemia (determined by myocardial perfusion imaging) and these studies have not supported the recommendation of the 1998 ADA consensus panel for screening asymptomatic patients with two or more risk factors (Rajagopalan et al., 2005; Scognamiglio et al., 2006). In asymptomatic patients with diabetes mellitus clinical features that help to identify the patient with increased risk for myocardial infarction or cardiac death include: evidence of other atherosclerotic disease, microalbuminuria and chronic renal disease, abnormal resting ECG, diabetes complications including autonomic neuropathy, rethinopathy, age, sex, unexplained dyspnoea and multiple both traditional and novel risk factors (Bax et al., 2007).

Atherosclerotic disease involving lower extremity, cerebral, renal or mesenteric arteries identifies a patient with diabetes who is at increased risk for adverse cardiovascular outcomes and might have advanced coronary atherosclerosis (Golomb et al., 2006). Other atherosclerotic location is of bad prognosis in asymptomatic diabetic patients leading to increased silent myocardial ischemia and cardiovascular event rates (Criqui et al., 1992). A diminished ankle-brachial index is sensitive indicator of increased risk for future cardiovascular events (Doobay & Anand, 2005). In patients with claudication or asymptomatic peripheral arterial disease, 90% of deaths are attributable to coronary artery disease (Mann et al., 2001).

Microalbuminuria predicts increased risk for vascular disease complications (Schuijf et al., 2006, Anand et al., 2006, Gerstein et al., 2001) as well as for the progression to overt nephropathy in patients with diabetes. Microalbuminuria has been a predictor of inducible ischemia in some (Rutter et al., 1999) but not all (Wackers et al., 2004) studies of asymptomatic patients with diabetes. An increased microalbuminuria predicts a high cardiovascular event rate with a two-time earlier mortality rate (Dinneen & Gerstein, 1997).

Asymptomatic patients with type 2 diabetes occasionally have evidence of previously unrecognized myocardial infarction on resting ECG, including abnormal Q waves or deep T-wave inversions or left bundle branch block. These findings should trigger evaluation for coronary artery disease and inducible ischemia. In a retrospective study of 1427 asymptomatic patients who were referred to the Mayo Clinic for stress testing, Rajagopalan and colleagues aimed to define the variables that would characterize which asymptomatic diabetic patients are most suitable for screening with stress myocardial perfusion imaging. They conducted multivariate analysis and found that high-risk scans were most strongly associated with seven independent variables, the most notable being electrocardiographic Q waves and peripheral arterial disease. Although this was a retrospective study and many have been influenced by verification bias, it provides additional support for identifying high-risk asymptomatic diabetic patients with electrocardiographic abnormalities, peripheral arterial disease, among other clinical variable. Nonspecific ST-T wave changes also are a strong predictor of inducible ischemia in asymptomatic diabetic patients (Rajagopalan et al., 2005).

Cardiovascular autonomic neuropathy is associated with poor overall prognosis in patients with type 2 diabetes (Vinik et al., 2003). That is probably due to impairment in ischemia awareness delaying the diagnosis of coronary artery disease or hemodynamic lability due to blunted parasympathetic activation. Autonomic neuropathy might also be a parallel consequence of cardiac risk factors including hyperglycaemia, dyslipidemia and renal disease. Several studies have implicated autonomic neuropathy as a contributing factor in the mechanism of silent ischemia (Marchant et al, 1993; O'Sullivan et al., 1991). Autonomic neuropathy was a major predictor of inducible ischemia in DIAD (Detection of Ischemia in Asymptomatic Diabetics) (Wackers et al., 2004) and has been associated with abnormal cardiac test findings in other (Valensi et al., 2001) but not all (MiSAD Group, 1997) studies. Cardiac autonomic neuropathy should be considered in the presence of unexplained tachycardia, orthostatic hypotension and other autonomic or peripheral neuropathies.

Diabetic retinopathy is a manifestation of microvascular disease but is also an indicator of risk for coronary artery disease. In clinical studies retinopathy has been associated with inducible ischemia in some (Akasaka et al., 1997) but not all screening studies. In a recent study that assessed the prevalence and risk factors predictors of true silent myocardial ischemia in asymptomatic type 2 diabetic patients, the prevalence of silent ischemia was 21, 9% and male gender and the presence of diabetic retinopathy were the risk factors related to its development (Hernandez et. al, 2011). Hyperglycaemia is a stronger predictor of microvascular disease than atherosclerotic macrovascular disease in people with diabetes (Laakso, 1999).

Although diabetes increases relative cardiovascular risk more in women than in men the absolute risk for cardiovascular events is still higher in men than in women (Abbott et al., 1988). Male sex and duration of diabetes were also strong predictors of silent ischemia in DIAD, but traditional risk factors, novel biomarkers (hs C reactive protein, homocysteine, lipid subtractions, and plasminogen activator inhibitor-10) and the number of risk factors were not predictive of abnormal myocardial perfusion (Wackers et al., 2004). Age is an important determinant of cardiovascular risk and the prevalence of inducible ischemia is significantly higher in patients with type 2 diabetes >65 years (Chaowalit et al., 2006). Patients with exertional symptoms as shortness of breath, generalized fatigue should be screened for ischemia. It is difficult to attribute these symptoms to myocardial ischemia (an angina equivalent) or to obesity and deconditioning. But however patients who are unable to exercise are at increased cardiac risk. The incidence of inducible ischemia is increased in these patients and when present is associated with poor prognosis (Vanzetto et al., 1999).

Patients with type 2 diabetes often have multiple cardiac risk factors including hypertension, dyslipidemia, inactivity, smoking and abdominal obesity. Multiple risk factors in the same patient substantially increase the overall cardiovascular risk (Multiple Risk Factor Intervention Trial, 1996). Also intervention directed at multiple risk factors significantly improves cardiovascular prognosis (Gaede et al., 2003). A prospective smaller study performed on 120 truly asymptomatic diabetic patients with one or more risk factors for coronary artery disease revealed that 33% had an abnormal myocardial perfusion stress study. Smoking, duration of diabetes and cholesterol/HDL ratio were identified as independent predictors of an abnormal stress myocardial perfusion imaging (Scholte et al., 2009).

Some recent prospective studies in type 2 diabetes have been unable to link the number of risk factors to inducible ischemia on perfusion imaging (Wackers et al., 2004). That is probably due to the fact that these studies did not account for the severity, duration, and effect of treatment of dyslipidemia and hypertension in patients with long-standing type 2 diabetes. It is important to improve the ability to identify based on clinical data those patients at highest risk for cardiovascular events. While simple categorical risk factor burden has not proven to effectively discriminate which asymptomatic diabetic patients will or will not have ischemia on stress testing it is possible that risk factor burden might predict risk of cardiovascular events in individual patients (Bax et al., 2007). Efforts have been made using data from Framingham, which included fewer than 400 diabetic subjects, the UKPDS (United Kingdom Prospective Diabetes Study) which included only newly diagnosed diabetic subjects and excluded patients with significant comorbidities and other populations (Guzder et al., 2005) to develop models that identify individuals at higher risk for cardiovascular events (Bax et al., 2007). It is necessary to define a subgroup of high risk asymptomatic patients that will benefit from silent ischemia screening.

A substantial body of evidence has established that coronary artery calcium measurement provides potent risk stratification for asymptomatic diabetics. Diabetic patients with a low coronary artery calcium score have a very favourable prognosis. Among diabetics with a CAC score <10, the 5 year all cause mortality rate was extremely low and was similar to rates for those without diabetes and similar coronary artery calcium score. For any category of coronary artery calcium over zero, there a stepwise increased mortality risk in individual with diabetes compared to those without diabetes (Raggi et al., 2004).

The study PREDICT (PRospective Evaluation of Diabetic Ischemic heart disease by Computed Tomography) a prospective cohort study on 589 asymptomatic type 2 diabetic patients showed that coronary artery calcium score was a highly significant independent predictor of cardiovascular events. A doubling in coronary artery calcium was associated with a 29% increase in risk of events (Elkeles et al., 2008). Coronary artery calcium provided greater predictive value for cardiac events than Framingham risk score and UKPDS risk scores, and than conventional and novel risk factors. In asymptomatic diabetic patients, the prevalence of stress induced ischemia increases the higher the coronary artery calcium score is on computed tomography scanning. From asymptomatic diabetic patients with coronary artery calcium score between 100 and 400, 23% had a positive stress SPECT scan, and 48% from those with coronary artery calcium score >400. This number increased to 71, 4% for asymptomatic diabetic patients with coronary artery calcium score >1000. The greater the extent of ischemia, the worse the clinical outcome and coronary artery calcium score was superior to established risk factors for predicting silent ischemia and cardiac events (Anand et al., 2006).

It is now possible to test a new paradigm for screening asymptomatic diabetic patients (Berman et al., 2004). This consist of using coronary artery calcium scanning rather than cardiac stress testing as the first line screening test. Above coronary artery calcium threshold (400 or 100) SPECT-myocardial perfusion imaging could be selectively used for identifying high-risk silent ischemia. In the presence of high-risk ischemia coronary angiography should be performed, this being the group that could benefit from revascularization (He et al., 2000). It is expected that approximately one-third of such patients would have no detectable coronary artery calcium and many others would have coronary artery calcium scores at levels which obviate the need for SPECT-myocardial perfusion imaging. The inclusion of various clinical parameters as suggested by Bax et al. could alter the threshold criteria used to guide referral to stress testing respectively selective use of a lower coronary artery calcium score threshold among those with high-risk clinical features. In patients with < 10% ischemia, repeat myocardial perfusion imaging might be appropriate in 3 years (Qu et al., 2003).

There are continuing controversies regarding the screening for coronary artery disease in asymptomatic diabetic patients. Given the growing threat posed by increasing prevalence of diabetes, testing of algorithms which cost-effectively select for the identification of high-risk asymptomatic individuals with diabetes is urgently warranted.

6. What are the implications of an early diagnosis of coronary atherosclerosis or ischemia? The detection of silent ischemia in diabetic patients impacts upon their treatment and outcome?

Several recent prospective studies have addressed the value of screening for coronary artery disease in asymptomatic diabetic patients. The DIAD (Detection of Ischemia in Asymptomatic Diabetics) study is a randomized controlled trial in which 1123 patients with type 2 diabetes and no symptoms of coronary artery disease were randomly assigned to be screened with adenosine-stress radionuclide myocardial perfusion imaging or not to be screened. The aim of the study was to test that systematic screening would identify higher-risk individuals and beneficially affect their risk of myocardial infarction or cardiac death. In DIAD although type 2 diabetes is considered to be a coronary artery disease equivalent patients had a low cardiac event rate (0, 6%/year) and the identification of patients with abnormal screening did not serve to eliminate their risk over 5 years of follow-up. The cardiac event rate is 3-4 folds lower than that reported in previous retrospective studies on asymptomatic diabetic patients referred to nuclear cardiology laboratories. But these patients had a higher incidence of peripheral arterial disease, renal insufficiency and many were referred to preoperative evaluation (Rajagopalan et al., 2005; Zellweger et al., 2004). The favourable outcomes of patients in DIAD likely reflect in part the impact of aggressive, guideline-driven management of cardiac risk factors. One of the surprises of the DIAD was that there was no evidence for more inducible ischemia in screened patients when myocardial perfusion imaging was repeated after 3 years. Rather than greater prevalence of abnormal myocardial perfusion there was significantly less inducible ischemia at repeated imaging: 12% vs. 20%. A remarkable 79% of participants with initially abnormal stress myocardial perfusion at recruitment had resolution of ischemia. This improvement was not restricted to small perfusion defects but rather occurred regardless of the initial magnitude of perfusion defect. Only 10% of participants with initially normal screening myocardial perfusion imaging developed new inducible ischemia after 3 years. This resolution of ischemia was unanticipated but can be explained after the review of the medical regimens of participants. In the course of three years there was a significant increase in the treatment of patients with aspirin, statins and angiotensin converting enzyme inhibitors. The observed resolution of inducible ischemia was also a harbinger of the low cardiac events that subsequently emerged (Young et al., 2009). Routine screening for inducibile ischemia in asymptomatic patients with type 2 diabetes is not recommended because: the yield of detecting inducible ischemia is relatively low (Wackers et al., 2004); the overall cardiac event rate is low, even in patients with moderate or large defects and the highest event rate are conventionally assigned to an intermediate risk category; routine screening does not appear to affect overall outcome and routine screening of millions of asymptomatic diabetic patients is prohibitively expensive. Although screening had no impact on outcomes in

DIAD it is noteworthy that stress myocardial perfusion imaging did effectively stratify patients into higher risk (moderate-large defects and ischemic ECG) and low-risk (small defects or normal myocardial perfusion imaging) subsets. On the other hand there were adverse cardiac events in both screened and unscreened patients. Thus DIAD results do not exclude the possibility that strategies to better identify patients at higher risk coupled with more effective treatment strategies might prove effective for screening in the future. A selective evaluation of asymptomatic diabetic patients will be a better approach for screening.

The COURAGE (Clinical Outcomes Utlizing Revascularization and Aggresive Drug Evaluation) (Boden et al., 2006) reported among 2.287 patients with stable angina, overall event rates nearly 5%/year indicating a significant residual risk in intensively medically treated patients as well as those undergoing percutaneous interventions. These findings seem to highlight the need for improved methods to stratify residual risk within populations undergoing intensive medical management. Many of these patients had multivessel or proximal left anterior descending coronary artery disease and intensive medical treatment was as effective as percutaneous intervention combined with intensive medical treatment in preventing overall mortality or myocardial infarction. Results were similar in the approximate one-third of the subjects with diabetes. It may be not appropriate to extrapolate the results of this trial in symptomatic patients (in which the event rate for diabetic subjects approached 5% per year) to somewhat lower-risk asymptomatic patients. In the treatment arm of the CARDS (Collaborative Atorvastatin Diabetes Study) trial (Colhoun et al., 2004) which included individuals with type 2 diabetes and no history of cardiovascular disease even after risk factor modification in the active treatment group in whom LDL cholesterol was lowered, still the cardiovascular mortality of diabetic patients remains high; 1, 54/100 person-years. These findings suggest that type 2 diabetic patients being treated according to intensive treatment guidelines likely have a residual, intermediate risk (1 2% per year) for cardiac events. This high mortality will be due in part to silent, prognostically important coronary artery disease (left main, proximal left anterior descending, three vessel disease). Detection and revascularization of this disease will improve this poor prognosis (Sorajja et al., 2005, The BARI Investigators, 1997). This is an important argument for screening high risk diabetic patients for silent ischemia. In diabetic patients autopsy studies observed a greater prevalence of severe multivessel coronary artery disease among patients with diabetes compared with nondiabetic patients even in the absence of prior symptoms or clinical evidence of disease (Goraya et al., 2002). Thus the presumed benefit of evaluation of the presence and extent of myocardial ischemia is to identify those patients with left main or severe multivessel disease with a large area of myocardium at risk and who would have a benefit from coronary revascularization. Diabetic patients have a significant risk for atherosclerotic vascular disease and aggressive treatment of risk factors is recommended in the absence of symptomatic or known coronary artery disease. The role of coronary imaging is not to document the presence of atherosclerosis but to identify those with more extensive disease. Patients with myocardial ischemia involving a large segment of left ventricular myocardium are candidates for coronary angiography and subsequent revascularization. Available data (Hachamovitch et al., 2003, Sorajja et al., 2005) suggests that patients with ischemia involving 10% or more of the left ventricle have a better outcome after myocardial revascularization compared with the results of medical therapy alone.

The hypothesis that asymptomatic patients with severe ischemia benefit from revascularization above aggressive medical was subject of several prospective randomized trials some specifically targeted to the diabetic population. The BARI (Bypass Angioplasty Revascularization Investigation) trial evaluated the effectiveness of percutaneous coronary intervention versus coronary artery bypass grafting in over 1800 patients with symptomatic multivessel coronary artery disease (The BARI Investigators, 2007). The primary outcome of survival was similar in both groups. In a subgroup of patients with diabetes and multivessel disease coronary artery bypass grafting conferred higher survival rates (57,8%) versus percutaneous coronary intervention (45,5%) (p=0,025). The BARI 2D study Group (A Randomized Trial of Therapies for Type 2 Diabetes and Coronary Artery Disease) (The BARI 2D Study Group, 2009) randomly assigned 2368 patients with type 2 diabetes and stable ischemic heart disease to undergo either prompt revascularization with intensive medical therapy or intensive medical therapy alone. Overall there was no significant difference in rates of death and major cardiovascular events between patients undergoing prompt revascularization and those undergoing medical therapy. Prompt revascularization significantly reduced cardiovascular events as compared to medical therapy among patients who were selected to undergo coronary artery bypass grafting but not among those who were selected to undergo percutaneous coronary intervention. The study suggest that patients with diabetes, evidence of myocardial ischemia and extensive multivessel disease would benefit from prompt surgical revascularization mainly because of a lower rate of nonfatal myocardial infarction. Accurate and early diagnosis of coronary artery disease is likely of benefit in those patients with severe anatomic disease, where revascularization has particular benefits. It is not recommended extensive and expensive diagnostic testing to define the presence of coronary artery disease before implementing medical therapy for established risk factors in diabetic patients. Negative screening tests in patients with diabetes do not uniformly confer a benign prognosis. Tests that detect inducible ischemia or assess atherosclerotic burden do not always identify patients at risk for plaque rupture and thrombosis which leads to acute coronary events. Further research focusing on the biological properties of the vessel wall and characterization of plaque structure and stability are warranted. Eventually, we will need better imaging techniques that can assess both plaque burden (soft and calcified) and the extent of vulnerable plaques. These techniques will require molecular imaging that permit delineation of plaque macrophage density and inflammatory markers, the thickness of the fibrous cap, the extent of the lipid-laden necrotic core, fibrin deposition, and the presence of neovessels (Davies et al., 2004; Jaffer et al., 2006; Waxman et al., 2006). If total plaque burden and some index of "vulnerability" could be detected noninvasively, at a reasonable cost, then this approach may be preferable to plaque coronary artery calcium imaging, which is merely reflective of the presence of atherosclerosis. Soft plaques, as previously mentioned, are missed, and no information on vulnerability to rupture is obtained (Beller, 2007).

7. Conclusion

Although the coronary artery disease asymptomatic patient with diabetes is by definition at least at intermediate risk for cardiovascular events it is difficult to support routine screening for these patients. As previous recommendations for stratifying diabetic patients based upon the number of risk factors have not proven effective the question remains whether there are individuals with diabetes in whom coronary artery imaging would seem particularly appropriate. The motivation of such testing would be the clinical suspicion that the individual is at high risk for having a coronary artery disease event in the short term. What would be the best strategy for identifying at-risk individuals is still under debate. In patients evaluated clinically to be at high risk coronary artery calcium scoring may be reasonable first test with subsequent functional imaging performed if the calcium scoring indicates a substantial atherosclerotic burden. The concept of screening asymptomatic subjects is heavily debated and the controversy can only be resolved by gathering evidence for or against screening, which requires data from a randomized clinical trial.

8. References

Abbott, RD., Donahue, RP., Kannel, WB., & Wilson, PW. (1988). The impact of diabetes on survival following myocardial infarction in men vs. women: the Framingham Study. *JAMA*, Vol. 260, No.23, (December 1988), pp. 3456–3460, ISSN 0098-7484.

Ahluwalia, G., Jain, P., Chugh, SK., Wasir, HS., & Kaul, U. (1995) Silent myocardial ischemia in diabetics with normal autonomic function. *Int J Cardiol*, Vol. 48, No.2, (February 1995) pp.147–153, ISSN: 0167-5273.

Albers, AR., Krichavsky, MZ., & Balady, GJ. (2006). Stress testing in patients with diabetes mellitus: Diagnostic and Prognostic value *Circulation*, Vol.113, No.4, (January 2006), pp.583-592, ISSN 1524-4539.

Akasaka, T., Yoshida, K., Hozumi, T., Takagi, T., Kaji, S., Kawamoto, T., Morioka, S., & Yoshikawa, J. (1997). Retinopathy identifies marked restriction of coronary flow reserve in patients with diabetes mellitus. *J Am Coll Cardiol*, Vol. 30, No.4, (October 1997), pp. 935–941, ISSN 0735-1097.

American Diabetes Association (1998). Consensus development conference on the diagnosis of coronary heart disease in people with diabetes. *Diabetes Care*, Vol.21, No.9, (September 1998), pp.1551-1559, ISSN 1935-5548.

Anand, DV., Lim, E., Hopkins, D., Corder, R., Shaw, LJ., Sharp, P., Lipkin, D., & Lahiri A, (2006). Risk stratification in uncomplicated type 2 diabetes: prospective evaluation of the combined use of coronary artery calcium imaging and selective myocardial perfusion scintigraphy. Eur Heart J, Vol.27, No. 6, (March 2006), pp.713-721, ISSN1522-9645.

Anand, DV., Lim, E., Lahiri ,A., & Bax, JJ. (2006). The role of non-invasive imaging in the risk stratification of asymptomatic diabetic subjects (review). *Eur Heart J*, Vol.27, No.8, (April 2006), pp. 905–12, ISSN 1522-9645.

Aronow, WS., Mercando, AD.,& Epstein, S. (1992). Prevalence of silent myocardial ischemia detected by 24-hour ambulatory electrocardiography, and its association with new coronary events at 40-month follow-up in elderly diabetic and nondiabetic patients with coronary artery disease. *Am J Cardiol*, vol.69, No.5, (February 1992), pp.555-556, ISSN 0002-9149.

Bacci, S., Villela, M., Villela, A., Langialonga, T., Grilli, M., Rauseo, A., Mastroianno, S., De Cosmo, S., Fannelli, R., & Trischitta, V. (2002). Screening for silent myocardial ischemia in type 2 diabetic patients with additional atherogenic risk factors: applicability and accuracy of the exercise stress test. *Eur J Endocrinol*, Vol. 147, No.5, (July 2002), pp. 649–654, ISSN 0804-4643.

Bax, JJ., Young, LH., Frye, RL., Bonow, RO., Steinberg, HO., & Barrett, EJ. (2007). Screening for coronary artery disease in patients with diabetes *Diabetes Care*, Vol.30, No.10, (October 2007), pp. 2729-2736, ISSN 1935-5548.

Beller, GA. Noninvasive screening for coronary atherosclerosis and silent ischemia in asymptomatic type 2 diabetic patients. Is it appropriate and cost-effective?. *J Am Coll Cardiol*, Vol.49, No.19, (May 2007), pp.1918-1923, ISSN 0735-1097.

Berman, DS., Wong, ND., Gransar, H.,Miranda-Peats, R., Dahlbeck, J., Hayes, SW., Friedman, JD., Kang, X., Polk, D., Hachamovitch, R., Shaw, L., & Rozanski, A. (2004). Relationship between stress-induced myocardial ischemia and atherosclerosis measured by coronary calcium tomography. *J Am Coll Cardiol*, Vol. 44, No. 4, (August 2004), pp.923-930, ISSN 0735-1097.

Bernard, S., Sérusclat, A., Targe, F., Charriere, S., Roth, O., Beaune, J., Berthezene, F., & Moulin, P. (2005) Incremental predictive value of carotid ultrasonography in the assessment of coronary risk in a cohort of asymptomatic type 2 diabetic subjects. *Diabetes Care*, Vol. 28, No.5, (May 2005), pp.1158–1162, ISSN 1935-5548.

Blandine, JD., Bernard, S., Habib, G., Bory, M., Vague, P., & Lassman-Vague, V. (1999). Silent myocardial ischemia in patients with diabetes: who to screen. *Diabetes Care*, Vol. 22, No. 9, (September 1999), pp. 1396–1400, ISSN 1935-5548.

Boden, WE., O'Rourke, RA., Teo, KK., Hartigan, PM., Maro, DJ., Kostuk, W., Knudtson,M., Dada, M., Casperson, P., Harris, CL., Spertus, JA., Shaw, L., Chaitman, BR., Mancini, GB., Berman, DS., & Weintraub, WS. (2006). Design and rationale of the Clinical Outcomes Utilizing Revascularization and Aggressive DruG Evaluation (COURAGE) trial Veterans Affairs Cooperative Studies Program no. 424. *Am Heart J*, Vol. 151, No.6, (June 2006), pp.1173–1179, ISSN 0002-8703.

Caracciolo, EA., Chaitman, BR., & Forman, SA. (1996) Diabetics with coronary disease have a prevalence of asymptomatic ischemia during exercise treadmill testing and ambulatory ischemia monitoring similar to that of nondiabetic patients. An ACIP database study. ACIP Investigators. Asymptomatic Cardiac Ischemia Pilot Investigators. *Circulation*, Vol.93, No.12, (June 1996), pp. 2097–2105. ISSN 1524-4539.

Chaowalit, N., Arruda, AL., McCully, RB., Bailey KR., & Pellikka, PA. (2006). Dobutamine stress echocardiography in patients with diabetes mellitus: enhanced prognostic prediction using a simple risk score. *J Am Coll Cardiol*, Vol. 47, No.5, (March 2006), pp.1029–1036, ISSN 0735-1097.

Chiariello, M., Indolfi, C., Cotecchia, MR., Sifola, C., Romano, M., & Condorelli, M. (1985) Asymptomatic transient ST changes during ambulatory ECG monitoring in diabetic patients. *Am Heart J*, Vol.110, No.3, (September 1985) pp.529–534, ISSN 0002-8703.

Colhoun, HM., Betteridge, DJ., Durrington, PN., Hitman, GA., Neil, AW., Livingstone, SJ., Thomason, MJ., Mackness, MI., Charlton-Menys, V. & Fuller, JH. CARDS investigators. (2004). Primary prevention of cardiovascular disease with atorvastatin in type 2 diabetes in the Collaborative Atorvastatin Diabetes Study (CARDS): multicentre randomised placebo-controlled trial. *Lancet*, Vol. 364, No.9435, (August 2004), pp. 685-696, ISSN 0140-6736.

Cortigiani, L., Bigi, R., Sicari, R., Landi, P., Bovenzi, F., & Picano, E. (2006). Prognostic value of pharmacological stress echocardiography in diabetic and nondiabetic patients with known or suspected coronary artery disease. *J Am Coll Cardiol* ,Vol. 47, No. 3, (February 2006), pp. 605–610, ISSN 1558-3597.

Cosson, E., Paycha, F., Paries, J. Cattan, S., Ramadan, A., Meddah, D., Attali, J-R., & Valensi, P. (2004) Detecting silent coronary stenoses and stratifying cardiac risk in patients with diabetes: ECG stress test or exercise myocardial scintigraphy? *Diabet Med,* Vol.21, No.4, (April 2004), pp. 342–348, ISSN 1464-5491.

Cosson, E., Nguyen, MT., Pham, I., Pontet, M., Nitenberg, A. & Valensi, P. (2009). N-terminal pro-B-type natriuretic peptide: an independent marker for coronary artery disease in asymptomatic diabetic patients. *Diabetic Medicine,* Vol.26, No.9, (September 2009), pp. 872-879, ISSN 1464-5491.

Criqui, MH., Langer, RD., Fronek, A., Feigelson, HS., Klauber, MR., Mc Cann, TJ., & Browner D. (1992). Mortality over a period of 10 years in patients with peripheral arterial disease. *N Engl J Med,* Vol. 326, No.6, (February 1992), pp. 381-386, ISSN 0028-4793.

Cruickshank, K., Riste, L., Anderson, SG., Wright, JS., Dunn, G., & Gosling, RG, (2002) Aortic pulse-wave velocity and its relationship to mortality in diabetes and glucose intolerance: an integrated index of vascular function? *Circulation,* Vol.106, No.16, (October 2002), pp.2085–2090, ISSN 1524-4539.

Davies, JR., Rudd, JH., & Weissberg, PL. (2004). Molecular and metabolic imaging of atherosclerosis (review). *J Nucl Med,* Vol.45, No.11, (November 2004), pp.1898 – 1907, ISSN 1071-3581.

De Lorenzo, A., Lima, RS., Siquiera-Filho, AG., & Pantoja, MR. Prevalence and prognostic value of perfusion defects detected by stress technetium-99m sestamibi myocardial perfusion single-photon emission computed tomography in asymptomatic patients with diabetes mellitus and no known coronary artery disease. *Am J Cardiol.,* Vol.90, No.8, (October 2002), pp.827-832, ISSN 0002-9149.

Dinneen, SF. & Gerstein, HC. (1997). The association of microalbuminuria and mortality in non-insulin-dependent diabetes mellitus. A systematic overview of the literature. *Arch Intern Med,* Vol. 157, No.13, (July 1997), pp.1413-1418, ISSN 1538-3679.

Djaberi, R., Beishuizen, ED., Pereira, AM., Rabelink, TJ., Smit, JW., Tamsma, JT., Huisman, MV., & Jukema, JW. (2008). Non-invasive cardiac imaging techniques and vascular tools for the assessment of cardiovascular disease in type 2 diabetes mellitus *Diabetologia,* Vol. 51, No.9, (September 2008), pp.1581–1593, ISSN1432-0428.

Doobay, AV., & Anand, SS. (2005). Sensitivity and specificity of the ankle-brachial index to predict future cardiovascular outcomes: a systematic review. *Arterioscler Thromb Vasc Biol,* Vol.25, No.7, (July 2005), pp. 1463–1469, ISSN: 1524-4636.

Elhendy, A., van Domburg, RT., Poldermans, D., Bax, JJ., Nierop, PR., Geleijnse, ML., & Roelandt, JR. (1998) Safety and feasibility of dobutamine-atropine stress echocardiography for the diagnosis of coronary artery disease in diabetic patients unable to perform an exercise stress test. *Diabetes Care,* Vol.21, No.11, (November 1998), pp. 1797–1802, ISSN 1935-5548.

Elkeles, RS., Godsland, IF., Feher, MD., Rubens, MB., Roughton, M., Nugara, F., Humphries, SE., Richmond, W., & Flather, MD., (2008). Coronary calcium measurement improves prediction of cardiovascular events in asymptomatic patients with type 2 diabetes: the PREDICT study. *Eur Heart J,* Vol. 29, No. 18, (September 2008), pp.2244-2251, ISSN1522-9645.

Faglia, E., Favales, F., Calia, P., Paleari, F., Segalini, G., Gamba, PL., Rocca, A., Musacchio, N., Mastropasquq, A., Testori, G., Rampini, P., Moratti, F., Braga, A., & Morabito, A. (2002). Cardiac Events in 735 Type 2 Diabetic Patients Who Underwent Screening for Unknown Asymptomatic Coronary Heart Disease: 5-year follow-up report from the Milan Study on Atherosclerosis and Diabetes (MiSAD). *Diabetes Care* ,Vol. 25, No. 11, (November 2002), pp. 2032-2036, ISSN 1935-5548.

Faglia, E., Manuela, M., Antonella, Q., Michela, G., Vincenzo, C., Maurizio, C., Roberto, M., & Alberto, M. (2005) Risk reduction of cardiac events by screening of unknown asymptomatic coronary artery disease in subjects with type 2 diabetes mellitus at high cardiovascular risk: an open-label randomized pilot study. *Am Heart J*, Vol. 149, No.2, (February 2005), pp.e1–6, ISSN 0002-8703.

Folsom AR, Chambless LE, Duncan BB, Gilbert AC,& Pankow JS, Atherosclerosis Risk in Communities Study Investigators (2003) Prediction of coronary heart disease in middle-aged adults with diabetes. *Diabetes Care*, Vol, 26, No.10. (October 2003), pp. 2777–2784, ISSN 1935-5548.

Fukui, M., Kitagawa, Y., Nakamura, N.,Mogami, S., Ohnishi, M., Hirata, C., Ichio, N., Wada, K., Kamuchi, K., Shigeta, M., Sawada, M., Hasegawa, G., & Yoshikawa, T. (2003) Augmentation of central arterial pressure as a marker of atherosclerosis in patients with type 2 diabetes. *Diabetes Res Clin Pract* (February 2003), Vol.59, No.2, (February 2003), pp.153–161, ISSN 0168-8227.

Gaede, P., Vedel, P., Larsen, N., Jensen, GV., Parving, HH., & Pedersen, O. (2003). Multifactorial intervention and cardiovascular disease in patients with type 2 diabetes. *N Engl J Med*, Vol.348, No.5, (January 2003, pp.383–393, ISSN 0028-4793.

Gerstein, HC., Mann, JF., Yi, Q., Zinman, B., Dinneen, SF., Hoogwerf, B., Halle, JP., Young, J., Rashkow, A., Joyce, C., Nawaz, S., & Yusuf, S. (2001). Albuminuria and risk of cardiovascular events, death, and heart failure in diabetic and nondiabetic individuals. *JAMA*, Vol.286, No.4, (July 2001), pp. 421–426, ISSN 0098-7484.

Giri, S., Shaw, LJ., Murthy, DR., Travin, MI., Miller, DD., Hachamovitch, R., Borges-Neto, S., Berman, DS, Waters, DD., & Heller, GV. (2002). Impact of diabetes on the risk stratification using stress single-photon emission computed tomography myocardial perfusion imaging in patients with symptoms suggestive of coronary artery disease. *Circulation*, Vol. 105, No.1, (January 2002), pp. 32– 40, ISSN 1524-4539.

Golomb, BA., Dang, TT., & Criqui, MH. (2006). Peripheral arterial disease: morbidity and mortality implications. *Circulation*, Vol.114, No.7, (August 2006), pp. 688–699, ISSN 1524-4539.

Goraya, T., Leibson, CL., Palumbo, PJ., Weston, SA., Killian, JM., Pfeifer, EA., Jacobsen, SJ., Frye, RL., & Roger, V, (2002). Coronary atherosclerosis in diabetes mellitus: A population based autopsy study. J Am Coll Cardiol, Vol. 40, No.5, (September 2002), pp. 946-953, ISSN 1558-3597.

Grundy, SM., Cleeman, JI., Merz, CN., Brewer, HB Jr., Clark LT., Hunninghake, DB., Pasternak, RC., Smith, SC., & Stone, NJ. for the Coordinating Committee of the National Cholesterol Education Program Endorsed by the National Heart, Lung, and Blood Institute; American College of Cardiology Foundation; American Heart Association (2004). Implications of recent clinical trials for the National Cholesterol

Education Program Adult Treatment Panel III guidelines (review). *Circulation*, Vol.110, No. 2, (July 2004), pp. 227–239, ISSN 1524-4539.

Guzder, RN., Gatling, W., Mullee, MA., Mehta, RL., & Byrne, CD. (2005). Prognostic value of the Framingham cardiovascular risk equation and the UKPDS risk engine for coronary heart disease in newly diagnosed type 2 diabetes: results from a United Kingdom study. *Diabet Med*, Vol.22, No.5, (May 2005), pp. 554–562, ISSN 1464-5491.

Hachamovitch, R., Berman, DS., Shaw, LJ., Kiat, H., Cohen, I., Cabico, AJ., Friedman, J., & Diamond, GA. (1998). Incremental prognostic value of myocardial perfusion single photon emission computed tomography for the prediction of cardiac death: differential stratification for risk of cardiac death and myocardial infarction. *Circulation*, Vol.97, No.6, (February 1998), pp.535–543, ISSN 1524-4539.

Hachamovitch, R., Hayes, SW., Friedman, JD., Cohen, I., & Berman, DS. (2003). Comparison of the short-term survival benefit associated with revascularization compared with medical therapy in patients with no prior coronary artery disease undergoing stress myocardial perfusion single photon emission computed tomography. *Circulation*, Vol.107, No.23, (July 2003), pp. 2900–2907, ISSN 1524-4539.

Haffner, SM., Lehto, S., Ronnemaa, T., Pyorala, K., & Laakso, M, (1998). Mortality from coronary heart disease in subjects with type 2 diabetes and in nondiabetic subjects with and without prior myocardial infarction. *N Engl J Med*, Vol. 339, No.4 , (July 1998), pp. 229-234, ISSN 1533-4406.

Hamano, K., Abe, M., Komi, R., & Kobayasi, S. (2010). N-terminal fragment of pro-brain natriuretic peptide (NT-proBNP) for predicting silent myocardial ischaemia in type 2 diabetes mellitus independent of microalbuminuria. *Diabetes/Metabolism Research and Reviews*, Vol. 26, No.7, (October 2010), pp. 534-539.ISSN 1520-7560.

Hammoud, T., Tanguay, J-F., & Bourassa, MG, (2000). Management of coronary artery disease: therapeutic options in patients with diabetes. *J Am Coll Cardiol*, Vol. 36, No. 2, (August 2000), pp. 355–365, ISSN 1558-3597.

Hatsuda, S., Shoji, T., Shinohara, K., Kimoto, E., Mori, K., Fukumoto, S., Koyama, H., Masanori, E., & Nishizava, Y. (2006). Regional arterial stiffness associated with ischemic heart disease in type 2 diabetes mellitus. *J Atheroscler Thromb*, Vol.13, No.2, (May 2006), pp.114–121, ISSN 1340-3478.

He, ZX., Hedrick, TD., Pratt, CM., (2000). Severity of coronary artery calcification by electron beam computed tomography predicts silent myocardial ischemia. *Circulation*, Vol. 101, No.3, (January 2000), pp.244-251, ISSN 1524-4539.

Hennessy, TG., Codd, MB., Kane, G., McCarthy, C,. McCann, HA., & Sugrue, DD. (1997). Evaluation of patients with diabetes mellitus for coronary artery disease using dobutamine stress echocardiography. *Coron Artery Dis*, Vol. 8, No.3-4, (March-April 1997), pp. 171–174, ISSN 1473-5830.

Hernandez, C., Candell-Riera, J., Ciudin, A., Francisco, G., Aguade-Bruix, S. & Simo, R. (2011). Prevalence and risk factors accounting for true silent myocardial ischemia: a pilot case-control study comparing type 2 diabetic with non-diabetic control subjects. *Cardiovascular Diabetology* 10:9 doi:10.1186/1475-2840-10-9, (January 2011), ISSN 1475-2840.

Hoff, JA., Quinn, L.,& Sevrukov, A., (2003) The prevalence of coronary artery calcium among diabetic individuals without known coronary artery disease. *J Am Coll Cardiol*, Vol. 41, No.6, (March 2003), pp. 1008–1012, ISSN 0735-1097.

http://www.nhlbi.nih.gov/giudelines/cholesterol/atp3_rpt.htm.

Iskander, S., & Iskandrian, AE. Risk assessment using single-photon emission computed tomographic technetium-99 m sestamibi imaging. *J Am Coll Cardiol*, Vol. 32, No.1, (July 1998), pp.57-62, ISSN 0735-1097.

Jaffer, FA., Libby, P., & Weissleder, R. (2006). Molecular and cellular imaging of atherosclerosis: emerging applications (review). *J Am Coll Cardiol*, Vol. 47, No.7, (April 2006), pp. 1328 -38. ISSN 0735-1097.

Khaleeli, E., Peters, SR., Bobrowsky, K., Oudiz, RJ., Ko, JY., & Budoff, MJ. (2001). Diabetes and the associated incidence of subclinical atherosclerosis and coronary artery disease: implications for management. *Am Heart J*, Vol.141, No. 4, (April 2001), pp. 637- 644, ISSN 0002-8703.

Laakso, M. (1999) Hyperglycemia and cardiovascular disease in type 2 diabetes. *Diabetes*, Vol.48, No.1, (January 1999), pp.937-942, ISSN: 1939-327X.

Lee CD, Folsom AR, Pankow JS, & Brancati FL, For the Atherosclerosis Risk in Communities (ARIC) Study Investigators (2004). Cardiovascular events in diabetic and nondiabetic adults with or without history of myocardial infarction. *Circulation*, Vol.109, No.7, (February 2004), pp.855-860, ISSN 1524-4539.

Mann, JF., Gerstein, HC., Pogue, J., Bosch, J., & Yusuf, S. (2001). Renal insufficiency as a predictor of cardiovascular outcomes and the impact of ramipril: the HOPE randomized trial. *Ann Intern Med*, Vol.134, No.8, (April 2001), pp. 629-636, ISSN 1539-3704.

Marchant, B., Umachandran, V., Stevenson, R., Kopelman, PG., & Timmis, AD. (1993). Silent myocardial ischemia: role of subclinical neuropathy in patients with and without diabetes. *J Am Coll Cardiol*, Vol.22, No.5, (November 1993), pp.1433-1437, ISSN 0735-1097.

Milan Study on Atherosclerosis and Diabetes (MiSAD) Group. (1997). Prevalence of unrecognized silent myocardial ischemia and its association with atherosclerotic risk factors in noninsulin-dependent diabetes mellitus. *Am. J. Cardiol.*, Vol.79, No.2, (January 1997), pp.134-139, ISSN 0002-9149.

Miller, TD., Rajagopalan, N., Hodge, DO., Frye, RL., & Gibbons, RJ. (2004). Yield of stress single-photon emission computed tomography in asymptomatic patients with diabetes. *Am Heart J*, Vol.147, No.5, (May 2004), pp.890-896, ISSN 0002-8703.

Miller, TD., Redberg, RF., & Wackers, FJ.(2006). Screening asymptomatic diabetic patients for coronary artery disease: why not? *J Am Coll Cardiol*, Vol.48, No. 4, (September 2006), pp.761- 764, ISSN1558-3597.

Mortality after 16 years for participants randomized to the Multiple Risk Factor Intervention Trial. *Circulation*, Vol.94, No.5, (September 1996), pp.946-951, ISSN 1524-4539.

Moser, KW., O'Keefe, JH., Jr, Baterman, TM., & McGhie, IA. (2003). Coronary calcium screening in asymptomatic patients as a guide to risk factor modification and stress myocardial perfusion imaging. *J Nucl Cardiol*, Vol. 10, No.6, (November 2003), pp.590-598, ISSN 1071-3581.

Nesto, RW., & Kowalchuk, GJ. (1987). The ischemic cascade: temporal sequence of hemodynamic, electrocardiographic and symptomatic expressions of ischemia. *Am J Cardiol.*, Vol.59, No.7, (March 1987), pp.23C-30C, ISSN 0002-9149.

Nesto, RW., Philips, RT., Kett, KG., Hill, T., Perper, E., Young, E., & Leland, OS Jr, (1988). Angina and exertional myocardial ischemia in diabetic and nondiabetic patients:

assessment by exercise thallium scintigraphy. *Ann Intern Med*, Vol.108, No. 1, (February 1998), pp. 170-175, ISSN 1539-3704.

Nitenberg, A., Pham, I., Antony, I., Valensi, P., Attali, JR., & Chemla, D. (2005) Cardiovascular outcome of patients with abnormal coronary vasomotion and normal coronary arteriography is worse in type 2 diabetes mellitus than in arterial hypertension: a 10 year follow-up study. *Atherosclerosis*, Vol.183, No.1, (November 2005), pp.113–120, ISSN 0021-9150.

O' Sullivan, JJ., Conroy, RM., MacDonald, K., Mc Kenna, TJ., & Maurer, Bj. (1991). Silent ischemia in diabetic men with autonomic neuropathy. *Br Health J*, Vol.66, No.4, (October 1991), pp.313-315, ISSN1687-5958.

Paillole, C., Ruiz, J., Juliard, JM., Leblanc, H., Gourgon, R., & Passa, P. (1995). Detection of coronary artery disease in diabetic patients. *Diabetologia*, Vol. 38, No.6, (June 1995), pp. 726–731, ISSN: 1432-0428.

Penfornis, A., Zimmerman, C., Boumal, D., Sabbah, A., Meneveau, N., Gaulteir-Bourgeois, S., Bassand, JP., & Bernard, Y. (2001). Use of dobutamine stress echocardiography in detecting silent myocardial ischaemia in asymptomatic diabetic patients: a comparison with thallium scintigraphy and exercise testing. *Diabet Med.*, Vol. 18, No.11, (November 2001), pp. 900–905, ISSN 1464-5491.

Prevalence of unrecognized silent myocardial ischemia and its association with atherosclerotic risk factors in noninsulindependent diabetes mellitus: Milan Study on Atherosclerosis and Diabetes (MiSAD) Group. *Am J Cardiol*, Vol.79, No.2, (January 1997), pp.134 –139, ISSN 0002-9149.

Prior, JO., Monbaron, D., Koehli, M., Calcagni, ML., Ruiz, J., & Bischof, DA. (2005). Prevalence of symptomatic and silent stress-induced perfusion defects in diabetic patients with suspected coronary artery disease referred for myocardial perfusion scintigraphy. *Eur J Nucl Med Mol Imaging*, Vol. 32, No. 1, (January 2005), pp.60-69, ISSN 1619-7070.

Pundziute, G., Schuijf, JD., Jukema, JW,. Boersma, E., Scholte, AJHA., Kroft, LJM., van der Wall, EE., & Bax, JJ. (2007). Noninvasive assessment of plaque characteristics with multislice computed tomography coronary angiography in symptomatic diabetic patients. *Diabetes Care*, Vol.30, No.5, (May 2007), pp.1113–1119, ISSN 1935-5548.

Qu, W., Le, TT., Azen, SP., Xiang, M., Wong, ND., Doherty, TM., & Detrano, RC. (2003).Value of coronary artery calcium scanning by computed tomography for predicting coronary heart disease in diabetic subjects. *Diabetes Care*, Vol. 26, No.3, (March 2003), pp.905-910, ISSN 1935-5548.

Raggi, P., Shaw, LJ., Berman, DS., & Callister, TQ. (2004). Prognostic value of coronary artery calcium screening in subjects with and without diabetes. *J Am Coll Cardiol*, Vol. 43, No. 9, (May 2004), pp. 1663–1669, ISSN 1558-3597.

Raggi, P., Cooil, B., Ratti, C., Callister, TQ., & Budoff, M. (2005). Progression of coronary artery calcium and occurrence of myocardial infarction in patients with and without diabetes mellitus. *Hypertension*, Vol.46, No.1, (July 2005), pp.238–243, ISSN: 1524-4563.

Rajagopalan, N., Miller, TD., Hodge, DO., Frye, RL., & Gibbons, RJ. (2005). Identifying high-risk asymptomatic diabetic patients who are candidates for screening stress single-photon emission computed tomography imaging. *J Am Coll Cardiol*, Vol. 45, No.1, (January 2005), pp.43-49, ISSN 1558-3597.

Rana,BS., Davies, JI, Band, MM., Pringle, SD., Morris, A., & Struthers, AD. (2006). B-type natriuretic peptide can detect silent myocardial ischaemia in asymptomatic type 2 diabetes *Heart*, Vol. 92, No.7, (July 2006), pp.916-920, ISSN 1355-6037.

Reaven, PD.,& Sacks, J., Investigators for the VADT (2005). Coronary artery and abdominal aortic calcification are associated with cardiovascular disease in type 2 diabetes. *Diabetologia*, Vol. 48, No.2, (February 2005), pp. 379–385, ISSN 1432-0428.

Rubler, S., Gerber, D., Reitano, J., Chokshi, V., & Fisher, VJ. (1987). Predictive value of clinical and exercise variables for detection of coronary artery disease in men with diabetes mellitus. *Am J Cardiol.* Vol. 59, No.15, (June 1987), pp 1310–1313, ISSN 0002-9149.

Rutter, MK., McComb, JM., Brady, S., & Marshall, SM. (1999). Silent myocardial ischemia and microalbuminuria in asymptomatic subjects with non-insulin-dependent diabetes mellitus. *Am J Cardiol*, Vol.83, No.1, (January 1999), pp.27–31, ISSN 0002-9149.

Rutter, MK., Wahid, ST., McComb, JM., & Marshall, SM. (2002). Significance of silent ischemia and microalbuminuria in predicting coronary events in asymptomatic patients with type 2 diabetes. *J. Am. Coll. Cardiol.* (July 2002), Vol.40, No.1, pp. 56-61, ISSN 1558-3597.

Schaper, J. (1988). Effects of multiple ischemic events on human myocardium: an ultrastructural study. *Eur Heart J*, Vol. 9, No suppl. A, (January 1988), pp. 141-149, ISSN1522-9645.

Schinkel, AFL., Bax, JJ., Geleijnse, ML., Boersma, E., Elhendy, A, Roelandt, JRTC., & Poldermans, D. (2003). Non-invasive evaluation of ischemic heart disease: myocardial perfusion imaging or stress echocardiography. Eur Heart J, Vol.24, No.9, (May 2003) pp.789–800.

Scholte, AHJA., Bax, JJ., Wackers, FJTh. (2006). Screening of asymptomatic patients with type 2 diabetes mellitus for silent coronary artery disease. Combined use of stress myocardial perfusion imaging and coronary calcium scoring *J Nucl Cardiol*, Vol.13, No.1, (January 2006), pp. 11-18, ISSN 1071-3581.

Scholte, AJHA., Schuijf, JD., Kharagjitsingh, AV., Dibbets-Schneider, P., Stokkel, MP., van der Wall, EE.,& Bax, JJ. (2009). Prevalence and predictors of an abnormal stress myocardial perfusion study in asymptomatic patients with type 2 diabetes mellitus. *Eur J Nucl Med Mol Imaging*, Vol.36, No.4, (April 2009), pp.567–575, ISSN 1619-7070.

Schuijf, JD., Bax, JJ., Jukema, JW., Lamb, HJ., Vliegen, HW., Salm, LP., de Ross, A., & van der Wall, EE. (2004). Noninvasive angiography and assessment of left ventricular function using multislice computed tomography in patients with type 2 diabetes. *Diabetes Care*, Vol.27, No.12, (December 2004), pp.2905–2910, ISSN 1935-5548.

Schuijf, JD., Pundziute, G., Jukema, JW., Lamb, HJ., van der Hoeven, BL., de Roos, A., van der Wall, EE., & Bax, JJ. (2006). Diagnostic accuracy of 64-slice multislice computed tomography in the noninvasive evaluation of significant coronary artery disease. *Am J Cardiol*, Vol.98, No.2, (July 2006), pp.145–148, ISSN 0002-9149.

Schuijf, JD., Bax, JJ., Jukema, JW., der Wall, EE., Lamb, HJ., de Roos, A., Mollet, NR., Cademartiri, F., & Feyter, PJ. (2006). Do risk factors influence the diagnostic accuracy of noninvasive coronary angiography with multislice computed tomography? *J Nucl Cardiol*, Vol.13, No.5, (September 2006), pp.635–641, ISSN 1071-3581.

Schurgin, S., Rich, S., & Mazzone, T. (2001). Increased prevalence of significant coronary artery calcification in patients with diabetes. *Diabetes Care*, Vol. 24, No.2, (February 2001), pp. 335–338, ISSN 1935-5548.

Scognamiglio, R., Negut, Christian., Ramondo, A., Tiengo, A., & Avogaro, A. (2006). Detection of coronary artery disease in asymptomatic patients with type 2 diabetes mellitus. *J Am Coll Cardiol*, Vol. 47, No.1, (January 2006), pp.65-71, ISSN 0735-1097.

Shaw, LJ., & Iskandrian, AE, (2004). Prognostic value of gated myocardial perfusion SPECT (review). *J Nucl Cardiol*, Vol. 11, No. 2, (March 2004), pp. 171– 185, ISSN: 1532-6551.

Sorajja, P., Chareonthaitawee, P., Rajagopalan, N., Miller, TD., Frye, RL., Hodge, DO., & Gibbons, RJ. (2005). Improved survival in asymptomatic diabetic patients with high-risk SPECT imaging treated with coronary artery bypass grafting. *Circulation*, Vol.112, No.9, (August 2005), Suppl. 1 pp. I-311–316, ISSN: 1524-4539.

Stamler, J., Vaccaro, O., Neaton, JD., & Wentworth, D, (1993). Diabetes, other risk factors, and 12-yr cardiovascular mortality for men screened in the Multiple Risk Factor Intervention Trial. *Diabetes Care*, Vol. 16, No.2, (February 1993), pp. 434-444, ISSN 1935-5548.

The BARI Investigators. Influence of diabetes on 5-year mortality and morbidity in a randomized trial comparing CABG and PTCA in patients with multivessel disease: the Bypass Angioplasty Revascularization Investigation. *Circulation*, Vol. 96, No.6, (September 1997), pp.1761-1769, ISSN 1524-4539.

The BARI Investigators: The Final 10 Year Follow-Up Results From the BARI Randomized Trial. *J Am Coll of Cardiol*, Vol. 49, No.15, (April 2007), pp. 1600-1606, ISSN 0735-1097.

The BARI 2D Study Group (2009). A randomized trial of therapies for type 2 diabetes and coronary artery disease. *N Engl J Med*, Vol. 360, No. 24, (June 2009), pp. 503-2514, ISSN 0028-4793.

Valensi, P., Sachs, R-N., Harfouche, B., Lormeau, B., Paries, J., Cosson, E., Paycha, F., Leutenegger, M., & Attali, J-R. (2001). Predictive value of cardiac autonomic neuropathy in diabetic patients with or without silent myocardial ischemia. *Diabetes Care*, Vol.24, No.2, (February 2001), pp. 339–343, ISSN 1935-5548.

Valensi, P., Paries, J., Brulport-Cerisier, V., Torremocha, F., Sachs, RN., Vanzetto, G., Cosson, E., Lormeau, B., Attali, JR., Marechaud, R, Estour, B, & Halimi, S. (2005). Predictive value of silent myocardial ischemia for cardiac events in diabetic patients: influence of age in a French multicenter study. *Diabetes Care*, Vol. 28, No.11, (November 2005), pp.2722–2727, ISSN 1935-5548.

van der Meer, IM., Iglesias del Sol, A, Hak, AE, Bots, ML., Hofman, A., & Witteman, JC. (2003). Risk factors for progression of atherosclerosis measured at multiple sites in the arterial tree: the Rotterdam Study. *Stroke*, Vol.34, No.10, (October 2003), pp.2374–2379, ISSN 0039-2199.

Vanzetto, G., Halimi, S., & Hammoud, T. Prediction of cardiovascular events in clinically selected high-risk NIDDM patients. Prognostic value of exercise stress test and thallium-201 single-photon emission computed tomography. *Diabetes Care*, Vol.22, No.1, (January 1999), pp.19-26, ISSN 1935-5548.

Vinik, AI., Maser, RE., Mitchell, BD., & Freeman, R. (2003). Diabetic autonomic neuropathy. *Diabetes Care*, Vol.26, No.5, (May 2003), pp.1553–1579, ISSN 1935-5548.

Wackers, FJ., Young, LH., Inzzuchi, SE., Chuyn, DA., Davey, JA., Barrett EJ., Taillefer, R., Wittlin, SD., Heller, GV., Filipchuck, N., Engel, S., Ratner, RE., & Iskandrian, AE. . For The Detection of Ischemia in Asymptomatic Diabetics Investigators (2004). Detection of silent myocardial ischemia in asymptomatic diabetic subjects; the DIAD study. *Diabetes Care,* Vol. 27, No.8, (August 2004), pp.1954-1961, ISSN 1935-5548.

Wagenknecht, LE., Zaccaro, D., Espeland, MA., Karter, AJ., O'Leary, DH., & Haffner, SM. (2003). Diabetes and progression of carotid atherosclerosis: the insulin resistance atherosclerosis study. *Arterioscler Thromb Vasc Biol,* Vol. 23, No.6, (June 2003), pp.1035–1041, ISSN: 1524-4636.

Waxman, S., Ishibashi, F., & Muller, JE. (2006). Detection and treatment of vulnerable plaques and vulnerable patients: novel approaches to prevention of coronary events (review). *Circulation,* Vol.114, No.28, (November 2006), pp. 2390–411, ISSN 1524-4539.

Weber, T., Auer, J., O'Rourke, MF., Kvas, E., Lassing, E., Berent, R., & Eber, B. (2004). Arterial stiffness, wave reflections, and the risk of coronary artery disease. *Circulation,* Vol.109, No.2, (January 2004), pp.184–189, ISSN 1524-4539.

Wild, S., Roglic, G., Green, A., Sicree, R., & King, H, (2004). Global prevalence of diabetes: Estimates for the year 2000 and projections for 2030. *Diabetes Care,* Vol. 27, No. 5, (May 2004), pp. 1047–1053, ISSN 1935-5548.

Wong, ND., Rozanski, A., Gransar, H., Miranda-Peats, R., Kang, X., Hayes, S., Shaw, L., Friedman, J., Polk, D., & Berman, DS. (2005). Metabolic syndrome and diabetes are associated with an increased likelihood of inducible ischemia among patients with subclinical atherosclerosis. *Diabetes Care,* Vol.28, No. 6, (June 2005), pp.1445-1450, ISSN 1935-5548.

Young, LH., Wackers, FJT., Chyun, DA., Davey, JA., Barrett, EJ., Taillefer, R., Heller, GV., Iskandrian, AE., Wittlin, SD., Filipchuk, N., Ratner, RE.,& Inzucchi, SE., for the DIAD Investigators (2009). Cardiac Outcomes After Screening for Asymptomatic Coronary Artery Disease in Patients With Type 2 Diabetes .The DIAD Study: A Randomized Controlled Trial. (Reprinted with Corrections) *JAMA,* Vol. 301, No. 15, (April 2009), pp.1547-1555, ISSN 0098-7484.

Zellweger, MJ., Hachamovitch, R., Kang, X., Hayes, SW., Friedman, JD., Germano, G., Pfisterer, ME., & Berman DS. (2004). Prognostic relevance of symptoms versus objective evidence of coronary artery disease in diabetic patients. *Eur Heart J,* Vol. 25, No.7, (April 2004), pp. 543-550, ISSN1522-9645.

10

Effects of Type 2 Diabetes on Arterial Endothelium

Arturo A. Arce-Esquivel, Aaron K. Bunker and M. Harold Laughlin
Department of Biomedical Sciences, University of Missouri, Columbia Missouri and Morningside College, Sioux City, Iowa United States of America

1. Introduction

The endothelium, the innermost layer of blood vessels, has many important biological functions which are responsible for regulating vascular tone and structure. One of the major functions of a healthy endothelium is to ensure adequate blood supply to the different tissues. This particular process is regulated by the release and interaction of different vasoactive substances (i.e. vasodilators and vasoconstrictors), which are under tight balance. On the other hand, it is well known that the chronic exposure to certain stresses (e.g. inflammation, oxidative stress, and hyperglycemia) promotes changes in the endothelium leading to endothelial dysfunction.

Type 2 diabetes mellitus (T2DM) is among those chronic diseases that are associated with endothelial dysfunction which may contribute to limited glucose uptake in skeletal muscle. In fact, diabetes-related endothelial dysfunction has been reported to lead to morphologic and structural vascular changes present throughout the course of diabetes (Taylor and Poston, 1994). There are around 17 million people in the United States who have diabetes, of whom close to 95% have T2DM. Cardiovascular disease (CVD) is the major cause of morbidity and mortality in people with T2DM (Ness et al., 1999), and coronary heart disease is the most common cause of death among those individuals. For instance, people with T2DM are two to four times more likely to develop CVD compared with people without the condition (Stamler et al., 1993).

Interestingly, physical activity is an important therapeutic tool to maintain endothelial function. In fact, regular physical exercise has been reported to be effective in the prevention and delay of onset of T2DM (Bassuk and Manson, 2005; Sanz et al., 2010; Stewart, 2002). Thus the primary purpose of this chapter is to summarize the current available literature concerning the effects of T2DM on arterial endothelium. In addition, this chapter is intended to summarize evidence of the beneficial effects of physical activity on the untoward cardiovascular effects of T2DM and/or the apparent ability of physical activity to prevent progression of diabetes-induced CVD.

2. Vascular endothelial function

2.1 Role of the endothelium in vasoregulation

All blood vessels in the systemic and pulmonary circulations are lined by a continuous single cell layer of endothelium. This layer of endothelial cells continues throughout the cardiac chambers as well. As a result of research over the past 30 years it is established that the endothelium constitutes a very important and exciting organ. The endothelium plays an important role in hemostasis, inflammation, lipid metabolism, vascular growth, cell migration, formation of (and interactions with) extracellular matrix molecules, as well as control of vascular permeability and vascular resistance (both vasodilator and vasoconstrictor responses) (Furchgott and Vanhoutte, 1989; Ganz and Vita, 2003). The endothelium can detect chemical substances within the blood and physical forces imparted to blood vessel walls (i.e. shear stress and distention) and initiate responses to these chemical and/or physical signals by releasing substances that modulate vascular tone and/or blood vessel structure (Adair et al., 1990; Furchgott and Vanhoutte, 1989). The vascular endothelium releases a variety of vasoactive substances, including vasodilator and vasoconstrictor substances such as endothelin, which contribute to vasomotor control in tissues throughout the body. As described below, the most common measure of the functional capacity of the endothelium is to measure endothelium-dependent dilation (EDD) primarily because of the potential to assess the health of the endothelium non-invasively. Usually, EDD is the result of release of endothelium-derived relaxing factors (EDRFs).

There appear to be at least three EDRF substances, two of which have been identified; prostacyclin (PGI_2) and nitric oxide (NO) (Furchgott and Vanhoutte, 1989; Palmer et al., 1988a; Palmer et al., 1987; Palmer et al., 1988b). The other EDRF, often referred to as endothelium-derived hyperpolarizing factor (EDHF) may not actually be a factor but perhaps represents electrical communication through the gap junctions between endothelial and vascular smooth muscle cells (Cohen and Vanhoutte, 1995; Feletou and Vanhoutte, 2004; Fichtlscherer et al., 2004; Triggle et al., 2003). The relative importance of endothelium-dependent control differs among the tissues of the body at least in part because the endothelial lining is not a homogeneous compartment. Rather the endothelium is characterized by significant structural and functional heterogeneity among tissues and within tissues (Aird, 2007a, b; Laughlin et al., 2008). Even within the vascular bed of a given skeletal muscle, the relative importance of endothelium-dependent vascular control mechanisms changes along the length of the arteriolar network (Laughlin et al., 2008; Laughlin et al., 2001; Laughlin et al., 2003; Laughlin et al., 2004).

NO is produced in endothelial cells by endothelial nitric oxide synthase (eNOS) from L-arginine and oxygen. In its role in vascular control, NO diffuses to the underlying smooth muscle cells, where it activates soluble guanylyl cyclase, resulting in production of cyclic guanosine monophosphate (cGMP) and activation of protein kinase G (PKG), which leads to vasodilation. eNOS is activated by phopshorylation stimulated by shear stress, chemical mediators, and/or by binding of calcium-calmodulin following increases in intracellular calcium signalled by mechanical forces (i.e. an increase in shear stress exerted by the blood flow on the endothelium, referred to as flow-induced dilation) and/or by a host of chemical factors (acetylcholine, bradykinin, substance P, noradrenaline)(Balligand et al., 2009; Barnes and Liu, 1995; Furchgott and Vanhoutte, 1989; Vanhoutte, 1989) acting on their respective receptors on the endothelium (Furchgott and Vanhoutte, 1989; Ganz and Vita, 2003). Flow-induced dilation has been demonstrated in conduit and resistance arteries in various vascular beds (Drexler et al., 1989; Miura et al., 1999; Miura et al., 2001; Sinoway et al., 1989). The weight of evidence suggests that an increase in wall shear stress, secondary to the increased flow, is the physical force that initiates dilation (Pohl et al., 1991). Selective removal or destruction of the endothelium typically abolishes the response (Hull et al., 1986;

Lie et al., 1970; Rubanyi et al., 1986) implicating the production and/or release of endogenous, transferable vascular smooth muscle relaxing factor(s) from endothelial cells (Kuo et al., 1991).

Prostanoid EDRFs are metabolites of arachidonic acid produced by the cyclooxygenase pathway. Arachidonic acid itself can produce vasoconstriction or vasodilation in some vascular beds such as the pulmonary vascular bed, depending on concentration and tone at the time of administration (Barnes and Liu, 1995; Furchgott and Vanhoutte, 1989; Vanhoutte, 1989). These effects of arachidonic acid on the vasculature are largely due to formation of prostanoids and/or thromboxane A_2 (Barnes and Liu, 1995; Furchgott and Vanhoutte, 1989; Palmer et al., 1988a; Palmer et al., 1987; Selig et al., 1986; Vanhoutte, 1989). There is evidence that the chemical identity of EDHF may vary across vascular beds (Laurindo et al., 1994; Miura et al., 2003; Sorop et al., 2003). The five leading candidates for the identity of EDHF include extracellular potassium (Edwards et al., 1998), hydrogen peroxide and/or superoxide anion, epoxygenase/cytochrome P450 metabolites, and electrical conduction of hyperpolarization through myoendothelial gap junctions (Feletou and Vanhoutte, 2004; Fichtlscherer et al., 2004; Fisslthaler et al., 1999; Triggle et al., 2003).

Endothelins are vasoactive peptides produced by vascular endothelial cells (Korth et al., 1999). Three different isoforms of endothelins (ET) have been identified, namely, ET-1, ET-2 and ET-3 (Haynes and Webb, 1998; Masaki, 2004). ET-1 is the most abundant isoform expressed and secreted in endothelial cells and it is one of the most potent vasoconstrictor agents described to date (Haynes and Webb, 1998). ET-1 is constitutively released by endothelial cells with the majority (~80%) released luminally towards vascular smooth muscle (Wagner et al., 1992). Thus ET-1 appears to act primarily in a local paracrine, rather than circulating endocrine, manner. ET receptors are expressed on endothelial and vascular smooth muscle cells of both arteries and veins throughout the pulmonary and systemic vascular trees (Loesch, 2005; Rubanyi and Polokoff, 1994). Binding of ET to the Gq-protein coupled endothelin type A (ET_A) and to endothelin type B (ET_B) receptors on vascular smooth muscle leads to vasoconstriction whereas activation of ET_B receptors on the endothelium leads to production of NO and prostacyclin, which induce vasodilation (Rubanyi and Polokoff, 1994; Schiffrin and Touyz, 1998; Webb and Haynes, 1995). Although the role of ET-1 in determination of regional blood flow remains unclear, it appears that ET-1 contributes to the control of blood flow to the heart, lungs, kidneys, visceral organs and skeletal muscle but likely not to the brain under normal conditions (Koedel et al., 1998; Maeda et al., 2002; Merkus et al., 2003). Also, there is evidence that alterations in the ET-1 system contribute to vascular dysfunction in T2DM (Lam, 2001; Schneider et al., 2007).

2.2 Endothelial function assessment

2.2.1 Non-invasive techniques

These techniques are mainly used to evaluate the vasomotor response to physical and/or pharmacological stimuli of the endothelium. For instance, flow-mediated vasodilation (FMD), using ultrasonography, is the classic technique used to detect changes in superficial arteries (e.g. brachial, radial or femoral), allowing the measurement of blood flow, blood flow velocity and vascular diameter changes (Corretti et al., 1995). The vasodilatory response, after a period of transient ischemia (~ 5 min), is dependent upon a series of neurologic, myogenic and chemical intermediates, which includes the release of NO. There is a good correlation between this post-ischemic vasodilation observed in the forearm (i.e.

FMD) and the coronary vasodilation caused by acetylcholine (Anderson et al., 1995). Thus FMD is used as a surrogate of endothelial health. In addition, strain gauge plethysmography is also used to determine blood flow.

2.2.2 Invasive *in vivo* techniques

These techniques are used to evaluate endothelial function of arteries and to determine the probable changes in their diameter, by ultrasonograhpy, or blood flow, by plethysmography, after cardiac catheterization to access the coronary circulation. These methods allow also the intra-arterial infusion of different drugs and/or neurohumoral factors to study the endothelial-dependent or independent properties. Finally, it is worth noting that the use of *in vitro* direct methods. For instance, cell culture allows the evaluation of the different vasoactive substances that can be secreted by the endothelium in response to changes in blood flow and/or shear stress (Malek et al., 1999). Isolated arteries, from different vascular beds, can be used to determine the specific responses to diverse endothelial-dependent dilators and/or inhibitors (Luscher and Noll, 1996).

3. Link between endothelial dysfunction and T2DM: Pathophysiology

3.1 Vascular inflammation

Endothelial dysfunction is characterized by a chronic, systemic pro-inflammatory state, reduced vasodilation (reduction in relaxing factors and an increase in contracting factors), and a pro-thrombotic state. T2DM is among the multiple diseases and conditions that are initiated or associated with endothelial dysfunction (Beckman et al., 2003; Laight et al., 1999; Schofield et al., 2002). In fact, it has been suggested that endothelial dysfunction is an important factor in the pathogenesis of vascular disease observed in patients with diabetes (De Caterina, 2000; Schalkwijk and Stehouwer, 2005). There is evidence that inflammatory states are associated with T2DM, obesity, and insulin resistance (Hotamisligil et al., 1993; Lehrke and Lazar, 2004).

The plasma concentrations of C-reactive protein (CRP), fibrinogen, interleukin-6, interleukin-1, and tumor necrosis factor alpha (TNFα) are increased in diabetes (Grau et al., 1996; Shurtz-Swirski et al., 2001). Hotamisligil et al. (Hotamisligil et al., 1993) reported that the expression of TNFα, a pro-inflammatory cytokine, was markedly increased in obese mice; and when TNFα was counterbalanced insulin resistance improved. Interestingly, the increased levels of CRP would mediate opposite actions on the vasculature. It promotes the increase of adhesion molecules (intracellular adhesion molecule; ICAM-1, vascular cell adhesion molecule; VCAM-1), E-selectin, monocyte chemotactic protein-1 (MCP-1), and ET-1. On the other hand it decreases eNOS expression, NO and prostacyclin bioavailability, and elevates the expression of angiotensin receptor type 1 in the vessel wall (Pasceri et al., 2000; Schalkwijk and Stehouwer, 2005; Venugopal et al., 2002). Insulin exerts anti-inflammatory effects at the cellular and molecular levels in vitro and in vivo. It has been shown that low-dose infusion of insulin reduces reactive oxygen species generation, and suppresses NADPH oxidase expression and plasma ICAM-1 and MCP-1 concentrations. Conversely, long-term insulin infusion (~ 4 hours) in healthy subjects was associated with an induction of endothelial dysfunction (Hartge et al., 2006).

Clearly, the increased levels of these inflammatory cytokines resulted in increased vascular permeability, change in the vasoregulatory responses, and increase in the adhesion of leucokytes to the endothelium. The diabetes-associated alterations on the endothelium that lead to endothelial dysfunction can be summarized as follows; a) impairment of NO production and/or bioavailability, b) reduced NO responsiveness, c) elevated expression and plasma levels of different vasoconstrictors, d) increased adhesion molecule expression, and e) associated enhanced adhesion of vascular cells (e.g. platelets and monocytes) to the endothelium.

3.2 The metabolic syndrome: Obesity and cardiovascular disease

The metabolic syndrome is a collection of risk factors for CVD, typically characterized by endothelial dysfunction. Metabolic syndrome is diagnosed if there are three of the five following components; a) increased abdominal adiposity, b) atherogenic dyslipidemia, c) elevated blood pressure, d) insulin resistance and/or glucose intolerance (i.e. T2DM), and e) a proinflammatory and prothrombotic state (Grundy et al., 2005; Kahn et al., 2005). Incidence of metabolic syndrome has been on the rise over the last decade both in the United States (Ford et al., 2002; Park et al., 2003) and world-wide (Gupta et al., 2004; Magi et al., 2005). Individuals with identified metabolic syndrome are at increased risk for CVD (Malik et al., 2004; Mottillo et al., ; Wilson et al., 2005), an observation independent of age (Ferreira et al., 2007; Lakka et al., 2002; McNeill et al., 2006). The key findings of these studies were that metabolic syndrome leads to a 2-fold increase in CVD and a 1.5-fold increase in all-cause mortality (Mottillo et al.), that increased risk for CVD is not gender specific (Wilson et al., 2005), and that children with metabolic syndrome possess high levels of multiple risk factors (e.g. hypertension, dyslipidemia, and glucose intolerance) for CVD (Ferreira et al., 2007; Taha et al., 2009).
Obesity and/or adipose tissue disorders are also recognized as a potential primary etiological origin for metabolic syndrome. However, independent of the metabolic syndrome, obesity has been increasing in incidence in both adults and children (Klein et al., 2004; Poirier et al., 2006), and is a risk factor for CVD (Hubert et al., 1983; Larsson et al., 1984). It is also well established that metabolic syndrome and obesity linked with metabolic syndrome promote endothelial dysfunction in adults and children (Aggoun, 2007; Singhal, 2005). More current studies over obesity have elucidated that adipose tissue is not just a simple reservoir for energy storage and thermoregulation but rather a complex, indispensable, active metabolic and endocrine organ (Rosito et al., 2008; Sacks and Fain, 2007). Recent studies have demonstrated that adipose tissue possesses the potential to undergo a phenotypic switch in inflammatory and obese like environments leading it to secrete "adipokines" that increase risk for CVD (Chatterjee et al., 2009; Payne et al., 2010; Sacks and Fain, 2007) and negatively impact endothelial function (Bunker and Laughlin, 2010; Ketonen et al., 2010; Ma et al., 2010; Payne et al., 2009).

3.3 Insulin resistance

In addition to possessing metabolic actions, it is also established that insulin exerts influence over vascular function via; a) stimulation NO production from endothelium, leading to vasodilation; b) increased skeletal muscle blood flow, and c) augmentation of glucose disposal in skeletal muscle (Baron and Clark, 1997). Insulin resistance is typically defined as decreased responsiveness to insulin's actions that stimulate glucose uptake in the tissues (Lebovitz, 2001). Endothelial dysfunction and insulin resistance often co-exist, however at present it remains unclear as to which one leads to/causes the other. A key characteristic of T2DM, insulin resistance is also an independent risk factor for endothelial dysfunction associated with various forms of CVD (Arcaro et al., 2002; Campia et al., 2004; Williams et al., 1996). Cross-sectional studies indicate endothelial dysfunction can independently predict incidence of insulin resistance/diabetes in humans (Meigs et al., 2004; Meigs et al., 2006; Thorand et al., 2006). Additionally, studies examining rodent models of endothelial dysfunction have demonstrated that even partial defects in endothelial function are sufficient to cause insulin resistance (Cook et al., 2004; Duplain et al., 2001). Taken together current evidence supports a causal role for endothelial dysfunction in the development of insulin resistance.

On the other hand a very recent study, the Women's Health Initiative Observational Study (WHIOS), was conducted calling into question the utility of using endothelial dysfunction biomarkers for insulin resistance and T2DM prediction (Chao et al., 2010). The WHIOS involved 1,584 incident T2DM cases and 2,198 matched controls to evaluate the utility of plasma markers of inflammation and endothelial dysfunction for T2DM risk prediction. Results indicated that none of the inflammatory and endothelial dysfunction markers improved T2DM prediction in a multiethnic cohort of postmenopausal women. Other recent studies have also shown that in humans with insulin resistance, a subsequent impairment occurs in insulin's ability to induce endothelium dependent vasodilation that is dramatically improved with insulin therapy (Franklin et al., 2008; Rask-Madsen et al., 2001; Vehkavaara et al., 2000). It was also demonstrated recently in rat model of T2DM that insulin resistance manifested prior to a dramatic (20-35%) progressive decline in endothelial function concurrent with T2DM disease development (Bunker et al., 2010). Collectively these studies suggest a potential causal role of insulin resistance in the development of endothelial dysfunction.

Whichever pathology manifests first, endothelial dysfunction or insulin resistance, it is demonstrably clear that development of either pathology rarely occurs without the subsequent development of the other pathology.

3.4 Hyperglycemia

Generally speaking, hyperglycemia can be divided into two broad categories; a) impaired fasting glucose, and b) impaired glucose tolerance. The latter is commonly characterized by 2-hour post-prandial hyperglycemic spikes of 140mg/dl to ≥200mg/dl (Node and Inoue, 2009). These post-prandial spikes in plasma glucose are known to contribute to endothelial dysfunction and CVD in humans, independent of the metabolic syndrome (Ceriello et al., 2002; Su et al., 2008; Title et al., 2000). Indeed, hyperglycemia is the major causal factor in the development of endothelial dysfunction in diabetes. Results from these studies and many others suggest that endothelial dysfunction is mediated through mechanisms that primarily involve generation of oxidative stress that subsequently lowers NO bioavailability.

Impaired fasting glucose is defined by an elevated fasting plasma glucose concentration of ≥100mg/dl and <126 mg/dl (Genuth et al., 2003), which is also an indication of chronically elevated plasma glucose levels. Evidence from recent human studies suggests that fasting hyperglycemia, independent of diabetes and the metabolic syndrome, contributes to endothelial dysfunction and CVD (Rodriguez et al., 2005; Su et al., 2008). However, evidence is slowly mounting from human and animal studies that suggest oscillating glucose levels seen with impaired glucose tolerance can have more deleterious effects than the constant high glucose levels seen with impaired fasting glucose on endothelial function and oxidative stress (Ceriello et al., 2008; Horvath et al., 2009; Monnier et al., 2006).

3.5 Oxidative stress

Elevated production of reactive oxide species (ROS) has been implicated in the development of T2DM (Avogaro et al., 2006; Irani, 2000; Liu et al., 2005; Tesfamariam and Cohen, 1992; Yang et al., 2010). The molecular basis for excessive mitochondrial ROS in diabetes has been extensively reviewed elsewhere (Irani, 2000; Yang et al., 2010; Avogaro et al., 2006). These free radicals also play a critical role in the pathogenesis of diabetes-associated vascular complications (macro-and microangiopathy) (Giugliano et al., 1996; Spitaler and Graier, 2002). In T2DM, the endothelium, due to glucose oxidation, promotes the increase of free radicals (e.g. superoxide and hydrogen peroxide) leading to enhanced intracellular production of hydroxyl radical which has been linked to diabetes-induced endothelial dysfunction (Giugliano et al., 1996; Pieper et al., 1997; Shi and Vanhoutte, 2009; Spitaler and Graier, 2002; Tesfamariam and Cohen, 1992). In that regard, animal models of diabetes have been associated not only with reduced NO bioavailability but also with impaired EDD (Durante et al., 1988; Rosen et al., 1995; Tesfamariam, 1994) as the result of the hyperproduction of superoxide and hydrogen peroxide. In addition, there is evidence that indicates that increased ROS plays an important role in the development of diabetic complications. Maejima et al. (Maejima et al., 2001) reported that the decrease EDD observed in patients with T2DM is linked to NO inactivation resulting from increased oxidative stress, and that abnormal NO metabolism is related to advanced diabetic microvascular complications. Furthermore, endothelial cells in patients with T2DM are not able to produce sufficient amount of NO and therefore fail to vasodilate in response to vasodilators (e.g. acetylcholine, bradykinin, shear stress) (Avogaro et al., 2006).
The increased glucose levels ("hyperglycemia") also promote mitochondrial formation of ROS. It has been reported that in aortic endothelial cells hyperglycemia induced increased superoxide production which prevents eNOS activity and expression (Srinivasan et al., 2004). The formation of peroxynitrite (superoxide and NO interaction) promotes blunted NO-mediated vasodilatory response and further induces cellular damage through depletion of tetrahydrobiopterin (BH4), an important co-factor for eNOS activity (Pannirselvam et al., 2002). In addition, there are reports indicating that glucose variability ("intermittent low and high glucose levels") is associated with an excessive production of ROS (Monnier et al., 2006; Piconi et al., 2004) which promotes even more detrimental effects to the endothelium (Ceriello et al., 2008; Piconi et al., 2004). Shi et al. (Shi et al., 2007; Shi and Vanhoutte, 2009) reported that elevated levels of ROS not only reduce NO bioavailability, but also facilitate the production and/or action of EDCFs in the course of T2DM. Finally, the augmented production of ROS in T2DM can also promote the inactivation of antioxidant proteins and therefore reduce the antioxidant defense mechanisms (Laight et al., 1999; Shi et al., 2007).

3.6 Dyslipidemia

T2DM promotes elevated total cholesterol, high levels of oxidized lipoproteins, especially low density lipoptotein (LDL), high triglycerides levels, and decreased high-density lipoprotein (HDL) (Watkins, 2003). It has been suggested that abnormal lipids and lipoproteins play a role in endothelial dysfunction in T2DM (McVeigh et al., 1992). For instance, endothelium-dependent vasodilation was negatively and significantly correlated with elevated triglyceride, LDL and low HDL cholesterol concentrations (Watts et al., 1996). In the same manner, it has been shown that only LDL size was inversely correlated with the

acetylcholine-induced brachial EDD (Makimattila et al., 1999). Clearly, we can infer from the above studies that LDL is one of the chief factors involved in endothelial dysfunction.
LDL and other lipoproteins are able to cross the endothelial cells layer by vascular transport, and later they are oxidatively modified at the sub-endothelial space into reactive oxygen species generated by macrophages, endothelial cells and smooth muscles (Steinberg, 1997). The accumulation of oxidized-LDL is toxic to endothelial cells, which in turn alters the function and structure of the endothelium (McVeigh et al., 1992; Tribe and Poston, 1996). Oxidized-LDL decreases NO production by reduction of NOS (Tribe and Poston, 1996) or by stimulating the synthesis of caveolin-I (Bist et al., 1997), consequently contributing to defective vasodilatation. In addition, there are indications that oxidized-LDL could also enhance the release of ET-1, a main endothelial constrictor peptide (Boulanger et al., 1992).

3.7 Mechanisms of endothelial dysfunction in T2DM

Over 170 million people in the world were affected by diabetes in 2000 and this is expected to increase to over 360 million by the year 2030 (Bakker et al., 2009; Ostergard et al., 2007). Type 1 diabetes is characterized by an absence of insulin while T2DM is characterized by insulin resistance followed in time with decreased plasma insulin. Vascular disease is the major cause of death in individuals with T2DM. The vascular complications of T2DM take two major forms; a) atherosclerosis in conduit arteries and b) microvascular dysfunction in skeletal muscle vascular beds. The vasodilatory effects of insulin account for up to 40% of insulin-mediated glucose disposal in skeletal muscle following a meal. In obesity and T2DM, the vasodilatory action of insulin is impaired. Insulin-stimulated NO production via the insulin-receptor substrate-1 (IRS-1) pathway is diminished, while vasoconstriction through the mitogen-activated protein kinase (MAPK) pathway, endothelin-converting enzyme (ECE) and subsequent secretion of the vasoconstrictor ET-1 may be augmented. As a result, microvascular blood flow and delivery of glucose to muscle tissue are diminished, contributing to reduced skeletal muscle glucose uptake and peripheral insulin resistance. Insulin resistance in T2DM appears to be the result of abnormal insulin-induced glucose uptake by skeletal muscle and microvascular dysfunction in skeletal muscle (blunted insulin-induced vasodilation).
Control of blood flow to skeletal muscle is abnormal in diabetes as muscle blood flow is less than normal during exercise in forearms of obese women (Hodnett and Hester, 2007), obese children (Ribeiro et al., 2005), in legs of diabetes subjects during cycle exercise (Hodnett and Hester, 2007; Kingwell et al., 2003), and in obese Zucker rats (Frisbee, 2003; Frisbee et al., 2006; Xiang et al., 2005). The abnormal control of vascular resistance in diabetes is associated with decreased arterial compliance, decreased microvascular density, altered smooth muscle dependent vascular reactivity and endothelial dysfunction (Frisbee et al., 2006; Hodnett and Hester, 2007). Local metabolic control of blood flow is abnormal and myogenic control of vascular smooth muscle tone is affected in diabetes as well. For instance, arterioles isolated from obese Zucker rat skeletal muscle exhibit increased spontaneous tone due to changes in vascular smooth muscle and to changes in an endothelium-derived factor (Frisbee et al., 2006). The endothelium of both conduit arteries and resistance arteries is dysfunctional in diabetes (Hodnett and Hester, 2007). Endothelial dysfunction in conduit arteries appears to be associated with decreased bio-availability of NO with sustained (or normal) eNOS content, decreased phospho-eNOS, deceased BH4 and cytochrome P450 expression as well as increased thromboxane (TXA_2) content. In the conduit arteries, endothelial dysfunction is

believed to contribute to development of atherosclerosis while in the resistance arteries endothelial dysfunction leads to disruptions in the control of blood flow as well as blunted angiogenesis and structural vascular remodeling (rarefaction)(Frisbee et al., 2006). In normal skeletal muscle insulin-mediated EDD-induced increases in blood flow are responsible for 25-50 % of the increase in glucose clearance stimulated by insulin administration (Kim et al., 2006). Thus, it appears that endothelial dysfunction of resistance arteries in muscle tissue includes blunted insulin-stimulated vasodilation (Mikus et al., 2010).

Endothelial dysfunction in T2DM is associated with glucotoxicity, lipotoxicity, and inflammation which impair insulin signaling (i.e. endothelial cell insulin resistance). These effects may be the result of cytokine signaling and/or increased ROS in the arteries. There are at least two sources of ROS believed to cause endothelial dysfunction in diabetes; a) hyperglycemia, and b) vascular inflammation (Kim et al., 2006; Luscher and Steffel, 2008). Kim et al (Kim et al., 2007) concluded that nutrient excess (excess glucose/lipid) stimulates cellular inflammatory responses that produce insulin resistance leading to decreased Akt and eNOS phosphorylation and increased NF-kB expression leading to expression of inflammatory cytokines in endothelial cells. For instance, Romero et al. (Romero et al., 2008) concluded that hyperglycemia plays a key role in increasing ROS in diabetes through stimulation of arginase activity/expresson in vascular cells. Insulin binding to its receptor signals through two distinct pathways in endothelial cells; a) activation of the IRS-1/phosphatidylinositol 3-kinase (PI3-kinase)/phosphor- Akt/phosphor-eNOS causing release of NO and EDD; b) increased release of ET-1through the mitogen-activated protein kinase (MAPK) pathway. Evidence indicates that T2DM produces an imbalance in the production of NO and ET-1 in response to insulin so that ET-1 release is up-regulated (Kim et al., 2006). It appears that when endothelium is insulin resistant, due to blunted signaling through the IRS-1/Akt/p-eNOS signaling pathway, ET-1 induced constriction leads to decreased muscle blood flow during insulin stimulation (Eringa et al., 2007).

4. Physical activity and type 2 diabetes: Focus on the endothelium

4.1 Benefits of physical activity

Physical activity may be beneficial in slowing the initiation and progression of T2DM and its cardiovascular sequelae through favorable effects on body weight, insulin sensitivity, glycemic control, blood pressure, lipid profile, fibrinolysis, inflammatory defense systems, and endothelial function. More comprehensive reviews regarding the beneficial effects and/or recommendations of physical activity in patients with T2DM have been previously published (Bassuk and Manson, 2005; Sanz et al., 2010; Stewart, 2002; Colberg, 2010). The following section is intended to present the available evidence of the beneficial effects of physical activity focusing on endothelial function. For instance, in clinical trials of patients with diabetes, physical activity (e.g. aerobic exercise) has been shown to increase vasodilator bioavailability (e.g. NO and prostacyclin) and to improve EDD (Moyna and Thompson, 2004, Roberts et al., 2002).

4.2 Acute effects of exercise

4.2.1 Aerobic exercise

Studies examining the acute effects of aerobic exercise training on endothelial function in T2DM are somewhat limited. A series of experiments examining the effects of a single bout of maximal (Colberg et al., 2003) and moderate (Colberg et al., 2006b) aerobic cycling exercise training found that baseline skin blood flow following local heating significantly increased following the exercise in subjects with T2DM (Colberg et al., 2003; Colberg et al., 2006b) and that this effect was independent of interstitial subcutaneous NO levels (Colberg et al., 2006b).

A study by Kingwell et al. (Kingwell et al., 2003) demonstrated that leg blood flow during aerobic cycling exercise and in response to acetylcholine infusion was significantly impaired in T2DM. Infusions of sodium nitroprusside were not different between diabetic subjects and weight-matched controls, suggesting that the impaired leg blood flow during aerobic exercise in T2DM was a result of endothelial dysfunction.

4.2.2 Resistance exercise

Even more limited are studies examining the acute effects of resistance exercise training on endothelial function in T2DM. Currently only one study has examined the acute effects of resistance exercise training on endothelial function in subjects with T2DM. Indeed, Colberg et al. (Colberg et al., 2006a) investigated whether 8-weeks of cycle-ergometery resistance exercise would affect cutaneous perfusion following local heating in T2DM subjects. Their results indicated that resistance exercise training does not significantly affect cutaneous perfusion, either at baseline or following local heating. This finding was independent of unchanged interstitial NO levels. More studies are needed in this area for a better understanding of how resistance exercise training affects the endothelium in T2DM.

4.3 Chronic effects of exercise training

4.3.1 Aerobic exercise

Very few studies exist examining the effects of chronic aerobic exercise training alone on endothelial function in T2DM. A positive association between aerobic status, skin blood flow, and endothelial function has been demonstrated in patients with T2DM (Colberg et al., 2002); however further studies from this same group revealed that 10 weeks of aerobic exercise training intervention does not improve impaired cutaneous perfusion (i.e. endothelial function) in patients with T2DM (Colberg et al., 2005).

Several human studies exist examining the combined effects of chronic aerobic and resistance exercise training on endothelial function in T2DM, but yield conflicting results. For instance, Mairoana et al. (Maiorana et al., 2001) found that 8 weeks of combined aerobic and resistance exercise training exerted a significant positive effect on conduit (i.e. brachial artery FMD) and resistance artery (i.e. forearm plethysmography) endothelial function in patients with diagnosed T2DM. Okada et al. (Okada et al., 2010) also found very recently that 3 months of combined chronic aerobic and resistance exercise training improved brachial FMD in patients with T2DM.

However, the study by Miche et al. (Miche et al., 2006) found that 4 weeks of combined aerobic and resistance exercise training had no effect on brachial artery endothelial function in patients with severe T2DM. Lastly Middlebrooke et al. (Middlebrooke et al., 2006) demonstrated in elderly patients with T2DM (60+ years of age) that 6 months of regular aerobic exercise training does not improve microvascular function (i.e. skin blood flow) or aerobic fitness. It should be noted that the patients in the Colberg et al. (Colberg et al., 2005), Miche et al. (Miche et al., 2006), and Middlebrooke et al. (Middlebrooke et al., 2006) studies had numerous other co-morbidities in addition to T2DM, thereby underscoring the importance of starting exercise training programs before the disease manifests into a complex, multidimensional condition that is difficult to treat. Further studies in humans are needed at this time to know whether chronic aerobic exercise training alone exerts beneficial effects on endothelial function during T2DM.

Current studies using the Otsuka Long-Evans Tokushima Fatty (OLETF) rat model of T2DM and obesity have revealed that chronic aerobic exercise training alone maintains endothelial function in conduit (i.e. aortic EDD) (Bunker et al., 2010) and resistance arteries (i.e. skeletal muscle arterioles) (Mikus et al., 2010) during the progression of T2DM. Other OLETF studies demonstrated the positive effect of chronic aerobic exercise training alone as a preventative measure for endothelial function (thoracic aorta and mesentery artery EDD) at single time-points during T2DM progression (Minami et al., 2002; Sakamoto et al., 1998). It is worth noting that the experimental design of the OLETF studies was such that aerobic exercise training served as a preventative measure for endothelial dysfunction associated with T2DM, whereas in the human studies discussed above it served as an interventional measure for endothelial dysfunction associated with T2DM. The findings thus far from long-term studies of aerobic exercise training alone collectively suggest that alterations in vascular NO bioavailability, due to direct or indirect changes in eNOS activity/expression, are contributing in part to endothelial dysfunction associated with T2DM.

4.3.2 Resistance exercise

The effects of chronic resistance exercise training on endothelial function are equally unclear at present. Chronic resistance exercise training alone has been shown to have little to no effect on skin blood flow and endothelial function in patients with T2DM (Colberg et al., 2006a). This study observed in ten individuals with T2DM and nine similar non-diabetic controls that 8 weeks of moderate-intensity resistance training did not enhance baseline skin blood perfusion or interstitial NO levels. Results from this study are in agreement with the studies by Miche et al. (Miche et al., 2006) and Middlebrooke et al. (Middlebrooke et al., 2006), discussed in the previous section (i.e. aerobic exercise), which showed that combined aerobic and resistance exercise training had no effect on endothelial function in T2DM.

However they conflict with a recent study conducted by Cohen et al. (Cohen et al., 2008) where 14-months of resistance exercise training alone significantly improved endothelial function in the skin of men and women with diagnosed T2DM. They also conflict with the Mairoana et al. (Maiorana et al., 2001) and Okada et al. (Okada et al., 2010) studies, discussed in the previous section, where combined aerobic and resistance exercise training was found to positively influence endothelial function in T2DM. At present it remains very unclear as to the effect of chronic resistance exercise training alone on endothelial function in T2DM and more studies are warranted in this area.

4.4 Physical activity: Mechanisms for its vascular benefits

The mechanisms responsible for the beneficial effects of physical activity on endothelium in T2DM are under intense investigation at this time. As for other forms of CVD, it is possible that exercise has beneficial effects on endothelial function directly due to the effects of shear stress or other hemodynamic effects of each exercise bout on the vascular wall or through effects of physical activity on systemic risk factors. For instance, exercise bouts influence circulating cytokines released by skeletal muscle and adipose tissues and can alter circulating lipid profiles. However, most in the field seem to consider that physical activity positively impacts the vascular wall directly via episodic increases in shear stress and

indirectly via reduction of comorbidities often associated with insulin resistance (i.e., hyperglycemia, hypercholesterolemia) (Joyner and Green, 2009).
It is known that endurance and interval sprint training enhance vascular function of the gastrocnemius, but not soleus, vasculature of healthy animals (Laughlin et al., 2004; McAllister, 2005) and that daily wheel running is sufficient to prevent the declines/changes in endothelial function associated with insulin resistance in feed arteries of skeletal muscles but effects in the aorta are less clear (Bunker et al, 2010). Physical activity also sustains insulin induced EDD (Mikus et al, 2010). Beneficial effects could also be the result of exercise-induced improvements in antioxidant systems in the vascular cells of the arteries, either endothelium or smooth muscle. It is important for research to establish the exact mechanisms so that exercise protocols can be designed to maximize these benefits.

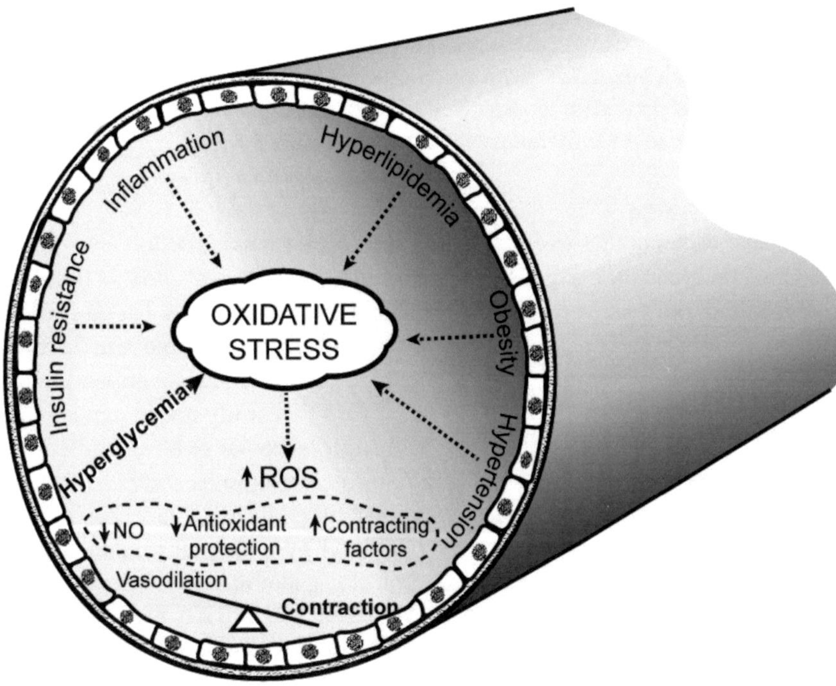

Fig. 1. Factors that participated in the pathogenesis of endothelial dysfunction in T2DM. NO; nitric oxide, ROS; reactive oxygen species.

5. Conclusion

Clearly, the information presented in this chapter emphasizes the major role of endothelial dysfunction in the development and/or progression of T2DM. However, the relationship of endothelial dysfunction and the many independent factors associated with T2DM (e.g. hyperglycemia, inflammation, hyperlipidemia, oxidative stress, insulin resistance, hypertension, obesity), presented in figure 1, is not completely understood. Furthermore, the precise mechanisms responsible for the beneficial effects of physical activity on the endothelium of individuals with T2DM are still under intense investigation. Obviously, more research is needed in this area, but we could speculate that the beneficial effects of exercise on endothelial function are due to the effects of shear stress and/or other hemodynamic effects acting directly on the vascular wall or through effects of physical activity on systemic risk factors.

6. Acknowledgment

This work was supported by National Institutes of Health Grant HL-35088.

7. References

Adair, T.H., Gay, W.J., Montani, J.P., 1990, Growth regulation of the vascular system: evidence for a metabolic hypothesis. Am J Physiol 259, R393-404.

Aggoun, Y., 2007, Obesity, metabolic syndrome, and cardiovascular disease. Pediatr Res 61, 653-659.

Aird, W.C., 2007a, Phenotypic heterogeneity of the endothelium: I. Structure, function, and mechanisms. Circ Res 100, 158-173.

Aird, W.C., 2007b, Phenotypic heterogeneity of the endothelium: II. Representative vascular beds. Circ Res 100, 174-190.

Anderson, T.J., Uehata, A., Gerhard, M.D., Meredith, I.T., Knab, S., Delagrange, D., Lieberman, E.H., Ganz, P., Creager, M.A., Yeung, A.C., et al., 1995, Close relation of endothelial function in the human coronary and peripheral circulations. J Am Coll Cardiol 26, 1235-1241.

Arcaro, G., Cretti, A., Balzano, S., Lechi, A., Muggeo, M., Bonora, E., Bonadonna, R.C., 2002, Insulin causes endothelial dysfunction in humans: sites and mechanisms. Circulation 105, 576-582.

Avogaro, A., Fadini, G.P., Gallo, A., Pagnin, E., de Kreutzenberg, S., 2006, Endothelial dysfunction in type 2 diabetes mellitus. Nutr Metab Cardiovasc Dis 16 Suppl 1, S39-45.

Bakker, W., Eringa, E.C., Sipkema, P., van Hinsbergh, V.W., 2009, Endothelial dysfunction and diabetes: roles of hyperglycemia, impaired insulin signaling and obesity. Cell and tissue research 335, 165-189.

Balligand, J.L., Feron, O., Dessy, C., 2009, eNOS activation by physical forces: from short-term regulation of contraction to chronic remodeling of cardiovascular tissues. Physiol Rev 89, 481-534.

Barnes, P.J., Liu, S.F., 1995, Regulation of pulmonary vascular tone. Pharmacol Rev 47, 87-131.

Baron, A.D., Clark, M.G., 1997, Role of blood flow in the regulation of muscle glucose uptake. Annu Rev Nutr 17, 487-499.

Bassuk, S.S., Manson, J.E., 2005, Epidemiological evidence for the role of physical activity in reducing risk of type 2 diabetes and cardiovascular disease. J Appl Physiol 99, 1193-1204.

Beckman, J.A., Goldfine, A.B., Gordon, M.B., Garrett, L.A., Keaney, J.F., Jr., Creager, M.A., 2003, Oral antioxidant therapy improves endothelial function in Type 1 but not Type 2 diabetes mellitus. Am J Physiol Heart Circ Physiol 285, H2392-2398.

Bist, A., Fielding, P.E., Fielding, C.J., 1997, Two sterol regulatory element-like sequences mediate up-regulation of caveolin gene transcription in response to low density lipoprotein free cholesterol. Proc Natl Acad Sci U S A 94, 10693-10698.

Boulanger, C.M., Tanner, F.C., Bea, M.L., Hahn, A.W., Werner, A., Luscher, T.F., 1992, Oxidized low density lipoproteins induce mRNA expression and release of endothelin from human and porcine endothelium. Circ Res 70, 1191-1197.

Bunker, A.K., Arce-Esquivel, A.A., Rector, R.S., Booth, F.W., Ibdah, J.A., Laughlin, M.H., 2010, Physical activity maintains aortic endothelium-dependent relaxation in the obese type 2 diabetic OLETF rat. Am J Physiol Heart Circ Physiol 298, H1889-1901.

Bunker, A.K., Laughlin, M.H., 2010, Influence of exercise and perivascular adipose tissue on coronary artery vasomotor function in a familial hypercholesterolemic porcine atherosclerosis model. J Appl Physiol 108, 490-497.

Campia, U., Sullivan, G., Bryant, M.B., Waclawiw, M.A., Quon, M.J., Panza, J.A., 2004, Insulin impairs endothelium-dependent vasodilation independent of insulin sensitivity or lipid profile. Am J Physiol Heart Circ Physiol 286, H76-82.

Ceriello, A., Esposito, K., Piconi, L., Ihnat, M.A., Thorpe, J.E., Testa, R., Boemi, M., Giugliano, D., 2008, Oscillating glucose is more deleterious to endothelial function and oxidative stress than mean glucose in normal and type 2 diabetic patients. Diabetes 57, 1349-1354.

Ceriello, A., Taboga, C., Tonutti, L., Quagliaro, L., Piconi, L., Bais, B., Da Ros, R., Motz, E., 2002, Evidence for an independent and cumulative effect of postprandial hypertriglyceridemia and hyperglycemia on endothelial dysfunction and oxidative stress generation: effects of short- and long-term simvastatin treatment. Circulation 106, 1211-1218.

Chao, C., Song, Y., Cook, N., Tseng, C.H., Manson, J.E., Eaton, C., Margolis, K.L., Rodriguez, B., Phillips, L.S., Tinker, L.F., Liu, S., 2010, The lack of utility of circulating biomarkers of inflammation and endothelial dysfunction for type 2 diabetes risk prediction among postmenopausal women: the Women's Health Initiative Observational Study. Arch Intern Med 170, 1557-1565.

Chatterjee, T.K., Stoll, L.L., Denning, G.M., Harrelson, A., Blomkalns, A.L., Idelman, G., Rothenberg, F.G., Neltner, B., Romig-Martin, S.A., Dickson, E.W., Rudich, S., Weintraub, N.L., 2009, Proinflammatory phenotype of perivascular adipocytes: influence of high-fat feeding. Circ Res 104, 541-549.

Cohen, N.D., Dunstan, D.W., Robinson, C., Vulikh, E., Zimmet, P.Z., Shaw, J.E., 2008, Improved endothelial function following a 14-month resistance exercise training program in adults with type 2 diabetes. Diabetes research and clinical practice 79, 405-411.

Cohen, R.A., Vanhoutte, P.M., 1995, Endothelium-dependent hyperpolarization. Beyond nitric oxide and cyclic GMP. Circulation 92, 3337-3349.

Colberg, S.R., Albright, A.L., Blissmer, B.J., Braun, B., Chasan-Taber, L., Fernhall, B., Regensteiner, J.G., Rubin, R.R., Sigal, R.J., 2010, Exercise and type 2 diabetes: American College of Sports Medicine and the American Diabetes Association: joint position statement. Exercise and type 2 diabetes. Medicine and science in sports and exercise 42, 2282-2303.

Colberg, S.R., Parson, H.K., Holton, D.R., Nunnold, T., Vinik, A.I., 2003, Cutaneous blood flow in type 2 diabetic individuals after an acute bout of maximal exercise. Diabetes Care 26, 1883-1888.

Colberg, S.R., Parson, H.K., Nunnold, T., Herriott, M.T., Vinik, A.I., 2006a, Effect of an 8-week resistance training program on cutaneous perfusion in type 2 diabetes. Microvasc Res 71, 121-127.

Colberg, S.R., Parson, H.K., Nunnold, T., Holton, D.R., Swain, D.P., Vinik, A.I., 2005, Change in cutaneous perfusion following 10 weeks of aerobic training in Type 2 diabetes. J Diabetes Complications 19, 276-283.

Colberg, S.R., Parson, H.K., Nunnold, T., Holton, D.R., Vinik, A.I., 2006b, Effect of a single bout of prior moderate exercise on cutaneous perfusion in type 2 diabetes. Diabetes Care 29, 2316-2318.

Colberg, S.R., Stansberry, K.B., McNitt, P.M., Vinik, A.I., 2002, Chronic exercise is associated with enhanced cutaneous blood flow in type 2 diabetes. J Diabetes Complications 16, 139-145.

Cook, S., Hugli, O., Egli, M., Menard, B., Thalmann, S., Sartori, C., Perrin, C., Nicod, P., Thorens, B., Vollenweider, P., Scherrer, U., Burcelin, R., 2004, Partial gene deletion of endothelial nitric oxide synthase predisposes to exaggerated high-fat diet-induced insulin resistance and arterial hypertension. Diabetes 53, 2067-2072.

Corretti, M.C., Plotnick, G.D., Vogel, R.A., 1995, Technical aspects of evaluating brachial artery vasodilatation using high-frequency ultrasound. Am J Physiol 268, H1397-1404.

De Caterina, R., 2000, Endothelial dysfunctions: common denominators in vascular disease. Curr Opin Lipidol 11, 9-23.

Drexler, H., Zeiher, A.M., Wollschlager, H., Meinertz, T., Just, H., Bonzel, T., 1989, Flow-dependent coronary artery dilatation in humans. Circulation 80, 466-474.

Duplain, H., Burcelin, R., Sartori, C., Cook, S., Egli, M., Lepori, M., Vollenweider, P., Pedrazzini, T., Nicod, P., Thorens, B., Scherrer, U., 2001, Insulin resistance, hyperlipidemia, and hypertension in mice lacking endothelial nitric oxide synthase. Circulation 104, 342-345.

Durante, W., Sen, A.K., Sunahara, F.A., 1988, Impairment of endothelium-dependent relaxation in aortae from spontaneously diabetic rats. Br J Pharmacol 94, 463-468.

Edwards, G., Dora, K.A., Gardener, M.J., Garland, C.J., Weston, A.H., 1998, K+ is an endothelium-derived hyperpolarizing factor in rat arteries. Nature 396, 269-272.

Eringa, E.C., Stehouwer, C.D., Roos, M.H., Westerhof, N., Sipkema, P., 2007, Selective resistance to vasoactive effects of insulin in muscle resistance arteries of obese Zucker (fa/fa) rats. Am J Physiol Endocrinol Metab 293, E1134-1139.

Feletou, M., Vanhoutte, P.M., 2004, EDHF: new therapeutic targets? Pharmacol Res 49, 565-580.

Ferreira, A.P., Oliveira, C.E., Franca, N.M., 2007, Metabolic syndrome and risk factors for cardiovascular disease in obese children: the relationship with insulin resistance (HOMA-IR). J Pediatr (Rio J) 83, 21-26.

Fichtlscherer, S., Dimmeler, S., Breuer, S., Busse, R., Zeiher, A.M., Fleming, I., 2004, Inhibition of cytochrome P450 2C9 improves endothelium-dependent, nitric oxide-mediated vasodilatation in patients with coronary artery disease. Circulation 109, 178-183.

Fisslthaler, B., Popp, R., Kiss, L., Potente, M., Harder, D.R., Fleming, I., Busse, R., 1999, Cytochrome P450 2C is an EDHF synthase in coronary arteries. Nature 401, 493-497.

Ford, E.S., Giles, W.H., Dietz, W.H., 2002, Prevalence of the metabolic syndrome among US adults: findings from the third National Health and Nutrition Examination Survey. JAMA 287, 356-359.

Franklin, V.L., Khan, F., Kennedy, G., Belch, J.J., Greene, S.A., 2008, Intensive insulin therapy improves endothelial function and microvascular reactivity in young people with type 1 diabetes. Diabetologia 51, 353-360.

Frisbee, J.C., 2003, Impaired skeletal muscle perfusion in obese Zucker rats. American journal of physiology 285, R1124-1134.

Frisbee, J.C., Samora, J.B., Peterson, J., Bryner, R., 2006, Exercise training blunts microvascular rarefaction in the metabolic syndrome. Am J Physiol Heart Circ Physiol 291, H2483-2492.

Furchgott, R.F., Vanhoutte, P.M., 1989, Endothelium-derived relaxing and contracting factors. FASEB J 3, 2007-2018.

Ganz, P., Vita, J.A., 2003, Testing endothelial vasomotor function: nitric oxide, a multipotent molecule. Circulation 108, 2049-2053.

Genuth, S., Alberti, K.G., Bennett, P., Buse, J., Defronzo, R., Kahn, R., Kitzmiller, J., Knowler, W.C., Lebovitz, H., Lernmark, A., Nathan, D., Palmer, J., Rizza, R., Saudek, C., Shaw, J., Steffes, M., Stern, M., Tuomilehto, J., Zimmet, P., 2003, Follow-up report on the diagnosis of diabetes mellitus. Diabetes Care 26, 3160-3167.

Giugliano, D., Ceriello, A., Paolisso, G., 1996, Oxidative stress and diabetic vascular complications. Diabetes Care 19, 257-267.

Grau, A.J., Buggle, F., Becher, H., Werle, E., Hacke, W., 1996, The association of leukocyte count, fibrinogen and C-reactive protein with vascular risk factors and ischemic vascular diseases. Thromb Res 82, 245-255.

Grundy, S.M., Cleeman, J.I., Daniels, S.R., Donato, K.A., Eckel, R.H., Franklin, B.A., Gordon, D.J., Krauss, R.M., Savage, P.J., Smith Jr, S.C., Spertus, J.A., Costa, F., 2005, Diagnosis and management of the metabolic syndrome. An American Heart Association/National Heart, Lung, and Blood Institute Scientific Statement. Executive summary. Cardiol Rev 13, 322-327.

Gupta, R., Deedwania, P.C., Gupta, A., Rastogi, S., Panwar, R.B., Kothari, K., 2004, Prevalence of metabolic syndrome in an Indian urban population. Int J Cardiol 97, 257-261.

Hartge, M.M., Kintscher, U., Unger, T., 2006, Endothelial dysfunction and its role in diabetic vascular disease. Endocrinol Metab Clin North Am 35, 551-560, viii-ix.

Haynes, W.G., Webb, D.J., 1998, Endothelin as a regulator of cardiovascular function in health and disease. J Hypertens 16, 1081-1098.

Hodnett, B.L., Hester, R.L., 2007, Regulation of muscle blood flow in obesity. Microcirculation 14, 273-288.

Horvath, E.M., Benko, R., Kiss, L., Muranyi, M., Pek, T., Fekete, K., Barany, T., Somlai, A., Csordas, A., Szabo, C., 2009, Rapid 'glycaemic swings' induce nitrosative stress, activate poly(ADP-ribose) polymerase and impair endothelial function in a rat model of diabetes mellitus. Diabetologia 52, 952-961.

Hotamisligil, G.S., Shargill, N.S., Spiegelman, B.M., 1993, Adipose expression of tumor necrosis factor-alpha: direct role in obesity-linked insulin resistance. Science 259, 87-91.

Hubert, H.B., Feinleib, M., McNamara, P.M., Castelli, W.P., 1983, Obesity as an independent risk factor for cardiovascular disease: a 26-year follow-up of participants in the Framingham Heart Study. Circulation 67, 968-977.

Hull, S.S., Jr., Kaiser, L., Jaffe, M.D., Sparks, H.V., Jr., 1986, Endothelium-dependent flow-induced dilation of canine femoral and saphenous arteries. Blood Vessels 23, 183-198.

Irani, K., 2000, Oxidant signaling in vascular cell growth, death, and survival : a review of the roles of reactive oxygen species in smooth muscle and endothelial cell mitogenic and apoptotic signaling. Circ Res 87, 179-183.

Joyner, M.J., Green, D.J., 2009, Exercise protects the cardiovascular system: effects beyond traditional risk factors. The Journal of physiology 587, 5551-5558.

Kahn, R., Buse, J., Ferrannini, E., Stern, M., 2005, The metabolic syndrome: time for a critical appraisal: joint statement from the American Diabetes Association and the European Association for the Study of Diabetes. Diabetes Care 28, 2289-2304.

Ketonen, J., Shi, J., Martonen, E., Mervaala, E., 2010, Periadventitial adipose tissue promotes endothelial dysfunction via oxidative stress in diet-induced obese C57Bl/6 mice. Circ J 74, 1479-1487.

Kim, F., Pham, M., Luttrell, I., Bannerman, D.D., Tupper, J., Thaler, J., Hawn, T.R., Raines, E.W., Schwartz, M.W., 2007, Toll-like receptor-4 mediates vascular inflammation and insulin resistance in diet-induced obesity. Circ Res 100, 1589-1596.

Kim, J.A., Montagnani, M., Koh, K.K., Quon, M.J., 2006, Reciprocal relationships between insulin resistance and endothelial dysfunction: molecular and pathophysiological mechanisms. Circulation 113, 1888-1904.

Kingwell, B.A., Formosa, M., Muhlmann, M., Bradley, S.J., McConell, G.K., 2003, Type 2 diabetic individuals have impaired leg blood flow responses to exercise: role of endothelium-dependent vasodilation. Diabetes Care 26, 899-904.

Klein, S., Burke, L.E., Bray, G.A., Blair, S., Allison, D.B., Pi-Sunyer, X., Hong, Y., Eckel, R.H., 2004, Clinical implications of obesity with specific focus on cardiovascular disease: a statement for professionals from the American Heart Association Council on Nutrition, Physical Activity, and Metabolism: endorsed by the American College of Cardiology Foundation. Circulation 110, 2952-2967.

Koedel, U., Lorenzl, S., Gorriz, C., Arendt, R.M., Pfister, H.W., 1998, Endothelin B receptor-mediated increase of cerebral blood flow in experimental pneumococcal meningitis. J Cereb Blood Flow Metab 18, 67-74.

Korth, P., Bohle, R.M., Corvol, P., Pinet, F., 1999, Cellular distribution of endothelin-converting enzyme-1 in human tissues. J Histochem Cytochem 47, 447-462.

Kuo, L., Chilian, W.M., Davis, M.J., 1991, Interaction of pressure- and flow-induced responses in porcine coronary resistance vessels. Am J Physiol 261, H1706-1715.

Laight, D.W., Carrier, M.J., Anggard, E.E., 1999, Endothelial cell dysfunction and the pathogenesis of diabetic macroangiopathy. Diabetes Metab Res Rev 15, 274-282.

Lakka, H.M., Laaksonen, D.E., Lakka, T.A., Niskanen, L.K., Kumpusalo, E., Tuomilehto, J., Salonen, J.T., 2002, The metabolic syndrome and total and cardiovascular disease mortality in middle-aged men. JAMA 288, 2709-2716.

Lam, H.C., 2001, Role of endothelin in diabetic vascular complications. Endocrine 14, 277-284.

Larsson, B., Svardsudd, K., Welin, L., Wilhelmsen, L., Bjorntorp, P., Tibblin, G., 1984, Abdominal adipose tissue distribution, obesity, and risk of cardiovascular disease and death: 13 year follow up of participants in the study of men born in 1913. Br Med J (Clin Res Ed) 288, 1401-1404.

Laughlin, M.H., Newcomer, S.C., Bender, S.B., 2008, Importance of hemodynamic forces as signals for exercise-induced changes in endothelial cell phenotype. J Appl Physiol 104, 588-600.

Laughlin, M.H., Pollock, J.S., Amann, J.F., Hollis, M.L., Woodman, C.R., Price, E.M., 2001, Training induces nonuniform increases in eNOS content along the coronary arterial tree. J Appl Physiol 90, 501-510.

Laughlin, M.H., Rubin, L.J., Rush, J.W., Price, E.M., Schrage, W.G., Woodman, C.R., 2003, Short-term training enhances endothelium-dependent dilation of coronary arteries, not arterioles. J Appl Physiol 94, 234-244.

Laughlin, M.H., Woodman, C.R., Schrage, W.G., Gute, D., Price, E.M., 2004, Interval sprint training enhances endothelial function and eNOS content in some arteries that perfuse white gastrocnemius muscle. J Appl Physiol 96, 233-244.

Laurindo, F.R., Pedro Mde, A., Barbeiro, H.V., Pileggi, F., Carvalho, M.H., Augusto, O., da Luz, P.L., 1994, Vascular free radical release. Ex vivo and in vivo evidence for a flow-dependent endothelial mechanism. Circ Res 74, 700-709.

Lebovitz, H.E., 2001, Insulin resistance: definition and consequences. Exp Clin Endocrinol Diabetes 109 Suppl 2, S135-148.

Lehrke, M., Lazar, M.A., 2004, Inflamed about obesity. Nat Med 10, 126-127.

Lie, M., Sejersted, O.M., Kiil, F., 1970, Local regulation of vascular cross section during changes in femoral arterial blood flow in dogs. Circ Res 27, 727-737.

Liu, H., Colavitti, R., Rovira, II, Finkel, T., 2005, Redox-dependent transcriptional regulation. Circ Res 97, 967-974.

Loesch, A., 2005, Localisation of endothelin-1 and its receptors in vascular tissue as seen at the electron microscopic level. Curr Vasc Pharmacol 3, 381-392.

Luscher, T.F., Noll, G., 1996, Endothelial function as an end-point in interventional trials: concepts, methods and current data. J Hypertens Suppl 14, S111-119; discussion S119-121.

Luscher, T.F., Steffel, J., 2008, Sweet and sour: unraveling diabetic vascular disease. Circ Res 102, 9-11.

Ma, L., Ma, S., He, H., Yang, D., Chen, X., Luo, Z., Liu, D., Zhu, Z., 2010, Perivascular fat-mediated vascular dysfunction and remodeling through the AMPK/mTOR pathway in high-fat diet-induced obese rats. Hypertens Res 33, 446-453.

Maeda, S., Miyauchi, T., Iemitsu, M., Tanabe, T., Irukayama-Tomobe, Y., Goto, K., Yamaguchi, I., Matsuda, M., 2002, Involvement of endogenous endothelin-1 in exercise-induced redistribution of tissue blood flow: an endothelin receptor antagonist reduces the redistribution. Circulation 106, 2188-2193.

Maejima, K., Nakano, S., Himeno, M., Tsuda, S., Makiishi, H., Ito, T., Nakagawa, A., Kigoshi, T., Ishibashi, T., Nishio, M., Uchida, K., 2001, Increased basal levels of plasma nitric oxide in Type 2 diabetic subjects. Relationship to microvascular complications. J Diabetes Complications 15, 135-143.

Magi, L., Stramenga, C., Morosini, P., 2005, [Prevalence of the metabolic syndrome among Italian adults. Findings from the SIMAP study]. Recenti Prog Med 96, 280-283.

Maiorana, A., O'Driscoll, G., Cheetham, C., Dembo, L., Stanton, K., Goodman, C., Taylor, R., Green, D., 2001, The effect of combined aerobic and resistance exercise training on vascular function in type 2 diabetes. J Am Coll Cardiol 38, 860-866.

Makimattila, S., Liu, M.L., Vakkilainen, J., Schlenzka, A., Lahdenpera, S., Syvanne, M., Mantysaari, M., Summanen, P., Bergholm, R., Taskinen, M.R., Yki-Jarvinen, H., 1999, Impaired endothelium-dependent vasodilation in type 2 diabetes. Relation to LDL size, oxidized LDL, and antioxidants. Diabetes Care 22, 973-981.

Malek, A.M., Alper, S.L., Izumo, S., 1999, Hemodynamic shear stress and its role in atherosclerosis. JAMA 282, 2035-2042.

Malik, S., Wong, N.D., Franklin, S.S., Kamath, T.V., L'Italien, G.J., Pio, J.R., Williams, G.R., 2004, Impact of the metabolic syndrome on mortality from coronary heart disease, cardiovascular disease, and all causes in United States adults. Circulation 110, 1245-1250.

Masaki, T., 2004, Historical review: Endothelin. Trends Pharmacol Sci 25, 219-224.

McAllister, R.M., Jasperse, J.L., Laughlin, M.H., 2005, Nonuniform effects of endurance exercise training on vasodilation in rat skeletal muscle. J Appl Physiol 98, 753-761.

McNeill, A.M., Katz, R., Girman, C.J., Rosamond, W.D., Wagenknecht, L.E., Barzilay, J.I., Tracy, R.P., Savage, P.J., Jackson, S.A., 2006, Metabolic syndrome and cardiovascular disease in older people: The cardiovascular health study. J Am Geriatr Soc 54, 1317-1324.

McVeigh, G.E., Brennan, G.M., Johnston, G.D., McDermott, B.J., McGrath, L.T., Henry, W.R., Andrews, J.W., Hayes, J.R., 1992, Impaired endothelium-dependent and independent vasodilation in patients with type 2 (non-insulin-dependent) diabetes mellitus. Diabetologia 35, 771-776.

Meigs, J.B., Hu, F.B., Rifai, N., Manson, J.E., 2004, Biomarkers of endothelial dysfunction and risk of type 2 diabetes mellitus. JAMA 291, 1978-1986.

Meigs, J.B., O'Donnell C, J., Tofler, G.H., Benjamin, E.J., Fox, C.S., Lipinska, I., Nathan, D.M., Sullivan, L.M., D'Agostino, R.B., Wilson, P.W., 2006, Hemostatic markers of endothelial dysfunction and risk of incident type 2 diabetes: the Framingham Offspring Study. Diabetes 55, 530-537.

Merkus, D., Houweling, B., Mirza, A., Boomsma, F., van den Meiracker, A.H., Duncker, D.J., 2003, Contribution of endothelin and its receptors to the regulation of vascular tone during exercise is different in the systemic, coronary and pulmonary circulation. Cardiovasc Res 59, 745-754.

Miche, E., Herrmann, G., Nowak, M., Wirtz, U., Tietz, M., Hurst, M., Zoller, B., Radzewitz, A., 2006, Effect of an exercise training program on endothelial dysfunction in diabetic and non-diabetic patients with severe chronic heart failure. Clin Res Cardiol 95 Suppl 1, i117-124.

Middlebrooke, A.R., Elston, L.M., Macleod, K.M., Mawson, D.M., Ball, C.I., Shore, A.C., Tooke, J.E., 2006, Six months of aerobic exercise does not improve microvascular function in type 2 diabetes mellitus. Diabetologia 49, 2263-2271.

Mikus, C.R., Rector, R.S., Arce-Esquivel, A.A., Libla, J.L., Booth, F.W., Ibdah, J.A., Laughlin, M.H., Thyfault, J.P., 2010, Daily physical activity enhances reactivity to insulin in skeletal muscle arterioles of hyperphagic Otsuka Long-Evans Tokushima Fatty rats. J Appl Physiol 109, 1203-1210.

Minami, A., Ishimura, N., Harada, N., Sakamoto, S., Niwa, Y., Nakaya, Y., 2002, Exercise training improves acetylcholine-induced endothelium-dependent hyperpolarization in type 2 diabetic rats, Otsuka Long-Evans Tokushima fatty rats. Atherosclerosis 162, 85-92.

Miura, H., Bosnjak, J.J., Ning, G., Saito, T., Miura, M., Gutterman, D.D., 2003, Role for hydrogen peroxide in flow-induced dilation of human coronary arterioles. Circ Res 92, e31-40.

Miura, H., Liu, Y., Gutterman, D.D., 1999, Human coronary arteriolar dilation to bradykinin depends on membrane hyperpolarization: contribution of nitric oxide and Ca2+-activated K+ channels. Circulation 99, 3132-3138.

Miura, H., Wachtel, R.E., Liu, Y., Loberiza, F.R., Jr., Saito, T., Miura, M., Gutterman, D.D., 2001, Flow-induced dilation of human coronary arterioles: important role of Ca(2+)-activated K(+) channels. Circulation 103, 1992-1998.

Monnier, L., Mas, E., Ginet, C., Michel, F., Villon, L., Cristol, J.P., Colette, C., 2006, Activation of oxidative stress by acute glucose fluctuations compared with sustained chronic hyperglycemia in patients with type 2 diabetes. JAMA 295, 1681-1687.

Mottillo, S., Filion, K.B., Genest, J., Joseph, L., Pilote, L., Poirier, P., Rinfret, S., Schiffrin, E.L., Eisenberg, M.J., The metabolic syndrome and cardiovascular risk a systematic review and meta-analysis. J Am Coll Cardiol 56, 1113-1132.

Moyna, N.M., Thompson, P.D., 2004, The effect of physical activity on endothelial function in man. Acta Physiol Scand 180, 113-123.

Ness, J., Nassimiha, D., Feria, M.I., Aronow, W.S., 1999, Diabetes mellitus in older African-Americans, Hispanics, and whites in an academic hospital-based geriatrics practice. Coron Artery Dis 10, 343-346.

Node, K., Inoue, T., 2009, Postprandial hyperglycemia as an etiological factor in vascular failure. Cardiovasc Diabetol 8, 23.

Okada, S., Hiuge, A., Makino, H., Nagumo, A., Takaki, H., Konishi, H., Goto, Y., Yoshimasa, Y., Miyamoto, Y., 2010, Effect of exercise intervention on endothelial function and incidence of cardiovascular disease in patients with type 2 diabetes. Journal of atherosclerosis and thrombosis 17, 828-833.

Ostergard, T., Jessen, N., Schmitz, O., Mandarino, L.J., 2007, The effect of exercise, training, and inactivity on insulin sensitivity in diabetics and their relatives: what is new? Applied physiology, nutrition, and metabolism = Physiologie appliquee, nutrition et metabolisme 32, 541-548.

Palmer, R.M., Ashton, D.S., Moncada, S., 1988a, Vascular endothelial cells synthesize nitric oxide from L-arginine. Nature 333, 664-666.

Palmer, R.M., Ferrige, A.G., Moncada, S., 1987, Nitric oxide release accounts for the biological activity of endothelium-derived relaxing factor. Nature 327, 524-526.

Palmer, R.M., Rees, D.D., Ashton, D.S., Moncada, S., 1988b, L-arginine is the physiological precursor for the formation of nitric oxide in endothelium-dependent relaxation. Biochem Biophys Res Commun 153, 1251-1256.

Pannirselvam, M., Verma, S., Anderson, T.J., Triggle, C.R., 2002, Cellular basis of endothelial dysfunction in small mesenteric arteries from spontaneously diabetic (db/db -/-) mice: role of decreased tetrahydrobiopterin bioavailability. Br J Pharmacol 136, 255-263.

Park, Y.W., Zhu, S., Palaniappan, L., Heshka, S., Carnethon, M.R., Heymsfield, S.B., 2003, The metabolic syndrome: prevalence and associated risk factor findings in the US population from the Third National Health and Nutrition Examination Survey, 1988-1994. Arch Intern Med 163, 427-436.

Pasceri, V., Willerson, J.T., Yeh, E.T., 2000, Direct proinflammatory effect of C-reactive protein on human endothelial cells. Circulation 102, 2165-2168.

Payne, G.A., Bohlen, H.G., Dincer, U.D., Borbouse, L., Tune, J.D., 2009, Periadventitial adipose tissue impairs coronary endothelial function via PKC-beta-dependent phosphorylation of nitric oxide synthase. Am J Physiol Heart Circ Physiol 297, H460-465.

Payne, G.A., Borbouse, L., Kumar, S., Neeb, Z., Alloosh, M., Sturek, M., Tune, J.D., 2010, Epicardial perivascular adipose-derived leptin exacerbates coronary endothelial dysfunction in metabolic syndrome via a protein kinase C-beta pathway. Arterioscler Thromb Vasc Biol 30, 1711-1717.

Piconi, L., Quagliaro, L., Da Ros, R., Assaloni, R., Giugliano, D., Esposito, K., Szabo, C., Ceriello, A., 2004, Intermittent high glucose enhances ICAM-1, VCAM-1, E-selectin and interleukin-6 expression in human umbilical endothelial cells in culture: the role of poly(ADP-ribose) polymerase. J Thromb Haemost 2, 1453-1459.

Pieper, G.M., Langenstroer, P., Siebeneich, W., 1997, Diabetic-induced endothelial dysfunction in rat aorta: role of hydroxyl radicals. Cardiovasc Res 34, 145-156.

Pohl, U., Herlan, K., Huang, A., Bassenge, E., 1991, EDRF-mediated shear-induced dilation opposes myogenic vasoconstriction in small rabbit arteries. Am J Physiol 261, H2016-2023.

Poirier, P., Giles, T.D., Bray, G.A., Hong, Y., Stern, J.S., Pi-Sunyer, F.X., Eckel, R.H., 2006, Obesity and cardiovascular disease: pathophysiology, evaluation, and effect of weight loss: an update of the 1997 American Heart Association Scientific Statement on Obesity and Heart Disease from the Obesity Committee of the Council on Nutrition, Physical Activity, and Metabolism. Circulation 113, 898-918.

Rask-Madsen, C., Ihlemann, N., Krarup, T., Christiansen, E., Kober, L., Nervil Kistorp, C., Torp-Pedersen, C., 2001, Insulin therapy improves insulin-stimulated endothelial function in patients with type 2 diabetes and ischemic heart disease. Diabetes 50, 2611-2618.

Ribeiro, M.M., Silva, A.G., Santos, N.S., Guazzelle, I., Matos, L.N., Trombetta, I.C., Halpern, A., Negrao, C.E., Villares, S.M., 2005, Diet and exercise training restore blood pressure and vasodilatory responses during physiological maneuvers in obese children. Circulation 111, 1915-1923.

Roberts, C.K., Vaziri, N.D., Barnard, R.J., 2002, Effect of diet and exercise intervention on blood pressure, insulin, oxidative stress, and nitric oxide availability. Circulation 106, 2530-2532.

Rodriguez, C.J., Miyake, Y., Grahame-Clarke, C., Di Tullio, M.R., Sciacca, R.R., Boden-Albala, B., Sacco, R.L., Homma, S., 2005, Relation of plasma glucose and endothelial function in a population-based multiethnic sample of subjects without diabetes mellitus. Am J Cardiol 96, 1273-1277.

Romero, M.J., Platt, D.H., Tawfik, H.E., Labazi, M., El-Remessy, A.B., Bartoli, M., Caldwell, R.B., Caldwell, R.W., 2008, Diabetes-induced coronary vascular dysfunction involves increased arginase activity. Circ Res 102, 95-102.

Rosen, P., Ballhausen, T., Bloch, W., Addicks, K., 1995, Endothelial relaxation is disturbed by oxidative stress in the diabetic rat heart: influence of tocopherol as antioxidant. Diabetologia 38, 1157-1168.

Rosito, G.A., Massaro, J.M., Hoffmann, U., Ruberg, F.L., Mahabadi, A.A., Vasan, R.S., O'Donnell, C.J., Fox, C.S., 2008, Pericardial fat, visceral abdominal fat, cardiovascular disease risk factors, and vascular calcification in a community-based sample: the Framingham Heart Study. Circulation 117, 605-613.

Rubanyi, G.M., Polokoff, M.A., 1994, Endothelins: molecular biology, biochemistry, pharmacology, physiology, and pathophysiology. Pharmacol Rev 46, 325-415.

Rubanyi, G.M., Romero, J.C., Vanhoutte, P.M., 1986, Flow-induced release of endothelium-derived relaxing factor. Am J Physiol 250, H1145-1149.

Sacks, H.S., Fain, J.N., 2007, Human epicardial adipose tissue: a review. Am Heart J 153, 907-917.

Sakamoto, S., Minami, K., Niwa, Y., Ohnaka, M., Nakaya, Y., Mizuno, A., Kuwajima, M., Shima, K., 1998, Effect of exercise training and food restriction on endothelium-dependent relaxation in the Otsuka Long-Evans Tokushima Fatty rat, a model of spontaneous NIDDM. Diabetes 47, 82-86.

Sanz, C., Gautier, J.F., Hanaire, H., 2010 Physical exercise for the prevention and treatment of type 2 diabetes. Diabetes Metab 36, 346-351.

Schalkwijk, C.G., Stehouwer, C.D., 2005, Vascular complications in diabetes mellitus: the role of endothelial dysfunction. Clin Sci (Lond) 109, 143-159.

Schiffrin, E.L., Touyz, R.M., 1998, Vascular biology of endothelin. J Cardiovasc Pharmacol 32 Suppl 3, S2-13.

Schneider, M.P., Boesen, E.I., Pollock, D.M., 2007, Contrasting actions of endothelin ET(A) and ET(B) receptors in cardiovascular disease. Annu Rev Pharmacol Toxicol 47, 731-759.

Schofield, I., Malik, R., Izzard, A., Austin, C., Heagerty, A., 2002, Vascular structural and functional changes in type 2 diabetes mellitus: evidence for the roles of abnormal myogenic responsiveness and dyslipidemia. Circulation 106, 3037-3043.

Selig, W.M., Noonan, T.C., Kern, D.F., Malik, A.B., 1986, Pulmonary microvascular responses to arachidonic acid in isolated perfused guinea pig lung. J Appl Physiol 60, 1972-1979.

Shi, Y., So, K.F., Man, R.Y., Vanhoutte, P.M., 2007, Oxygen-derived free radicals mediate endothelium-dependent contractions in femoral arteries of rats with streptozotocin-induced diabetes. Br J Pharmacol 152, 1033-1041.

Shi, Y., Vanhoutte, P.M., 2009, Reactive oxygen-derived free radicals are key to the endothelial dysfunction of diabetes. J Diabetes 1, 151-162.

Shurtz-Swirski, R., Sela, S., Herskovits, A.T., Shasha, S.M., Shapiro, G., Nasser, L., Kristal, B., 2001, Involvement of peripheral polymorphonuclear leukocytes in oxidative stress and inflammation in type 2 diabetic patients. Diabetes Care 24, 104-110.

Singhal, A., 2005, Endothelial dysfunction: role in obesity-related disorders and the early origins of CVD. Proc Nutr Soc 64, 15-22.

Sinoway, L.I., Hendrickson, C., Davidson, W.R., Jr., Prophet, S., Zelis, R., 1989, Characteristics of flow-mediated brachial artery vasodilation in human subjects. Circ Res 64, 32-42.

Sorop, O., Spaan, J.A., Sweeney, T.E., VanBavel, E., 2003, Effect of steady versus oscillating flow on porcine coronary arterioles: involvement of NO and superoxide anion. Circ Res 92, 1344-1351.

Spitaler, M.M., Graier, W.F., 2002, Vascular targets of redox signalling in diabetes mellitus. Diabetologia 45, 476-494.

Srinivasan, S., Hatley, M.E., Bolick, D.T., Palmer, L.A., Edelstein, D., Brownlee, M., Hedrick, C.C., 2004, Hyperglycaemia-induced superoxide production decreases eNOS expression via AP-1 activation in aortic endothelial cells. Diabetologia 47, 1727-1734.

Stamler, J., Vaccaro, O., Neaton, J.D., Wentworth, D., 1993, Diabetes, other risk factors, and 12-yr cardiovascular mortality for men screened in the Multiple Risk Factor Intervention Trial. Diabetes Care 16, 434-444.

Steinberg, D., 1997, Low density lipoprotein oxidation and its pathobiological significance. J Biol Chem 272, 20963-20966.

Stewart, K.J., 2002, Exercise training and the cardiovascular consequences of type 2 diabetes and hypertension: plausible mechanisms for improving cardiovascular health. JAMA 288, 1622-1631.

Su, Y., Liu, X.M., Sun, Y.M., Wang, Y.Y., Luan, Y., Wu, Y., 2008, Endothelial dysfunction in impaired fasting glycemia, impaired glucose tolerance, and type 2 diabetes mellitus. Am J Cardiol 102, 497-498.

Taha, D., Ahmed, O., bin Sadiq, B., 2009, The prevalence of metabolic syndrome and cardiovascular risk factors in a group of obese Saudi children and adolescents: a hospital-based study. Ann Saudi Med 29, 357-360.

Taylor, P.D., Poston, L., 1994, The effect of hyperglycaemia on function of rat isolated mesenteric resistance artery. Br J Pharmacol 113, 801-808.

Tesfamariam, B., 1994, Free radicals in diabetic endothelial cell dysfunction. Free Radic Biol Med 16, 383-391.

Tesfamariam, B., Cohen, R.A., 1992, Free radicals mediate endothelial cell dysfunction caused by elevated glucose. Am J Physiol 263, H321-326.

Thorand, B., Baumert, J., Chambless, L., Meisinger, C., Kolb, H., Doring, A., Lowel, H., Koenig, W., 2006, Elevated markers of endothelial dysfunction predict type 2 diabetes mellitus in middle-aged men and women from the general population. Arterioscler Thromb Vasc Biol 26, 398-405.

Title, L.M., Cummings, P.M., Giddens, K., Nassar, B.A., 2000, Oral glucose loading acutely attenuates endothelium-dependent vasodilation in healthy adults without diabetes: an effect prevented by vitamins C and E. J Am Coll Cardiol 36, 2185-2191.

Tribe, R.M., Poston, L., 1996, Oxidative stress and lipids in diabetes: a role in endothelium vasodilator dysfunction? Vasc Med 1, 195-206.

Triggle, C.R., Hollenberg, M., Anderson, T.J., Ding, H., Jiang, Y., Ceroni, L., Wiehler, W.B., Ng, E.S., Ellis, A., Andrews, K., McGuire, J.J., Pannirselvam, M., 2003, The endothelium in health and disease--a target for therapeutic intervention. J Smooth Muscle Res 39, 249-267.

Vanhoutte, P.M., 1989, Endothelium and control of vascular function. State of the Art lecture. Hypertension 13, 658-667.

Vehkavaara, S., Makimattila, S., Schlenzka, A., Vakkilainen, J., Westerbacka, J., Yki-Jarvinen, H., 2000, Insulin therapy improves endothelial function in type 2 diabetes. Arterioscler Thromb Vasc Biol 20, 545-550.

Venugopal, S.K., Devaraj, S., Yuhanna, I., Shaul, P., Jialal, I., 2002, Demonstration that C-reactive protein decreases eNOS expression and bioactivity in human aortic endothelial cells. Circulation 106, 1439-1441.

Wagner, O.F., Christ, G., Wojta, J., Vierhapper, H., Parzer, S., Nowotny, P.J., Schneider, B., Waldhausl, W., Binder, B.R., 1992, Polar secretion of endothelin-1 by cultured endothelial cells. J Biol Chem 267, 16066-16068.

Watkins, P.J., 2003, Cardiovascular disease, hypertension, and lipids. BMJ 326, 874-876.

Watts, G.F., O'Brien, S.F., Silvester, W., Millar, J.A., 1996, Impaired endothelium-dependent and independent dilatation of forearm resistance arteries in men with diet-treated non-insulin-dependent diabetes: role of dyslipidaemia. Clin Sci (Lond) 91, 567-573.

Webb, D.J., Haynes, W.G., 1995, The role of endothelin-1 in cardiovascular physiology and pathophysiology. Scott Med J 40, 69-71.

Williams, S.B., Cusco, J.A., Roddy, M.A., Johnstone, M.T., Creager, M.A., 1996, Impaired nitric oxide-mediated vasodilation in patients with non-insulin-dependent diabetes mellitus. J Am Coll Cardiol 27, 567-574.

Wilson, P.W., D'Agostino, R.B., Parise, H., Sullivan, L., Meigs, J.B., 2005, Metabolic syndrome as a precursor of cardiovascular disease and type 2 diabetes mellitus. Circulation 112, 3066-3072.

Xiang, L., Naik, J., Hester, R.L., 2005, Exercise-induced increase in skeletal muscle vasodilatory responses in obese Zucker rats. American journal of physiology 288, R987-991.

Yang, G., Lucas, R., Caldwell, R., Yao, L., Romero, M.J., Caldwell, R.W., 2010 Novel mechanisms of endothelial dysfunction in diabetes. J Cardiovasc Dis Res 1, 59-63.

Part 3

Hypertension, Nephropathy and Diabetes

11

Antihypertensive Treatment in Type 2 Diabetic Patients

Angelo Michele Carella
Department of Internal Medicine "T. Masselli-Mascia" Hospital
San Severo (Foggia)
Italy

1. Introduction

Hypertension is an heterogeneous disease in which both genetic and environmental factors play a relevant role. Among the major environmental determinants of essential hypertension are high alcohol consumption, physical inactivity, overweight, smoking and dietary factors, in particular animal fats, salt, and potassium intake (Binder A, 2007; Staessen et al, 2003). Worldwide prevalence estimates for hypertension may be as much as 1 billion individuals, and approximately 7.1 million deaths per year may be attributable to hypertension (World Health Report, 2002).

Hypertension is a highly prevalent risk factor for cardiovascular diseases throughout the industrialized world; data from several studies show that Hypertension plays a relevant etiologic role in the development of cerebrovascular attack, ischemic heart disease, cardiac and renal failure (Yusuf et al., 2001). The relationship between high blood pressure and cardiovascular events is continuous, consistent, and independent of other risk factors. It is becoming an increasingly common health problem worldwide because of growing longevity and prevalence of contributing factors such as obesity, physical inactivity and an unhealthy diet.

High blood pressure often coexists with other cardiovascular risk factors, such as obesity, dyslipidemia, impaired glucose tolerance, and type 2 diabetes, which compound the cardiovascular risk attributable to hypertension. The concordance of hypertension and type 2 diabetes is increased in the population; hypertension is disproportionately higher in diabetics, while persons with elevated blood pressure are two and a half times more likely to develop diabetes within 5 years (Gress et al., 2000; Sowers & Bakris, 2000).

The present chapter focuses on the most recent and significant literature that explored the possible pathogenetic links between essential hypertension and type 2 diabetes, and it reviews the evidences for "optimal" antihypertensive treatment in type 2 diabetic patients and concomitant hypertension, discussing in detail some areas of uncertainty, such as the selection of antihypertensive drugs of choice in these patients.

2. High blood pressure and type 2 diabetes

The association of hypertension with diabetes is particularly bad for the health and the evidences that the association of type 2 diabetes with hypertension markedly increases cardiovascular and renal risk are incontrovertible (Fagan & Sowers, 1999): it has been shown that hypertension in type 2 diabetic patients increases the risk for macrovascular and microvascular complications (Adler et al., 2000), thus predisposing patients to stroke, cardiac death, congestive heart failure, coronary heart disease, peripheral vascular diseases, progression of nephropathy and retinopathy (Sowers & Haffner, 2002; Adler et al., 2000; Kohner et al., 1998). Hypertension in type 2 diabetes is one of the most widespread, important, and treatable cardiovascular risk factors in clinical practice; thus, good management of hypertensive diabetic patients is essential.

2.1 Pathogenetic links

Although there is a large evidence that shows the relationship between essential hypertension and type 2 diabetes, the precise mechanism of this link is still unclear. In 1966, Welborn and colleagues studied 19 normoglycemic patients with essential hypertension and demonstrated that these individuals had significantly higher plasma insulin concentrations compared with a normotensive control group (Welborn et al., 1966). This observation suggested that the prevalence of resistance to insulin would be increased in patients with essential hypertension. The relationship between essential hypertension, insulin resistance, and compensatory hyperinsulinemia, that occurs as a response to insulin resistance, has been extensively studied in the following years. Several research groups supported the hypothesis that insulin resistance, well known cause of type 2 diabetes, could play a key role in the pathogenesis of essential hypertension (Ferrannini et al., 1987; Shen et al., 1988; Swislocki et al., 1989; Pollare T, 1990). In 1992, the European Group for the Study of Insulin Resistance revealed that, in normotensives, blood pressure was directly related to both insulin resistance and insulin concentration; these relationships were independent of differences in age, gender, and degree of obesity (Ferrannini et al., 1992).

Several studies showed that the relation between insulinemia and/or insulin resistance and blood pressure appears to vary among ethnic groups. Nearly all studies showing a strong association between insulin and blood pressure were conducted among non-Hispanic whites (Saad et al., 1991); studies in African Americans (Mbanya et al., 1988; Falkner B et al., 1990), Hispanics (Haffner et al., 1988), Pima Indians (Saad et al., 1990), and Asian Indians (Nagi et al., 1990) showed a weak or no association. At the same time, Shamiss et al. demonstrated that the prevalence of insulin resistance was not increased in patients with secondary forms of hypertension (Shamiss et al., 1992); in addition, other studies revealed insulin resistance and hyperinsulinemia in normotensive, first-degree relatives of patients with essential hypertension (Ferrari P, 1992; Allemann Y, 1993).

Furthermore, results of several prospective studies support the view that insulin resistance and compensatory hyperinsulinemia are causally linked to the development of essential hypertension (Lissner et al., 1992; Zavaroni et al., 1994; Raitakari et al., 1995). In this regard, the most relevant study was performed by Skarfors et al., who evaluated risk factors for the development of hypertension in 2130 men observed over a 10-yr period; in individuals who subsequently developed hypertension, the analysis showed that independent predictors of the progression to hypertension were overweight, fasting and post-glucose challenge plasma insulin concentrations, and a family history of hypertension (Skarfors et al., 1991).

Recently, in some studies carried out in Japanese (Kanauchi et al., 2004), Indian (Sathiyapriya et al., 2006) and American (Player et al., 2007) populations has been reported the association between insulin resistance and prehypertension. Prehypertension is a new category of blood pressure classification, introduced by The Seven Joint National Commission on the Prevention, Detection, Evaluation and Treatment of Hypertension to identify individuals with systolic blood pressure in the range of 120–139 mmHg or diastolic blood pressure between 80 and 89 mmHg (The Seventh Report of the Joint National Committee [JNC 7], 2004); it is not a benign condition, as it is strong predictor for the development of hypertension (Wang W, et al., 2006).

Prehypertension is not a disease category, but it is a condition at high risk of developing hypertension; so that both patients and clinicians are alerted to this risk and encouraged to prevent or delay hypertension. Prehypertensive individuals don't need drug therapy, however they should practice lifestyle modification in order to reduce their risk of developing hypertension in the future. Instead, individuals with prehypertension, who also have diabetes or kidney disease, should be considered candidates for appropriate drug therapy, if a trial of lifestyle modification fails (JNC-7).

Although some population-based studies have not been able to discern a significant relationship between insulin resistance and hyperinsulinemia, or showed only a weak association, at present there is substantial evidence that a large number of patients with essential hypertension are insulin resistant and hyperinsulinemic compared with normotensive individuals.

The mechanism through insulin resistance is associated with hypertension and blood pressure is not known. Skeletal muscle appears to be the primary site of insulin resistance in essential hypertension (Cepaldo et al., 1991; Natali et al., 1991); other organs, such as the kidney (Zheng et al., 2005; Strazzullo et al., 2006) may respond abnormally to insulin and adipocytes also appear to be a site of insulin resistance (Sironi et al., 2004). Thus, the putative interrelationship between insulin resistance and high blood pressure may involve organ-specific insulin resistance.

It is thought that insulin resistance could cause hypertension through compensatory hyperinsulinemia (Reaven & Hoffman, 1987). Insulin has been shown to increase renal sodium retention, stimulate the sympathetic nervous system, modulate membrane cation transport, and induce hypertrophy of vascular smooth muscle cells (Passa, 1992; Edelson & Sowers, 1993). In addition, insulin resistance has been associated with impaired endothelium-dependent vasodilatation, which could contribute to increased blood pressure (Wheatcroft et al., 2003). Moreover, there is a growing body of evidence indicating that Angiotensin II is also involved in the development of insulin resistance in vascular and skeletal muscle tissue, possibly by oxidative stress production (Sowers, 2004). It is plausible that insulin resistance, through the concomitant compensatory hyperinsulinemia, could contribute to the pathogenesis of hypertension by one or more of these mechanisms.

It has been hypothesized that insulin can increase renal sodium reabsorption in the proximal tubules and stimulate sympathetic tone, thus hyperinsulinemia could increase the blood pressure by inducing salt retention and central sympathetic overactivity (Galleti et al., 1997; Strazzullo et al., 2006). This hypothesis is strengthened by a interesting ex vivo study using the proximal tubules of both insulin receptor substrate-1 and insulin receptor substrate-2 deficient mice, in which while both mice showed insulin resistance and hyperinsulinemia, only the former showed hypertension. Administration of insulin, probably, increased the sodium reabsorption in the proximal tubules of the insulin receptor substrate-1 deficient mice, by the activation of $NaHCO_3^-$ co-transport, but not in the proximal tubules of the insulin receptor substrate-2 deficient mice, suggesting that the renal action of insulin is mediated by insulin receptor substrate-2. Consequently, insulin receptor substrate-1 deficient mice showed higher blood pressure than insulin receptor substrate-2 deficient mice, possibly mediated by the greater sodium retention in the body. Thus, insulin resistance in the muscle, which is attributable to derangements of insulin receptor substrate-1, induces glucose intolerance and dyslipidemia; in turn, hyperinsulinemia induces sodium retention via insulin receptor substrate-2 phosphorylation in the kidney, resulting in volume-dependent salt-sensitive hypertension (Zheng et al., 2005). Lending support to this concept, the Olivetti Heart Study revealed that obese insulin-resistant individuals with metabolic syndrome showed a higher fractional sodium reabsorption in the proximal tubules (Strazzullo et al., 2006).

In this regard it has been supposed that high-salt intake could be a common cause of hypertension and insulin resistance. Actually, several experimental studies, involving various species and genetically modified animals, have demonstrated that a prolonged increase in salt intake leads to an increase in blood pressure (Denton et al., 1995; Elliott et al., 2007). Evidence of a positive association between sodium intake and the level of blood pressure has been also obtained in humans (Rose & Stamler, 1989; Frost et al., 1991; Khaw et al., 2004). Moreover, it has been shown that a high-salt diet not only increases the blood pressure, but also decreases the insulin sensitivity in Dahl salt-sensitive rats (Ogihara et al., 2002). In this regard, several studies showed an intimate relationship between salt-sensitivity and insulin sensitivity in hypertensive patients (Galleti et al., 1997; Suzuki et al., 2000); accordingly, the Finnish epidemiological study showed that the prevalence of diabetes was higher among obese people on a high-salt diet (Hu et al., 2005). It has been hypothesized that salt-induced insulin resistance might be attributable to the overproduction of reactive oxygen species (Aviv, 2002); in contrast to sodium, potassium possesses antihypertensive and anti-oxidant effects (Ogihara et al., 2002) associated with the normalization of reactive oxygen species overproduction.

In addition, in Dahl salt-sensitive rats, a high salt intake induced cardiac diastolic dysfunction, because of increased reactive oxygen species production in the heart, but potassium supplementation could reverse this abnormality through the inhibition of reactive oxygen species production (Matsui et al., 2006). At the vascular level, increased sodium intake has been reported to induce pronounced structural alterations of arteries, such as cerebral or renal arteries, independently of blood pressure levels; through changes in shear stress and endothelial function, high sodium intake can induce pressure-independent effects on the vascular wall, affecting the vascular content of collagen and elastin fibres (Tobian, 1991; Avolio, 1985). Thus, dietary salt and potassium stimulate and inhibit reactive oxygen species production, respectively; in turn, overproduction of reactive oxygen species might induce insulin resistance and cardiac dysfunction. Taken together, reactive oxygen species might play a critical role not only in the development of insulin resistance and hypertension, but also in that of salt-induced cardiovascular damage (Aviv, 2002).

Insulin has been also shown to stimulate sympathetic nervous system activity (Reaven et al., 1996); however, the neural mechanisms and pathways that mediate the sympathoexcitatory effects of insulin are poorly understood. These actions could be mediated by a central mechanism, because intracerebroventricular administration of insulin causes a similar selective increase in lumbar sympathetic nerve activity (Muntzel et al., 1994). It is well known that the rostral ventrolateral medulla plays a pivotal role in the regulation of sympathetic nerve activity and blood pressure (Guyenet, 2006). Rostral neurons support basal sympathetic activity and its excitability is regulated by a number of neurotransmitters including L-glutamate. Injection of L-glutamate into the rostral ventrolateral medulla increases neuronal discharge, sympathetic activity, and blood pressure, while blockade of local glutamate receptors eliminates many sympathoexcitatory reflexes and lowers blood pressure in multiple experimental models of hypertension (Bergamaschi et al., 1995; Ito et al., 2000; Guyenet, 2006). Based on this evidence, it has been hypothesized that glutamate receptor activation in the rostral ventrolateral medulla mediates the sympathoexcitatory response to hyperinsulinemia. In addition to glutamate, several evidences suggest that the brain renin-angiotensin and melanocortin systems mediate the sympathoexcitatory response to insulin (Song et al., 1991; Adan et al., 2000). In this regard, rostral neurons express Angiotensin II-AT_1 receptors, and injection of Angiotensin II into the rostral ventrolateral medulla increases sympathetic activity and blood pressure (Dampney et al., 2002), whereas blockade of brain AT_1 receptors blunts the pressor response to hyperinsulinemia (Nakata et al., 1998); thus, blockade of the renin-angiotensin system could prevent insulin-induced hypertension (Brands et al., 1997). On the other hand, rostral neurons express melanocortin receptors (Adan et al., 2000), and injection of a melanocortin agonist into the rostral ventrolateral medulla increases sympathetic activity and blood pressure (Kawabe et al., 2006). Interestingly, the sympathoexcitatory effect to insulin is abolished in melanocortin knockout mice (Rahmouni et al., 2003). Therefore, it is plausible that one or more of these systems may contribute to the sympathoexcitatory response during hyperinsulinemia.

Altered cation transport is another of several mechanisms by which insulin resistance might raise blood pressure. Both sodium/potassium-ATPase (Ewart & Klip, 1995; Sweeney & Klip, 1998) and calcium-ATPase pumps (Levy et al., 1989; Zemel et al., 1993) are insulin sensitive; thus, when insulin resistance is present, the activity of these pumps in the smooth muscle of the arterial wall might be reduced. This would lead to an intracellular accumulation of sodium and calcium, thereby sensitizing the vascular wall to pressor substances (Resnick, 1993). Nevertheless, several data have demonstrated a significant vasodilating effect of insulin (Zemel et al., 1990; Kim & Zemel, 1993; Kahn et al., 1993); to reconcile these discordant observations, it was suggested that vascular smooth muscle resistance to this action may be the cause of hypertension in insulin resistance. This concept is supported by the observation that pharmacological amplification of peripheral insulin sensitivity results in reduced arterial pressure (Morgan et al., 1992; Dubey et al., 1993) Therefore, although insulin attenuates vasoconstrictor responses to pressor agonists and accelerates vascular smooth muscle relaxation, these effects are blunted in obesity and insulin resistance (Laakso et al., 1990). In addition, insulin is also a growth factor and therefore might have a trophic effect on the vessel wall, one that could initiate and sustain hypertension as well as atherosclerosis (DeFronzo & Ferrannini, 1991).

There are several lines of evidence showing that also endothelial function is compromised in situations of reduced sensitivity to endogenous insulin. For example, the increase of blood flow in the legs in response to methacholine, a measure of endothelium-dependent vasorelaxation, is reduced in non diabetic insulin-resistant individuals (Steinberg et al., 1996); moreover, nitric oxide–dependent flow-mediated dilatation of the brachial artery is impaired in hypertensive (Higashi et al., 1997) and normotensive (Balletshofer et al., 2000) subjects with insulin resistance. It is well established that a decreased bioavailability of nitric oxide contributes to endothelial dysfunction (Singh et al., 2010); furthermore, nitric oxide may modulate insulin sensitivity (Pitocco et al., 2010). Activation of nitric oxide synthase augments blood flow to insulin-sensitive tissues, such as skeletal muscle, liver, and adipose tissue, and its activity is impaired in insulin resistance; whereas inhibition of nitric oxide synthase reduces the microvascular delivery of nutrients and blunts insulin-stimulated glucose uptake in skeletal muscle (Shi & Vanhoutte, 2009; Roberts & Sindhu, 2009). It has been shown that increased levels of asymmetric dimethylarginine, an endogenous inhibitor of nitric oxide synthase, are associated with endothelial vasodilator dysfunction and increased risk of cardiovascular diseases; moreover it has been found that plasma levels of asymmetric dimethylarginine are positively correlated with insulin resistance in non diabetic, normotensive people (Toutouzas et al., 2008).

However, the findings that plasma concentrations of plasminogen activator inhibitor 1 and endothelin 1 are elevated in the metabolic syndrome may indicate a more generalized endothelial dysfunction strongly related to insulin resistance (Ferri et al., 1997; Abbasi et al., 1999). Along the same lines, it has been shown that plasma concentrations of soluble adhesion molecules are increased in proportion to the degree of insulin resistance in healthy volunteers (Chen et al., 1999).

Angiotensin II, which is generated from angiotensinogen, is also well known to be a key substance influencing endothelial function and involved in the development of cardiovascular disease, through the activation of NADPH oxidase; oxidative stress may play an important role also in Angiotensin II-induced insulin resistance (Houstis et al., 2006). It has been reported that Angiotensin II-induced reactive oxygen species up-regulation affects several levels of the intracellular insulin signaling pathways (Ogihara et al., 2002). In vitro, reactive oxygen species has been shown to impair insulin receptor substrate-1 phoshorylation and insulin receptor substrate-1-induced phosphatidylinositol 3-kinase activation in cultured adipocytes, leading to impaired translocation of GLUT-4 glucotransporters to the membrane and consequently insulin resistance (Ogihara et al., 2004). Angiotensin II may also influence the development of type 2 diabetes via direct effects on the endocrine pancreas (Leung & de Gasparo, 2006; Leung, 2007). Local rennin-angiotensin system is known to be present in the pancreas, and AT1 receptors are expressed in islet beta-cells and upregulated in states of insulin resistance. By reducing blood flow to the pancreas and its islet cells, angiotensin II has the potential to alter the first phase of glucose-stimulated insulin secretion. Additionally, angiotensin II-promoted reactive oxygen species synthesis has been shown to induce islet cell fibrosis and apoptosis and ultimately beta-cell dysfunction (Leung & de Gasparo, 2006).

At last, in hypertensive obese patients, visceral obesity plays a critical role in the development of insulin resistance; in support of this contention, there is a growing body of evidence indicating that adipocytes produce several cytokines, the so-called adipokines, such as leptin, tumor necrosis factor-alpha, non esterified fatty acids, adiponectin, resistin and angiotensinogen, which can influence insulin sensitivity (Galic et al., 2010). According to the contribution of visceral fat to insulin resistance, a recent study revealed that mice fed with a high-fat diet showed up-regulation of the angiotensinogen gene expression in the visceral fat (Rahmouni et al., 2004). In obese humans the levels of the circulating components of the renin-angiotensin system are elevated, however weight loss is associated with a decrease in the levels of these components (Engeli et al., 2005). Therefore, the adipocyte-related renin-angiotensin system may fill an important role in the pathogenesis of insulin resistance. Several other adipokines, such as tumor necrosis factor-α, resistin, leptin

and non esterified fatty acids have the potential to decrease insulin sensitivity (Houstis et al., 2006), while adiponectin (Ziemke & Mantzoros, 2010) and adrenomedullin (Shimosawa et al., 2002) produced by adipocytes increase insulin sensitivity.
Alternatively, insulin resistance and hypertension may be linked indirectly through mechanisms of an inherited or acquired nature. Ethnic or racial differences in sympathetic nervous system activity might explain the differences in the relation of insulin resistance to blood pressure; a further possibility is that a cellular or structural defect, genetic or acquired, may constitute the link between insulin resistance and blood pressure. Racial differences in cation regulation have been described and could account for the observed variation in the relation of insulin resistance to blood pressure (Aviv & Gardner, 1989).
In conclusion, there is a large body of experimental evidence that the prevalence of insulin resistance and compensatory hyperinsulinemia is increased in patients with essential hypertension, and similar changes can be seen in normotensive first-degree relatives of patients with essential hypertension. In addition, insulin resistance and hyperinsulinemia have also been shown in several large, prospective, population-based studies to be independent predictors of the development of essential hypertension. However, not all patients with essential hypertension are insulin resistant/hyperinsulinemic, and it is obvious that the increase in blood pressure in these individuals is unrelated to any change in insulin action. The fact that insulin resistance does not provide an unitarian hypothesis to account for the etiology of essential hypertension should not obscure the wide evidences of the importance of insulin resistance, and its metabolic consequences, in the pathogenesis of perhaps as many as half of the patients with essential hypertension.

2.2 Therapeutic blood pressure target and treatment

Treating high blood pressure has been associated with about a 40% reduction in the risk of stroke, about a 20-25% reduction in the risk of myocardial infarction, and heart failure, averaging 50% (Collins et al., 1990).
Although the treatment of hypertension has been shown to prevent cardiovascular diseases and to extend and enhance life, hypertension remains inadequately managed everywhere (Trilling & Froom, 2000; Berlowitz et al., 1998). The World Health Organization reports that suboptimal blood pressure is responsible for 62% of cerebrovascular disease and 49% of ischemic heart disease, with little variation by sex. For this reason, suboptimal blood pressure is recognized the number one attributable risk factor for death throughout the world (World Health Organization, 2002).
Thus, International Guidelines for the management of hypertension provides that, in hypertensive patients, the treatment should be initiated before significant cardiovascular damage develops, and the primary goal of treatment is to achieve maximum reduction in the long-term total risk of cardiovascular diseases; in order to this aim systolic/diastolic blood pressure should be reduced to at least below 140/90mmHg, and to lower values if tolerated, in all hypertensive patients.
In individuals with high blood pressure and additional risk factors, is essential the effective management for controlling the coexisting problems that contribute to overall cardiovascular risk (JNC-7, 2004; Mancia et al., 2007).
The United Kingdom Prospective Diabetes Study (Adler et al, 2000) demonstrated that each 10 mmHg decrease in systolic blood pressure was associated with average reductions in rates of diabetes-related mortality, myocardial infarction, and microvascular complications

of retinopathy or nephropathy. Moreover, randomized controlled trials (Mann et al., 2001; Hansson et al., 1998; Tuomilehto et al., 1999) including large diabetic populations have demonstrated that adequate blood pressure control improves cardiovascular outcomes, especially stroke, when aggressive blood pressure targets are achieved (Arauz-Pacheco et al., 2003; Psaty et al., 2003).

Recommendations from both American Diabetes Association (Arauz-Pacheco et al., 2003) and International Diabetes Federation (IDF Clinical Guidelines Task Force; 2006) are consistent with International Guidelines for the management of hypertension which have provided that in hypertensive patients with type 2 diabetes and in high or very high risk patients, such as those with associated clinical conditions (stroke, myocardial infarction, renal dysfunction, proteinuria), target blood pressure should be at least < 130/80mmHg.

The treatment for hypertensive patients with type 2 diabetes should aim at achieving blood pressure target, reducing cardiovascular risk and at improving insulin resistance (Giles & Sander, 2005).

The therapeutic lifestyle change is the first step for treatment of hypertensive patients with type 2 diabetes; it includes: diet, regular aerobic physical activity such as brisk walking at least 30 minutes daily, weight loss, if the patients are obese, and behavioural treatment. Both smoking cessation and alcohol intake reduction - no more than 30 mL of ethanol per day - are also need. These non pharmacological interventions can decrease blood pressure and improve insulin sensitivity; they should be more strongly recommended to diabetic and non diabetic hypertensive patients, on account of their positive impact on cardiovascular diseases prevention (Wagh & Stone, 2004; JNC-7, 2004).

In several studies weight reduction has been shown to improve insulin resistance in obese patients, apparently associated with the reduction of visceral fat (Park & Lee, 2005; Buchwald et al., 2004; Busetto, 2001); benefits of moderate weight loss include decreased blood glucose, insulinemia, lipid levels, and blood pressure. In particular, the loss of one kilogram in body weight has resulted in decreases in mean arterial blood pressure of 1 mmHg (Wagh & Stone, 2004). However the role of very low calorie diets and pharmacologic agents that induce weight loss in the management of hypertension in diabetic patients has not been adequately studied.

Lifestyle change cannot leave aside dietary intervention, promoting salt restriction and increasing potassium intakes, that should be more systematically considered in the management and prevention of essential hypertension. In recent years, the benefits of lowering sodium and increasing potassium intakes have been reinforced by the demonstration that these non-pharmacological approaches to hypertension management enable the lowering of blood pressure and the reduction of target organ damage as well as cardiovascular events (Lawes et al., 2008).

A restriction in dietary salt intake reduced pulse pressure, suggesting an improvement in arterial distensibility (Gates et al., 2004); moreover, several interventional studies have been conducted to investigate the clinical impact of lowering dietary sodium intake on blood pressure and cardiovascular events (Elmer et al., 1991; Lasser et al., 1995; Whelton et al., 1998). Systolic and diastolic blood pressure resulted significantly reduced among individuals assigned to reduced sodium intake group; accordingly, a meta-analysis of randomized studies, which took into account only studies with a duration of at least one month and modest reductions of sodium intake (mean 4.4–4.6 g of salt daily), demonstrated that a reduction in salt intake is associated with a significant decrease in blood pressure, both in normotensive and hypertensive individuals (He & MacGregor, 2002). In addition, based on the changes in blood pressure from the meta-analysis of randomized salt-reduction trials and the relationship between blood pressure and stroke and ischemic heart disease, it has been estimated that a 3 g daily reduction of dietary salt intake would reduce stroke by 13% and ischemic heart disease by 10% (He & MacGregor, 2003). Experimentally, a low sodium diet prevents also renal alterations in several models of hypertension and renal diseases (Lax et al., 1992; Bank, 1988). In humans, the long-term benefits of a low sodium intake on the progression of non-diabetic or diabetic nephropathies are less well documented; the most significant impact of dietary salt intake on renal function could be its effect on urinary albumin excretion. (Du Cailar et al., 2002; Verhave et al., 2004).

Regarding potassium, its supplementation not only attenuated salt-induced elevation of blood pressure, but also improved salt-induced insulin resistance in salt-sensitive hypertensive patients (Fujita & Ando, 1984) and animals (Fujita & Sato, 1983). Consistent with this, in the DASH study, the "dietary approaches to stop hypertension" eating plan (DASH diet), consisting of low-fat dairy products, vegetables and fruits rich in potassium, which could lower lipid-induced oxidative stress in obesity, decreased not only blood pressure, but also the fasting blood sugar in hypertensive patients (Lopes et al., 2003; Azadbakht et al., 2005). In the subsequent DASH-sodium trial, three different dietary sodium intakes were compared, 150, 100, and 50 mmol/24 h, corresponding to approximately 8.8, 5.8, and 2.9 g. of salt per day respectively, with and without DASH diet. Blood pressure was significantly lower when going to a lower group of dietary salt intake in both the control diet or the DASH diet groups. The results of low sodium-DASH diet trial further strengthen the conclusion that reduction of dietary sodium intake through low-salt diet lowers blood pressure effectively and adds to the benefits conferred by the DASH diet (Sacks et al., 2001). Therefore, salt restriction and dietary intake of potassium should be prescribed as a first-line lifestyle therapy for hypertensive patients, especially in coexisting type 2 diabetes; dietary sodium should be reduced to no more than 100 mmol per day, corresponding to 2.4 g of sodium (Sacks et al., 2001; Vollmer et al., 2001).

The therapeutic lifestyle change should be instituted with adequate behavioural and expert support, and reinforced periodically; nevertheless it often is inadequate to achieve blood pressure target. In this case drug therapy is necessary; moreover, most patients can require two or more antihypertensive drugs (Cushman et al., 2002; Black et al., 2001).

A large number of drugs are currently available for reducing blood pressure, five major classes of commonly used antihypertensive agents - diuretics, calcium antagonists, angiotensin converting enzyme Inhibitors (ACE inhibitors), angiotensin receptor blockers (ARBs) and beta blockers - are suitable for the initiation and maintenance of antihypertensive treatment, alone or in combination (JNC-7, 2004; Mancia et al., 2007).

There are a number of intervention trials demonstrating benefits in the treatment of hypertension in type 2 diabetics in reducing outcomes including cardiovascular events and microvascular complications of retinopathy and progression of nephropathy. These studies used different drug classes, including ACE inhibitors, ARBs, diuretics, and beta blockers, as the initial step in therapy; all of these agents were superior to placebo.

In the Systolic Hypertension in the Elderly Program (SHEP) low-dose, chlorthalidone-based treatment was found to be effective compared with placebo in preventing cardiovascular complications in elderly patients with type 2 diabetes mellitus and isolated systolic hypertension (Curb et al., 1996). Later, the Hypertension Optimal Treatment Study (HOT) investigated the efficacy of antihypertensive treatment using a dihydropyridine calcium antagonist, felodipine, as baseline therapy in hypertensive patients averaging 62 years of age and 170/105 mm Hg in baseline blood pressure, including 1501 patients with type 2 diabetes. In this study the incidence of major cardiovascular events was lowered ($p = 0.005$) from 24.4 to 18.6 and 11.9 events/100 patient-years, respectively, in the randomised tertiles of diabetes patients who had achieved 85, 83, and 81 mm Hg, respectively, in diastolic blood pressure. Approximately twenty patients needed to be treated for 5 years to prevent one major cardiovascular event when blood pressure was further lowered from 84 to 81 mm Hg (Hansson et al., 1998). Similarly, the Systolic Hypertension in Europe Trial (Syst-Eur) compared another dihydropyridine calcium antagonist, nitrendipine, with placebo in elderly patients with isolated systolic hypertension and in a subgroup with type 2 diabetes; the treatment for five years prevented 178 major cardiovascular events in every 1000 diabetic patients treated; approximately six patients had to be treated for five years to prevent one major cardiovascular event (Tuomilehto et al., 1999).

The results of the Heart Outcomes Prevention Evaluation (HOPE) Study and the MIcroalbuminuria, Cardiovascular, and Renal Outcomes (MICRO-HOPE) substudy showed that treatment with the ACE inhibitor ramipril, compared with placebo, significantly lowered the risk of cardiovascular events and overt nephropathy in type 2 diabetic patients with a previous cardiovascular event or at least one other risk factor. Although 56% of the HOPE diabetics (n=3577) had a history of hypertension, uncontrolled diabetic hypertensives (blood pressure >160/90 mmHg) were not randomized; thus, the cardiovascular benefit of ramipril was greater than that attributable to the decrease in blood pressure (Heart Outcomes Prevention Evaluation (HOPE) Study Investigators, 2000).

The Reduction of Endpoints in NIDDM with the Angiotensin II Receptor Antagonist Losartan (RENAAL) study is a randomized, double-blind clinical trial that studied 1513 patients with type 2 diabetes and nephropathy for a mean of 3.4 years. Patients were administered either losartan or placebo, each in addition to conventional antihypertensive therapy, with dosage adjustments as necessary to achieve a target blood pressure of less than 140/90 mm Hg. The study showed a significant benefit of losartan, beyond the effects of lowering blood pressure, on the primary composite end point of doubling serum creatinine level and end-stage renal disease; however, losartan had no effect on rate of death. In addition, losartan was associated with a 21% risk reduction for the composite cardio-renal outcome (Brenner et al., 2001).

In 2007, in the ADVANCE trial it was shown that addition of the combination of ACE inhibitor perindopril and diuretic indapamide to type 2 diabetic patients, irrespective of initial blood pressure levels or the use of other blood pressure lowering drugs, was associated with substantial clinical benefits versus placebo treatment. Routine administration of a fixed combination of perindopril and indapamide was well tolerated and reduced the risks of major vascular events, including death. Although the confidence limits were wide, the results suggest that over 5 years, one death due to any cause would be averted among every 79 patients assigned active therapy (Patel et al., 2007).

Other several trials found an improvement in renal outcomes in patients with type 2 diabetes and overt nephropathy through antihypertensive treatment with other ARBs such as irbesartan (Lewis et al., 2001) and telmisartan (Barnett et al., 2004; Mann et al., 2008). Moreover, recent results of the Nateglinide and Valsartan in Impaired Glucose Tolerance Outcomes Research (NAVIGATOR) trial showed that the addition of valsartan to lifestyle

modification reduced the risk of diabetes but did not improve cardiovascular outcomes. (McMurray et al., 2010). Finally, in the recent Aliskiren in the Evaluation of Proteinuria inDiabetes (AVOID) study, it has been shown that aliskiren, a new antihypertensive drug, added to losartan reduced albuminuria and renal dysfunction and it was well tolerated. The AVOID study was the first double-blind, randomized controlled trial to demonstrate the antiproteinuric ability of aliskiren, an oral direct renin inhibitor, as add-on to standard treatment including an ARB, in patients with type 2 diabetes, hypertension and nephropathy (Persson et al., 2010).
Regarding the selection of medications, the most suitable antihypertensive drug to reduce the risk of cardiovascular disease in patients with hypertension and diabetes is unclear, also because the majority of patients requires two or more drugs to achieve blood pressure target (Sowers & Reed, 2000; Sowers & Haffner, 2002). In order to this purpose numerous comparative studies have been carried out to define the question of which class of antihypertensive agents is superior for lowering blood pressure in diabetic patients.
After more than 8 years of follow-up of 1148 hypertensive patients in the United Kingdom Prospective Diabetes Study (UKPDS), a tight blood pressure control was successful to prevent macro- and micro-vascular complications, especially for prevention of stroke and retinopathy (UK Prospective Diabetes Study Group, 1998). However, no significant effect difference was found between captopril and atenolol, but the patients on atenolol needed significantly more oral anti-glycaemic drugs due to weight increase and dysmetabolic effects of beta blocker agent (UK Prospective Diabetes Study Group, 1998).
Subsequently, in the Swedish Trial in Old Patients with Hypertension-2 (STOP-2) study all patients were above the age of 70 years, and as many as 719 of them had type-2 diabetes at baseline; the prevention of cardiovascular mortality was similar on conventional standard therapy (diuretics, beta-blockers, or both), ACE inhibitor, or calcium-antagonist treatment and the reduction in blood pressure was also the same in the three treatment groups of diabetics. There were, however, significantly fewer ($P = 0.025$) myocardial infarctions during ACE inhibitor treatment than during calcium antagonist treatment (Lindholm et al., 2000).
In 2001, the Collaborative Study Group randomly assigned 1715 hypertensive patients with nephropathy, due to type 2 diabetes, to treatment with irbesartan 300 mg daily, amlodipine - a dihydropyridine calcium antagonist - 10 mg daily, or placebo. The target blood pressure was 135/85 mm Hg or less in all groups. It was compared the groups with regard to the time to the primary composite end point of a doubling of the base-line serum creatinine concentration, the development of end stage renal disease, or death from any cause. Treatment with irbesartan was associated with a risk of the primary composite end point that was 20% lower than that in the placebo group (P=0.02) and 23% lower than that in the amlodipine group (P=0.006). The risk of a doubling of the serum creatinine concentration was 33% lower in the irbesartan group than in the placebo group (P=0.003) and 37% lower in the irbesartan group than in the amlodipine group (P<0.001). Treatment with irbesartan was associated with a relative risk of end-stage renal disease that was 23% lower than that in both other groups (P=0.07 for both comparisons). These differences were not explained by differences in the blood pressure that were achieved. The serum creatinine concentration increased 24% more slowly in the irbesartan group than in the placebo group (P=0.008) and 21% more slowly than in the amlodipine group (P=0.02). There were no significant differences in the rates of death from any cause or in the secondary cardiovascular

composite end point (Lewis et al., 2001). Another comparative study between an ARB and other antihypertensive drugs was the Losartan Intervention For Endpoint reduction (LIFE) trial; in this study a subgroup of 1195 patients with diabetes, hypertension, and left-ventricular hypertrophy on electrocardiograms were randomised to either losartan-based or atenolol-based treatment; losartan was more effective than beta blocker atenolol in reducing cardiovascular morbidity and mortality, as well as mortality from all causes. Losartan seemed to have benefits beyond blood pressure reduction. (Lindholm et al., 2002).

In the Antihypertensive and Lipid-Lowering Treatment to Prevent Heart Attack Trial (ALLHAT) a subgroup of patients (36%) with diabetes were randomised to treatment with thiazide-type diuretic chlorothalidone, calcium channel blocker amlodipine, or ACE inhibitor lisinopril; the primary composite cardiovascular outcome was combined fatal coronary heart disease or nonfatal myocardial infarction. There were no differences between these three drugs, used in a very heterogeneous study population; likewise, all-cause mortality did not differ between groups (The ALLHAT Collaborative Research Group, 2002). A similar result of equity between treatment arms for the primary composite cardiovascular end-point was found in the International Nifedipine GITS Study: Intervention as a Goal in Hypertension Treatment (INSIGHT), based on a sub-analysis of 1302 patients with hypertension and diabetes randomised to either dihydropyridine calcium antagonist nifedipine slow-release or hydrochlorothiazide plus amiloride (Mancia et al., 2003).

In 2004, the groundbreaking Diabetics Exposed to Telmisartan And enalaprIL (DETAIL) study revealed that telmisartan, an ARBs, conferred comparable renoprotection to enalapril, an ACE inhibitor; moreover, telmisartan was associated with a low incidence of mortality. The DETAIL study was designed to compare the long-term renal outcome of treatment with telmisartan versus enalapril in patients with type 2 diabetes, mild-to-moderate hypertension and albuminuria. The primary endpoint was the change in glomerular filtration rate after 5 years. The secondary endpoints are annual changes in glomerular filtration rate, serum creatinine and urinary albumin excretion, as well as incidences of end-stage renal disease, cardiovascular events, all-cause mortality and adverse events (Barnett et al., 2004). Similar results were obtained recently in the ONgoing Telmisartan Alone and in combination with Ramipril Global Endpoint Trial (ONTARGET) study. In this multicentre, randomised, double-blind, controlled trial it was investigated the renal effects of ramipril, telmisartan, and their combination in patients aged 55 years or older with established atherosclerotic vascular disease or with diabetes with end-organ damage. The primary renal outcome was a composite of dialysis, doubling of serum creatinine, and death. The number of events for the composite primary outcome was similar for telmisartan and ramipril; and also the secondary renal outcome, dialysis or doubling of serum creatinine, was similar between two drugs (Mann et al., 2008).

The Anglo-Scandinavian Cardiac Outcome Trial (ASCOT) has shown substantial benefits for the reduction of stroke and total mortality in patients randomised to a treatment based on amlodipine, adding perindopril as required, versus atenolol-based treatment, with thiazide as add-on therapy if needed; moreover, in this study the incidence of developing diabetes was significantly ($p<0.0001$) less on the amlodipine-based regimen (Dahlöf et al., 2005).

In the Shiga Microalbuminuria Reduction Trial (SMART) the objective of the study was to assess the effect of an angiotensin receptor blocker, valsartan, on microalbuminuria in comparison with that of a calcium channel blocker, amlodipine, in patients with the targeting blood pressure level < 130/80 mmHg. The reductions in blood pressure were similar between the valsartan group and the amlodipine group. However, valsartan was more effective than amlodipine for reducing microalbuminuria. In addition, the reduction of the urinary albumin creatinine ratio was significantly greater in the valsartan group with uncontrolled systolic blood pressure than that in the amlodipine group with controlled systolic blood pressure. These findings showed that the antiproteinuric effect of valsartan may be independent of its effect on blood pressure (Uzu et al., 2007). Moreover, data from the recent VALUE trial revealed that the angiotensin receptor blocker valsartan, compared with calcium-channel antagonist amlodipine, reduces the risk of developing diabetes mellitus, particularly in hypertensive patients with the highest susceptibility for development of diabetes (Kjeldsen et al. 2008). However, in 2004 a subanalysis of the Captopril Prevention Project (CAPPP) revealed a similar result assessing the effects of an ACE inhibitor, captopril, with a conventional antihypertensive treatment, including diuretic and/or beta blockers, in middle-aged hypertensive patients; for each tertile of risk, captopril therapy was associated with a reduced risk of diabetes development compared with conventional treatment. (Niklason et al., 2004).

Finally, in the ACCOMPLISH (Avoiding Cardiovascular Events Through COMbination Therapy in Patients Living With Systolic Hypertension) trial a total of 6946 diabetic patients were randomized to treatment with fixed combination of a renin-angiotensin system blocker, benazepril, and amlodipine, or fixed combination of benazepril and hydrochlorothiazide; it was shown that combining benazepril with amlodipine, compared with hydrochlorothiazide, was superior in reducing relative risk of cardiovascular events (Weber et al., 2010).

There are no significant long-term studies regarding the effect of other classes of antihypertensive agents, such as alpha-1 antagonists, for instance doxazosin, or centrally alpha-2 agonist drugs, like clonidine, on long-term cardiovascular complications of diabetes. The alpha-1 antagonists arm of the ALLHAT study was stopped by the safety monitoring committee because of an increase in cases of new-onset heart failure in patients assigned to the doxazosin (Davis et al., 2002). While this could merely represent unmasking of heart failure in patients previously treated with an ACE inhibitor or a diuretic, it seems reasonable to use these antihypertensives as second-line agents.

In summary, the benefits of treating hypertension in type 2 diabetic patients, in terms of reductions in cardiovascular morbidity and mortality, have been documented in several trials, but the optimal first-step therapy remains unknown. It has been shown that most of commonly used antihypertensive agents have nearly similar efficacy; however is well established that renin-angiotensin system blockade lowers significantly the frequency of various diabetic complications, including diabetic nephropathy. Furthermore, in the high risk group of diabetic patients, blockade of the renin-angiotensin system reduces cardiovascular mortality and morbidity. ACE inhibitors and ARBs have also been shown to lower cardiovascular events in diabetic patients and to delay or avoid the onset of type 2 diabetes. Both drug classes are believed to improve endothelial function by increasing nitric oxide bioavailability, and rennin-angiotensin system blockade has demonstrated protective effects on pancreatic beta-cells attributed, in part, to a reduction in oxidative stress (Lupi et al., 2006; Nakayama et al., 2005). Strong evidences indicate that oxidative stress plays a key role in the pathogenesis of diabetic microvascular and macrovascular complications; thus, abrogation of oxidative stress through inhibition of angiotensin II production and enhancement of antioxidant activity with rennin-angiotensin blockers would be expected to reduce this risk. Recently, it has been shown that aliskiren, a new oral antihypertensive drug, by direct renin inhibition reduces albuminuria and renal dysfunction in hypertensive type 2 diabetic patients; however, as for aliskiren, further research are warranted to build on the favourable effects that have been observed with ACE inhibitors and ARBs in high-risk diabetic patients, with the goal of achieving cardiovascular outcomes benefits.

Finally, regarding the selection of medications, the therapeutic choices must also consider the potential adverse metabolic effects of some antihypertensive drugs (Black, 1991).

There is a large evidence that both ARBs and ACE inhibitors could be considered first-line antihypertensive drugs in type 2 diabetic patients. Calcium channel blockers, peripheral alpha-1 antagonists and central alpha-2 agonist drugs are metabolically neutral, while diuretics, except for indapamide and anti-aldosterone drugs, can reduce insulin sensitivity (Ramsay et al., 1992; McCarty, 2004; Bousquet at al., 2000) thus they are not first-line therapy, yet they are recommended in selected cases only. Beta blockers, especially non-selective and without intrinsic sympathomimetic activity, also reduce insulin sensitivity and they have adverse effects on carbohydrate and lipid metabolism; moreover an higher incidence of new onset diabetes was observed in patients with hypertension taking beta-blocking drugs (Lithell, 1991; Lind et al., 1994). For these reasons, beta blockers are not considered first-line therapy in hypertensive diabetic patients and are recommended only in selected cases as heart failure, acute or previous myocardial infarction and ischemic heart disease (Black, 1991). However, two large studies have revealed that third generation beta blockers with vasodilating properties, such as nebivolol and especially carvedilol, have not shown negative effects on blood lipids, carbohydrate metabolism and insulin sensitivity in hypertensive patients with type 2 diabetes mellitus (Bakris et al., 2004; Schmidt et al., 2007). The vasodilating and antioxidant properties of these beta blockers could play a key-role in mediating their favourable metabolic profile (Agabiti Rosei & Rizzoni, 2007; Feuerstein & Ruffolo; 1995). It can be supposed that the vasodilation, improving the blood flow in the skeletal muscle, allows more adequate, opportune and efficacious release of insulin and glucose to myocytes. Moreover, the antioxidant action, reducing oxidative stress, could improve both the insulin sensitivity of peripheral tissue and the pancreatic beta cell dysfunction (Jacob et al., 1999). The metabolic advantages of vasodilating third-generation beta blockers highlight the importance of dissociating older conventional agents from newer agents. These are a class of antihypertensive drugs that could be a valuable aid for hypertensive patients with type 2 diabetes because of increased cardiovascular risk of these patients and the high proportion of concomitant cardiac diseases, such as congestive heart failure and coronary heart disease. Thus, Carvedilol and Nebivolol could be a valuable tool for hypertension treatment in patients with metabolic syndrome too.

3. Conclusion

The association of hypertension and type 2 diabetes is increased in the population and there is a strong epidemiological link between hypertension and cardiovascular outcomes of diabetes. Clinical trials have demonstrated the efficacy of the antihypertensive treatment in reducing these outcomes. The general consensus for treatment of hypertension in type 2 diabetes is to aim for a well controlled blood pressure of 130/80 mm Hg. In order to this purpose, lifestyle measures should be instituted in all patients, including those who require drug treatment; where applicable, intense non-pharmacological measures should be encouraged, with particular attention to weight loss and reduction of salt intake. Drug therapy is necessary if lifestyle change is inadequate, and it is very clear that many patients need two or more drugs to achieve the recommended blood pressure target. Regarding the selection of medications, clinical trials with major classes of antihypertensives have demonstrated the efficacy of drug therapy versus placebo in reducing cardiovascular outcomes. The question of which class of agents is superior for lowering blood pressure in diabetic patients is somewhat moot, thus to reduce blood pressure values, all effective and well tolerated antihypertensive drugs can be used. However, ACE inhibitors and ARBs, because of their considerable cardiovascular and nephroprotective properties could be considered first-line antihypertensive drugs in type 2 diabetic patients with high blood pressure.

4. References

Abbasi F, McLaughlin T, Lamendola C, Lipinska I, Tofler G, Reaven GM. Comparison of plasminogen activator inhibitor-1 concentration in insulin-resistant versus insulin-sensitive healthy women. Arterioscler Thromb Vasc Biol. 1999;19:2818-2821.

Adan RA, Gispen WH. Melanocortins and the brain: from effects via receptors to drug targets. Eur J Pharmacol. 2000;405:13–24.

Adler AI, Stratton IM, Neil HA, Yudkin JS, Matthews DR, Cull CA, et al. Association of systolic blood pressure with macrovascular and microvascular complications of type 2 diabetes (UKPDS 36): Prospective observational study. BMJ 2000;321:412-9.

Adler AI, Stratton IM, Neil HA, Yudkin JS, Matthews DR, Cull CA, et al. Association of systolic blood pressure with macrovascular and microvascular complications of type 2 diabetes (UKPDS 36): Prospective observational study. BMJ 2000;321:412-9.

Agabiti Rosei E, Rizzoni D. Metabolic profile of nebivolol, a beta-adrenoceptor antagonist with unique characteristics. Drugs 2007; 67(8): 1097-107.

Allemann Y, Horber FF, Colombo M, Ferrari P, Shaw S, Jaeger P, Weidman P. Insulin sensitivity and body fat distribution in normotensive offspring of hypertensive parents. Lancet 1993;341:327-331.

Aviv A, Gardner J. Racial difference in ion regulation and their possible links to hypertension in Blacks. Hypertension. 1989; 14: 584–589

Aviv A. Salt consumption, reactive oxygen species and cardiovascular ageing: a hypothetical link. J Hypertension 2002;20:555-559.

Avolio AP, Deng FQ, Li WQ, et al. Effects of aging on arterial distensibility in populations with high and low prevalence of hypertension: comparison between urban and rural communities in China. Circulation 1985; 71: 202–210

Azadbakht L, Mirmiran P, Esmaillzadeh A, Azizi T, Azizi F. Beneficial effects of a dietary approaches to stop hypertension eating plan on features of the metabolic syndrome. Diabetes Care 2005;28:2823 2831.

Bakris GL, Fonseca V, Katholi RE, *et al*; GEMINI Investigators. Metabolic effects of carvedilol vs metoprolol in patients with type 2 diabetes mellitus and hypertension: a randomized controlled trial. JAMA 2004; 292(18): 2227-36.

Balletshofer BM, Rittig K, Enderle MD, et al. Endothelial dysfunction is detectable in young normotensive first-degree relatives of subjects with type 2 diabetes in association with insulin resistance. Circulation. 2000;101:1780-1784

Bank N, Lahorra G, Aynedjian HS, et al. Sodium restriction corrects hyperfiltration of diabetes. Am J Physiol 1988; 254: F668–F676.

Barnett AH, Bain SC, Bouter P, Karlberg B, Madsbad S, Jervell J, Mustonen J; Diabetics Exposed to Telmisartan and Enalapril Study Group. Angiotensin-receptor blockade versus converting-enzyme inhibition in type 2 diabetes and nephropathy. N Engl J Med. 2004 Nov 4;351(19):1952-61.

Bergamaschi C, Campos RR, Schor N, Lopes OU. Role of the rostral ventrolateral medulla in maintenance of blood pressure in rats with Goldblatt hypertension. Hypertension. 1995;26:1117–1120.

Berlowitz DR, Ash AS, Hickey EC, Friedman RH, Glickman M, Kader B, et al. Inadequate management of blood pressure in a hypertensive population. N Engl J Med 1998;339:1957-63.

Binder A. A review of the genetics of essential hypertension. Curr Opin Cardiol 2007 May;22(3):176-84.

Black HR. Metabolic considerations in the choice of therapy for the patient with Hypertension. Am Heart J 1991;121:707-15.

Black HR, Elliott WJ, Neaton JD, Grandits G, Grambsch P, Grimm R, et al. Baseline characteristics and early blood pressure control in the CONVINCE trial. Hypertension 2001;37:12-8.

Bousquet P, Dontenwill M, Greney H, at al. Imidazoline receptors in cardiovascular and metabolic diseases. J Cardiovasc Pharmacol 2000;35:S21-5.

Brands MW, Harrison DL, Keen HL, Gardner A, Shek EW, Hall JE. Insulin-induced hypertension in rats depends on an intact renin-angiotensin system. Hypertension. 1997;29:1014–1019.

Brenner BM, Cooper ME, de Zeeuw D, Keane WF, Mitch WE, Parving HH, Remuzzi G, Snapinn SM, Zhang Z, Shahinfar S; RENAAL Study Investigators: Effects of losartan on renal and cardiovascular outcomes in patients with type 2 diabetes and nephropathy. N Engl J Med 345: 861–869, 2001.

Buchwald H, Avidor Y, Braunwald E, et al. Bariatric surgery: a systematic review and meta-analysis. JAMA 2004;292:1724-1737.

Busetto L. Visceral obesity and the metabolic syndrome: effects of weight loss. Nutr Metab Cardiovascular Dis 2001;11:195-204

Cepaldo B, Lembo G, Napoli R, Rendina V, Albano G, Sacc L, Trimarco B. Skeletal muscle is a primary site of insulin resistance in essential hypertension. Metabolism 1991; 40:1320–1322.

Chen NG, Holmes M, Reaven GM. Relationship between insulin resistance, soluble adhesion molecules, and mononuclear cell binding in healthy volunteers. J Clin Endocrinol Metab. 1999;84:3485-3489.

Collins R, Peto R, MacMahon S, Hebert P, Fiebach NH, Eberlein KA. Blood pressure, stroke, and coronary heart disease. Part 2: Short-term reductions in blood pressure:

overview of randomized drug trials in their epidemiological context. Lancet 1990; 335:827-838.

Curb JD, Pressel SL, Cutler JA, et al. Effect of diuretic-based antihypertensive treatment on cardiovascular disease in older diabetic patients with isolated systolic hypertension. JAMA 1996; 276: 1886.1892.

Cushman WC, Ford CE, Cutler JA, Margolis KL, Davis BR, Grimm RH, et al. Success and predictors of blood pressure control in diverse North American settings: The Antihypertensive and Lipid-Lowering Treatment to Prevent Heart Attack Trial (ALLHAT). J Clin Hypertens (Greenwich) 2002;4:393-404.

Dahlöf B, Sever P, Poulter NR, et al. Prevention of cardiovascular events with an antihypertensive regimen of amlodipine adding perindopril as required versus atenolol adding bendroflumethiazide as required, in the Anglo-Scandinavian Cardiac Outcomes Trial-Blood Pressure Lowering Arm (ASCOT-BPLA): a multicentre randomised controlled trial. Lancet 2005; 366: 895.906

Dampney RA, Fontes MA, Hirooka Y, Horiuchi J, Potts PD, Tagawa T. Role of angiotensin II receptors in the regulation of vasomotor neurons in the ventrolateral medulla. Clin Exp Pharmacol Physiol. 2002;29:467–472.

Davis BR, et al. Relationship of antihypertensive treatment regimens and change in blood pressure to risk for heart failure in hypertensive patients randomly assigned to doxazosin or chlorthalidone: further analyses from the antihypertensive and lipid-lowering treatment to prevent heart attack trial. Ann Intern Med. 2002;137:313–320

DeFronzo RA, Ferrannini E. Insulin resistance. A multifaceted syndrome responsible for NIDDM, obesity, hypertension, dyslipidemia, and atherosclerotic cardiovascular disease. Diabetes Care. 1991;14(3):173-94.

Denton D, Weisinger R, Mundy NI, et al. The effect of increased salt intake on blood pressure of chimpanzees. Nat Med 1995; 1: 1009–1016

Dubey RK, Zhang HY, Reddy SR, Buegehold MA, Kotchen TA. Pioglitazone attenuates hypertension and growth of renal arteriolar smooth muscle cells in rats. Am J Physiol 1993;265:R726-R732.

Du Cailar G, Ribstein J, Mimran A. Dietary sodium and target organ damage in essential hypertension. Am J Hypertens 2002; 15: 222–229.

Edelson GW, Sowers JR. Insulin resistance in hypertension: a focused review.Am J Med Sci 1993;306(5):345-7.

Elliott P, Walker LL, Little MP, et al. Change in salt intake affects blood pressure of chimpanzees: implications for human populations. Circulation 2007; 116: 1563–1568.

Elmer PJ, Grimm RH Jr, Flack J, Laing B. Dietary sodium reduction for hypertension prevention and treatment. Hypertension. 1991 Jan;17(1 Suppl):I182-9.

Engeli S, Bohnke J, Gorzelniak K, et al . Weight loss and the renin-angiotensin-aldosterone system. Hypertension 2005;45:356-362.

Ewart HS, Klip A. Hormonal regulation of the Na(+)-K(+)-ATPase: mechanisms underlying rapid and sustained changes in pump activity. Am J Physiol. 1995;269(2 Pt 1):C295-311.

Fagan TC, Sowers J. Type 2 diabetes mellitus: Greater cardiovascular risks and greater benefits of therapy. Arch Intern Med 1999;159:1033-4.

Falkner B, Hulman S, Tannenbaum J, Kushner H. Insulin resistance and blood pressure in young black men. Hypertension. 1990; 16: 706–711.

Ferrannini E, Buzzigoli G, Bonadona R. Insulin resistance in essential hypertension. N Engl J Med 1987; 317:350–357.

Ferrannini E, Natali A, Capaldo B, Lehtovirta M, Jacob S, Yki-Järvinen H, for the European Group for the Study of Insulin Resistance (EGIR). Insulin resistance, hyperinsulinemia, and blood pressure. Role of age and obesity. Hypertension 1992;30:1144–1149.

Ferrari P, Chen Y-DI, Clinkingbeard C, Jeppesen J, Reaven GM. Insulin resistance, hyperinsulinemia, and dyslipidemia in nonobese individuals with a family history of hypertension. Am J Hypertens 1992;5:694–699.

Ferri C, Bellini C, Desideri G, et al. Circulating endothelin-1 levels in obese patients with the metabolic syndrome. Exp Clin Endocrinol Diabetes. 1997;105(suppl 2):38-40.

Feuerstein GZ, Ruffolo RR Jr. Carvedilol, a novel multiple action antihypertensive agent with antioxidant activity and the potential for myocardial and vascular protection. Eur Heart J 1995; 16 Suppl F: 38-42.

Frost CD, Law MR, Wald NJ. By how much does dietary salt reduction lower blood pressure? Analysis of observational data within populations. Br Med J 1991; 302: 815–818.

Fujita T, Sato Y. Natriuretic and antihypertensive effects of potassium in DOCA-salt hypertensive rats. Kidney Int 1983;24:731-739.

Fujita T, Ando K. Hemodynamic and endocrine changes associated with potassium supplementation in sodium-loaded hypertensives. Hypertension 1984;6:184-192.

Galic S, Oakhill JS, Steinberg GR. Adipose tissue as an endocrine organ. Mol Cell Endocrinol. 2010;316(2):129-39.

Galleti F, Strazzullo P, Ferrara I, et al. NaCl sensitivity of essential hypertensive patients is related to insulin resistance. J Hypertension 1997;15:1485-91.

Gates PE, Tanaka H, Hiatt WR, Seals DR. Dietary sodium restriction rapidly improves large elastic artery compliance in older adults with systolic hypertension. Hypertension 2004; 44: 35–41.

Giles TD, Sander GE. Pathophysiologic, diagnostic, and therapeutic aspects of the metabolic syndrome. J Clin Hypertens 2005;7(11):669-78.

Gress TW, Nieto FJ, Shahar E, Wofford MR, Brancati FL. Hypertension and antihypertensive therapy as risk factors for type 2 diabetes mellitus. Atherosclerosis Risk in Communities Study. N Engl J Med 2000;342:905-12.

Guyenet PG. The sympathetic control of blood pressure. Nat Rev Neurosci. 2006;7:335–346.

Haffner SM, Fong D, Hazuda HP, Pugh JA, Patterson JK. Hyperinsulinemia, upper body adiposity, and cardiovascular risk factors in non-diabetics. Metabolism. 1988; 37: 338–345.

Hansson L, Zanchetti A, Carruthers SG, Dahlof B, Elmfeldt D, Julius S, et al. Effects of intensive blood-pressure lowering and low-dose aspirin in patients with hypertension: Principal results of the Hypertension Optimal Treatment (HOT) randomised trial. HOT Study Group. Lancet 1998;351:1755-62.

Heart Outcomes Prevention Evaluation (HOPE) Study Investigators. Effects of ramipril on cardiovascular and microvascular outcomes in people with diabetes mellitus: results of the HOPE study and MICRO-HOPE substudy. Lancet 2000;355:253-9.

He FJ, MacGregor GA. Effect of modest salt reduction on blood pressure: a meta-analysis of randomized trials. Implications for public health. J Hum Hypertens 2002; 16: 761–770.

He FJ, MacGregor GA. How far should salt intake be reduced? Hypertension 2003; 42:1093–1099.

Higashi Y, Oshima T, Sasaki N, et al. Relationship between insulin resistance and endothelium-dependent vascular relaxation in patients with essential hypertension. Hypertension. 1997;29(1 pt 2):280-285.

Houstis N, Rosen ED, Lander ES. Reactive oxygen species have a causal role in multiple forms of insulin resistance. Nature 2006;440:944-948.

Hu G, Jousilahti P, Peltonen M, Lindstrom J, Tuomilehto J. Urinary sodium and potassium excretion and the risk of type 2 diabetes: a prospective study in Finland. Diabetologia 2005;48:1477-1483.

IDF Clinical Guidelines Task Force. Global Guideline for Type 2 Diabetes: recommendations for standard, comprehensive, and minimal care. Diabet Med. 2006 Jun;23(6):579-93.

Ito S, Komatsu K, Tsukamoto K, Sved AF. Excitatory amino acids in the rostral ventrolateral medulla support blood pressure in spontaneously hypertensive rats. Hypertension. 2000;35:413–417.

Jacob S, Balletshofer B, Henriksen EJ, et al. Beta-blocking agents in patients with insulin resistance: effects of vasodilating beta-blockers. Blood Press 1999; 8(5-6): 261-8.

Kahn AM, Seidel CL, Allen JCS, O'Neil RG. Insulin reduces contraction and intracellular calcium concentration in vascular smooth muscle. Hypertension 1993;22:735-742.

Kanauchi M, Kanauchi K, Hashimoto T, Saito Y. Metabolic syndrome and new category 'pre-hypertension' in a Japanese population. Curr Med Res Opin 2004;20:1365-70.

Kawabe T, Chitravanshi VC, Kawabe K, Sapru HN. Cardiovascular effects of adrenocorticotropin microinjections into the rostral ventrolateral medullary pressor area of the rat. Brain Res. 2006;1102:117 126.

Khaw KT, Bingham S, Welch A, et al. Blood pressure and urinary sodium in men and women. the Norfolk Cohort of the European Prospective Investigation into Cancer (EPIC-Norfolk). Am J Clin Nutr 2004; 80: 1397–1403.

Kim YC, Zemel MB. Insulin increases vascular smooth muscle recovery from intracellular calcium loads. Hypertension 1993;22:74-77.

Kjeldsen SE, McInnes GT, Mancia G, Hua TA, Julius S, Weber MA, Coca A, Girerd X, Jamerson K, Larochelle P, Macdonald T, Schmieder RE, Anthony Schork M, Viskoper R, Widimsky J, Zanchetti A. Progressive effects of valsartan compared with amlodipine in prevention of diabetes according to categories of diabetogenic risk in hypertensive patients: the VALUE trial. Blood Press. 2008;17(3):170-7.

Kohner EM, Aldington SJ, Stratton IM, Manley SE, Holman RR, Matthews DR, et al. United

Kingdom Prospective Diabetes Study, 30: Diabetic retinopathy at diagnosis of non-insulin-dependent diabetes mellitus and associated risk factors. Arch Ophthalmol 1998;116:297-303.

Laakso M, Edelman SV, Brechtel G, Baron AD. Decreased effect of insulin to stimulate skeletal muscle blood flow in obese men: a novel mechanism for insulin resistance. J Clin Invest 1990;85:1844–1852.

Lasser VI, Raczynski JM, Stevens VJ, Mattfeldt-Beman MK, Kumanyika S, Evans M, Danielson E, Dalcin A, Batey DM, Belden LK, et al.Trials of Hypertension Prevention, phase II. Structure and content of the weight loss and dietary sodium reduction interventions. Trials of Hypertension Prevention (TOHP) Collaborative Research Group. Ann Epidemiol. 1995;5(2):156-64.

Lawes CM, Vander HS, Rodgers A. Global burden of blood-pressure-related disease, 2001. Lancet 2008; 371: 1513–1518.

Lax DS, Benstein JA, Tolbert E, et al. Effects of salt restriction on renal growth and glomerular injury in rats with remnant kidneys. Kidney Int 1992; 41: 1527–1534.

Leung PS. The physiology of a local renin-angiotensin system in the pancreas. J Physiol. 2007;580:31-37.

Leung PS, de Gasparo M. Involvement of the pancreatic renin-angiotensin system in insulin resistance and the metabolic syndrome. J Cardiometab Syndr. 2006;1:197-203.

Levy J, Zemel MB, Sowers JR. Role of cellular calcium metabolism in abnormal glucose metabolism and diabetic hypertension. Am J Med 1989;87(suppl 6A): 15S-16S.

Lewis EJ, Hunsicker LG, Clarke WR, Berl T, Pohl MA, Lewis JB, Ritz E, Atkins RC, Rohde R, Raz I; Collaborative Study Group: Renoprotective effect of the angiotensin-receptor antagonist irbesartan in patients with nephropathy due to type 2 diabetes. N Engl J Med 345: 851–860, 2001.

Lind L, Pollare T, Berne C, et al. Long-term metabolic effects of antihypertensive drugs. Am Heart J 1994; 128(6 Pt 1): 1177-83.

Lindholm LH, Hansson L, Ekbom T, et al. Comparison of antihypertensive treatments in preventing cardiovascular events in elderly diabetic patients: results from the Swedish Trial in Old Patients with Hypertension-2. STOP Hypertension-2 Study Group. J Hypertens 2000; 18:1671-5.

Lindholm LH, Ibsen H, Dahlöf B, et al; LIFE Study Group. Cardiovascular morbidity and mortality in patients with diabetes in the Losartan Intervention For Endpoint reduction in hypertension study (LIFE): a randomised trial against atenolol. Lancet 2002; 359: 1004-1010.

Lissner L, Bengtsson C, Lapidus L, Kristjansson K, Wedel H. Fasting insulin in relation to subsequent blood pressure changes and hypertension in women. Hypertension 1992;20:797–801.

Lithell HO. Effect of antihypertensive drugs on insulin, glucose, and lipid metabolism. Diabetes Care 1991; 14: 203-9.

Lopes HF, Martin KL, Nashar K, Morrow JD, Goodfriend TL, Egan BM. DASH diet lowers blood pressure and lipid-induced oxidative stress in odbesity. Hypertension 2003;41:422-430.

Lupi R, Del Guerra S, Bugliani M, et al. The direct effects of the angiotensinconverting enzyme inhibitors, zofenoprilat and enalaprilat, on isolated human pancreatic islets. Eur J Endocrinol. 2006;154:355-361.

Mancia G, Brown M, Castaigne A, et al.; INSIGHT. Outcomes with nifedipine GITS or Co-amilozide in hypertensive diabetics and nondiabetics in Intervention as a Goal in Hypertension (INSIGHT). Hypertension 2003; 41: 431-436.

Mancia G, De Backer G, Dominiczak A, Cifkova R, Fagard R, Germano G, Grassi G, Heagerty AM, Kjeldsen SE, Laurent S, Narkiewicz K, Ruilope L, Rynkiewicz A, Schmieder RE, Boudier HA, Zanchetti A; ESH-ESC Task Force on the Management of Arterial Hypertension. 2007 ESH-ESC Practice Guidelines for the Management of Arterial Hypertension: ESH-ESC Task Force on the Management of Arterial Hypertension. J Hypertens. 2007 Sep;25(9):1751-62.

Mann JF, Gerstein HC, Pogue J, Bosch J, Yusuf S. Renal insufficiency as a predictor of cardiovascular outcomes and the impact of ramipril: The HOPE randomized trial. Ann Intern Med 2001;134:629-36.

Mann JF, Schmieder RE, McQueen M, Dyal L, Schumacher H, Pogue J, Wang X, Maggioni A, Budaj A, Chaithiraphan S, Dickstein K, Keltai M, Metsärinne K, Oto A, Parkhomenko A, Piegas LS, Svendsen TL, Teo KK, Yusuf S. The ONgoing Telmisartan Alone and in combination with Ramipril Global Endpoint Trial (ONTARGET®) Investigators. Renal outcomes with telmisartan, ramipril, or both, in people at high vascular risk (the ONTARGET® study): a multicentre, randomised, double-blind, controlled trial. Lancet. 2008;372:547–53.

Matsui H, Shimosawa T, Uetake Y, et al. Protective effect of potassium against the hypertensive cardiac dysfunction: association with reactive oxygen species reduction. Hypertension 2006;48:225-231.

Mbanya J-CN, Thomas TH, Wilkinson R, Alberti KGMM, Taylor R. Hypertension and hyperinsulinemia: a relation in diabetes but not essential hypertension. Lancet. 1988; 1: 733–734.

McCarty MF. Elevated sympathetic activity may promote insulin resistance syndrome by activating alpha-1 adrenergic receptors on adipocytes. Med Hypoteses 2004;62:830-8.

McMurray JJ, Holman RR, Haffner SM, Bethel MA, Holzhauer B, Hua TA, Belenkov Y, Boolell M, Buse JB, Buckley BM, Chacra AR, Chiang FT, Charbonnel B, Chow CC, Davies MJ, Deedwania P, Diem P, Einhorn D, Fonseca V, Fulcher GR, Gaciong Z, Gaztambide S, Giles T, Horton E, Ilkova H, Jenssen T, Kahn SE, Krum H, Laakso M, Leiter LA, Levitt NS, Mareev V, Martinez F, Masson C, Mazzone T, Meaney E, Nesto R, Pan C, Prager R, Raptis SA, Rutten GE, Sandstroem H, Schaper F, Scheen A, Schmitz O, Sinay I, Soska V, Stender S, Tamás G, Tognoni G, Tuomilehto J, Villamil AS, Vozár J, Califf RM. NAVIGATOR Study Group. N Engl J Med. 2010 Apr 22;362(16):1477-90.

Morgan DA, Ray CA, Balon TW, Mark AL. Metformin increases insulin sensitivity and lowers arterial pressure in spontaneously hypertensive rats. Hypertension 1992;20:421.

Muntzel MS, Morgan DA, Mark AL, Johnson AK. Intracerebroventricular insulin produces nonuniform regional increases in sympathetic nerve activity. Am J Physiol Regul Integr Comp Physiol. 1994;267:R1350–1355.

Nagi DK, Hendra TJ, Ryle AJ, Cooper TM, Temple RC, Clark PMS, Eschneider AE, Hales CN, Yudkin JS. The relationship of concentrations of insulin, intact proinsulin and 32–33 split proinsulin with cardiovascular risk factors in type 2 (non-insulin-dependent) diabetic subjects. Diabetologia. 1990; 33: 532–537.

Nakata T, Takeda K, Hatta T, Kiyama M, Moriguchi J, Miki S, Kawa T, Morimoto S, Nakamura K, Uchida A, Itoh H, Sasaki S, Nakagawa M. Blockade of angiotensin II receptors inhibits the increase in blood pressure induced by insulin. J Cardiovasc Pharmacol. 1998;31:248–252.

Natali A, Santoro D, Palombo C, Cerri M, Ghione S, Ferrannini E. Impaired insulin action on skeletal muscle metabolism in essential hypertension. Hypertension 1991; 17:170–178.

Niklason A, Hedner T, Niskanen L, Lanke J; Captopril Prevention Project Study Group. Development of diabetes is retarded by ACE inhibition in hypertensive patients--a subanalysis of the Captopril Prevention Project (CAPPP). J Hypertens 2004; 22: 645.652

Ogihara T, Asano T, Ando K, et al. High-salt diet enhances insulin signaling and induces insulin resistance in Dahl salt-sensitive rats. Hypertension 2002;40:83-89.

Ogihara T, Asano T, Ando K, et al . Angiotensin II-induced insulin resistance is associated with enhanced insulin signaling. Hypertension 2002;40:872-879.

Ogihara T, Asano T, Katagiri H, et al . Oxidative stress induces insulin resistance by activating the nuclear factor-kappa B pathway and disrupting normal subcellular distribution of phosphatidylinositol 3-kinase. Diabetologia 2004;47:794-805.

Park HS, Lee K. Greater beneficial effects of visceral fat reduction compared with subcutaneous fat reduction on parameters of the metabolic syndrome: a study of weight reduction programmes in subjects with visceral and subcutaneous obesity. Diabet Med 2005;22:266-72.

Passa P. Hyperinsulinemia, insulin resistance and essential hypertension. Horm Res 1992;38(1-2):33-8.

Patel A; ADVANCE Collaborative Group, MacMahon S, Chalmers J, Neal B, et al. Effects of a fixed combination of perindopril and indapamide on macrovascular and microvascular outcomes in patients with type 2 diabetes mellitus (the ADVANCE trial): a randomised controlled trial. Lancet. 2007; 370:829-840.

Persson F, Lewis JB, Lewis EJ, Rossing P, Hollenberg NK, Parving HH; AVOID Study Investigators. Impact of baseline renal function on the efficacy and safety of aliskiren added to losartan in patients with type 2 diabetes and nephropathy. Diabetes Care 2010;33(11):2304-9.

Pitocco D, Zaccardi F, Di Stasio E, Romitelli F, Santini SA, Zuppi C, Ghirlanda G. Oxidative stress, nitric oxide, and diabetes. Rev Diabet Stud. 2010;7(1):15-25.

Player MS, Mainous AG 3rd, Diaz VA, Everett CJ. Prehypertension and insulin resistance in a nationally representative adult population. J Clin Hypertens (Greenwich) 2007;9:424-9.

Pollare T, Lithell H, Berne C. Insulin resistance is a characteristic feature of primary hypertension independent of obesity. Metabolism 1990;39:167–174.

Psaty BM, Lumley T, Furberg CD, Schellenbaum G, Pahor M, Alderman MH, et al. Health outcomes associated with various antihypertensive therapies used as first-line agents: A network meta-analysis. *JAMA* 2003;289:2534-44.

Rahmouni K, Haynes WG, Morgan DA, Mark AL. Role of melanocortin-4 receptors in mediating renal sympathoactivation to leptin and insulin. J Neurosci. 2003;23:5998–6004.

Rahmouni K, Mark AL,Haynes WG, et al. Adipose depot-specific modulation of angiotensinogen gene expression in diet-induced obesity. Am J Physiol Endocrinol Metab 2004;286:E891-E895.

Raitakari OT, Porkka KVK, Rönnemaa T, Knip M, Uhari M, Akerblom HK, Viikari JSA. The role of insulin in clustering of serum lipids and blood pressure in children and adolescents. Diabetologia 1995; 38:1042–1050.

Ramsay LE, Yeo WW, Jackson PR. Influence of diuretics, calcium antagonists, and alpha-blockers on insulin sensitivity and glucose tolerance in hypertensive patients. J Cardiovasc Pharmacol 1992; 20 Suppl 11:S49-53.

Reaven GM, Hoffman BB. A role for insulin in the aetiology and course of hypertension. Lancet 1987;2:435–436.

Reaven GM. Hyperinsulinemia in a normal population as a predictor of non-insulin-dependent diabetes mellitus, hypertension, and coronary heart disease: The Barilla factory revisited. Metabolism 1994;48:989–994.

Reaven GM, Lithell H, Landsberg L. Hypertension and associated metabolic abnormalities–the role of insulin resistance and the sympathoadrenal system. N Engl J Med 1996;334:374-381.

Resnick LM. Ionic basis of hypertension, insulin resistance, vascular disease, and related disorders. The mechanism of "syndrome X". Am J Hypertens 1993;6(4):123S-134S.

Roberts CK, Sindhu KK. Oxidative stress and metabolic syndrome. Life Sci. 2009;84(21-22):705-12.

Rose G, Stamler J.The INTERSALT study: background, methods and main results. INTERSALT Co-operative Research Group. J Hum Hypertens. 1989 Oct;3(5):283-8.

Saad MF, Knowler WC, Pettitt DJ, Nelson RG, Mott DM, Bennett PH. Insulin and hypertension: relationship to obesity and glucose intolerance in Pima Indians. Diabetes 1990; 39: 1430 1435.

Saad MF, Lillioja S, Nyomba BL, Castillo C, Ferraro R, DeGregorio M, Ravussin E, Knowler WC, Bennett PH, Howard BV, Bogardus C. Racial differences in the relation between blood pressure and insulin resistance. N Engl J Med. 1991; 324: 733–739.

Sacks FM, Svetkey LP, Vollmer WM, Appel LJ, Bray GA, Harsha D, et al. Effects on blood pressure of reduced dietary sodium and the Dietary Approaches to Stop Hypertension (DASH) diet. DASH-Sodium Collaborative Research Group. N Engl J Med 2001;344 :3-10.

Sathiyapriya V, Nandeesha H, Bobby Z, Pavithran P, Selvaraj N, Rattina Dasse N. Insulin resistance and enhanced protein glycation in men with prehypertension. Clin Chem Lab Med 2006;44:1457-61.

Schmidt AC, Graf C, Brixius K, *et al.* Blood pressure-lowering effect of nebivolol in hypertensive patients with type 2 diabetes mellitus: the YESTONO study._Clin Drug Investig 2007; 27(12): 841-9.

Shamiss A, Carroll J, Rosenthall T. Insulin resistance in secondary hypertension. Am J Hypertens 1992;5:26–28.

Shen D-C, Shieh S-M, Fuh M, Wu D-A, Chen Y-DI, Reaven GM. Resistance to insulin-stimulated glucose uptake in patients with hypertension. J Clin Endocrinol Metab 1988;66:580–583.

Shi Y, Vanhoutte PM. Reactive oxygen-derived free radicals are key to the endothelial dysfunction of diabetes. J Diabetes. 2009;1(3):151-62.

Shimosawa T, Shibagaki Y, Ishibashi K, et al . Adrenomedullin, an endogenous peptide, counteracts cardiovascular damage. Circulation 2002;105:106-111.

Singh M, Mensah GA, Bakris G. Pathogenesis and clinical physiology of hypertension. Cardiol Clin 2010;28(4):545-59.

Sironi AM, Gastaldelli A, Mari A, et al. Visceral fat in hypertension: influence on insulin resistance and beta-cell function. Hypertension 2004;44:127-133.

Skarfors ET, Lithell HO, Selinus I. Risk factors for the development of hypertension: a 10-year longitudinal study in middle-aged men. J Hypertens 1991;9:217–223.

Song K, Allen AM, Paxinos G, Mendelsohn FA. Angiotensin II receptor subtypes in rat brain. Clin Exp Pharmacol Physiol. 1991;18:93–96.

Sowers JR, Bakris GL. Antihypertensive therapy and the risk of type 2 diabetes mellitus. N Engl JMed 2000;342:969-70.

Sowers JR, Reed J. 1999 Clinical Advisory Treatment of Hypertension and Diabetes. J Clin Hypertens (Greenwich) 2000;2:132-3.

Sowers JR, Haffner S. Treatment of cardiovascular and renal risk factors in the diabetic hypertensive. Hypertension 2002;40:781-8.

Sowers JR. Insulin resistance and hypertension. Am J Physiol Heart Circ Physiol 2004;286(5):H1597-602.

Staessen JA, Wang J, Bianchi G, Birkenhäger WH. Essential hypertension. Lancet 2003 May 10;361(9369):1629-41.

Steinberg HO, Chaker H, Leaming R, Johnson A, Brechtel G, Baron AD. Obesity/insulin resistance is associated with endothelial dysfunction: implications for the syndrome of insulin resistance. J Clin Invest. 1996;97:2601-2610.

Strazzullo P, Barbato A, Galletti F, et al. Abnormalities of renal sodium handling in the metabolic syndrome. Results of Olivetti heart study. J Hypertension 2006;24:*1633-1639.*

Suzuki M, Kimura Y, Tsushima M, Harano Y. Association of insulin resistance with salt sensitivity and nocturnal fall of blood pressure. Hypertension 2000;35:864-868.

Sweeney G, Klip A. Regulation of the Na+/K+-ATPase by insulin: why and how? Mol Cell Biochem. 1998;182(1-2):121-33.

Swislocki ALM, Hoffman BB, Reaven GM. Insulin resistance, glucose intolerance and hyperinsulinemia in patients with hypertension. Am J Hypertens 1989;2:419–423.

The ALLHAT Officers and Coordinators for the ALLHAT Collaborative Research Group. Major outcomes in high-risk hypertensive patients randomized to angiotensin-converting enzyme inhibitor or calcium channel blocker vs diuretic: The Antihypertensive and Lipid-Lowering Treatment to Prevent Heart Attack Trial (ALLHAT). JAMA 2002;288:2981-97.

The Seventh Report of the Joint National Committee on Prevention, Detection, Evaluation, and Treatment of High Blood Pressure. National High Blood Pressure Education Programm. Bethesda (MD): National Heart, Lung, and Blood Institute (US); 2004 Aug. Report No.: 04-5230.

Tobian L. Salt and hypertension: lessons from animal models that relate to human hypertension. Hypertension 1991; 17 (Suppl I): I52–I58.

Toutouzas K, Riga M, Stefanadi E, Stefanadis C. Asymmetric dimethylarginine (ADMA) and other endogenous nitric oxide synthase (NOS) inhibitors as an important cause of vascular insulin resistance. Horm Metab Res. 2008;40(9):655-9.

Trilling JS, Froom J. The irgent need to improve hypertension care. Arch Fam Med 2000; 9:794-801.

Tuomilehto J, Rastenyte D, Birkenhager WH, Thijs L, Antikainen R, Bulpitt CJ, et al. Effects of calcium-channel blockade in older patients with diabetes and systolic hypertension. Systolic Hypertension in Europe Trial Investigators. N Engl J Med 1999;340:677-84.

UK Prospective Diabetes Study Group. Tight blood pressure control and risk of macrovascular and microvascular complications in type 2 diabetes: UKPDS 38. BMJ 1998;317:703-13.

UK Prospective Diabetes Study Group. Efficacy of atenolol and captoril in reducing risk of macrovascular and microvascular complications in type 2 diabetes. UKPDS 39. BMJ 1998; 317: 713-720.

Uzu T, Sawaguchi M, Maegawa H, Kashiwagi A, Shiga Microalbuminuria Reduction Trial (SMART) Group. Reduction of microalbuminuria in patients with type 2 diabetes: the Shiga Microalbuminuria Reduction Trial (SMART). Diabetes Care. 2007;30(6):1581-3.

Verhave JC, Hillege HL, Burgerhof JG, et al. Sodium intake affects urinary albumin excretion especially in overweight subjects. J Intern Med 2004; 256: 324–330.

Vollmer WM, Sacks FM, Ard J, Appel LJ, Bray GA, Simons-Morton DG, et al. Effects of diet and sodium intake on blood pressure: Subgroup analysis of the DASH-sodium trial. Ann Intern Med 2001;135:1019-28.

Wagh A, Stone NJ. Treatment of metabolic syndrome. Expert Rev Cardiovasc Ther 2004;2(2):213 28.

Wang W, Lee ET, Fabsitz RR, Devereux R, Best L, Welty TK, Howard BV. A longitudinal study of hypertension risk factors and their relation to cardiovascular disease. The Strong Heart Study. Hypertension 2006;47:403-9.

Weber MA, Bakris GL, Jamerson K, Weir M, Kjeldsen SE, Devereux RB, Velazquez EJ, Dahlöf B, Kelly RY, Hua TA, Hester A, Pitt B; ACCOMPLISH Investigators. Cardiovascular events during differing hypertension therapies in patients with diabetes. J Am Coll Cardiol. 2010;56(1):77-85.

Welborn TA, Breckenridge A, Rubinstein AH, Dollery CT, Fraser TR. Serum-insulin in essential hypertension and in peripheral vascular disease. Lancet 1966;1:1136–1137.

Wheatcroft SB, Williams IL, Shah AM, Kearney MT. Pathophysiological implications of insulin resistance on vascular endothelial function. Diabet Med. 2003; 20: 255–268.

Whelton PK, Appel LJ, Espeland MA, et al. Sodium reduction and weight loss in the treatment of hypertension in older persons: a randomized controlled trial of nonpharmacologic interventions in the elderly (TONE). TONE Collaborative Research Group. JAMA 1998; 279:839–846.

World Health Report 2002: Reducing risks, promoting healthy life. Geneva, Switzerland: World Health Organization. 2002. http://www.who.int/whr/2002/.

World Health Organization. The World Health Report 2002: Risk to Health 2002. Geneva: World Health Organization. http://www.who.int/whr/2002/.

Yusuf S, Reddy S, Ounpuu S, Anand S. Global burden of cardiovascular diseases. Part I: General considerations, the epidemiologic transition, risk factors, and impact of urbanization. Circulation 2001; 104:2746-2753.

Zavaroni I, Bonini L, Gasparini P, Barilli AL, Zuccarelli A, Dall'Aglio E, Delsignore R.,

Zemel MB, Reddy S, Shehin S, Lockette W, Sowers JR. Vascular reactivity in Zucker obese rats. Role of insulin resistance. J Vase Med Biol 1990;2:81-85.

Zemel MB, lannucci A, Moore JW. Role of insulin in regulating vascular smooth muscle CaI+-ATPase expression. J Vase Med Biol 1993;4:79-84.

Zheng Y, Yamada H, Sakamoto K, et al. Roles of insulin receptor substrates in insulin-induced stimulation of renal proximal bicarbonate absorption. J Am Soc Nephrol 2005;16:2288-2295.

Ziemke F, Mantzoros CS. Adiponectin in insulin resistance: lessons from translational research. Am J Clin Nutr. 2010;91(1):258S-261S.

12

Managing Hypertension in Patients with Diabetes

Arthur L.M. Swislocki[1,2] and David Siegel[1, 2]
[1]*Medical Service, Department of Veterans Affairs, Northern California Health Care System, Mather, CA*
[2]*Department of Medicine, School of Medicine, University of California, Davis USA*

1. Introduction

Cardiovascular disease remains the leading cause of death in industrialized nations. Type 2 diabetes confers cardiovascular risk comparable to a previous myocardial infarction, and is the most common cause of chronic kidney disease. Diabetes and hypertension account for 2/3 of cardiovascular risk [1]. Over 75% of adults with diabetes are hypertensive, or being treated with hypertensive medications [2] In patients with type 1 diabetes, the presence of hypertension signals significant kidney damage whereas in patients with type 2 diabetes, hypertension is usually present at the time of diagnosis [2]. On the other hand, many hypertensive treatments, specifically diuretics, worsen glucose control; the overall implications of this are as yet unclear [2]. Because of the singular risk resulting from the combination of diabetes and hypertension, significant effort has been expended to improve patient outcome. While several recent excellent reviews address different aspects of this issue [1-3], we will evaluate the management of hypertension in diabetes, particularly from the perspective of managing hypertension in metabolic syndrome. We will evaluate the metabolic effects of different agents used for blood pressure control, consider specific patient-related issues, discuss shortcomings of recent trials, and consider possible future directions in genetic analyses.

There are over 65 million hypertensives in the United States [4]. Unfortunately, the pharmacological treatment of these individuals has had less than the predicted benefit on coronary heart disease (CHD) mortality [5-7]. For many years, It has been postulated that treatment with some antihypertensives might have metabolic and other untoward effects that negate some of the benefits of blood-pressure lowering [5, 8]. This may be particularly true for individuals with the metabolic syndrome, a constellation of anthropometric and metabolic abnormalities that includes central obesity, hypertension, elevated levels of fasting glucose and triglycerides, low concentrations of high-density lipoprotein cholesterol (HDL-C), and insulin resistance which is associated with increased cardiovascular disease morbidity and mortality [9-11]. Of the five diagnostic criteria for metabolic syndrome, hypertension and central obesity are most frequently present [12, 13].

Why is this increasingly important in the US? The prevalence of obesity has doubled in the US in the past 20 years [14]; the number of extremely obese individuals with a BMI >35 kg/m^2 is almost 5% of the population. Obese compared with normal weight individuals have a 3.5 fold increased risk of developing hypertension while up to 60% of obese individuals have hypertension [15, 16]. The association between obesity and hypertension may be related to greater insulin resistance, leptin-mediated enhancement of sympathetic activity, sodium and fluid retention, and adipocyte-mediated effects on angiotensin II and atrial natriuretic peptide levels [17]. Patients with hypertension have an increased prevalence of type 2 diabetes mellitus and impaired glucose tolerance [18, 19]. Patients with mild hypertension also have lower HDL-cholesterol concentrations and higher HDL catabolic rates; these findings appear to correlate with insulin resistance [20]. With hypertension, obesity and diabetes mellitus increasing in frequency, it is not surprising that the age-adjusted prevalence of metabolic syndrome in the general US population is 24.0% for men and 24.3% for women [21].

Lifestyle therapies for patients with metabolic syndrome, including weight reduction, increased physical activity, decreased sodium and alcohol reduction, reduced consumption of saturated and trans fats and cholesterol, and increased consumption of fresh fruits and vegetables are extremely important. Studies have shown that dietary changes can lower blood pressure and improve other metabolic syndrome components [22, 23]. Increased exercise can also lower blood pressure [24].

Despite the benefits of lifestyle changes, pharmacological treatment of hypertension is frequently needed. However, the choice of an antihypertensive is controversial. Studies suggest that treatment with different antihypertensive drug classes may have varied effects on glucose and lipid metabolism [25]. Changes in insulin sensitivity are associated with adverse effects on glucose control [26, 27]. Increases in blood glucose during antihypertensive treatment have been found to be a predictor of myocardial infarction [28]. Insulin resistance is also associated with endothelial dysfunction, which is also predictive of future cardiovascular events [29]. Lind et al. have reported that these metabolic effects persist with long-term (> 2-3 years) antihypertensive treatment [30]. In this context, it would be important to choose antihypertensives that have the least adverse metabolic effects, particularly in patients with the metabolic syndrome.

In addition, to the choice of antihypertensive agent, the degree of blood pressure lowering is important. The lower the goal, the greater the number of antihypertensive agents needed, the cost of these agents and the potential for side effects. Patient adherence declines with the number of medications required. It is important to balance these drawbacks with improvement in clinical outcomes.

2. Evidence for blood pressure goals

By some standards, the Action to Control Cardiovascular Risks in Diabetes Study (ACCORD) was a disappointment. ACCORD was a large well-designed trial that attempted to study the effects of tight control of blood sugar, hypertension, and lipids in patients with type 2 diabetes mellitus [31]. In the original report, published in the *New England Journal of Medicine* in 2008, 10,251 patients (mean age, 62.2 years and median glycated hemoglobin level of 8.1%) were assigned to receive intensive therapy targeting a glycated hemoglobin level below 6 % or standard therapy targeting a level from 7.0 to 7.9% [31]. Of these patients, 38% were women and 35% had had a previous cardiac event. The primary outcome was a composite of nonfatal myocardial infarction, nonfatal stroke or death from cardiovascular causes. Details of the glycemic and lipid control arms have been presented [31, 32], and analyzed [33] elsewhere. The results of the blood pressure arm will be focused on below.

4,733 participants in ACCORD were randomly assigned to intensive blood pressure therapy, targeting a systolic pressure of <120 mm Hg or standard therapy targeting a systolic pressure of <140 mm Hg [34]. Again, the primary composite outcome was nonfatal myocardial infarction, nonfatal stroke, or death from cardiovascular causes. The mean follow-up was 4.7 years. The annual rate of the primary outcome was 1.87% in the intensive therapy group and 2.09% in the standard therapy group (P=0.20). The annual death rates from any cause were 1.28% and 1.19% in the two groups, respectively (P=0.55). The annual stroke rate, a pre specified secondary outcome, were 0.32% and 0.53% in the two groups, respectively (P=0.01). Serious adverse events attributed to antihypertensive treatment occurred in 77 of the 2,362 participants in the intensive therapy group (3.3%) and 30 of the 2,371 participants in the standard therapy group (1.3%) (P <0.01). There were more subjects with a decrease of their estimated glomerular filtration rate to less than 30 ml per minute per 1.73 m^2 of body surface area in the intensive therapy group than in the standard therapy group (99 versus 52 events, P <0.01).

The interpretation of the ACCORD blood pressure results is complicated by a number of factors. The event rate observed in the standard therapy group was almost 50% lower than expected. This result may have been a consequence of the frequent use of statins and inclusion criteria that directed participants with dyslipidemia into the ACCORD lipid trial, leaving participants who were at lower risk in the blood pressure trial. Additionally, ACCORD may have been under powered and of too short of duration to discern a benefit [35]. In ACCORD the confidence intervals were wide and do not exclude a 27% benefit for the intensively treated group for the primary end point at 5 years. It is also possible that the effects of intensive blood pressure control in the setting of good lipid and glucuose control may differ for cerebrovascular and coronary events. That is, intensive blood pressure control is more likely to prevent strokes than myocardial infarctions. In a classic meta analysis, Collins and colleagues found that the decrease in stroke from antihypertensive therapy in clinical trials was what would be predicted based on epidemiologic studies [5]. However the decrease in coronary artery disease (CAD) was about one-half of what would be predicted.

The ACCORD blood pressure study population was relatively healthy and thus unlikely to have a high proportion of events. The 5,000 patients pre study mean systolic blood pressure was 140 mm Hg of mercury. Their mean age was 62 years and nearly one-half were women. The mean serum creatinine of this group was 0.9 mg per deciliter and 87% were receiving antihypertensive medication at the time of enrollment. The average glycated hemoglobin level was 8.3% and the mean body mass index was 32 kg/m^2. The mean urinary albumin/creatinine ratio was 14.3. Although these middle-aged patients were overweight and had type 2 diabetes, they had no substantial evidence of kidney disease and appeared to have good blood pressure control. At the 12 month visit, nearly 90% of patients were receiving a drug that blocks the renin angiotensin system, while more than 50% received β-blockers, about 40% received a calcium channel blocker, and nearly 60% received statins and platelet inhibitors. One might conclude that at 5 years, people with type 2 diabetes who have good quality cardiovascular care and no evidence of kidney disease do not have a major therapeutic advantage from lowering systolic blood pressure to <120 mm Hg. A longer follow-up time might be necessary to see a benefit of lowering blood pressure to this degree.

The negative outcome in ACCORD in the intensely treated blood pressure arm might also be attributed to the lack of effect on ischemic heart disease events that are included in the composite end point. In the intensive treatment arm, investigators were advised to begin a regimen of an ACE inhibitor or angiotensin receptor blocker (ARB) plus a thiazide-like diuretic, chlorthalidone [36]. The same requirements were not given to the less intensively treated group. This resulted in the intensively treated group receiving roughly twice as much chlorthalidone as the less intensively treated group. That is, diuretics were used 83% and 89% of the time at 12 months and at the last visit, respectively, in the intensively treated group while in the standard care group, the usage was 52% and 56%. This amount of diuretic usage could account for the greater prevalence of hypokalemia seen in the intensive treatment group (P=.01) [8]. Data from the Systolic Hypertension in the Elderly Program (SHEP Trial), suggest that this degree of hypokalemia would essentially eliminate the projected benefit on ischemic heart disease events from the blood pressure reduction achieved in ACCORD [37].

The United Kingdom Prospective Diabetes Study (UKPDS) was a randomized, prospective, multicenter trial that, in addition to its attention to glycemic control, randomized patients to a "tight" blood pressure control regimen including ACE inhibition (captopril) or β-blocker therapy (atenolol), or "less-tight" blood pressure control that excluded these agents [38]. For tight compared to less-tight control of blood pressure, there were dramatic and significant improvements in risk reduction in any diabetes-related end point (24%), diabetes-related death (32%), stroke (44%), and microvascular disease (37%) [39]. In UKPDS, the goal blood pressure for the tight group was <150/85, and for the less-tight, <180/105. The mean achieved blood pressures were 144/82 and 154/87 mm Hg for the tight and less-tight groups, respectively. Of note, the mean blood pressure, at entry, was 160/94.

The Steno-2 Study reported a post interventional benefit for micro- and macrovascular complications of diabetes that persisted after risk factor intervention, although within-trial differences in risk factors for these complications (e.g., blood pressure) diminished, suggesting a persistent effect of earlier improvement in risk factors—a so-called legacy effect [40]. The diminishment in the difference of risk factors resulted from different phenomena: In the intensively-treated group, systolic blood pressure rose slightly in follow-up, while it remained stable in the conventionally-treated group. On the other hand, diastolic blood pressure remained low in the intensively-treated group, while it continued to fall in the conventional group. Recently, the survivor cohort of UKPDS was evaluated after a 10-year post-interventional follow-up that examined whether a continued benefit of improved blood pressure control could be demonstrated [41]. In contrast to the Steno-2 Study, the benefits of previously-attained improved blood pressure control were not sustained when between-group differences were lost. There were no differences in blood pressure control in patients treated with captopril or atenolol. Again, in contrast to the Steno-2 findings, in both "tight" and "less-tight" groups, blood pressures actually improved in follow-up and were indistinguishable, in the mid-140's/high 70's range. Thus, it may be that it was the improved blood pressure control in the "less-tight" group, as opposed to treatment failure in the "tight" group that decreased treatment differences.

INVEST (INternational VErapamil-SR/Trandolapril STudy) studied patients with multiple risk factors [42]. Of the 22576 participants (who were recruited because they had both coronary disease and hypertension), 6400 (28%) had diabetes. These patients were evaluated for the effects of achieved systolic blood pressure on the risk of cardiovascular events. Patients were categorized into three groups on this basis: tight (<130), usual (130-<140), and

uncontrolled (≥140) mm Hg achieved systolic blood pressure. Tight control was not associated with improved cardiovascular outcome compared to usual control. Uncontrolled patients did worse. A similar post hoc analysis of INVEST compared participants with and without peripheral arterial disease (PAD) [43]. 41.4% of PAD patients and 26.6% of those without PAD had diabetes (P<0.001). A J-shaped relationship was observed for patients with PAD: the hazard ratio for the primary outcome (all-cause death, nonfatal myocardial infarction, or nonfatal stroke), when plotted against achieved blood pressure, showed fewest events at blood pressures of 135-145/60-90); this was more pronounced for systolic blood pressure. Patients without PAD did not manifest this J-shaped association with systolic blood pressure. Patients with or without diabetes were not analyzed separately.
What lessons can be drawn about goal blood pressure for patients with metabolic syndrome from the studies cited above? It does not appear that the notion "the lower the better" applies to blood pressure in patients with type 2 diabetes, especially in those who are nonsmokers, have reasonable glycemic control and are taking statins and anti-platelet therapy. In ACCORD, lowering systolic blood pressure from the mid-130s to 120 mm Hg did not further reduce cardiovascular events, with the possible exception of stroke, which should be a pre-specified primary endpoint in future blood pressure clinical trials that aim for such low blood pressures. The price of lowering blood pressure to this degree in ACCORD was generally one additional antihypertensive and it was accompanied by a significantly higher rate of serious adverse events. Thus, it appears that lowering systolic blood pressure to 120 mm Hg is not warranted and recommendations to aim for a systolic blood pressure of <140 mm Hg and a diastolic blood pressure, based on the HOT and UKPDS results presented above, of <80 mm Hg are best supported by current evidence. However, it must be remembered that longer term follow-up of ACCORD may lead to different conclusions.

3. Effect of different classes of antihypertensive on components of the metabolic syndrome

Thiazide diuretics

Several studies have suggested an association between thiazide use and the development of glucose intolerance and diabetes. In the Antihypertensive and Lipid-Lowering Treatment to Prevent Heart Attack Trial (ALLHAT), the group randomized to chlorthalidone had a higher proportion of patients who developed diabetes than those randomized to either amlodipine or lisinopril [44]. In the Systolic Hypertension in the Elderly Program (SHEP), there was not a statistically significant increased rate of diabetes comparing chlorthalidone with placebo after 3 years, but in a later 14.3 year follow-up, 13% of patients given chlorthalidone versus 8.7% of those given placebo (P < 0.0001) developed diabetes [45, 46]. In a large study of hypertensive men and women, after adjustment for BMI, those taking compared with those not taking thiazide diuretics had an increased risk of developing diabetes [47]. We studied 2624 patients who were initiated on thiazide diuretics [48]. Increasing values of fasting blood glucose (FBG) were associated with increasing baseline BMI and there was a positive association between a new diagnosis of diabetes after thiazide initiation and increasing BMI that ranged from 2.7% in the first quartile of BMI to 6.5 % in the heaviest quartile. Studies have also found an association between blood glucose and thiazide dose [49, 50]. A review of nine studies using a relatively low dose (12.5 mg) of hydrochlorothiazide as monotherapy found that increases in glucose levels were nether clinically nor statistically different from baseline levels [51]. Interestingly, in most of these studies, there was little relationship between blood pressure effects and diuretic dose. An association between hypokalemia and glucose intolerance, even in euglycemic subjects, has been described [48, 52, 53]. In patients on thiazides, hypokalemia has been associated with higher FBG that improved after replacement of potassium [54].

Thiazide diuretics may impair glucose metabolism by decreasing peripheral insulin sensitivity, resulting in increasing insulin secretion [55-57]. Our results suggest that the probability of developing new diabetes after thiazide initiation is associated with increasing BMI [48]. This association is supported by our previous work (DS). In 139 patients randomized to 50 mg of hydrochlorothiazide for 2 months, there was an increasing change from baseline serum insulin levels as a consequence of increasing body mass index [18].

Diuretics may also affect lipid metabolism. In general, high dose diuretics have been reported to increase serum total cholesterol by about 4% and serum LDL-cholesterol by 10% [51]. In ALLHAT, the group randomized to chlorthalidone had a higher total cholesterol levels at 2 years by about 3 mg/dL (~1.5%) than those randomized to either amlodipine or lisinopril ($P<.001$ for both); this difference diminished at 4 years for amlodipine, although not for lisinopril [44]. In SHEP, there was a small but significant increase of total cholesterol ($P<.01$) and decrease of HDL-cholesterol ($P<.01$) comparing chlorthalidone to placebo after 3 years. In another study, there was a 10% increase ($P<.05$) in fasting triglycerides from baseline after 16 weeks of treatment with hydrochlorothiazide compared with those treated with valsartan [58]. In a cross-sectional study from Brazil, hypertensive patients treated with diuretic monotherapy had a more atherogenic lipid profile (increased total- and LDL-cholesterol and apolipoprotein B) than patients on combined diuretic-based medication regimes, suggesting that the nondiuretic therapy had a mitigating effect on the lipid profile [59]. The mechanism of diuretic induced dyslipidemia may be related to increased hepatic production, in part mediated by a reduction in insulin sensitivity [51].

The impact of the ALLHAT findings on clinical recommendations is controversial [44]. On the one hand, are the metabolic abnormalities associated with chlorthalidone noted above. On the other hand, is the fact that those patients randomized to chlorthalidone had virtually identical clinical outcomes compared with lisinopril and amlodipine in terms of the primary outcome: the occurrence of coronary heart disease and nonfatal myocardial infarction. For secondary outcomes, chlorthalidone was superior to amlodipine in preventing heart failure, and compared with lisinopril, chlorthalidone was superior as a means to lower blood pressure and prevent stroke, as well as to prevent combined cardiovascular disease and perhaps heart failure. At present, we believe that thiazide diuretics (especially chlorthalidone) are alternative first choice agents in nondiabetic patients with metabolic syndrome but should be used carefully in patients with elevated BMI. In those instances where patients become diabetic after initiation of thiazides, we recommend that an alternative antihypertensive class be used rather than treat the metabolic consequences of thiazides with diabetic medications. In diabetics, thiazides diuretics may also be used. However, in those instances where initiation of these agents results in a worsening of glucose control, again, we would recommend the use of alternative agents.

β-Blockers

The place of β-blockers in the treatment of hypertension is controversial. This is partly based on the finding that these agents are less effective in reducing the incidence of stroke [60, 61], myocardial infarction and death than are other antihypertensives [61, 62]. These findings are complicated by the diversity of β-blockers that have varying pharmacological properties. The mechanisms of action and pathophysiological effects vary widely among the nonselective, selective, and vasodilating β-blockers. Added to this variation are the effects of agents such as carvedilol that have both non-selective β-blocker and α_1-blocking properties.

In several studies of non-selective [63] or β_1 selective [64-66] β-blockers, there was a significant decrease in insulin sensitivity in hypertensive patients. This decrease in insulin sensitivity may have a deleterious effect on glycemic control in patients with hypertension or in those with type 2 diabetes mellitus. In patients with the metabolic syndrome, decreases in insulin sensitivity may be initially compensated for by increases in insulin secretion by pancreatic β-cells. However, after a period of time, the β-cells are no longer able to keep up with the increasing insulin demands and increase in blood glucose, and potentially overt diabetes, may result.

In the Atherosclerosis Risk in Communities Study (ARIC), hypertensives treated with β-blockers had a 28% increased risk of developing type 2 diabetes compared with patients taking no medication [67]. In INVEST, hypertensives randomized to verapamil-based therapy had a 15% lower incidence of new onset diabetes than subjects in the atenolol group [68]. Other studies have found similar results comparing β-blockers to either the angiotensin-converting enzyme (ACE) inhibitors [69] or angiotensin receptor blockers (ARBs) [70] .

Several actions of β-blockers may affect insulin sensitivity and glycemic control. β-blockers block pancreatic β_2 receptors resulting in an inhibition of insulin secretion that results in an impairment of glucose metabolism leading to hyperglycemia [55]. This effect is more pronounced with nonselective β-blockers, but can also be seen with higher doses of selective β-blockers [71]. β-blockers have been associated with weight gain leading to the metabolic syndrome due to the weight gain itself as well as through obesity mediated impairment of insulin sensitivity [72, 73]. Insulin promotes vasodilatation resulting in increased blood flow in skeletal muscles [74]. During treatment with nonselective β-blockers, unopposed α_1-activity causes vasoconstriction leading to decreased blood flow to muscles [75]. This may result in decreased insulin-stimulated glucose uptake and insulin resistance. In insulin-resistant states such as type 2 diabetes and obesity, endothelium-dependent insulin-mediated vasodilatation is impaired which may also lead to insulin resistance [74, 76]. In the metabolic syndrome, the interaction of obesity and hyperglycemia with β-blockers may lead to more severe skeletal vasoconstriction resulting in worsening insulin resistance.

Newer β-blockers that cause vasodilatation appear to not have the deleterious effects on insulin sensitivity and glucose metabolism described above. Carvedilol, as noted above, a non-selective β-blocker with α_1-blocking properties has been found to improve insulin sensitivity. In 72 hypertensive patients without diabetes, carvedilol compared with metoprolol resulted in a 14% increase in insulin sensitivity while metoprolol led to a decrease [77]. A study comparing carvedilol with atenolol had similar results [78]. In two trials comparing carvedilol with metoprolol, the Glycemic Effects in Diabetes Mellitus: Carvedilol-Metoprolol Comparison in Hypertensives (GEMINI) trial and the Carvedilol or Metoprolol European Trial (COMET), the carvedilol group had decreases in both insulin resistance and HbA_{1c} while the metoprolol group had an increase in HbA_{1c} and no change from baseline in insulin resistance (GEMINI) [79], and improved rates of survival and cardiovascular hospitalizations (COMET). In GEMINI, although blood pressure was similar between groups, progression to microalbuminuria was less frequent with carvedilol than with metoprolol. This may reflect an antioxidant effect specific to carvedilol [80]. Findings from GEMINI also suggest that the use of vasodilating β-blockers may not result in weight gain [81]. In addition to carvedilol, vasodilating β-blockers available in the US are labetalol and nebivolol.

The effects of β-blockers on lipid metabolism are modest, but also vary according to β-blocker type. Nonselective β-blockers increase serum triglycerides and tend to lower HDL-cholesterol, while cardioselective β_1-blockers and β-blockers without intrinsic sympathomimetic activity have qualitatively similar but less pronounced effects. These effects may be, at least in part, mediated by weight gain. In the Losartan Intervention for Endpoint (LIFE) reduction study, HDL- cholesterol decreased more and remained lower during the first 2 years of the study in those treated with the β_1-selective blocker atenolol compared with those randomized to losartan [82]. In a study comparing atenolol with metoprolol, treatment increased serum triglycerides by 21% and 29%, respectively, compared with placebo, and decreased HDL-cholesterol by about 7% [65]. In a recent study comparing the effects of carvedilol and metoprolol on serum lipids in diabetic hypertensive patients, both drugs decreased HDL-cholesterol and increased triglycerides [83]. Comparing the two drugs, there was no difference in HDL-cholesterol levels but carvedilol resulted in statistically significant lower levels of total cholesterol, triglycerides and non-HDL cholesterol.

Based on the above, it appears logical in patients with the metabolic syndrome, who require a β-blocker, to treat them with one of the newer vasodilating agents that have neutral or beneficial metabolic effects. That said, at present, there are few studies that directly compare the different types of β-blockers on hard clinical outcomes, especially total mortality. Adding to this uncertainty is the fact that newer β-blockers are far more expensive than older agents such as atenolol and metoprolol.

ACE inhibitors and angiotensin receptor blockers

Over20 years ago, the ACE inhibitor captopril was shown to benefit glucose metabolism and insulin resistance, particularly in comparison to thiazides [55]. ACE inhibitors and ARBs may exert beneficial effects on glycemic control through a variety of mechanisms related to the inhibition of angiotensin II. Angiotensin II activates the sympathetic nervous system resulting in impairment of insulin secretion and peripheral glucose uptake [84]. Angiotensin II also impairs pancreatic blood flow and enhances insulin resistance, while ACE inhibitors directly improve insulin sensitivity primarily in skeletal muscle [85].

The magnitude of the beneficial effect of ACE inhibitors on glucose metabolism is demonstrated by clinical trials such as the HOPE (Heart Outcomes Prevention Evaluation) Study, which demonstrated a reduced rate of new onset diabetes mellitus in patients taking the ACE inhibitor ramipril [86]. Angiotensin II has a central role in glucose metabolism, in addition to its effect on the sympathetic nervous system and aldosterone release, that includes activation of insulin-stimulated mitogenic pathways that promote vascular smooth muscle proliferation (MAPK), but suppression of pathways involved in glucose transport (PI-3K) [87-91]. Nitric oxide synthase may play a key role in mediating angiotensin effects [92], as might oxidative stress [93, 94]. In an animal model of atherosclerosis, (the Watanabe Heritable Hyperlipidemic Rabbit), the combination of the aldosterone antagonist eplerenone with the ACE inhibitor enalapril led to additive protective effects on endothelial function and atherosclerotic changes [95]. In patients with documented atherosclerosis, ramipril lowered highly sensitive C-reactive protein [96]. This "crosstalk" between vascular growth and metabolic pathways may explain many of the defects in the metabolic syndrome. In patients with cardiac allograft vasculopathy, ACE inhibitors appear to be associated with plaque reduction [97].

While many of the studies reviewed above have grouped ACE inhibitors and ARBs together as generally having similar mechanisms of action, there are differences both among ACE inhibitors and between ACE inhibitors and ARBs. The ACE inhibitors enalapril and perindopril were compared in normotensive patients with coronary artery disease; neither agent lowered blood pressure, but perindopril was superior in terms of anti-oxidant, antithrombotic, and profibrinolytic activities [98]. In mild hypertensive patients, zofenopril (a sulfhydryl-containing ACE inhibitor) lowered LDL-cholesterol, oxidized LDL, peroxide, and increased flow-mediated dilation (a marker of endothelial function) compared to ramipril (a carboxylic-containing ACE inhibitor), and atenolol. Blood pressure was comparable in all three groups [99].

ARBs do not appear to be active on these pathways. Furthermore, there may be differences among ARBs. Telmisartan, for example, seems to activate insulin-sensitizing PPAR-γ pathways [100], with benefit in preclinical and clinical studies [101, 102]. Studies in nondiabetic hypertensive patients shown improvement in insulin sensitivity, measured by the homeostasis model assessment (HOMA) technique, when telmisartan was used alone; this effect was blunted when the drug was used in combination with the dihydropyridine calcium channel blocker nisoldipine [103]. This benefit occurred without changes in serum values of the adipose tissue-derived cytokine, adiponectin. Similar results on insulin sensitivity, also assessed by HOMA, were reported in a study of hypertensive type 2 diabetic patients [104]. Other investigators have found that telmisartan is associated with decreased vascular inflammation, reduced visceral fat, and increased adiponectin [105], while others have reported that telmisartan, compared to candesartan lowered fasting plasma glucose and body weight, and increased adiponectin. Diastolic blood pressure was comparably reduced in both treatment groups compared to control [106]. Losartan, another ARB, has an uricosuric effect that may be of benefit in cardiovascular risk [107].

A recent development in this treatment approach includes renin inhibitors, that improve blood pressure but have not been studied for their metabolic effects [108, 109], although recent data suggests an improvement (reduction) in atherosclerosis progression with aliskerin [109].

Calcium Channel Blockers

Calcium channel blockers (CCBs) may impair insulin release, but this effect on glucose metabolism appears to be balanced by their action to increase peripheral glucose uptake [110, 111]. CCBs have been shown to have no significant adverse metabolic effect [112, 113], or a slight negative effect [114]. Some short-term studies have even suggested a slight positive effect on glucose and insulin metabolism [66]. In one study, long-acting CCBs have been reported to have no significant metabolic effect [115], while an early study comparing short-acting nifedipine to atenolol showed improvement in postprandial glucose (suggesting improved insulin action since concurrent insulin concentrations were unaffected) and triglyceride values, as well increased HDL values, with the former agent [66].

Dihydropyridine CCBs (i.e., nifedipine) have no antiproteinuric effect, unlike the benzothiazepine diltiazem and the phenylalkylamine verapamil, and do not slow the progression of diabetic nephropathy [116]. This may have particular relevance in these high-risk patients. In a study of 12 550 nondiabetic hypertensives, subjects taking β -blockers, but not those taking thiazides, ACE inhibitors or calcium channel blockers, were at increased risk of developing diabetes [67]. In a study of 16176 coronary patients with hypertension, CCB-based therapy (verapamil SR) was less likely to result in the development of newly diagnosed diabetes mellitus than β-blocker (atenolol) based treatment [68]. In this study, addition of the ACE inhibitor trandolapril to verapamil SR decreased diabetes mellitus risk and the addition of hydrochlorothiazide to atenolol increased risk. In hypertensive patients with chronic kidney disease (stage not defined, but baseline creatinine ~1.6), treated with either telmisartan or amlodipine, creatinine, proteinuria, IL-6, MMP-9, and total cholesterol all declined, while 24 hour urinary creatinine clearance improved with telmisartan but not with amlodipine, despite comparable blood pressure reduction [117]. In another trial, treatment with the ARB valsartan was associated with a greater reduction in new onset diabetes compared with amlodipine [118].

CCBs appear to have systemic antiinflammatory effects that may be additive with other antihypertensive agents [119-121]; there may also be improvement (reduction) in oxidized LDL-cholesterol levels [122].

α-Antagonists

Prazosin, using fasting and postprandial glucose and insulin data, has been found to improve insulin sensitivity in patients with essential hypertension [123]. Pollare, et al. similarly reported that prazosin directly improved insulin sensitivity [124]. Prazosin has also been reported to improve HDL kinetics [125]. Terazosin appears to have no effect on glucose tolerance or insulin sensitivity [126], although men with benign prostatic hypertrophy treated with terazosin have improved lipid values [127]. No data is available for tamsulosin.

Doxazosin improved glucose and lipid metabolism in diabetic patients and in patients with impaired glucose tolerance [128, 129]. It has also been reported to improve insulin resistance, and increase LDL particle size [130, 131]. Doxazosin has also been described as acting synergistically with acarbose in patients with impaired glucose tolerance [132]. When doxazosin was added to existing therapies in patients with inadequately treated hypertension and impaired glucose metabolism, blood pressure control was improved in over 1/3 of cases, with concomitant improvement in glucose and lipid parameters and a reduction in atherosclerotic cardiovascular disease risk [133]. Similar metabolic benefit occurred when doxazosin was compared to bendrofluazide in hypertensive patients [134], and when doxazosin was compared to atenolol [135]. Doxazosin also reduced serum concentrations of oxidized LDL-cholesterol (a more atherogenic lipid fraction) in hypertensives [136]. Urapidil has no major effect on glucose metabolism, but favorably affects another cardiovascular risk marker, fibrinogen [137].

Central-acting α-agonists

Clonidine, which acts by binding to central α-2-adrenergic and imidazoline receptors, appears to be metabolically neutral in terms of glucose and insulin effects [138]; more recently developed imidazoline agonists have not been widely studied from this perspective [139]. However, rilmenidine has recently been reported to have similar blood pressure, lipid, and glucose effects to lisinopril in hypertensive women with metabolic syndrome [140].

The metabolic effects of antihypertensives are summarized in the Table.

Class of agent	Glucose and insulin effects		Lipid effects			
	Glucose	IR	Total Chol	HDL-C	LDL-C	TG
Thiazide (inc. chlorthalidone)[1]	↑	↑	↑	↓	↑	↑
β-blockers (nonselective)	↑	↑		↓		↑
Cardioselective β-blockers (β1)	↑	↑		↓		↑
Vasodilating β-blockers	↓	↓	↓	↓	↓	↓
ACEI/ARBs	↓	↓			↓	
Renin inhibitors	Unk.	Unk.	Unk.	Unk.	Unk.	Unk.
Calcium channel blockers	↓	↓	↓	↑	↓	↓
α-antagonists	↓	↓	↓	↑	↓	↓
Central α-agonists (e.g., clonidine)	neutral	neutral	neutral	neutral	neutral	neutral

Where IR=insulin resistance, and Total Chol, HDL-C, LDL-C, and TG are total cholesterol, HDL-cholesterol, LDL-cholesterol, and triglycerides, respectively. Unk=unknown. ACEI refers to angiotensin converting enzyme inhibitors, and ARBs refer to angiotensin receptor blockers.

[1] Thiazide diuretics (especially chlorthalidone) are alternative first choice agents in nondiabetic patients but should be used carefully in patients with elevated BMI. In those instances where patients become diabetic after initiation of thiazides, an alternative antihypertensive class should be used. For details, see text.

Table 1. Metabolic effects of antihypertensive agents.

Current treatment recommendations for blood pressure control in patients with diabetes are based on these considerations of balancing metabolic, blood pressure, renal, neurologic (dizziness) and electrolyte effects. Initial treatment should include RAS blockers (either ACE inhibitors or ARBs), followed with a calcium channel blocker or thiazide-like diuretic as 2nd line. Current data suggests that the deleterious metabolic effects that may result do not override the benefit of blood pressure reduction [3], although the recent ACCOMPLISH study (Avoiding Cardiovascular Events Through COMbination Therapy in Patients Living With Systolic Hypertension) pointed out that combining the ACE inhibitor benazepril with amlodipine, compared to benazepril with hydrochlorothiazide, resulted in benefit in terms of reduction in cardiovascular events such as acute clinical events and revascularizations; blood pressure was comparable between the two groups [141].

Lifestyle changes (weight loss, exercise, reduction of alcohol intake, smoking cessation,) should not be ignored. Glucose control, while laudable conceptually, may be problematic (see elsewhere). Potassium monitoring should continue, and potassium-containing foods and use of nonsteroidal antiinflammatories may need to be limited [3]. Combination agents, where available, might improve adherence [3]. α-blockers, while powerful in terms of blood pressure and prostate effects, may contribute to orthostatic dizziness and may need to be limited or avoided [3]. We should not forget that microalbuminuria is a marker of early diabetic nephropathy as well as a risk factor for microvascular and macrovascular cardiovascular disease [142] and should be monitored, with efforts expended to mitigate it. These overall recommendations are summarized in current American Diabetes Association (ADA) guidelines [143]. The Figure represents a treatment strategy derived from ADA (143) and other (2) guidelines.

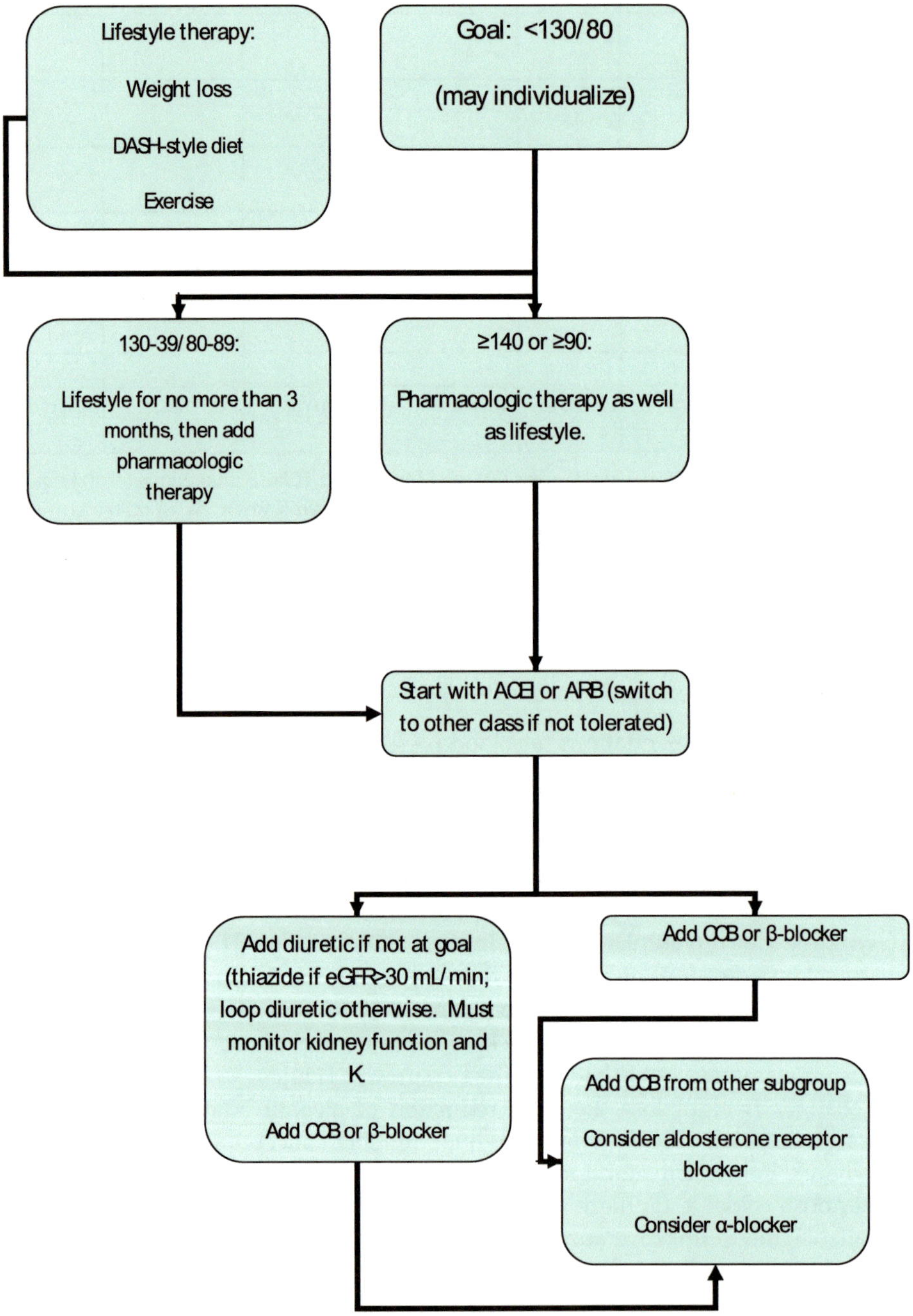

Fig. 1. Recommendations for blood pressure control in patients with diabetes (2, 143)

4. Genetic markers and treatment of hypertension in patients with the metabolic syndrome

As noted above, treatment of hypertension in the metabolic syndrome can exacerbate other of its components (e.g., glucose and lipid control). Further, hypertensive treatment in diabetics, may have less than the expected benefit in terms of preventing coronary disease and mortality. Is it possible that evolving genetic markers can help guide therapy more precisely?

The INVEST study observed that patients with more severe vascular disease, particularly those of Hispanic ethnicity, were at greater risk for developing diabetes, especially with hydrochlorothiazide treatment. This risk was attenuated by more aggressive BP control and use of a verapamil-trandolapril combination [144]. There is developing data that suggests that the CYP3A5 genotype, which does not appear to contribute importantly to the risk of hypertension, may influence response to calcium channel blockers [145]. Similarly, the KCNMB1 genotype (which contributes to polymorphisms in the large-conductance calcium and voltage-dependent potassium channel β1 subunit) may influence response to verapamil and potentially adverse outcomes [146].

Other data from Beitelshees and colleagues suggests that polymorphisms in the CACNA1C gene may help identify groups that benefit most from calcium channel blocker therapy, a group that benefits from β-blocker therapy, and a third group in which calcium channel blocker and β-blocker therapy are equivalent [147]. Similar analyses leading to possible future predictions are available for β-blocker treatment outcomes based on β-adrenergic receptor gene polymorphisms [148], and promoter polymorphisms in angiotensin-converting enzyme [149]. This last group of analyses may explain the variation between populations in cardiovascular risk and treatment outcomes, since certain alleles are more frequent in African-Americans than in either Hispanics or Caucasians [149]. Adducin is a ubiquitously expressed cytoskeleton protein that is coded by ADD1. Polymorphisms in this gene may lead to increased renal tubular sodium reabsorption and hypertension; certain alleles have been shown to manifest an excess risk for a cardiovascular event or death, particularly in African-Americans [150].

5. Conclusions

The prevalence of obesity, hypertension and type 2 diabetes mellitus, and, as a consequence, the metabolic syndrome, is increasing in the US. In this setting, it is important to individualize antihypertensive therapy and to monitor its metabolic consequences so that potential adverse effects that would negate some of the benefits of blood-pressure lowering are minimized. Strategies to improve blood pressure control in patients with metabolic syndrome, including decisions concerning the best pharmacological treatment for these patients, will have major morbidity and mortality consequences. The predominance of evidence favors a strategy to lower blood pressure to a level approaching the criteria for this syndrome (<130/80) [151, 152]. However, a goal blood pressure of <130/80 is not supported by current evidence. In hypertensives whose blood pressure is more than 20/10 above target, this frequently will require the initiation of a combination of antihypertensives [153].

Treatment with different antihypertensive drug classes has varied effects on glucose and lipid metabolism. Thiazide use in hypertensives has been associated with the development of glucose intolerance and diabetes. Studies suggest that the probability of worsening glucose metabolism and the development of new diabetes after thiazide initiation is associated with increasing body mass index. Thiazide use also results in small increases in total and LDL-cholesterol and triglycerides and decreases in HDL-cholesterol. These changes are more pronounced with high dose thiazides.

Non-selective or β_1 selective β-blockers may also lead to decreased insulin sensitivity in hypertensive patients. On the other hand, β-blockers, such as carvedilol, that cause vasodilatation may not have these deleterious effects on insulin sensitivity and glucose metabolism. The effects of β-blockers on lipid metabolism may also vary according to β-blocker type. Nonselective β-blockers modestly increase serum triglycerides and tend to lower HDL-cholesterol, while cardioselective β_1-blockers and those without intrinsic sympathomimetic activity have qualitatively similar but less pronounced effects. Vasodilating β-blockers appear to have even smaller deleterious effects on lipids.

ACE inhibitors and ARBs may exert beneficial effects on glycemic control through a variety of mechanisms related to the inhibition of angiotensin II. These agents may be particularly useful in patients with microalbuminuria to slow the progression of renal disease. While there may be some small differences among different classes of CCBs, there is little net effect of these agents on glucose or lipid metabolism. The α-antagonists generally appear to improve glucose and lipid metabolism in diabetic and non-diabetic patients but the increase in cardiovascular endpoints in the ALLHAT study with doxazosin suggests that until there is evidence to the contrary, this class of antihypertensive should not be used as first line agents.

The choice of an antihypertensive also has important implications for the cost of medical care. Thiazide diuretics and β-blockers are considerably less expensive than most other antihypertensive medications and have been shown to be effective antihypertensive treatment in several major studies [6, 7, 44]. However, some of the medication cost savings would be negated if thiazide and β-blocker use is complicated by an increased probability of developing glucose intolerance and even diabetes with its attendant medication and other costs associated with its treatment and manifestations. Most of the studies we have reviewed have focused on one agent in comparison to another; there is scant data on net metabolic effects of combining drug classes. Furthermore, individual patient responses may vary from the expected.

The coexistence of hypertension, dyslipidemia and glucose intolerance increases the risk of coronary artery disease, stroke, peripheral vascular disease, nephropathy, neuropathy and retinopathy [154-156]. The metabolic syndrome is associated with cardiovascular disease and the development of diabetes [157-159]. In treated hypertensive patients, occurrence of new diabetes portends a risk for subsequent cardiovascular disease that is similar to that of other diabetics [160]. The use of an antihypertensive that results in improvements in dyslipidemia, insulin sensitivity and glucose metabolism would be a logical choice in patients with metabolic syndrome, but this recommendation needs to be supported with clinical trials with hard clinical outcomes, especially total mortality.

6. References

[1] Bakris G, Vassalotti J, Ritz E, Wanner C, Stergiou G, Molitch M, Nesto R, Kaysen GA, Sowers JR; CKD Consensus Working Group. National Kidney Foundation consensus conference on cardiovascular and kidney diseases and diabetes risk: an integrated therapeutic approach to reduce events. Kidney Int. 2010;78:726-36.

[2] Bakris GL, Sowers JR, Glies TD, Black HR, Izzo JL Jr, Materson BJ, Oparil S, Weber MA. Treatment of hypertension in patients with diabetes--an update. J Am Soc Hypertens. 2010;4:62-7.

[3] Bakris GL, Sowers JR; American Society of Hypertension Writing Group. ASH position paper: treatment of hypertension in patients with diabetes-an update. J Clin Hypertens (Greenwich). 2008;10:707-13; discussion 714-5.

[4] Ong KL, Cheung BMY, ManYB, Lau CP, Lam KSL. Prevalence, awareness, treatment and control of hypertension among United States adults 1999-2004. *Hypertension* 2007;49:69-75.

[5] Collins R, Peto R, MacMahon S, Hebert P, Fiebach NH, Eberlein KA, et al. Blood pressure, stroke, and coronary heart disease part 2: short-term reductions in blood pressure: overview of randomised drug trials in their epidemiological context. *Lancet* 1990;335:827-838.

[6] Chobanian AV, Bakris GL, Black HR, Cushman WC, Green LA, Izzo JL Jr, et al. Joint National Committee on Prevention, Detection, Evaluation, and Treatment of High Blood Pressure. National Heart, Lung, and Blood Institute, National High Blood Pressure Education Program Coordinating Committee: The seventh report of the joint national committee on prevention, detection, evaluation, and treatment of high blood pressure: the JNC 7 report. *Hypertension* 2003;42:1206-1252.

[7] Blood pressure lowering treatment trialists' collaboration. Effects of different blood-pressure-lowering regiments on major cardiovascular events: results of prospectively-designed overviews of randomised trials. *Lancet* 2003, 362:1527-1535

[8] Siegel D, Hulley SB, Black DM, Cheitlin MD, Sebastian A, Seeley DG, Hearst N, Fine R. Diuretics, serum and intracellular electrolyte levels, and ventricular arrhythmias in hypertensive men. *JAMA* 1992;267:1083-1089.

[9] Malik C, Wong ND, Franklin SS, Kamath TV, L'Italien GJ, Pio JR, et al.Impact of the metabolic syndrome on mortality from coronary heart disease, cardiovascular disease, and all causes in United States adults. *Circulation* 2004;110:1245-50.

[10] Manrique C, Lastra G, Whaley-Connell A, Sowers JR. Hypertension and the cardiometabolic syndrome. *J Clin Hypertens* (Greenwich) 2005;7:471-6.

[11] Grundy SM, Cleeman JI, Daniels SR, Donato KA, Eckel RH, Franklin BA, et al. American Heart Association; National Heart, Lung, and Blood Institute. Diagnosis and management of the metabolic syndrome: an American Heart Association/National Heart, Lung, and Blood Institute Scientific Statement. *Circulation* 2005;112:2735-2752.

[12] Ishizaka N, Ishizaka Y, Toda E, Hashimoto H, Nagai R, Yamakado M. Hypertension is the most common component of metabolic syndrome and the greatest contributor to carotid arteriosclerosis in apparently healthy Japanese individuals. *Hypertens Res* 2005;28:27-34.

[13] Bener A, Siric M, Musallam M, Khader, Y, Al-Hamaq, A. Prevalence of Metabolic Syndrome According to Adult Treatment Panel III and International Diabetes Federation Criteria: A Population-Based Study. *Metab Syndr Relat Disord* 2008;7:221-228.

[14] Flegal KM, Carroll MD, Ogden CL, Johnson CL. Prevalence and trends in obesity among US adults, 1999-2000. *JAMA* 2002;288:1723-1727.

[15] Must A, Spadano J, Coakley EH, Field AE, Coldz G, Dietz W. The disease burden associated with overweight and obesity. *JAMA* 1999;282:1523-1529.

[16] Mokdad AH, Ford ES, Bowman BA, Vinicor F, Giles WH. Prevalence of obesity, diabetes, and obesity-related health risk factors, 2001. *JAMA* 2003;289:76-79.

[17] Sharma AM, Engeli S, Pischon T. New developments in mechanisms of obesity-induced hypertension: role of adipose tissue. *Curr Hypertens Rep* 2001;3:152-156.

[18] Siegel D, Saliba P, Haffner S. Glucose and insulin levels during diuretic therapy in hypertensive men and their association with serum and intracellular potassium and magnesium. *Hypertension* 1994;23[part 1]:688-694.

[19] Sowers JR, Bakris GL. Antihypertensive therapy and the risk of type 2 diabetes mellitus [editorial]. *N Engl J Med* 2000;342:969-970.

[20] Chen YD, Sheu WH, Swislocki AL, Reaven GM. High density lipoprotein turnover in patients with hypertension. *Hypertension* 1991;17:386-93.

[21] Ford ES, Giles WH, Dietz WH. Prevalence of the metabolic syndrome among US adults: findings from the third National Health and Nutrition Examination Survey. *JAMA* 2002;287:356-359.

[22] Appel LJ, Moore TJ, Obarzanek E, Vollmer WM, Svetkey LP, Sacks FM, et al. A clinical trial of the effects of dietary patterns on blood pressure. DASH collaborative Research Group. *N Engl J Med* 1997;336:1117-1124.

[23] Azadbakht L, Mirmiran P, Esmailzadeh A, Azizi T, Azizi F. Beneficial effects of a Dietary Approaches to Stop Hypertension eating plan on features of the metabolic syndrome. *Diabetes Care* 2005;28: 2823-2831.

[24] Whelton SP, Chin A, Exin X, He J. Effect of aerobic exercise on blood pressure: a meta-analysis of randomized, controlled trial. *Ann Intern Med* 2002;136:493-503.

[25] Padwal R, Laupacis A. Antihypertensive therapy and incidence of type 2 diabetes: a systematic review. *Diabetes Care* 2004;27:247-255.

[26] Reaven GM, Lithell H, Landsberg L. Hypertension and associated metabolic abnormalities-the role of insulin resistance and the sympathoadrenal system. *N Engl J Med* 1996;334:374-381.

[27] Swislocki AL, Hoffman BB, Reaven GM. Insulin resistance, glucose intolerance and hyperinsulinemia in patients with hypertension. *Am J Hypertens* 1989;2:419-423.

[28] Dunder K, Lind L, Zethelius B, Berglund L, Lithell H. Increase in blood glucose concentration during antihypertensive treatment as a predictor of myocardial infarction: population based cohort study. *BMJ* 2003;326:681.

[29] Hsueh WA, Lyon CJ, Quinones MJ. Insulin resistance and the endothelium. *Am J Med* 2004;117:109-117.

[30] Lind L, Pollare T, Berne C, Lithell H. Long-term metabolic effects of antihypertensive drugs. *Am Heart J* 1994;128:1177-1183.

[31] Action to Control Cardiovascular Risk in Diabetes Study Group. Effects of intensive glucose lowering in type 2 diabetes. *N Engl J Med* 2008;358:2545-59.

[32] ACCORD Study Group. Effects of combination lipid therapy in type 2 diabetes mellitus. *N Engl J Med* 2010;362:1563-74.

[33] Siegel D, Swislocki AL. The ACCORD Study: The Devil is in the Details. Metab Syndr Relat Disord. 2010 Dec 18. [Epub ahead of print]

[34] ACCORD Study Group. Effects of intensive blood-pressure control in type 2 diabetes mellitus. *N Engl J Med* 2010;362:1575-85.

[35] Bloch MJ, Basile JN. Is there accord in ACCORD? Lower blood pressure targets in type 2 diabetes does not lead to fewer cardiovascular events except for reductions in stroke. *J Clin Hypertens (Greenwich).* 2010;12:472-7.

[36] Giles TD, Houston MC. Do diuretics diminish the predicted benefits on ischemic heart disease events of lowering blood pressure in hypertension? Messages from ALLHAT, ACCOMPLISH, and ACCORD. *J Clin Hypertens (Greenwich).* 2010;12:469-71.

[37] Franse LV, Pahor M, Di Bari M, Somes GW, Cushman WC, Applegate WB. Hypokalemia associated with diuretic use and cardiovascular events in the Systolic Hypertension in the Elderly Program. *Hypertension* 2000;35:1025-30.

[38] UK Prospective Diabetes Study (UKPDS). VIII. Study design, progress and performance. *Diabetologia* 1991;34:877-90.

[39] UKPDS: Tight blood pressure control and risk of macrovascular and microvascular complications in type 2 diabetes. UKPDS 38. UK Prospective Diabetes Study Group. *BMJ* 1998;317:703-13.

[40] Gaede P, Lund-Andersen H, Parving HH, Pedersen O. Effect of a multifactorial intervention on mortality in type 2 diabetes. *N Engl J Med* 2008;358:580-91.

[41] Holman RR, Paul SK, Bethel MA, Neil HA, Matthews DR. Long-term follow-up after tight control of blood pressure in type 2 diabetes. *N Engl J Med* 2008;359:1565-76.

[42] Cooper-DeHoff RM, Gong Y, Handberg EM, Bavry AA, Denardo SJ, Bakris GL, Pepine CJ. Tight blood pressure control and cardiovascular outcomes among hypertensive patients with diabetes and coronary artery disease. *JAMA* 2010;304:61-8

[43] Bavry AA, Anderson RD, Gong Y, Denardo SJ, Cooper-DeHoff RM, Handberg EM, Pepine CJ. Outcomes among hypertensive patients with concomitant peripheral and coronary artery disease. Findings from the INternational Verapamil-SR/Trandolapril STudy. *Hypertension* 2010;55:48-53.

[44] ALLHAT Officers and Coordinators for the ALLHAT Collaborative Research Group. The Antihypertensive and Lipid-Lowering Treatment to Prevent Heart Attack Trial. Major outcomes in high-risk hypertensive patients randomized to angiotensin-converting enzyme inhibitor or calcium channel blocker vs diuretic; the Antihypertensive and Lipid-Lowering Treatment to Prevent Heart Attack Trial (ALLHAT). *JAMA* 2002;88:2981-2997.

[45] Savage PJ, Pressel SL, Curb JD, Schron EB, Applegate WB, Black HR, et al. Influence of long-term, low-dose, diuretic-based, antihypertensive therapy on glucose, lipid, uric acid, and potassium levels in older men and women with isolated systolic hypertension: The Systolic Hypertension in the Elderly Program. SHEP Cooperative Research Group. *Arch Intern Med* 1998;158:741-751.

[46] Kostis JB, Wilson AC, Freudenberger RS, Cosgrove NM, Pressel SL, Davis BR; SHEP Collaborative Research Group. Long-term effect of diuretic-based therapy on fatal

outcomes in subjects with isolated systolic hypertension with and without diabetes. *Am J Cardiol* 2005;95:29-35.

[47] Taylor EN, Hu FB, Curhan GC. Antihypertensive medications and the risk of incident type 2 diabetes. *Diabetes Care* 2006;29:1065-1070.

[48] Siegel D, Meier J, Maas C, Lopez J, Swislocki ALM, The effect of body mass index on fasting blood glucose after initiation of thiazide therapy in hypertensive patients. *Am J Hypertens* 2008;21:438-42.

[49] Tweeddale MG, Ogilvie RI, Ruedy J. Antihypertensive and biochemical effects of chlorthalidone. *Clin Pharmacol Ther* 1977;22:519-527.

[50] Carlsen JE, Kober L. Torp-Pedersen C, Johansen P. Relation between dose of bendrofluazide, antihypertensive effect, and adverse biochemical effects. *BMJ* 1990;300:975-978.

[51] Neutel JM. Metabolic manifestations of low-dose diuretics. *Amer J Med* 1996;101:71S-82S.

[52] Conn JW. Hypertension, the potassium ion and impaired carbohydrate tolerance. *N Engl J Med* 1965;273:1135-1143.

[53] Rowe JW, Tobin JD, Rosa RM, Andres R. . Effect of experimental potassium deficiency on glucose and insulin metabolism. *Metabolism* 1980;29:498-502.

[54] Rapoport MI, Hurd HF. Thiazide-induced glucose intolerance treated with potassium. *Arch Intern Med* 1964;113:405-408.

[55] Pollare T, Lithell H, Berne C. A comparison of the effects of hydrochlorothiazide and captopril on glucose and lipid metabolism in patients with hypertension. *N Engl J Med* 1989;321:868-873.

[56] Reaven GM, Clinkingbeard C, Jeppesen J, Maheux P, Pei D, Foote J, et al. Comparison of the hemodynamic and metabolic effects of low dose hydrochlorothiazide and lisinopril treatment in obese patients with high blood pressure. *Am J Hypertens* 1995;8:461-466.

[57] Bramlage P, Pittrow D, Wittchen HU, Kirch W, Boehler S, Lehnert H, et al. Hypertension in overweight and obese primary care patients is highly prevalent and poorly controlled. *Am J Hypertens* 2004;17:904-910.

[58] Zappe DH, Sowers JR, Hsueh WA, Haffner SM, Deedwania PC, Fonseca VA, et al. Metabolic and Antihypertensive Effects of Combined Angiotensin Receptor Blocker and Diuretic Therapy in Prediabetic Hypertensive Patients with the Cardiometabolic Syndrome. *J Clin Hypertens* (Greenwich) 2008;10:894-902.

[59] Martins RD, Alves Rde S, Silva GG, Martins N, Vasconcelos S, Assreuy A, et al. Antihypertensive treatment and its implications on lipoprotein metabolism of patients in care by a hypertension and diabetes program in Brazil. *Acta Med Port.* 2008;21(6):567-574.

[60] Lindholm LH, Carlbert B, Samuelsson O. Should beta blockers remain first choice in the treatment of primary hypertension? A meta-analysis. *Lancet* 2005;366:1545-1553.

[61] Bradley HA, Wiysonge CS, Volmink JA, Mayosi BM, Opie LH. How strong is the evidence for use of beta-blockers as first-line therapy for hypertension? Systematic review and meta-analysis. *J Hypertens* 2006;24:2131-2141.

[62] Khan N, McAlister FA. Re-examining the efficacy of beta-blockers for the treatment of hypertension: A meta-analysis *CMAJ* 2006;174:1737-1742.
[63] Lithell H, Pollare T, Vessby B. Metabolic effects of pindolol and propranolol in a double-blind cross-over study in hypertensive patients. *Blood Press* 1992;1:92-101.
[64] Pollare T, Lithell H, Mörlin C, Präntare H, Hvarfner A, Ljunghall S. Metabolic effects of diltiazem and atenolol: results from a randomized, double-blind study with parallel groups. *J Hypertens* 1989;7:551-559.
[65] Pollare T, Lithell HO, Selinus I, Brnce C. Sensitivity to insulin during treatment with atenolol and metoprolol: a randomized, double blind study of effects on carbohydrate and lipoprotein metabolism in hypertensive patients. *BMJ* 1989;298:1152-1157.
[66] Sheu WHH, Swislocki AL, Hoffman B, Chen, YDI, Reaven, GM. Comparison of the effects of atenolol and nifedipine on glucose, insulin, and lipid metabolism in patients with hypertension. *Am J Hypertens* 1991;4:199-205.
[67] Gress TW, Nieto FJ, Shahar E, Wooford MR, Brancati FL. Hypertension and antihypertensive therapy as risk factors for type 2 diabetes mellitus. Atherosclerosis Risk in Communities study. *N Engl J Med* 2000;342:905-912.
[68] Cooper-Dehoff R, Cohen JD, Bakris GL, Messerli FH, Erdine S, Hewkin AC, et al, INVEST Investigators. Predictors of development of diabetes mellitus in patients with coronary artery disease taking antihypertensive medications (Findings from the International VErapamil SR-Trandolapril Study [INVEST]). *Am J Cardiol* 2006;98:890-894.
[69] Hansson L, Lindholm LH, Niskanen L, Lanke J, Hedner T, Niklason A, et al. Effect of angiotensin-converting-enzyme inhibition compared with conventional therapy on cardiovascular morbidity and mortality in hypertension: the Captopril Prevention Project (CAPPP) randomized trial. *Lancet* 1999;353:611-616.
[70] Dahlöf B, Devereux RB, Kjeldsen SE, Julius S, Beevers G, de Faire U, et al; LIFE Study Group. Cardiovascular morbidity and mortality in the Losartan Intervention For Endpoint reduction in hypertension study (LIFE): a randomized trial against atenolol. *Lancet* 2002;359:995-1003.
[71] Wicklmayr M, Rett K, Dietze G, Mehnert H. Effects of beta-blocking agents on insulin secretion and glucose disposal. *Horm Metab Res Suppl* 1990;22:29-33.
[72] UK Prospective Diabetes Study Group. Efficacy of atenolol and captopril in reducing risk of macrovascular and microvascular complications in type 2 diabetes: UKPDS 39. *BMJ* 1998;317:713-720.
[73] Rossner S, Taylor CL, Byington RP, Furberg CD. Long term propranolol treatment and changes in body weight after myocardial infarction. *BMJ* 1990;300:902-903.
[74] Steinberg HO, Baron AD. Vascular function, insulin resistance and fatty acids. *Diabetologia* 2002;45:623-634.
[75] Lithell H, Pollare T, Berne C, Saltin B. The metabolic and circulatory response to beta-blockade in hypertensive men is correlated to muscle capillary density. *Blood Press* 1992;1:20-26.

[76] Sartori C, Scherrer U. Insulin, nitric oxide and the sympathetic nervous system; at the crossroads of metabolic and cardiovascular regulation. *J Hypertens* 1999;17:1517-1525.

[77] Jacob S, Rett K, Wicklmayr M, Agrawal B, Augustin HJ, Dietze GJ. Differential effect of chronic treatment with two beta-blocking agents on insulin sensitivity: the carvedilol-metoprolol study. *J Hypertens* 1996;14:489-494.

[78] Giugliano D, Acampora R, Marfella R, De Rosa N, Ziccardi P, Ragone R, et al. Metabolic and cardiovascular effects of carvedilol and atenolol in non-insulin-dependent diabetes mellitus and hypertension: a randomized, controlled trial. *Ann Intern Med* 1997;126:955-959.

[79] Bakris GL, Fonseca V, Atholi RE, McGill JB, Messerli FH, Phillips RA, et al. Metabolic effects of carvedilol vs metoprolol in patients with type 2 diabetes mellitus and hypertension, a randomized controlled trial. *JAMA* 2004;292:2227-2236.

[80] Bakris GL, Fonseca V, Katholi RE, McGill JB, Messerli F, Phillips RA, et al; GEMINI Investigators. Differential effects of beta-blockers on albuminuria in patients with type 2 diabetes. *Hypertension* 2005;46:1309-1315.

[81] Jacob S, Henriksen EJ. Metabolic properties of vasodilating beta blockers: management considerations for hypertensive diabetic patients and patients with the metabolic syndrome. *J Clin Hypertens* (Greenwich) 2004;6:690-696

[82] Olsen MH, Wachtell K, Beever G, Dahlöf B, de Simone G, Devereux RB, et al. Effects of losartan compared with atenolol on lipids in patients with hypertension and left ventricular hypertrophy: the Losartan Intervention For Endpoint reduction in hypertension study. *J Hypertens* 2009;27:567-574.

[83] Bell DS, Bakris GL, McGill JB. Comparison of carvedilol and metoprolol on serum lipid concentration in diabetic hypertensive patients. *Diabetes Obes Metab* 2009; 11:234-238

[84] Padwal R, Mamdani M, Alter DA, Hux JE, Rothwell DM, Tu K, et al. Antihypertensive therapy and incidence of type 2 diabetes in an elderly cohort. *Diabetes Care* 2004;27:2458-2463.

[85] Jandeleit-Dahm KA, Tikelis C, Reid CM, Johnston CI, Cooper ME. Why blockage of the renin-angiotensin system reduces the incidence of new-onset diabetes. *J Hypertens* 2005;23:463-473.

[86] Yusuf S, Sleight P, Pogue J, Bosch J, Davies R, Dagenais G. Effects of an angiotensin-converting-enzyme inhibitor, ramipril, on cardiovascular events in high-risk patients. The Heart Outcomes Prevention Evaluation Study Investigators. *N Engl J Med* 2000;342:145-153.

[87] Moule SK, Denton RM. Multiple signaling pathways involved in the metabolic effects of insulin. *Am J Cardiol* 1997;80:41A-49A.

[88] Nascimben L, Bothwell JH, Dominguez DY, et al. Angiotensin II stimulates insulin-independent glucose uptake in hypertrophied rat hearts. Abstract. *J Hypertens* 1997;15 (Suppl 4):S84.

[89] Schorb W, Peeler TC, Madigan NN, Conrad KM, Baker KM. Angiotensin II-induced protein tyrosine phosphorylation in neonatal rat cardiac fibroblasts. *J Biol Chem*1994; 269: 19626-19632.

[90] Wan Y, Kurosaki T, Huang XY. Tyrosine kinases in activation of the MAP kinase cascade by G-protein-coupled receptors. *Nature* 1996;380:541-544.

[91] Saad MJ, Velloso LA, Carvalho CR. Angiotensin II induces tyrosine phosphorylation of insulin receptor substrate 1 and its association with phosphatidylinositol 3-kinase in rat heart. *Biochem J* 1995;310:741-744.

[92] Miatello R, Risler N, Gonzalez S, Castro C, Ruttler M, Cruzado M. Effects of enalapril on the vascular wall in an experimental model of syndrome X. *Am J Hypertens* 2002;15:872-878.

[93] Khan BV, Sola S, Lauten WB, Natarajan R, Hooper WC, Menon RG, et al. Quinapril, an ACE inhibitor, reduces markers of oxidative stress in the metabolic syndrome. *Diabetes Care* 2004;27:1712-1715.

[94] Ferder L, Inserra F, Martinez-Maldonado M. Inflammation and the metabolic syndrome: role of angiotensin II and oxidative stress. *Curr Hypertens Rep* 2006;8:191-198.

[95] Imanishi T, Ikejima H, Tsujioka H, Kuroi A, Kobayashi K, Muragaki Y, Mochizuki S, Goto M, Yoshida K, Akasaka T. Addition of eplerenone to an angiotensin-converting enzyme inhibitor effectively improves nitric oxide bioavailability. *Hypertension* 2008;51:734-741.

[96] Mitrovic V, Klein HH, Krekel N, Kreuzer J, Fichtlscherer S, Schirmer A, Paar WD, Hamm CW. Influence of the angiotensin converting enzyme inhibitor ramipril on high-sensitivity C-reactive protein (hs-CRP) in patients with documented atherosclerosis. *Z Kardiol* 2005;94:336-342.

[97] Bae JH, Rihal CS, Edwards BS, Kushwaha SS, Mathew V, Prasad A, Holmes DR Jr, Lerman A. Association of angiotensin-converting enzyme inhibitors and serum lipids with plaque regression in cardiac allograft vasculopathy. *Transplantation* 2006;82:1108-1111.

[98] Krysiak R, Okopień B. Pleiotropic effects of angiotensin-converting enzyme inhibitors in normotensive patients with coronary artery disease. *Pharmacol Rep* 2008;60:514-523.

[99] Pasini AF, Garbin U, Nava MC, Stranieri C, Pellegrini M, Boccioletti V, Luchetta ML, Fabrizzi P, Lo Cascio V, Cominacini L. Effect of sulfhydryl and non-sulfhydryl angiotensin-converting enzyme inhibitors on endothelial function in essential hypertensive patients. *Am J Hypertens* 2007;20:443-450.

[100] Kurtz TW, Pravenec M. Antidiabetic mechanisms of angiotensin-converting enzyme inhibitors and angiotensin II receptor antagonists: beyond the renin-angiotensin system. *J Hypertens* 2004;22:2253-2261.

[101] Kurtz TW. Treating the metabolic syndrome: telmisartan as a peroxisome proliferator-activated receptor-gamma activator. *Acta Diabetol* 2005;42 Suppl 1:S9-S16.

[102] Karagiannis A, Mikhailidis DP, Athyros VG, Kakafika AI, Tziomalos K, Liberopoulos EN, Florentin M, Elisaf M. The role of renin-angiotensin system inhibition in the treatment of hypertension in metabolic syndrome: are all the angiotensin receptor blockers equal? *Expert Opin Ther Targets* 2007;11:191-205.

[103] Benndorf RA, Rudolph T, Appel D, Schwedhelm E, Maas R, Schulze F, et al. Telmisartan improves insulin sensitivity in nondiabetic patients with essential hypertension. *Metabolism* 2006;55:1159-1164.

[104] Negro R, Hassan H. The effects of telmisartan and amlodipine on metabolic parameters and blood pressure in type 2 diabetic, hypertensive patients. *J Renin Angiotensin Aldosterone Syst* 2006;7:243-246.

[105] Chujo D, Yagi K, Asano A, Muramoto H, Sakai S, Ohnishi A, Shintaku-Kubota M, Mabuchi H, Yamagishi M, Kobayashi J. Telmisartan treatment decreases visceral fat accumulation and improves serum levels of adiponectin and vascular inflammation markers in Japanese hypertensive patients. *Hypertens Res* 2007;30:1205-1210.

[106] Makita S, Abiko A, Naganuma Y, Moriai Y, Nakamura M. Effects of telmisartan on adiponectin levels and body weight in hypertensive patients with glucose intolerance. *Metabolism* 2008;57:1473-1478.

[107] O'Brien E, Barton J, Nussberger J, Mulcahy D, Jensen C, Dicker P, et al. Aliskiren reduces blood pressure and suppresses plasma renin activity in combination with a thiazide diuretic, an angiotensin-converting enzyme inhibitor, or an angiotensin receptor blocker. *Hypertension* 2007;49:276-284.

[108] Azizi M. Renin inhibition. *Curr Opin Nephrol Hypertens* 2006;15:505-510.

[109] Nussberger J, Aubert JF, Bouzourene K, Pellegrin M, Hayoz D, Mazzolai L. Renin inhibition by aliskiren prevents atherosclerosis progression: comparison with irbesartan, atenolol, and amlodipine. *Hypertension* 2008;51:1306-1311.

[110] Trost BN, Weidmann P. Effects of calcium antagonists on diabetic subjects: a review. *J Hypertens Suppl* 1987;5:S81-S104.

[111] Houston MC. The effects of antihypertensive drugs on glucose intolerance in hypertensive nondiabetics and diabetics. *Am Heart J* 1988;115:640-656.

[112] Ramsay LE, Yeo WW, Jackson PR. Influence of diuretics, calcium antagonists, and alpha-blockers on insulin sensitivity and glucose tolerance in hypertensive patients. *J Cardiovasc Pharmacol* 1992;20 Suppl 11:S49-S53; discussion S53-S54.

[113] Russell RP. Side effects of calcium channel blockers. *Hypertension* 1988;11:II42-II44.

[114] Lind L, Berne C, Pollare T, Lithell H. Metabolic effects of anti-hypertensive treatment with nifedipine or furosemide: a double-blind, cross-over study. *J Hum Hypertens* 1995;9:137-141.

[115] Zhang R, Thakur V, Morse S, Reisin E. Renal and cardiovascular considerations for the nonpharmacological and pharmacological therapies of obesity-hypertension. *J Hum Hypertens* 2002;16:819-827.

[116] Nathan S, Pepine CJ, Bakris GL. Calcium antagonists: effects on cardio-renal risk in hypertensive patients. *Hypertension.* 2005;46:637-642.

[117] Nakamura T, Inoue T, Suzuki T, Kawagoe Y, Ueda Y, Koide H, Node K. Comparison of renal and vascular protective effects between telmisartan and amlodipine in hypertensive patients with chronic kidney disease with mild renal insufficiency. *Hypertens Res* 2008;31:841-850.

[118] Julius S, Kjeldsen SE, Weber M, Brunner HR, Ekman S, Hansson L, et al; VALUE trial group . Outcomes in hypertensive patients at high cardiovascular risk treated with

regimens based on valsartan or amlodipine; the VALUE randomised trial. *Lancet* 2004;363:2022-2031.

[119] Farah R, Shurtz-Swirski R. The combined effect of calcium channel blocker Lercanidipine and antioxidants on low-grade systemic inflammation parameters in essential hypertension patients. *Minerva Cardioangiol* 2008;56:467-476.

[120] Fogari R, Preti P, Zoppi A, Lazzari P, Corradi L, Fogari E, Ciccarelli L, Derosa G. Effects of amlodipine-atorvastatin combination on inflammation markers and insulin sensitivity in normocholesterolemic obese hypertensive patients. *Eur J Clin Pharmacol* 2006;62:817-822.

[121] Martín-Ventura JL, Muñoz-Garcia B, Blanco-Colio LM, Martín-Conejero A, Madrigal-Matute J, Vega M, Ortega L, Serrano J, Egido J. Treatment with amlodipine and atorvastatin has additive effect on blood and plaque inflammation in hypertensive patients with carotid atherosclerosis. *Kidney Int Suppl* 2008;111:S71-74.

[122] Muda P, Kampus P, Teesalu R, Zilmer K, Ristimäe T, Fischer K, Zilmer M. Effects of amlodipine and candesartan on oxidized LDL level in patients with mild to moderate essential hypertension. *Blood Press* 2006;15:313-318.

[123] Swislocki AL, Hoffman BB, Sheu WH, Chen YD, Reaven GM. Effect of prazosin treatment on carbohydrate and lipoprotein metabolism in patients with hypertension. *Am J Med* 1989;86(1B):14-18.

[124] Pollare T, Lithell H, Selinus I, Berne C. Application of prazosin is associated with an increase of insulin sensitivity in obese patients with hypertension. *Diabetologia* 1988;31:415-420.

[125] Sheu WH, Swislocki AL, Hoffman BB, Reaven GM, Chen YD. Effect of prazosin treatment on HDL kinetics in patients with hypertension. *Am J Hypertens* 1990;3:761-768.

[126] Ferrari P, Rosman J, Neuner N, Shaw S, Riesen W, Weidmann P. Postsynaptic alpha 1-blockade with terazosin does not modify insulin sensitivity in nonobese normotensive subjects. *J Cardiovasc Pharmacol* 1991;18:106-110.

[127] Akbay E, Bozlu M, Doruk E, Akbay E, Cayan S, Ulusoy E. Effect of terazosin on the lipid profile in patients with symptomatic benign prostatic hyperplasia. *Urol Int* 2001;67:156-159.

[128] Inukai T, Inukai Y, Matsutomo R, Okumura K, Takanashi K, Takebayashi K, Tayama K, Aso Y, Takemura Y. Clinical usefulness of doxazosin in patients with type 2 diabetes complicated by hypertension: effects on glucose and lipid metabolism. *J Int Med Res* 2004;32:206-213.

[129] Shionoiri H, Ashino K, Yamanaka K, Shindo K, Hiroto S, Arita T. Effect of doxazosin therapy on glucose tolerance and lipid metabolism in hypertensive patients with impaired glucose tolerance. *Clin Ther* 1997;19:527-536.

[130] Ueshiba H, Miyachi Y. Effect of doxazosin on insulin resistance in hypertensive patients with obesity. *Horm Metab Res* 2003;35:532-536.

[131] Tamasawa N, Matsui J, Ogawa Y, Gotoh T, Hinata T, Murakami H, Zhi GJ, Suda T. Effect of doxazosin on the size of LDL particle in the type 2 diabetic patients with hypertension. *J Diabetes Complications* 2000;14:135-139.

[132] Derosa G, Cicero AF, D'Angelo A, Ragonesi PD, Ciccarelli L, Fogari E, Salvadeo SA, Ferrari I, Gravina A, Fassi R, Fogari R. Synergistic effect of doxazosin and acarbose in improving metabolic control in patients with impaired glucose tolerance. *Clin Drug Investig* 2006;26:529-539.

[133] Pessina AC, Ciccariello L, Perrone F, Stoico V, Gussoni G, Scotti A, Muggeo M. Clinical efficacy and tolerability of alpha-blocker doxazosin as add-on therapy in patients with hypertension and impaired glucose metabolism. *Nutr Metab Cardiovasc Dis* 2006;16:137-147.

[134] Hobbs FR, Khan T, Collins B. Doxazosin versus bendrofluazide: a comparison of the metabolic effects in British South Asians with hypertension. *Br J Gen Pract* 2005;55:437-443.

[135] Rabkin SW, Huff MW, Newman C, Sim D, Carruthers SG. Lipids and lipoproteins during antihypertensive drug therapy. Comparison of doxazosin and atenolol in a randomized, double-blind trial: the Alpha Beta Canada Study. *Hypertension* 1994;24:241-248.

[136] Kinoshita M, Shimazu N, Fujita M, Fujimaki Y, Kojima K, Mikuni Y, Horie E, Teramoto T. Doxazosin, an alpha1-adrenergic antihypertensive agent, decreases serum oxidized LDL. *Am J Hypertens* 2001;14:267-270.

[137] Haenni A, Lithell H. Urapidil treatment decreases plasma fibrinogen concentration in essential hypertension. *Metabolism* 1996;45:1221-1229.

[138] Swislocki AL, Vestal RE, Reaven GM, Hoffman BB. Acute metabolic effects of clonidine and adenosine in man. *Horm Metab Res* 1993;25:90-95.

[139] Prichard BN, Graham BR. I1 imidazoline agonists. General clinical pharmacology of imidazoline receptors: implications for the treatment of the elderly. *Drugs Aging* 2000;17:133-159. Review.

[140] Anichkov DA, Shostak NA, Schastnaya OV. Comparison of rilmenidine and lisinopril on ambulatory blood pressure and plasma lipid and glucose levels in hypertensive women with metabolic syndrome. *Curr Med Res Opin* 2005;21:113-9.

[141] Weber MA, Bakris GL, Jamerson K, Weir M, Kjeldsen SE, Devereux RB, Velazquez EJ, Dahlöf B, Kelly RY, Hua TA, Hester A, Pitt B; ACCOMPLISH Investigators. Cardiovascular events during differing hypertension therapies in patients with diabetes. J Am Coll Cardiol. 2010;56:77-85.

[142] Ruilope L, Izzo J, Haller H, Waeber B, Oparil S, Weber M, Bakris G, Sowers J. Prevention of microalbuminuria in patients with type 2 diabetes: what do we know? J Clin Hypertens (Greenwich). 2010;12:422-30. Review.

[143] American Diabetes Association. Standards of medical care in diabetes. Diabetes Care, 2011; 34 (suppl 1): S11-S61.

[144] Cooper-Dehoff R, Cohen JD, Bakris GL, Messerli FH, Erdine S, Hewkin AC, Kupfer S, Pepine CJ; INVEST Investigators. Predictors of development of diabetes mellitus in patients with coronary artery disease taking antihypertensive medications (findings from the INternational VErapamil SR-Trandolapril STudy [INVEST]). *Am J Cardiol.* 2006;98:890-4.

[145] Langaee TY, Gong Y, Yarandi HN, Katz DA, Cooper-DeHoff RM, Pepine CJ, Johnson JA. Association of CYP3A5 polymorphisms with hypertension and antihypertensive response to verapamil. *Clin Pharmacol Ther*. 2007; 81:386-91.

[146] Beitelshees AL, Gong Y, Wang D, Schork NJ, Cooper-Dehoff RM, Langaee TY, Shriver MD, Sadee W, Knot HJ, Pepine CJ, Johnson JA; INVEST Investigators. KCNMB1 genotype influences response to verapamil SR and adverse outcomes in the INternational VErapamil SR/Trandolapril STudy (INVEST). *Pharmacogenet Genomics*. 2007;17:719-29.

[147] Beitelshees AL, Navare H, Wang D, Gong Y, Wessel J, Moss JI, Langaee TY, Cooper-DeHoff RM, Sadee W, Pepine CJ, Schork NJ, Johnson JA. CACNA1C gene polymorphisms, cardiovascular disease outcomes, and treatment response. *Circ Cardiovasc Genet*. 2009; 2:362-70. Epub 2009 Jun 3.

[148] Pacanowski MA, Gong Y, Cooper-Dehoff RM, Schork NJ, Shriver MD, Langaee TY, Pepine CJ, Johnson JA; INVEST Investigators. beta-adrenergic receptor gene polymorphisms and beta-blocker treatment outcomes in hypertension. *Clin Pharmacol Ther*. 2008; 84:715-21. Epub 2008 Jul 9.

[149] Johnson AD, Gong Y, Wang D, Langaee TY, Shin J, Cooper-Dehoff RM, Schork NJ, Binkley P, Pepine CJ, Johnson JA, Sadee W. Promoter polymorphisms in ACE (angiotensin I-converting enzyme) associated with clinical outcomes in hypertension. *Clin Pharmacol Ther*. 2009; 85:36-44. Epub 2008 Oct 22.

[150] Gerhard T, Gong Y, Beitelshees AL, Mao X, Lobmeyer MT, Cooper-DeHoff RM, Langaee TY, Schork NJ, Shriver MD, Pepine CJ, Johnson JA; INVEST Investigators. Alpha-adducin polymorphism associated with increased risk of adverse cardiovascular outcomes: results from GENEtic Substudy of the INternational VErapamil SR-trandolapril STudy (INVEST-GENES). *Am Heart J*. 2008;156:397-404. Epub 2008 Jun 20.

[151] Hansson L, Zanchetti A, Carruthers SG, Dahlöf B, Elmfeldt D, Julius S, Menard J, Rahn KH, Wedel H, Westerling S. Effects of intensive blood-pressure lowering and low-dose aspirin in patients with hypertension: principal results of the Hypertension Optimal Treatment (HOT) randomised trial. HOT Study Group. *Lancet* 1998;351:1755-1762.

[152] Tight blood pressure control and risk of macrovascular and microvascular complication in type 2 diabetes: UKPDS38. UK Prospective Diabetes Study Group (no authors listed). *BMJ* 1998;317:703-713

[153] Staessen JA, Fagard R, Thijs L, Celis H, Arabidze GG, Birkenhäger WH, et al. Randomised double-blind comparison of placebo and active treatment for older patients with isolated systolic hypertension. The Systolic Hypertension in Europe (syst-Eur) Trial Investigator. *Lancet* 132.1997;350:757-764.

[154] Sowers JR, Haffner S. Treatment of cardiovascular and renal risk factors in the diabetic hypertensive. *Hypertension* 2002;40:781-788.

[155] Sowers JR. Treatment of hypertension in patients with diabetes. *Hypertension* 2004;164:1850-1857.

[156] Ninomiya JK, L'Italien G, Criqui MH, Whyte JL, Gamst A, Chen RS. Association of the metabolic syndrome with history of myocardial infarction and stroke in the Third National Health and Nutrition Examination Survey. *Circulation* 2004;109:42-46.
[157] Wilson PW, Kannel WB, Silbershatz H, D'Agostino RB. Clustering of metabolic factors and coronary heart disease. *Arch Intern Med* 1999;159:1104-1109.
[158] Isomaa B, Almgren P, Tuomi T, Forsén B, Lahti K, Nissén M, et al. Cardiovascular morbidity and mortality associated with the metabolic syndrome. *Diabetes Care* 2001;24:683-689.
[159] Stern MP, Williams K, González-Villalpando C, Hunt KJ, Haffner SM. Does the metabolic syndrome improve identification of individuals at risk of type 2 diabetes and/or cardiovascular disease? *Diabetes Care* 2004;27:2676-2681.
[160] Verdecchia P, Reboldi G, Angeli F, Borgioni C, Gattobigio R, Filippucci L, et al. Adverse prognostic significance of new diabetes in treated hypertensive subjects. *Hypertension* 2004;43:963-969.

13

Treatments for Hypertension in Type 2 Diabetes-Non-Pharmacological and Pharmacological Measurements

Kazuko Masuo[1,2] and Gavin W. Lambert[2,3]
[1]*Nucleus Network Ltd.,*
[2]*Human Neurotransmitters Laboratory Baker IDI Heart & Diabetes Institute,*
[3]*Faculty of Medicine, Nursing and Health Sciences, Monash University, Melbourne Australia*

1. Introduction

Type 2 diabetes and hypertension are becoming a major worldwide health problem, besing associated with increasing prevalence of obesity and excess morbidity and mortality. Furthermore, hypertensive patients with diabetes or obesity are more predisposed to target organ damage, resulting stringent targets for blood pressure control [1-4]. Focusing on the close associations between obesity, hypertension and diabetes, the NHANES [5, 6] and the Behavioral Risk Factor Surveillance System (BRFSS) [7] studies showed very close relationships between the prevalence of obesity, hypertension, and diabetes **(Figure 1)**. The Framingham Heart Study [8] demonstrated that diabetic subjects were at 2-fold higher risk mortality, comprising both cardiovascular and non-cardiovascular mortality. Evidence from these epidemiological studies indicates that obesity and weight gain are associated with an increased risk of hypertension [5-7, 9] and type 2 diabetes [7, 9, 10], and that intentional weight loss reduces the risk that currently overweight individuals will develop hypertension [11, 12] or type 2 diabetes [13] .

The clustering of cardiovascular risk factors associated with (abdominal) obesity is well established. Type 2 diabetes, itself, contributes strongly to mortality, morbidity, and cardiovascular risk, including myocardial infarction [14], cardiac events [15-18], stroke, atherosclerosis [19-21] and cardiovascular and renal complication [22, 23] Hypertension is observed twice as frequently in diabetic patients than in the general population, and its prevalence is higher in type 2 diabetes than in type 1 diabetes. Diabetes accompanying cardiovascular diseases such as hypertension is associated with higher mortality and morbidity [24]. The World Health Organization Multinational Study of Vascular Disease in diabetes [17, 18] showed that even in the absence of proteinuria and hypertension, standardized mortality rates were significantly higher in patients with both type 1 and type 2 diabetes compared to those in the general population. Standardized mortality was higher in those with type 1 diabetes compared with type 2 diabetes. Both hypertension and proteinuria in diabetes were associated with a markedly high mortality risk by 11-fold for men with type 1 diabetes, and 5 fold for men with type 2 diabetes. A longer duration of diabetes and hypertension was a stronger predictor of mortality among diabetic and hypertensive patients. Therefore, those hypertensive patients with concomitant diabetes mellitus, or strong lifestyle or dietary factors to predict the development of type 2 diabetes such as obesity, should be treated as a matter of priority in order to prevent subsequent cardiovascular complications [25]. Importantly, the blood pressure goals of antihypertensive treatments is much lower in hypertensive patients with diabetes (<130/80 mmHg) compared to hypertensive patients without complications [1, 4] **(Table 1)**.

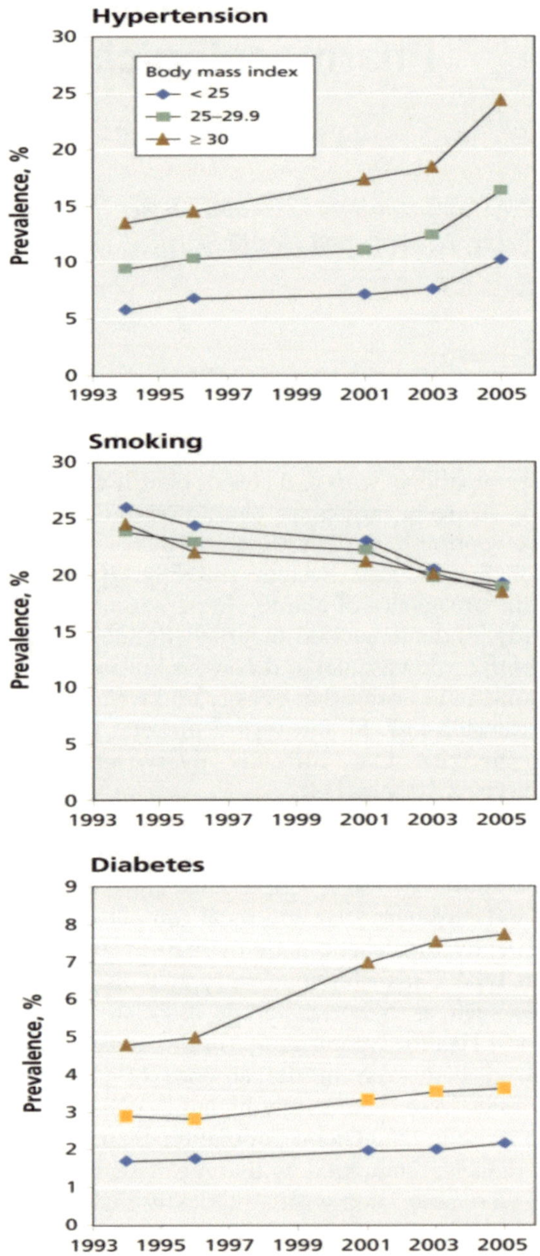

Fig. 1. Increased prevalence of diabetes and hypertension. [Reference 7]

	Clinic blood pressure	Home blood pressure
Young/middle-aged persons	<130/85 mmHg	<125/80 mmHg
Elderly persons	<140/90 mmHg	<135/85 mmHg
Diabetic patients with kidney disease	<130/80 mmHg	<125/75 mmHg
Diabetic Patients after myocardial infarction	<130/80 mmHg	<125/75 mmHg
Diabetic patients with cerebrovascular disorders	<140/90 mmHg	<136/85 mmHg

Note: As the criteria for hypertension include a clinic blood pressure (BP) of 140/90 mm Hg and a home BP of 135/85 mm Hg, the differences between clinic and home BP (5 mm Hg) were simply applied to the clinic BP in each condition and derived provisional target home BP levels.BP, blood pressure. [Reference 2]

Table 1. Expected target blood pressure levels of antihypertensive treatment

The selection of the most suitable pharmacological treatments for those hypertensive patients with type 2 diabetes is governed to a degree by the knowledge of the physiological mechanisms underpinning the specifics of the conditions. Insulin resistance, stimulated renin-angiotensin-aldosterone system (RAAS), sympathetic nervous activation, and leptin resistance (hyperleptinemia) [26-29] are observed very frequently in type 2 diabetes, hypertension and obesity, and these factors appears to play an important role on the onset and developments of these conditions [23, 30, 31].

The first line of treatments for obesity, type 2 diabetes, and hypertension are weight loss with a lifestyle modification such as low caloric diet and exercise [32-34], or, in those with more severe obesity or inability to undertake an exercise program, or bariatric surgery. Perhaps the most important and difficult aspect in controlling obesity is avoiding weight regain [35, 36]. Anti-obesity drugs such as orlistat, sibtramine, rimonabant, and contrave [37-40] have been developed, however these drugs were recently withdrawn from the markets in Europe, the United States and Australia due to serious side effects. Additionally, leptin administration (pegtlatyed recombinant leptin, PEG-OB; recombinant methionyl human leptin, r-metHu Leptin) has been investigated for effects of weight loss and their mechanisms, however, it has not yet been used clinically.

Despite the benefits of lifestyle modifications, additional pharmacological treatment for the management of hypertension is frequently needed. However, the choice of an antihypertensive drug is controversial for patients with associated with diabetes. Lind *et al.* [41] have previously summarized these metabolic effects with long-term antihypertensive treatments. Studies suggest that treatment with different antihypertensive drug classers may have varied effects on glucose and lipid metabolism [42]. In this context, it would be important to choose more beneficial antihypertensive drugs that have less adverse metabolic effects and to achieve stricter blood pressure goals for hypertension associated with type 2 diabetes and obesity.

An integrated cardiovascular risk management approach should be adopted. Aggressive blood pressure control is important, particularly in patients at high cardiovascular disease risk such as those with diabetes. Moreover, well-tolerated antihypertensive agents with protective benefits beyond blood pressure lowering, if this can be achieved, should be

adopted [43]. Recently, many large scale clinical studies have shown that angiotensin II receptor blockers (ARBs) and angiotensin converting enzyme inhibitors (ACE inhibitors) are highly efficacious, well-tolerated antihypertensive agents [44, 45]. More disputed is whether there are additional benefits, beyond blood pressure lowering, leading to greater cardiovascular protection in obesity-related hypertension, metabolic syndrome, and diabetes. Recently, renin-inhibition with Aliskiren has been reported to impart an ameliorative effect on insulin resistance in type 2 diabetic mice [46]. Calcium channel blockers (CCBs), especially newer longer-acting dihydropyridines, may also provide favourable metabolic effects by improving insulin sensitivity and stimulated RAAS and sympathetic nervous activation in diabetes patients [47-49].
In this review, we discuss i) mechanisms of hypertension in type 2 diabetes; ii) the importance of weight loss as a non-pharmacological treatments for type 2 diabetes and hypertension; iii) achieving blood pressure reduction goals for hypertension with diabetes (JNC-7 and JSH 2009), and iv) pharmacological treatments for hypertension in type 2 diabetes.

2. Characteristics of hypertension in obesity and type 2 diabetes: insulin resistance, elevated sympathetic nervous activity, and stimulated the renin-angiotensin-aldosterone system (RAAS) (Figure 2)

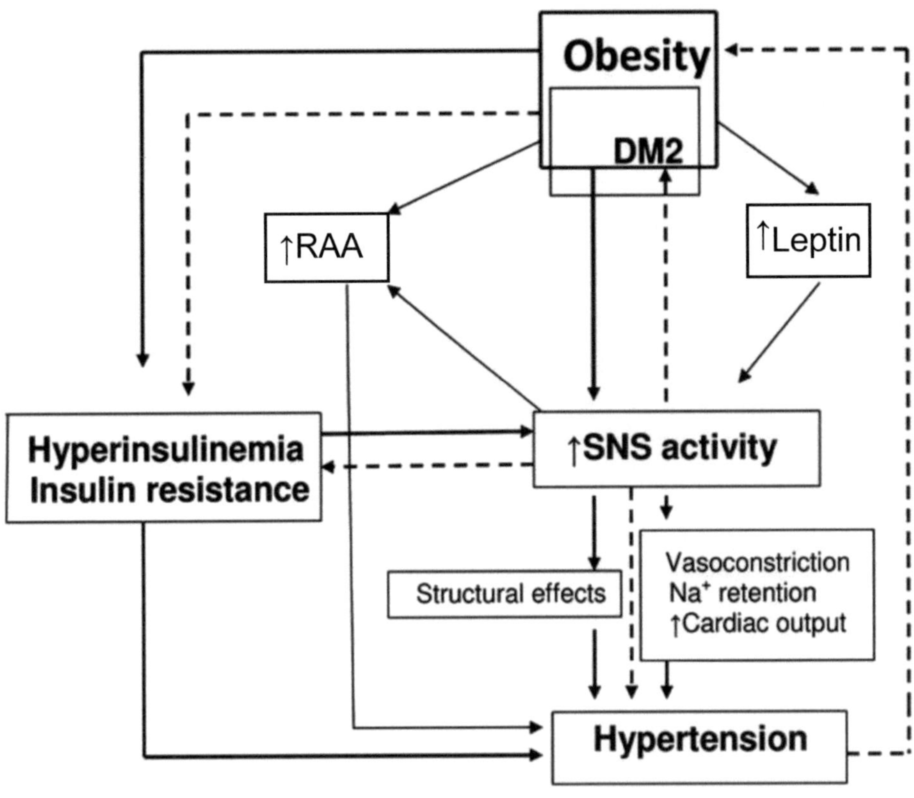

Fig. 2. Relationships between insulin resistance, sympathetic activation and stimulated renin-angiotensin-aldosterone system (RAA) in type 2 diabetes and hypertension. [Reference 22]

Data from many epidemiological and clinical studies has identified a close relationship between elevated sympathetic nervous system activity and insulin resistance / hyperinsulinemia in obesity **(Figure 2)** [22, 30, 50]. Several studies of longitudinal design have examined the effect of body weight changes (weight loss or weight gain) on sympathetic nervous system activity and insulin sensitivity (fasting plasma insulin levels and homeostatic model assessments of insulin resistance (HOMA-IR)). Elevations in sympathetic nervous activity and insulin levels during weight gain [51, 52] and reductions of sympathetic nerve activity and insulin levels during weight loss [11, 33, 53] have been observed. These longitudinal studies have clearly shown that elevated sympathetic activity and insulin resistance are closely linked to obesity (weight gain), the onset of obesity and the maintenance of obesity. Similarly, sympathetic activation and insulin resistance are strongly linked to the onset and development of hypertension [51, 52] and diabetes [54]. Furthermore, stimulation of the renin-angiotensin-aldosterone system (RAAS) is frequently demonstrated in obesity and hypertension [55, 56], and may be related to insulin resistance either via direct or indirect mechanisms [57, 58].

2.1 Insulin resistance

Ferrannini *et al.* was the first investigator who reported insulin resistance or hyperinsulinemia in obese hypertensive patients [59, 60] as well as lean hypertensive subjects [61] over 20 years ago. They observed in obese subjects that the insulin response to oral glucose was twice as high in the hypertensive patients as in the normotensive subjects, yet the glucose incremental area was 3-fold higher in the former than in the latter, thus indicating more severe insulin resistance in obese hypertensive patients. In the hypertensive group, 2-hrs plasma insulin was strongly correlated with systolic BP levels [61]. In obese hypertensive patients, the occurrence of hypertension marks the presence of additional hyperinsulinemia and insulin resistance, independent of any impairment of glucose tolerance [60].

The EGIR-RISC study (The European group for the study of insulin resistance: relationship between insulin sensitivity and cardiovascular disease risk) studied insulin resistance and cardiovascular disease risk in 1500 healthy, middle-aged individuals over a 3-10 year period. Glucose tolerance and insulin sensitivity were measured with using an oral glucose tolerance test and the euglycemic insulin clamp. The EGIR-RISC Study demonstrated the importance of insulin resistance in the development of cardiovascular disease and diabetes, and has implications for the development of prevention and treatment strategies [62]. The EGIR-RISC study's documentation of strong relationships of blood pressure to both insulin action and circulating insulin levels is compatible with the distinct influences on BP by insulin resistance and compensatory hyperinsulinemia [63].

2.2 Stimulated renin-angiotensin-aldosterone system

Angiotension II (Ang II) produced in vessel walls disrupts the regulation of physiologically active substances by impairment of endothelium cell function [56]. Ang II mediated production of reactive oxygen species (ROS) promotes growth factors, cytokines and chemotactic factors relating to atherosclerosis [65]. A high level of insulin, as occurs in insulin resistance states, induces the activation of the tissue RAAS in blood vessels and the heart, and leads to an overproduction of Ang II in these tissues [33, 58]. High levels of insulin directly activate the expression and production of angiotensin, cell growth through the angiotensin I receptor and the conversion of Ang I to Ang II in vascular smooth muscle cells. Although the mechanisms leading to the initial activation of tissue Ang II in high-risk conditions such as type 2 diabetes and hypertension, RAAS blocking agents such as angiotensin converting enzyme inhibitors (ACE inhibitors) and Ang II receptor blockers (ARBs), inhibits the multi-factorial effects of Ang II and reduce the frequency of cardiovascular events as observed in the HOPE and LIFE studies [58, 66, 67]. The HOPE Study (the Heart Outcomes Prevention Evaluation study) showed that high plasma rennin activity is an independent predictor of major vascular events and mortality in a stable population of high-risk patients with atherosclerosis and/or diabetes [58]. The RAAS associated with insulin resistance and sympathetic nerve activation plays an important role of hypertension in type 2 diabetes.

2.3 Sympathetic nervous activation

Energy intake stimulates hyperinsulinemia and sympathetic nerve activity resulting in blood pressure elevation.. Insulin-mediated sympathetic nerve stimulation in obese subjects is a compensatory mechanism aimed at restoring the energy balance by increasing the metabolic rate [22, 30]. Masuo *et al.* [51, 52] have shown in a longitudinal study that heightened sympathetic nervous activity (as indicated by plasma norepinephrine levels) may be a prime mover for future weight gain and blood pressure elevations in originally nonobese, normotensive subjects, and that insulin resistance may be an ancillary factor. During weight loss studies, reductions in plasma norepinephrine followed by reductions in HOMA-IR were observed [33, 34, 53]. These observations show, at least, that the sympathetic nervous system activity associated with insulin resistances play a major role in the onset and development of hypertension with type 2 diabetes associated with obesity.

3. Treatments for obesity

3.1 Lifestyle modification for weight loss

Weight loss is recommended as the first-line treatment for obesity-induced hypertension and type 2 diabetes. The objective of treatment for obesity is both to reduce the high risk of cardiovascular events and to prevent the developments of hypertension and type 2 diabetes [68]. A limited number of epidemiological studies have shown that intentional weight loss and fat loss may reduce the all-cause mortality rate [69]. The US Diabetes Prevention Program [70]and the Oslo Diet and Exercise Study [71] have shown marked clinical benefits with lifestyle intervention, and modest weight loss, on the resolution of the metabolic syndrome and type 2 diabetes . Cohort studies with lifestyle modifications [72] and case control studies with bariatric surgeries [73, 74] provide some evidence that intentional weight loss has long-term benefits on all cause mortality in overweight adults. In a cohort of patients enrolled in a cardiac rehabilitation program, weight loss was associated with favourable long-term outcomes on the composite end-point of mortality and acute cardiovascular events (fatal and nonfatal myocardial infarction, fatal and nonfatal stroke, emergent revascularization for unstable angina pectoris, and congestive heart failure) [75]. Maintaining weight loss is often the greatest challenge, but, many clinical studies have demonstrated that weight loss associated with life-style modification adds to the efficacy of antihypertensive pharmacological treatment [11].

Ribeiro *et al.* [76], Trombetta *et al.* [77] and Tonacio *et al.* [78] compared the blood pressure lowering effects and forearm blood flow between a low caloric diet and exercise, and they observed that only exercise significantly increased forearm blood flow. Recently, Straznicky *et al.* [79] and Masuo *et al.*[80 have shown that a low caloric diet and exercise exert different effects on insulin resistance, the RAAS, and sympathetic nervous activity in obese hypertensive subjects, even though similar weight loss were observed.

3.2 Bariatric surgery

Gastric bypass and adjustable gastric banding are the two most commonly performed bariatric procedures for the treatment of morbid obesity or obesity which is resistant to lifestyle modification such as a low caloric diet plus exercise. Dixon *et al.* [74] showed that a gastric banding induced significant weight loss and resulted in better glucose control and less need for diabetes medication than conventional approaches to weight loss and diabetes control in a randomized controlled study in obese subjects with recently diagnosed type 2 diabetes. Nguyen *et al.* [81] and other investigators [82, 83] compared the effects on weight loss, mortality, morbidity and changes in quality of life in subjects with either gastric banding or gastric banding. The percent of excess weight loss at 4 years was higher in the gastric bypass group compared to the gastric banding group. Postoperative HOMA-IR correlated with % weight loss [84]. Concurrent with restoration of insulin sensitivity and decreases in plasma leptin were dramatic decreases in skeletal muscle transcript levels of stearoyl coenzyme-A desaturase and pyruvate dehydrogenase kinase-4 at 3 and 9 months after gastric banding and a significant decrease in peroxisome proliferation activated receptor-alpha-regulated genes at 9 months. Gumbs *et al.* [84] speculated that decrease in fat mass caused by bariatric surgery significantly affected circulating adipocytokines, which favourably impact on insulin resistance. Improvements in glucose metabolism and insulin resistance following bariatric surgery result in the short-term from decreased stimulation of the entero-insular axis by restricted caloric intake and in the long-term by decreased fat mass resulting changes in release of adipocytokines. Leptin levels drop and adiponectin levels rise following laparoscopic adjustable gastric banding, gastric bypass and biliopancreatic diversion. These changes correlate with weight loss and improvement in insulin sensitivity [84].

All forms of weight loss surgery (bariatric surgery) lead to calorie restriction, weight loss, decrease in fat mass, improvement in insulin resistance and type 2 diabetes mellitus [84]. Left ventricular relaxation impairment, assessed by tissue Doppler imaging, normalized 9 months after surgery [85]. Laparoscopic gastric bypass and gastric banding are both safe and effective approaches for the treatment of morbid obesity, but gastric bypass surgery seems to have better early weight loss and more rapid ameliorative effects on insulin resistance and adipocytokines, muscle metabolism and left ventricular function, however effects the long term effects with similar sustained weight loss are unknown.

3.3 Pharmacological treatments for obesity (Orlistat, Sibtramine, and Rimonabant-Currently withdrawn in Europe, United States and Australia)

Pharmacological treatment for the management of obesity is primarily aimed at weight loss, weight loss maintenance and risk reduction. Anti-obesity agents decrease appetite, reduce absorption of fat or increase energy expenditure. Recently, anti-obesity drugs such as orlistat, sibtramine and rimonabant have been developed placed on markets, however, the latter two were withdrawn from markets in Europe and in the United States due to serious adverse events including psychiatric and cardiovascular related concerns. Lorcaserin, taranabant, topiramate and bupropion with naltrexone are currently on phase III trials with demonstrated significant weight loss compared to placebo at more than 12 months. Some pharmacotherapies have also demonstrated clinical benefits without any side effects, however, further studies are required for a long-term safety [86]. Recently, contrave, a combination of two approved drugs of bupropio and naltrexone, completed Phase III trials with significant weight loss and was approved by FDA in 2010, but FDA declined to approve contrive due to serious cardiovascular adverse events in 2011 [86]. Importantly, obesity is, at least, in part, determined by genetic backgrounds [87], suggesting that a genetic approach to limiting obesity may find a place in the future.

3.4 Leptin administration (pegylated recombinant leptin; PEG-OB, and recombinant methionyl human leptin; r-metHu Leptin)

Lejeune *et al.* [88], Hukshorn *et al.* [89] and Westerterp-Plantenga, *et al.* [90] investigated the effect of weight loss and dietary restraint during and following weekly subcutaneous pegylated recombinant leptin (PEG-OB protein) administration in overweight men. Although treatment with PEG-OB protein led to a significantly greater body weight loss, energy expenditure, and dietary restraint, weight regain (rebound) was faster and stronger in subjects treated with PEG-OB compared to placebo. Asakawa *et al.* [91] administrated leptin intraperitoneally for 5 days in ob/ob mice. Intraperitoneal leptin administration caused significantly body weight loss of 13.2%. Further, an additional ameliorative effect on anxiety was found with leptin administration. This finding, in ob/ob mice, appears not be relevant to the human condition. PEG-OB protein may theoretically work on human for weight loss, however, at this juncture there are few clinical studies available.

4. Pharmacological treatments for the metabolic syndrome as a precursor of type 2 diabetes

The metabolic syndrome, which may be considered to be the precursor of type 2 diabetes ,increases the risk of cardiovascular and renal events in hypertension. It has been associated with a wide range of classical and new cardiovascular risk factors as well as with early signs of subclinical cardiovascular and renal damage. The National Cholesterol Education Program's Adult Treatment Panel III definition uses easily measured clinical findings of increased abdominal circumference, elevated triglycerides, low high-density lipoprotein-cholesterol, elevated fasting blood glucose and/or elevated blood pressure. Three of these five are required for diagnosis. It should be noted that other definitions of metabolic syndrome focus more on insulin resistance and its key role in this syndrome [22] **(Table 2)**.
Metformin has been shown to be helpful in subjects with metabolic syndrome or diabetes [92]. Atabek *et al.* [93] examined whether metformin treatment for 6 months was effective in reducing body weight and hyperinsulinemia, whilst also ameliorating insulin sensitivity indices in 120 obese adolescents with hyperinsulinemia. Before treatment, there were no significant differences between the metformin group and control group in terms of anthropometric data, metabolic parameters, and blood pressure levels. After metformin, there was a significant decline in body mass index, fasting insulin, 120 min insulin levels and HOMA-IR and a significant increase in the fasting glucose/insulin ratio. With regards

to insulin sensitivity indices between the metformin treated and control groups, the metformin group displayed significantly improved metabolic control at the end of the study. These findings show the efficacy of metformin for obesity and insulin resistance (metabolic syndrome) in obese adolescents. While metformin has also been shown to prevent weight gain and improve blood glucose levels in hypertensive patients who received combination therapy of calcium antagonist (nitrendipine) and beta-blocker (atenolol) [94], in combination with drugs blocking the rennin-angiotensin system (ACEI or ARB), metformin may be associated with lactic acidosis and acute renal failure in patients with reduced renal function [95].

Whilst thiazolidinedione drugs (TZDs) may prove useful in the metabolic syndrome, or type 2 diabetes, a large concern has been expressed over the cardiovascular risks associated with rosiglitazone and pioglitazone [96]. Hsiao *et al.* [97] performed retrospective cohort study of 473,483 newly diagnosed patients with type 2 diabetes in order to evaluate the associations between oral antihyperglycemics (TZDs including rosiglitazone and pioglitazone, sulfonylureas, and metformin) with myocardial infarction, congestive heart failure, angina pectoris, stroke and transient ischemic attack. The findings extend the evidence provided further support to data derived from clinical trials that suggested that the disadvantages or harm caused by TZDs, especially rosiglitazone, may outweigh their benefits in patients with type 2 diabetes due to high risk for cardiac events. In addition, although the glycemic efficacy of TZDs are comparable to metformin, adverse effects and higher costs make TZDs less appealing for initial therapy. Among the TZDs, based on cardiovascular safety data, pioglitazone is the preferred choice. In combination with metformin, pioglitazone may be particularly beneficial for patients with metabolic syndrome and diabetes. In those patients who are achieving glycemic goals and tolerating the therapy without apparent complications, rosiglitazone may be continued [97]. Pioglitazone, but not metformin, in patients with type 2 diabetes significantly reduced hepatic lipid and increased adiponectin independent of weight change [98].

5. Pharmacological treatments for hypertension (Figure 3)

Although diabetes mellitus is associated with increased risks of death and cardiovascular events, in the Framingham Heart Study much of this excess risk wass attributable to coexistent hypertension [99]. Tight control of blood pressure (BP) significantly reduces cardiovascular morbidity and mortality in hypertensive patients with diabetes. In the United Kingdom Prospective Diabetes Study [100], a 10 mmHg reduction in systolic blood pressure was superior to a 0.7% decrease in glycosylated haemoglobin A1c (HbA1c) with regards to reducing morbidity and mortality [101]. In the Hypertension Optimal Treatment Study [102, 103] , the risk of cardiovascular events was decreased by 51% in those patients with type 2 diabetes randomized to the lower BP level. The HOT study demonstrated that monotherapy was successful in only 25-40% of patients, according to the target diastolic blood pressure in diabetic patients, and they wee needed at least 2 drugs, average 2.5-3 additional antihypertensive drugs to control blood pressure. [104, 105]. Based on these findings, contemporary treatment guidelines recommend a target blood pressure of <130/80 mmHg for patients with diabetes [106], however, evidence shows that most hypertensive patients with diabetes are very resistant to controlling hypertension and frequently require two or more types of antihypertensive medications in order to achieve blood pressure goals [103, 104, 107, 108].

2. Criteria for Metabolic Syndrome including Insulin Resistance

	WHO	EGIR	NCEP AT III (Expert Panel On Detection Evaluation and Treatment Of High Blood Cholesterol in Adults)	American Heart Association Updated NCEP III
Insulin resistance	Top 25% of population Distribution	Top 25% of population distribution	Not considered	Not considered
Hyperinsulinemia	Not considered	Top 25% of population distribution	Not considered	Not considered
Fasting glucose (mmol/L)	impaired fasting glucose, or impaired glucose tolerance or diabetes	>6.1, but not diabetic	≥6.1	≥5.6 (100 mg/dL) or medications for hyperglycemia
Hypertension (mmHg)	≥160/≥ 90	≥140/≥ 90 or on meds. for hypertension	≥130/85 or meds. for hypertension	≥130/85 or medications for hypertension
Central obesity	waist/hip ratio >0.9 (men), >0.85 (women) and/or BMI≥30kg/m^2	---	---	---
Waist circumference (cm)	Not considered	≥94 (men), ≥ 80 (women)	>102 (men), >88 (women)	≥102 (men), ≥88 (women)
HDL-cholesterol (mmol/L)	<1.0 or medications for dyslipidemia	<1.0 or medications for dyslipidemia	<1.07 (40 mg/dL, men), <1.25 (50 mg/dL , women	<1.07 (40 mg/dL, men) <1.25 (50 mg/dL, women)
Triglyceride (mmol/L)	<1.0 or medications for Dyslipidemia	>2.0 or medications for dyslipidemia	≥1.695 (150 mg/dL)	≥1.695 (150 mg/dL)
Micro-albuminemia	Present	Not considered	Not considered	Not considered
Criteria	1 of the first two + 2 of other features	1of the first two + 2 of other features	3 of above	3 of above

BMI, body mass index; EGIR, European Group of the study of Insulin Resistance; NCEP ATPIII, 3rd Recommendations of the Adult Treatment Panel of the National Cholesterol Education Program; HDL-cholesterol, high-density lipoprotein cholesterol. Values in NECP definition and American Heart Association/ Updated NCEP are approximations of values in mg/dL [Reference 31]

Fig. 3. The Guideline for Hypertension Treatments by the Seventh Report of the Joint National Committee on Prevention, Detection, Evaluation, and Treatment of High Blood Pressure (JNC-7) : Algorithm for Treatment of Hypertension [Reference 1]

Class differences in the effects of antihypertensive medications on metabolic indices may therefore be an important consideration when choosing treatment for hypertensive patients with type 2 diabetes. Prospective, randomized studies with antihypertensive drugs have demonstrated differences between classes of drugs regarding effects on insulin resistance. Treatment with some beta-blockers or high-dose diuretics may be associated with impairment in insulin sensitivity,

- Principal Hypertension Treatment
    1. Treat to BP <140/90 mmHg or BP < 130/80 mmHg in patients with diabetes or chronic kidney disease
    2. Majority of patients will require two medications to reach goal.
- Algorithm for Treatment of Hypertension

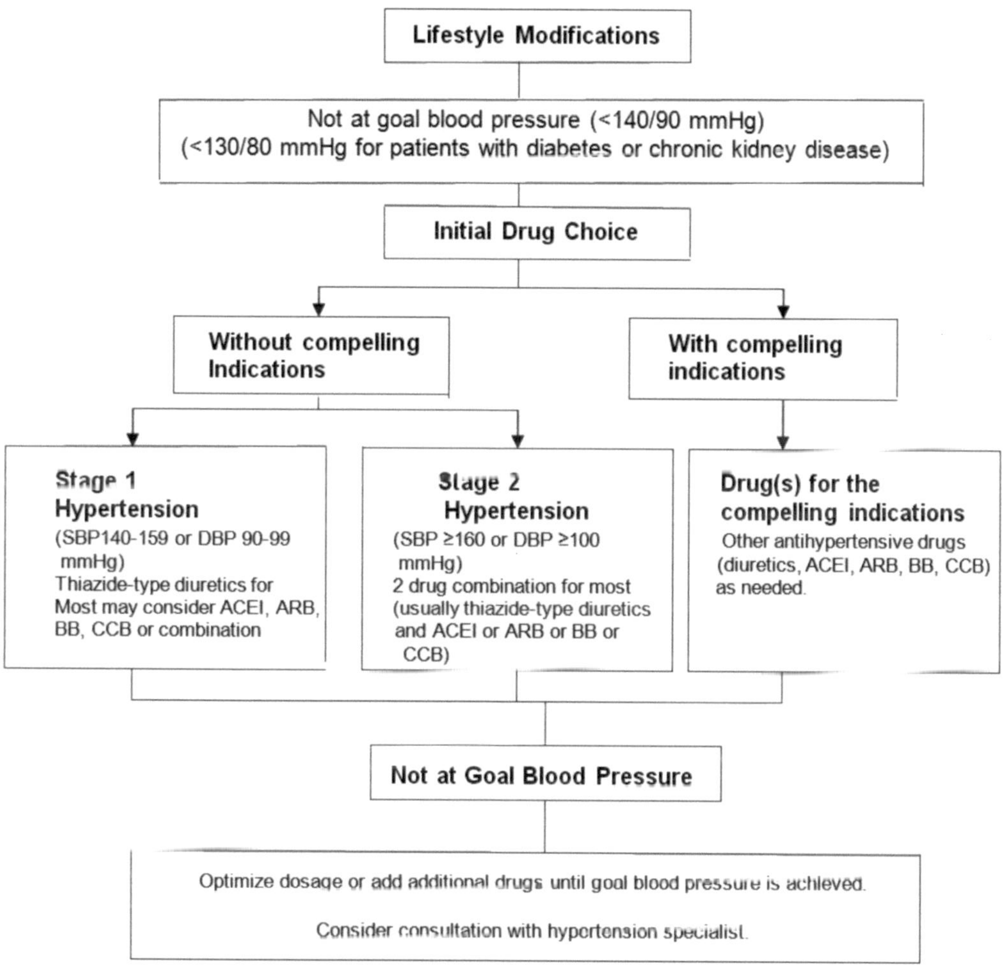

Fig. 3. The Guideline for Hypertension Treatments by the Seventh Report of the Joint National Committee on Prevention, Detection, Evaluation, and Treatment of High Blood Pressure (JNC-7) : Algorithm for Treatment of Hypertension [Reference 1]

whereas angiotensin converting enzyme (ACE) inhibitors, angiotensin receptor blockers (ARBs), renin inhibitors, and calcium channel blockers (CCBs) are ameliorative or neutral. The most pronounced improvements have been obtained with alpha1-blockers. In a recent study, data indicated that moxonidine, an imidazoline1 receptor agonist, was effective in lowering blood pressure and improving insulin sensitivity in insulin-resistant patients. In populations at high risk of diabetes development, it may be justified to select drugs that improve insulin sensitivity when treating hypertension in insulin-resistant individuals [109].

The most important factor for choosing antihypertensive medications for hypertensive patients with diabetes is the prevention of the progression of renal damage [105, 110], which impacts drastically on mortality and morbidity in diabetic patients. Experience from clinical trials suggests that drugs that target the RAAS may have metabolic advantages over drugs such as beta-blockers and diuretics, but this conclusion has not been proved definitively. The number of antihypertensive medications needed for blood pressure control in patients with diabetes is largely dependent on the estimated glomerular filtration rate (renal function) rather than hyperglycemia control [110].

5.1 Angiotensin-Converting Enzyme inhibitors (ACE inhibitors)

The stimulation of the RAAS is a key factor in the development of hypertension in obesity. Pharmacological blockade of the RAAS not only improve blood pressure, but also has a beneficial effect on inflammation, oxidative stress, insulin sensitivity, glucose homeostasis, and resultant renal and cardio-protection. Several strategies are available for RAAS blockade, including angiotensin-converting enzyme inhibitors (ACE inhibitors), angiotensin II receptor blocker (ARBs), renin inhibitors (Aliskiren) and mineralocorticoid-receptor blockers, which have been proven in the clinical studies to result in improvements in cardiovascular disease and chronic kidney disease outcomes. Likewise, while hypertension in obesity, metabolic syndrome or type 2 diabetes, benefits from therapeutic lifestyle change, recently, clinical and epidemiological studies have shown that ACE inhibitors and ARBs are highly efficacious, persistent and well-tolerated antihypertensive agents, due to their cardio-and renal-protective benefits [58, 66, 67] . Moreover they have further beneficial effects in preventing complications of obesity and diabetes, such as progression of diabetic nephropathy, metabolic syndrome. Renin inhibitor may also exert favourable effects on insulin resistance [46]. In other words, the use of the RAAS blockers as initial treatment (both ARBs and ACEIs) in several cardiovascular, metabolic, obesity, and renal disorders (*i.e.* diabetes, ischemic heart disease, heart failure, and proteinuria) is now well-established.

The Heart Outcomes Prevention Evaluation (HOPE) study established that the significant effect of ACE inhibition (ramipril) on cardiovascular morbidity and mortality occurred through mechanisms beyond pure blood pressure control [58, 66]. Additionally, a recent analysis from the Blood Pressure Lowering Treatment Trialist's Collaboration showed that ARBs-based and ACE inhibitors -based treatment regimens were comparable in terms of the odds ratio for stroke and heart failure, independent of blood pressure reduction [111]. There is an emerging body of evidence suggesting that a combination approach to RAAS blockade with an ARB and an ACE inhibitor may further improve cardiovascular outcomes compared with mono-therapy with either agent alone [67]. In addition, some but not all clinical studies have shown that ACE inhibitors exert a favourable effect on insulin resistance [41, 49], lower plasma leptin, suppress the sympathetic nervous overactivity in obesity [11] and provide renal protection especially in diabetic patients with renal injury [43]. The sympathetic inhibition, however, is much less than that achieved with centrally acting imidazoline anti-hypertensive agents. Therefore, ACE inhibitors have s been recommended for use in special patients such as those with obesity, metabolic syndrome, diabetes, renal injury, or high risk of cardiovascular disease before the developments of ARBs [112]. The Irbesartan/HCTZ combination therapy and Blood Pressure Reductions in Diverse Patient Populations (INCLUSIVE) trial [113, 114] showed comparable antihypertensive efficacy and tolerability regardless of BMI or diabetes status.

5.2 Angitension II receptor blockers (ARBs)

The Ongoing Telmisartan Alone and in Combination with Ramipril Global Endpoint Trial (ONTARGET) program compared the efficacy of the angiotensin II receptor blocker (ARB) telmisartan, the angiotensin-converting enzyme (ACE) inhibitor ramipril, and combination therapy with telmisartan plus ramipril for reducing cardiovascular events [115, 116]. The ONTARGET trial involved 25,588 high-risk cardiovascular or diabetic patients with organ damage and compared the effectiveness of telmisartan with that of ramipril and showed that the two drugs were 'therapeutically equivalent'. Telmisartan is now the only ARB with clinical trial evidence of cardiovascular protection equivalent to that of ramipril, which is widely regarded as the 'reference' drug for RAAS blockade in patients at increased cardiovascular risk [116, 117]. The ONTARGET program consists of 2 randomized, double-blind, multicenter international trials: the principal trial, ONTARGET, and a parallel trial, Telmisartan Randomized Assessment Study in ACE-I Intolerant Patients with Cardiovascular Disease (TRANSCEND) [115]. Results of ONTARGET and the TRANSCEND have allowed us to better define the therapeutic approach in high-risk patients showing the favorable effects of either ramipril or telmisartan on blood pressure control and cardiovascular risk [115]. The results of the ONTARGET and TRANSEND studies in patients with high risk cardiovascular disease as well as a number of recent meta-analyses of randomized trials comparing the efficacy and safety of ACE inhibitors to ARBs and their combination in patients with heart failure, hypertension, and chronic kidney disease focused attention on the RAAS.

Emerging data from experimental studies indicates a variety of beneficial effects of telmisartan [118]. In addition to blocking the angiotensin II type 1 receptor, telmisartan activates the peroxisome proliferator-activated receptor (PPAR)-gamma, a well-known target for treatment of the metabolic syndrome and diabetes. Few studies have analysed intra-class differences in ARBs with respect to anti-diabetic or metabolic effects. Makita *et al.* [119] examined a prospective randomized study comparing a PPAR gamma-activating ARB (telmisartan) with a non-activating ARB (candesatrtan), to delineate the effects on metabolic factors associated with cardiovascular disease in 153 hypertensive patient with glucose intolerance. Telmisartan decreased body weight while increasing serum adiponectin levels in hypertensive patients with glucose intolerance. Candesartan did not achieve similar improvements in these patients. Among ARBs, telmisartan may have a greater impact on obesity-related diseases.

5.3 Renin inhibitors

Recent pharmaceutical developments have shown that direct inhibition ofrenin results in decreased angiotensin I and II production and decreased urinary aldosterone excretion. Like

ACE inhibitors and ARBs, treatment with a direct renin inhibitor increases plasma renin concentration, but unlike the other RAAS inhibitors, treatment with a direct renin inhibitor decreases plasma renin activity. This unique combination of effects on the RAAS makes a direct renin inhibitor an attractive option to combine with other antihypertensive agents for the management of hypertension and its comorbidities [124]. Aliskiren/hydrochlorothiazide (HCTZ) therapy provides substantial BP reductions and may thus be a useful treatment option for older patients with stage 2 hypertension [125]. Clinical studies [126-128] including the ACTION study [125] have shown that combining aliskiren, with drugs representing each of the major classes of antihypertensive agents (thiazide diuretics, beta blockers, ACE inhibitors, ARBs, and CCBs) reduces blood pressure and improves markers of cardiovascular outcomes. Importantly, aliskiren had an ameliorative effect on insulin resistance in type 2 diabetic mice [46]. Persson *et al.* [129] investigated the effects of aliskiren on renal function and showed that aliskiren added to losartan reduced albuminuria and renal dysfunction and was well tolerated. In patients with type 2 diabetes, hypertension and albuminuria, aliskiren improved proteinuria [130]. Recently, Gao *et al.* [128] compared the efficacy between aliskiren and ARBs (losartan, valsartan and irbesartan) in 10 reports comprising 3,732 subjects and found that systolic and diastolic blood pressure reduction were similar. Results of several ongoing randomized clinical trials should provide additional insights into the potential of therapeutic combinations that include aliskiren to improve cardiovascular morbidity and mortality in patients with hypertension and related comorbidities. These studies have provided some further insight into the most effective strategy to prevent the adverse effects of RAAS activation. These insights may however need to be modified as the results of new strategies to block/inhibit the RAAS become available [131].

5.4 Calcium Channel Blockers (CCBs)

Calcium channel blockers (CCBs), especially newer long-acting dihydropyridines, may provide favourable metabolic effects by improving insulin sensitivity [49, 132, 133] and dampening the RAAS and sympathetic nervous activation in diabetes patients [47-49].

ACCOMPLISH (The Avoiding Cardiovascular events through COMbination therapy in Patients LIving with Systolic Hypertension) trial was designed in order to evaluate the indications for CCBs [108, 132-135]. The ACCOMPLISH study compare the cardiovascular outcomes between combination of ACE inhibitor (benazepril)/CCB (amlodipine) and ACE inhibitor (benazepril)/diuretic (hydrochlorothiazide, HCTZ) therapy in patients with hypertension and high risk of cardiovascular events. The primary end point of cardiovascular morbidity and mortality was reduced by 20% in the benazepril/CCB arm and was superior to benazepril/HCTZ during the 30 months-follow-up. For 2,842 diabetic patients at very high risk given previous cardiovascular or stroke events, benazepril/CCB had significantly lower prevalence of albuminuria or microalbuminuria compared to benazepri/HCTZ [108]. In the whole cohort, there were less coronary events including acute coronary events and revascularization in the group with the benazepril/CCB. Side effects were generally more frequent with CCB than with the HCTZ combinations. Furthermore, the ACCOMPLISH study also showed that benazepril/CCB demonstrated a marked ameliorative effect on serum creatinine and end-stage renal disease than benazepril/HCTZ [135]. Therefore, the ACCOMPLISH study provided evidence indicating that ACEI/CCB combinations are more effective in selected high-risk patients than are ACEI/HCTZ combinations [108, 132-135]. The AMANDHA Study [136] compared the effects on albuminuria between manidipine and amlodipine, as an additional medication on RAAS blockers. Both manidipine and amlodipine decreased blood pressure values to a similar extent. Urinary albumin excretion was reduced by 65.5% with manidipine versus 20% with amlodipine ($p < 0.01$) at 6 months and 62.7 versus 16.6% ($p < 0.01$) at 18 months. Thus, the addition of manidipine, but not amlodipine, resulted in a large reduction in the urinary albumin excretion rate despite similar blood pressure reductions [136].

Wiener *et al.* [137] showed that a combined therapy with an ACE inhibitor (benazepril) and a CCB (amlodipine) over 12 weeks hadadditive benefits on large-vessel compliance at similar levels of blood pressure lowering, compared with monotherapy with an ACE inhibitor (enalapril) in hypertensive patients with type 2 diabetes (52% vs. 32%, $P<0.05$) [137]. In addition, sub-studies to The International Nifedipine GITS study, Intervention as a Goal in Hypertension Treatment (INSIGHT), showed that nifedipine GITS was significantly more effective at preventing an increase in intima-media thickness in the carotid artery and significantly slowed the progression of coronary calcification, compared with diuretics, oamilozide, which are frequently observed in diabetes and atherosclerotic c patients [138]. The results from INSIGHT support incorporating nifedipine GITS in the management of high-risk hypertensive patients to prevent atherosclerosis-related illness and death [138]. These observations suggest CCBs has an ameliorative effects on atherosclerotic damage.

Interestingly, in the Valsartan Antihypertensive Long-Term Use Evaluation (VALUE) trial, the risk of new-onset diabetes was reported to be 23% lower among patients initiating therapy with valsartan versus amlodipine [139]. Unadjusted absolute risks of diabetes were 21.4 (95% confidence interval (CI) 18.9-24.3) and 26.3 (95% CI 24.3-28.3) per 1000 patient-years for valsartan and amlodipine, respectively; the corresponding relative risk (RR) for valsartan was 0.82 (95% CI 0.70-0.94). The meta-analysis including 1.721 trials and 99,006 patients showed that CCBs were associated with a reduced incidence of new-onset type 2 diabetes (odds ratio 0.81; 95% confidence interval [CI] 0.73-0.90; $p = 0.0001$) compared with diuretic or beta-blocker therapy [140]. The reduction in new-onset type 2 diabetes was maintained when CCB were compared to only thiazide diuretics (OR 0.86; 95% CI 0.75-0.99; $p = 0.0346$). Thus, CCBs may have benefits for treatments for hypertension in type 2 diabetes due to an ameliorative effect on insulin resistance and reductions in new-onset of type 2 diabetes.

5.5 Imidazoline-receptor agonists (moxonidine)

Class differences in the effects of antihypertensive agents on metabolic indices may therefore be an important consideration when choosing treatment for patients who exhibit these characteristics [109]. Moxonidine, which selectively targets imidazoline type-1 receptors in the sympathetic vasomotor centres of the rostral-ventrolateral medulla, is an effective antihypertensive and has been reported to exert favourable metabolic effects in preclinical and clinical studies [141]. In obese hypertensive rats, chronic, but not acute, moxonidine treatment partially restored insulin sensitivity [142]. Moxonidine reduced blood pressure associated with insulin sensitivity in obese hypertensive patients [143]. Moreover, although moxonidine and amlodipine were associated with comparable reductions in blood pressure, only moxonidine significantly decreased sympathetic nervous activity, improved insulin resistance and reduced plasma leptin levels [144]. A small dosage of moxonidine was effective to lowering blood pressure when it was used as a combination therapy with low-dose hydrochlorothiazides in hypertension with type 2 diabetes [145].

The MARRIAGE study (Moxonidine And Ramipril Regarding Insulin And Glucose Evaluation) has extended these preliminary observations by comparing the effects of moxonidine and the ACE inhibitor ramipril--and the combination of both drugs--on metabolic and haemodynamic parameters in patients with hypertension and impaired fasting glycaemia [146].

Both moxonidine and rilmenidine, were shown to exert beneficial effects, not only on blood pressure, but also lipid (reducing free fatty acids, triglycerides) [147, 148] and carbohydrate metabolism (improving glucose tolerance), and neurohormonal parameters such as plasma levels of norepinephrine, leptin, BNP, and ANP [149].

Moxonidine and rimenidine activates I_1 receptors in the RVLM, reducing the activity of the sympathetic nervous system [150, 151]. These I_1-agonists have been shown to produce pronounced and long-lasting BP reduction in different animal models of hypertension, including the spontaneously hypertensive rats [152, 153]. Blood pressure reduction with moxonidine is usually accompanied by a reduction in heart rate which, however, is of shorter duration and lesser magnitude compared to the blood pressure reduction. Chronic administration of moxonidine to SHRs causes normalization of the heart and kidney damage (myocardial fibrosis, capillarization, regressive changes in myocytes, ventricular arrhythmia, left ventricular hypertrophy and renal glomerulosclerosis) in parallel with the reduction of blood pressure [152, 153]. Direct injection of moxonidine into the vertebral artery of cats elicits a more pronounced fall in blood pressure compared with intravenous injection of an equivalent dose, indicating the centrally origins of the antihypertensive effects [153]. In addition, drugs of this class appear to have the capacity to favorably modify insulin sensitivity, which has particular relevance in the treatment of hypertensive diabetic patients and obese hypertensive patients who may be insulin resistant. In the hypertension accompanying maturity onset diabetes and obesity, with recent recommendations from advisory bodies setting lower BP goals, and with these lower targets often being reached only with combinations of antihypertensive agents, it is advisable that all drugs used in combination therapy exert a favorable, or at least a neutral effect on insulin resistance .

Sharma *et al.* [154] showed the efficacy of moxonidine in treating hypertension in those with metabolic syndrome or obesity. A post-marketing surveillance study (CAMUS) involving 772 obese hypertensive patients with hypertension with and without the metabolic syndrome was conducted in Germany. Approximately 50% of subjects had metabolic syndrome and patients were treated with moxonidine and followed for 8 weeks. Reductions in BP were similar between subjects with and without the metabolic syndrome (both from 168/97 to 141/83 mmHg), but the BP reduction was particularly pronounced in patients with severe hypertension at baseline. The response rate (diastolic blood pressure < or =90 mmHg or reduction > or =10 mmHg) of antihypertensive treatment with moxonidine was also similar (94.0% for all patients versus 93.8% for patients with metabolic syndrome). After 8 weeks of treatment, patients achieved a mean weight loss of 1.4 kg, which was not surprisingly, particularly pronounced in obese patients. Moxonidine effectively reduced blood pressure in patients with the metabolic syndrome while simultaneously reducing body weight in obese patients.

In a study examining 77 obese hypertensive patients, Haenni *et al.* [155] used the hyperinsulinemia euglycemic glucose clamp technique and observed that treatment with moxonidine for 8-9 weeks significantly improved insulin sensitivity in insulin-resistant obese hypertensive patients, but not in insulin-sensitive obese hypertensive patients. Sanjuliani *et al.* [144] compared the responses of blood pressure, sympathetic nerve activity and plasma levels of insulin and leptin to moxonidine and amlopdipine treatment over a 24-week period. Blood pressure reductions were of similar magnitude between both treatments. Moxonidine significantly reduced arterial plasma epinephrine and norepinephrine concentrations, orthostatic venous plasma norepinephrine and plasma insulin and leptin levels 120 minutes subsequent to an oral glucose loading, whereas amlodipine did not change any of those parameters. This study clearly demonstrated a comparable reduction in blood pressure with both antihypertensive drugs, but the neurohormonal and metabolic effects were different between the antihypertensive drugs.

5.6 Low dose diuretics

Low-dose of diuretics as a first agent in treatment of patients with hypertension and diabetes is well documented and widely recommended [156-160]. This treatment has beneficial effects on both morbidity and mortality while, previous general concern on the negative impact of diuretics on the different lipid parameters and metabolic effects appear not justified as, all long-term studies with low-dose diuretics have not been shown to affect lipid and glucose profiles in a negative way [161-163]. Moreover, in studies of a year or more duration, diuretics have been shown to reduce cardiovascular risk [145, 164-166]. Very recently, it was reported that Chlorthalidone reduced cardiovascular events more than Hydrochlorothiazide, suggesting that Chlorthalidone may be the preferred thiazide-type diuretics for hypertension in patients at a high risk of cardiovascular risk such as in diabetic or obese patients [167].

5.7 Combination therapies

The clinical combination of hypertension and diabetes carries a particular poor diagnosis. Achievement of target blood pressure (<130/80 mmHg) in this patient category is crucial in decreasing premature morbidity and mortality. Thus, management of subjects with type 2 diabetes and associated hypertension needs to be early and aggressive, and must utilize a global approach. Now, especially for hypertensive patients with diabetes and obesity, multiple-medications are common [168].

6. Conclusions

Hypertension and type 2 diabetes are frequently associated with obesity. Life style modification with diet and exercise remains the initial treatment. Many subjects, however, fail to normalize/lose body weight, to maintain their weight loss, to control hyperglycemia, or to normalize blood pressure. Although diabetes mellitus is associated with increased risk of death and cardiovascular or renal events, much of this excess risk is attributable to coexistent hypertension.

Several large cohort trials have demonstrated that tight control of blood pressure significantly reduces cardiovascular morbidity and mortality and cardio-and renal complications in hypertensive patients with diabetes [101-103]. Based on these findings, contemporary treatment guidelines recommend a target systolic blood pressure/diastolic blood pressure of <130/80 mmHg for patients with diabetes, however, evidence shows that most hypertensive patients with diabetes are very resistant to controlling hypertension and frequently require two or more types of antihypertensive medications to achieve blood pressure goals [103, 110].

Class differences in the effects of antihypertensive medications on metabolic indices and renal protective effects may therefore be an important consideration when choosing treatment for patients who exhibit these characteristics. Hypertension in type 2 diabetes is characterized as insulin resistance, which is associated with cardiovascular morbidity and mortality, and cardiac- and renal complications. Another important factor for choosing antihypertensive medications for hypertensive patients with diabetes is the prevention of the progression of renal damage, which impacts the mortality and morbidity in diabetic patients. While antihypertensive agents such as beta-adrenoceptor antagonists may worsen insulin resistance and impair glucose tolerance, ACE inhibitors or ARBs exert positive metabolic effects and renoprotection. Experience from clinical trials suggests the renal protective drugs that target the RAAS and CCBs and beneficial.

This article provides a synthesis of current findings with non-pharmacological and pharmacological treatments for hypertension in type 2 diabetes. Treatment of hypertension in type 2 diabetes is important with regards to the prevention of cardiovascular complications. To this stage, the preferred antihypertensive drug classes are somewhat uncertain, and disputed, however, smaller dosage of each class of drugs might lead less side events. Currently a combination therapy with 2 or more different classes of antihypertensive drugs is recommended [1, 4, 168]. Use of ACEIs and ARBs as the initial treatment in hypertension in type 2 diabetes is usually advocated as these agents exert favourable effects on insulin sensitivity and provide renal protection. A strong case for wider use of CCBs and the imidazoline drugs (moxonidine, rilmenidine) can also be made

There are many aspects of the pathogenesis, prevention and treatment of type 2 diabetes that still need to be uncovered before a complete strategy to reduce the ongoing epidemic and burden of type 2 diabetes may be offered.

7. References

[1] Chobanian, A.V.; Bakris, G.L.; Black, H.R.; Cushman, W.C.; Green,. L.A.; Izzo, J.L. Jr.; Jones, D.W.; Materson, B.J.; Opari,l S.; Wright, J.T.; Roccella, E.J. Joint National Committee in Prevention, Detection, Ecaluation, and Treatment of High Blood Pressure. National Heart, Lung, and Blood Institute; National High Blood Pressure Education Program Coodinating Committee. Seventh Report of the Joint National Committee on Prevention, Detection, Evaluation, and Treatment of High Blood Pressure. *Hypertension.* **2003,** 42(6), 1208-1252. www.nhlbi.nih.gov/guidelines/hypertension/; www.nhlbi.nih.gov/guidelines/hypertension/phycard.pdf;

[2] Whiteworth JA; World Health Organization, International Socity of Hypertension Writing Group. 2003 World Health Organization (WHO)/International Socity of Hypertension (ISH) statement on management of hypertension. J Hypertens. 2003; 21: 1983-1992.

[3] Olsen MH, Mallion JM, Rahn KM, Erdine S, Viigimae M, Laurent S, Agabiti-Rosei E, Mancia G, Schmieder RE, Cifkova R, Dominiczak A, Kjeldsen SE, Redon J, Zanchetti A, Nilsson P, Narkiewicz K: ESH Council. Agreement within Europe

about antihypertensive treatment and education - results from the European Society of Hypertension questionnaire. J Hypertens. 2010; 28: 1593-1594.

[4] Ogihara, T.; Kikuchi, K.; Matsuoka, H.; Fujita, T.; Higaki, J.; Horiuchi, M, Imai, Y.; Imaizumi, T.; Ito, S.; Iwao, H.; Kario, K.; Kawano, Y.; Kim-Matsuyama, S.; Kimura, G.; Matsubara, H.; Matsuura, H.; Naruse, M.; Saito, I.; Shimada, K.; Shimamoto, K.; Suzuki, H.; Takishita, S.; Tanahashi, N.; Tsuchihashi, T.; Uchiyama, M.; Ueda, S.; Ueshima, H.; Umemura, S.; Ishimitsu, T.; Rakugi, H. Japanese Society of Hypertension Committee. The Japanese Society of Hypertension Guidelines for the Management of Hypertension (JSH 2009). *Hypertens. Res.* **2009,** 32(1), 3-107.

[5] Phillips LK, Prins JB. The link between abdominal obesity and the metabolic syndrome. Curr Hypertens Rep. 2008; 10: 156-164.

[6] Ogden CL, Fryar CD, Carroll MD, Flegal KM. Advance Data from Vital and Health Statics. CDC. 2004; 347: 1-20.

[7] Mokdad AH, Ford ES, Bowman BA, Dietz WH, Vinicor F, Bales VS, Marks JS. Prevalence of obesity, diabetes, and obesity-related health risk factors, 2001. JAMA, 2003; 289: 76-79.

[8] Preis SR, Hwang SJ, Coady S, Pencina MJ, D'Agostino RB Sr, Savage PJ, Levy D, Fox CS. Trends in all-cause and cardiovascular disease mortality among women and men with and without diabetes mellitus in the Framingham Heart Study, 1950 to 2005. Circulation. 2009; 119: 1728-1735.

[9] Ford ES, Williamson DF, Liu S. Weight change and diabetes incidence: findings from a national cohort of US adults. Am J Epidemiolo. 1997; 146: 214-222.

[10] Resnick HE, Valsania P, Halter JB, Lin X. Relation of weight gain and weight loss on subsequent diabetes risk in overweight adults. J Epidemiol Communuty Health. 2000; 54: 596;602.

[11] Masuo K, Mikami H, Ogihara T, Tuck ML. Weight reduction and pharmacological treatment in obese hypertensives. Am J Hypertens. 2001; 14: 530-538.

[12] Straznicky NE, Lambert GW, McGrane MT, Masuo K, Dawood T, Nestle PJ, Eikelis N, Schlaich MP, Esler MD, Socratous F, Chopra R, Lambert EA. Weight loss may reserve blunted sympathetic neural responsiveness to glucose ingestion in obese subjectrs with metabolic syndrome. Diabetes. 2009; 58: 1126-11342.

[13] Will JC, Williamson DF, Ford ES, Calle EE, Thun MJ. Intentional weight loss and 13-year diavetes incidence in overweight adults. Am J Public Healthy. 2002; 92: 1245-1248.

[14] Cho E, RimmEB, Stampfer MJ, Willett WC, Hu FB. The impact of diabetes mellitus and prior myocardial infarction on mortality from all causes and from coronary heart disease in men. J Am Coll Cardiol. 2002; 40: 954-960.

[15] Heidmann C, Boeing H, Pischon T, Nothlings U, Joost HG, Schulze MB. Association of a diabetes risk score with risk of myocardial infarction, stroke, specific types of cancer, and mortality: a prospective study in the European Prospective Investigation into Cancer and Nutrition (EPIC)-Potsdam cohort. Eur J Epidemiol. 2009; 24: 281-288.

[16] Young LH, Wackers FJ, Chyun DA, *et al.* for DIAD Investigators. Cardiac outcomes after screening for asymptomatic coronary artery disease in patients with type 2 diabetes: the DIAD study: a randomized controlled trial. JAMA. 2009; 301: 1547-1555.

[17] Wang SL, Head J, Steven L, Fuller JH. Excess mortality and its relation to hypertension and proteinuria in diabetic patients. The World health organization multinational study of vascular disease in diabetes. Diabetes Care. 1996; 19: 305-312.

[18] Morrish NJ, Wang SL, Stevens LK, Fuller JH, Keen H. Mortality and causes of death in the WHO multinational study of vascular disease in diabetes. Diabetologia. 2001; 44 Suppl 2: S14-S21.

[19] Iglseder B, Cip P, Malaimare L, Ladurner G, Paulweber B. The metabolic syndrome is a stronger risk factor for early carotid atherosclerosis in women than in men. Stroke. 2005; 36: 1212-1217.

[20] Kawamoto R, Tomita H, Ohtsuka N, Inoue A, Kamitani A. Metabolic syndrome, diabetes and subclinical atherosclerosis as assessed by carotid intima-media thickness. J Atheroscler Thromb. 2007; 14: 78-85.

[21] Bertoni A, Wong ND, Shea S, *et al.* Insulin resistance, metabolic syndrome, and subclinical atherosclerosis. The Multi-Ethnic Study of Atheroclerosis (MESA). Diabetes Care. 2007; 30: 2951-2956.

[22] Masuo K, Rakugi H, Ogihara T, Esler MD, Lambert GW. Cardiovascular and renal complications of type 2 diabetes in obesity: role of sympathetic nerve activity and insulin resistance. Curr Diab Rev. 2010; 6: 58-67.

[23] Straznicky NE, Grima MT, Lambert EA, Eikelis N, Dawood T, Lambert GW, Nestel PJ, Masuo K, Sari CI, Chopra R, Mariani JA, Schlaich MP. J Hypertens. Exercise augments weight loss induced improvement in renal function in obese metabolic syndrome individuals. 2011; 29: 553-564.

[24] Held C, Gerstein HC, Yusuf S, *et al.* for the ONTARGET/TRANSCEND investigators. Glucose levels predict hospitalization for congestive heart failure in patients at high cardiovascular risk. Circulation. 2007; 115: 1371-1375.

[25] Schulze MB, Hoffmann K, Boeing H, *et al.* An accurate risk score based on anthropometric, dietary, and lifestyle factors to predict the development of type 2 diabetes. Diabetes Care. 2007; 30: 510-515.

[26] Bandaru P, Shankar A. Association between plasma leptin levels and diabetes mellitus. Metab Syndr Relat Disord. 2011; 9: 19-23.

[27] Shankar A, Xiao J. Positive relationship beterrn plasma leptin level and hypertension. Hypertension. 2011; 56: 623-628.

[28] Sari R, Balci MK, Apaydin C. The relationship between plasma leptin levels and chronic complication in patients with type 2 diabetes mellitus. Metab Syndr Relat Disord. 2010; 8: 499-503.

[29] Masuo K, Katsuya T, Ogihara T, Tuck ML. Acute hyperinsulinemia reduces plasma leptin levels in insulin-sensitive Japanese men. Am J Hypertens. 2005; 18: 235-243.

[30] Esler M, Straznicky N, Eikelis N, Masuo K, Lambert G, Lambert E. Mechanisms of sympathetic activation in obesity-related hypertension. Hypertension. 2006; 48: 787-796.

[31] Masuo K, Esler MD. Role of sympathetic nerve activity in obesity, hypertension, and metabolic syndrome. Curr Hypertens Rev. 2010; 6: 83-91.

[32] Straznicky NE, Lambert EA, Lambert Gw, Masuo K, Esler MD, Nestel PJ. Effects of dietary weight loss on sympathetic activity and cardiac risk factors associated with the metabolic syndrome. J Clin Endocrinol Metab. 2006; 90: 5998-6005

[33] Weir MR, Dzau VJ. The renin-angiotensin-aldosterone system: a specific target for hypertension management. Am J Hypertens. 1999; 12 (Pt 3):205S-213S.

[34] Masuo K, Mikami H, Ogihara T, Tuck ML. Different mechanisms between weight loss-sensitove and –resistant blood pressure reduction in obese subjects. Hypertens Res. 2001; 24: 371-374.

[35] Ross R. The challenge of obesity treatment: avoiding weight regain. CMAJ. 2009; 180: 997-998.

[36] Masuo K, Katsuya T, Kawaguchi H, Fu Y, Rakugi H, Ogihara T, Tuck ML. Rebound weight gain as associated with high plasma norepinephrine levels that are mediated through polymorphism in beta 2-adrenoceptor. Am J Hypertens. 2005; 18: 1508-1516.

[37] Whiltlock EA, O'Connor EP, Williams SB, Beil TL, Lutz KW. Evid Rep Technol Assess (Full Rep). 2008; 170: 1-308.

[38] Willemen MJ, Mantel-Teeuwisse AK, M Straus SM, Leufkens HG, Egberts AC, M Sturkenboom MC. Pharmacolepidemiol Drug Safe. 2009; May 5. [Epub ahead of print].

[39] Siebenhofer A, Horvath K, Jeitler K, Berghold A, Stich AK, Matyas E, Pignitter N, Siering U. Long-term effects of weight-reducing drugs in hypertensive patients. Cochrane Database Syst Rev. 2009; 8: CD007654.

[40] Czernichow S, Lee CM, Barzi F, Greenfield JR, Baur LA, Chalmers J, Woodward M, Huxley RR. Efficacy of weight loss drugs on obesity and cardiovascular risk factors in obese adolescents: a meta-analysis of randomized controlled trials. Obes Rev. 2009; Jun 1 [Epub a head of print].

[41] Lind L, Pollare T, Berne C, Lithell H. Long-term metabolic effects of antihypertensive drugs. Am Heart J. 1994; 128: 1177-1183.

[42] Padwal R, Laupacis A. Antihypertensive therapy and incidence of type 2 diabetes: a systemic review. Diabetes Care. 2004; 27: 247-255.

[43] Shammas NW, Sica DA, Toth PP. A guide to the management of blood pressure in the diabetic hypertensive patients. Am J Cardiovasc Drugs. 2009; 9: 149-162.

[44] Verma S, Gupta M, Holmes DT, Xu L, Tech H, Gupta S, Yusuf S, Lonn EM. Plasma renin activity predicts cardiovascular mortality in the Heart Outcomes Prevention Evaluation (HOPE) study. Eur Heart J. 2011. March 17. [Epub ahead of print].

[45] Nosadini R, Tonolo G. Cardiovascular and renal protection in type 2 diabetes mellitus: the role of calcium channel blockers. J Am Soc Nephrol. 2002; 13 Suppl 3: S216-S223.

[46] Iwai M, Kanno H, Tomono Y, Inaba S, Senmba I, Furuno M, Mogi M, Horiuchi M. Direct renin inhibition improved insulin resistance and adipose tissue dysfunction in type 2 diabetic KK-A9y) mice. J Hypertens. 2010; 28: 1471-1481.

[47] Masuda T, Ogura MN, Moriya T, Takahira N, mMatsumoto T, Kuysuna T, Hara M, Aibe N, Noda C, Izumi T. Beneficial effects of L- and N-type calcium channel blocker on glucose and lipids metabolism and renal function in patients with hypertension and type II diabetes mellitus. Cardiovasc Ther. 2011; 29: 46-53.

[48] Toba H, Yoshida M, Yojo C, Nakano A, Oshima Y, Kojima Y, Noda K, Kobara M, Nakata T. L/N-type calcium channel blocker cilinidipine ameliorates proteinuria and inhibits the renal renin-angiotensin-aldosterone system in deoxycorticosterone acetate-salt hypertensive rats. Hypertens Res. 2011; Jan 27. [Epub ahead of print].

[49] Masuo K, Mikami H, Ogihara T, Tuck ML. Metabolic effects of long-term treatments with nifedipine-retard and captopril in young hypertensive patients. Am J Hypertens. 1997; 10: 600-610.

[50] Masuo K. Obesity-related hypertension: role of the sympathetic nervous system, insulin, and leptin. Curr Hypertens Rep. 2002; 4: 112-118.

[51] Masuo K, Mikami H, Ogihara T, Tuck ML. Weight gain-induced blood pressure elevation. Hypertension. 2000; 35: 1135-1140.

[52] Masuo K, Katsuya T, Fu Y, Rakugi H, Ogihara T, Tuck ML. Beta2- and beta3-adrenoceptor polymorphisms are related to the onset of weight gain and blood pressure elevation over 5 years. Circulation. 2005; 111; 3429-3434.

[53] Masuo K, Kstsuya T, Kawaguchi H, Fu Y, Rakugi H, Ogihara T. Rebound weight gain as associated with high plasma norepinephrine levels that are mediated through polymorphisms in the beta2-adrenoceptor. Am J Hypertens. 2005; 18: 1508-1516.

[54] Huggett RJ, Scott EM, Gilbey SG, Stoker JB, Mackintosh AF, Mary DA. Impact of type 2 diabetes mellitus on sympathetic neural mechanisms in hypertension. Circulation. 2003; 108: 3097-3101.

[55] Stump CS, Henriksen EJ, Wei Y, Sowers JR. The metabolic syndrome: role of skeletal muscle metabolism. Ann Med. 2006; 38: 389-402.

[56] Kamide K, Rakugi H, Ogihara T. Insulin resistance and the renin-angiotensin-aldosterone system in metabolic syndrome and obesity-related hypertension. Curr Hypertens Rev. 2010; 6: 100-103.

[57] Matayoshi T, Kamide K, Takiuchi S, Horio T, Yoshihara F, Nakamura S, Nakahara H, Kawano Y. Relationship between insulin resistance and the renin-angiotensin system: analysis for patients with essential and renovascular hypertension. Clin Exp Hypertens. 2007; 29: 479-487.

[58] Kamide K, Rakugi H, Ogihara T, Nagai M, Takiuchi S, Matsukawa N, Higaki J, Kawano Y, Ogihara T, Tuck ML. Insulin-mediated modulation of the endothelial renin-angiotensin system and vascular cell growth. J Hypertens. 2004; 22: 121-127.

[59] Ferrannini E. Physiological and metabolic consequence of obesity. Metabolism. 1995; 44 (Suppl 3): 15-17.

[60] Manicardi V, Camellini L, Bellodi G, Coscelli C, Ferrannini E. Evidence for an association of high blood pressure and hyperinsulinemia in obese man. J Clin Endocrinol Metab. 1988; 62: 1302-1304.

[61] Ferrannini E, Buzzigoli G, Bonadonna R, Giorico MA, Oleggini M, Graziadei L, Pedrinelli R, Brandi L, Bevilacqua S. Insulin resistance in essential hypertension. N Engl J Med. 1987; 317: 350-357.

[62] Hills SA, Balkau B, Coppack SW, Dekker JM, Mari A, Natali A, Walker M, Ferrannini E; EGIR-RISC Study Group. The EGIR-RISC Study (The European Group for the study of insulin resistance: relationship between insulin sensitivity and cardiovascular disease risk): I. Methodology and objectives. Diabetologia 2004; 47: 566-570.

[63] Ferrannini E, Natali A, Capaldo B, Lehtovirta M, Jacob S, Yki-Jarvinen H. Insulin resistance, hypertensulinemia, and blood pressure: role of age and obesity. European Group for the Study of Insulin Resistance (EGIR). Hypertension. 1997; 30: 1144-1149.

[64] Ferranninini E. Analysis of data on insulin resistance from the European group for the study of insulin resistance: focus on obesity and hypertension. Endocr Pract. 2003; 9 suppl 2: 43-49.
[65] Harrison DG, Gongora MC. Oxidative stress and hypertension. Med Clin North Am. 2009; 93: 621-635.
[66] Van Mieghem W. Prevention of major cardiovascular events with an angiotensin-converting enzyme inhibitor or an angiotensin receptor blocker early or late after stroke. J Hypertens Suppl. 2009; 27: S26-S31.
[67] Slight P, Jakobsen A, Heroys J, Ralph A, Ress T, Shaw M. No HOPE without proof: do ARBs meet the standard for cardiovascular protection? Medscape J Med. 2008; 10 Suppl: S6.
[68] Redon J, Cifkova R, Laaurent Sm, Nilsson P, Narkiewicz K, Erdine S, Mancia G; Scientific Council of the European Society of Hypertension. J Hypertens. 2008; 26: 1891-1900.
[69] Allison DB, Zannolli R, Faith MS, Heo M, Pietrobelli A, VanItallie TB, Pi-Sunyer FX, Heymsfield SB. Weight loss increases and fat loss decreases all-cause mortality rate: results from two independent cohort studies. Int J obes Relat Metab Disord. 1999; 23: 603-611.
[70] Orchard TJ, Temprosa M, Goldberg R, Haffner S, Ratner R, Marcovina S, Fowler S. The effect of metformin and intensive lifestyle intervention on the metabolic syndrome: The Diabetes Prevention Program randomized trial. Am Intern Med. 2005; 142: 611-619.
[71] Anderssen SA, Carroll S, Urdal P, Holme I. Combined diet and exercise intervention reverses the metabolic syndrome in middle-aged males: results from the Oslo Diet and Exercise Study. Scand J Med Sci Sports. 2007; 17: 687-695.
[72] Poobalan AS, Aucott LS, Smith WCS, Avenell A, Jung R, Broom J. Long-term weight loss effects on all cause mortality in overweight/obese populations. Obes Rev. 2007; 8: 503-513.
[73] Sjostrom L, Narbro K, Sjostrom CD< et al. Effects of bariatric surgery on mortality in Swedish obese subjects. N Engl J Med. 2007; 357: 741-752.
[74] Dixon JB, O'Brien PE, Playfair J, Chapman L, Schachter LM, Skinner S, Proietto J, Bailey M, Anderson M. Adjustable gastric banding and conventional therapy for type 2 diabetes: a randomized controlled trial. JAMA. 2008; 299: 316-323.
[75] Sierra-Johnson J, Romeo-Corral A, Somers VK, Lopez-Jimenez F, Thomas RJ, Squires RW, Allison TG. Prognostic importance of weight loss in patients with coronary heart disease regardless of initial body mass index. Eur J Cardiovasc Prev Rehabil. 2008; 15: 336-340.
[76] Ribeiro MM, Silva AG, Santos NS, Guazzelle I, Matos LN, Trombetta IC, Halpern A, Negrao CE, Villares SM. Diet and exercise training restore blood pressure and vasodilatory responses during physiological maneuvers in obese children. Circulation. 2005; 111; 1915-1923.
[77] Trombetta IC, Batalha LT, Rondon MU, Laterza MC, Kuniyoshi FH, Gowdak MM, Barretto AC, Halpern A, Villares SM, Negrao CE. Weight loss improves neurovascular and muscle metaboreflex control in obesity. Am J Physiol Heart Circ Physiol. 2003; 11: H974-H982.

[78] Tonacio AC, Trombetta IC, Rondon MU, Batalha LT, Kuniyoshi FH, Laterza MC, Suzuki PH, Gowdak MM, Barretto AC, Halpern A, Villares SM, Negrao CE. Effects of diety and exercise training on neurovascular control during mental stress in obese women. Braz J Med Biol Res. 2006; 39: 53-62.
[79] Straznicky N, Grima MT, Eikelis N, Nestel PJ, Dawood T, Schlaich MP, Chopra R, Masuo K, Esler MD, Sari CI, Lambert GW, Lambert EA. The effects of weight loss versus weight loss maintenance on sympathetic nervous system activity and metabolic syndrome components. JCEM 2011; 96: 6503-8
[80] Masuo K, Rakugi H, Ogihara T, Lambert GW. Different mechanisms in weight loss-induced blood pressure reduction between a calorie restricted diet and exercise. Hypertens Res. 2011 {in press).
[81] Nguyen NT, slone JA, Nguyen XM, Hartman JS, Hoyt DB. A prospective randomized trial of laparoscopic gastric bypass versus laparoscopic adjustable gastric banding for the treatment of morbid obesity: outcomes, quality of life and costs. Ann Surg. 2009; Aug 27 [Epub ahead of print]
[82] Ballantyne GH, Wasielewski A, Saunders JK. The surgical treatment of type II diabetes mellitus: Changes in HOMA insulin resistance in the first year following laparoscopic Rou-en-Y gastric bypass (LRYGB) and laparoscopic adjustable gastric banding (LAGB). Obes Surg. 2009; 19: 1297-1303.
[83] Trakhenbroit MA, Leichman JG, Algahim MF, Miller CC 3rd, Moody FG, Lux TR, Taegtmeyer H. Body weight, insulin resistance, and serum adipokine levels 2 years after 2 types of bariatric surgery. Am J Med. 2009; 122: 435-442.
[84] Gumbs AA, Modlin IM, Ballantyne GH. Changes in insulin resistance following bariatric surgery: role of caloric restriction and weight loss. Obes Surg. 2005; 15: 462-73.
[85] Leichman JG, Wilson EB, Scarborough T, Aguilar D, Miller CC 3rd, Yu S, Algahim MF, Reyes M, Moody FG, Taegtmeyer H. Dramatic reversal of derangements in muscle metabolism and left ventricular function after bariatric surgery. Am J Med. 2008; 121: 966-973.
[86] Ioannides-Demos LI, Piccenna L, McNeil JJ. Pharmacotherapies for obesity: Past, currect, and future therapies. J Obes. 2011, Article ID 179674. Doi: 10.1155/2011/79674.
[87] Masuo K, Lambert GW. Relations of adrenoceptor polymorphisms with obesity. J Obes. 2011. Article ID 609485. Doi:10.1155/2011/609485
[88] Lejeune MP, Hukshorn CJ, Saris WH, Westerterp-Plantenga MS. Effect of dietary restraint during and following pegylated recombinant leptin (PEG-OB) treatment of overweight men. Int J Obes Relat Metab Disord. 2003; 27: 1494-1499.
[89] Hukshorn CJ, Westerterp-Plantenga MS, Saris WMH. Pegylated human recombinant leptin (PEG-OB) causes additional weight loss in severely energy-restricted, overweight men. Am J Clin Nutr. 2003; 77: 771-776.
[90] Westerterp-Plantenga MS, Saris WH, Hukshorn CJ, Campfield LA. Effects of weekly administration of pegylated recombinant human OB protein on appetite profile and energy metabolism in obese men. Am J Clin Nutr. 2001; 74: 426-434.
[91] Asakawa A, Inui A, Inui T, Katsuura G, Fujino MA, Kasuga M. Leptin treatment ameliorates anxiety in ob/ob mice. J Diabetes Complications. 2003; 17: 105-107.

[92] Drown DJ. Metformin: effective in the prevention of new-onset type 2 diabetes?Prog Cardiovasc Nurs. 2008; 23: 93-94.
[93] Atabek ME, Pirgon O. Use of metformin in obese adolescents with hyperinsulinemia: a 6-month, randomized, double-blind, placebo-controlled clinical trial. J Pediatr Endocrinol Metab. 2008; 21: 339-348.
[94] Zhang JL, Zheng X, Zou DJ, Qiu JL, Zhao XX, Qin YW. Effect of metformin on weight gain during antihypertensive treatment with a beta-blocker in Chinese patients. Am J Hypertens. 2009; Jul 2. [Epub ahead of print].
[95] Gudmundsdottir H, Aksnes H, Heldal K, Krogh A, Froyshov S, Rudberg N, Os I. Metformin and antihypertensive therapy with drugs blocking the renin angiotensin system, a cause of concern? Clin Nephrol. 2006; 66: 380-385.
[96] Khanderia U, Pop-Busui R, Eagle KA. Thiazolidinediones in type 2 diabetes: a cardiology perspective. Ann Pharmacother. 2008; 42: 1466-1474.
[97] Hsiao FY, Huang WF, Wen YW, Chen PF, Kuo KN, Tsai YW. Thiazolidinediones and cardiovascular events in patients with type 2 diabetes mellitus: A retrospective cohort study of over 473 000 patients using the national health insurance database in Taiwan. Drug Saf. 2009; 32: 675-690.
[98] Gupta AK, Bray GA, Greenway FL, Martin CK, Johnson WD, Smith SR. Pioglitazone, but not metformin, reduces liver fat in Type-2 diabetes mellitus independent of weight changes. J Diabetes Complications. 2009; Jul 3 [Epub ahead of print].
[99] Chen G, McAlister FA, Walker RL, Hemmelgam BR, Campbell NR. Cardiovascular outcomes in Framingham Participants with diabetes: the importance of blood pressure. Hypertension. 2011; Mar 14. [Epub ahead of print].
[100] Klonoff DC. United Kingdom Prospective Diabetes Study follow-up studies establish a legacy effect of therapy for hyoerglycemia but not hypertension. J Diabetes Sci Thechnol. 2008: 2: 922-924.
[101] Kalaitzidis R, Bakris G. Management of hypertension in patients with diabetes: the place of angiotensin-II receptor blockers. Diabetes Obes Metab. 2009; 11: 757-769.
[102] Hansson L. The Hypertension Optimal Treatment study and the importance of lowering blood pressure. J Hypertens. Suppl. 1999; 17: S9-S13.
[103] Mancia G. Optimal control of blood pressure in patients with diabetes reduces the incidence of macro and microvascular events. J Hypertens. Suppl. 2007; 25: S7-S12.
[104] Brenner BM, Cooper ME, De Zeeuw D, Keane WF, Mitch WE, Parving HH. Effects of Losartan on renal and cardiovascular outcomes in patients with type 2 diabetes and nephropathy. N Engl J Med. 2001; 345: 861-869.
[105] Lewis EJ, Hunsicker LG, Rodby RA; Collaborative study group. A clinical trial in type 2 diabetic nephropathy. Am J Kidney 2001; 38 (Suppl 1): S191-S194.
[106] Zanchetti A, Ruilope LM. Antihypertensive treatment in patients with type-2 diabetes mellitus: what guidance from recent controlled randomized trials? J Hypertens. 2002; 20: 2099-2110.
[107] Gradman AH. Rationale for triple-combination therapy for management of high blood pressure. J Clin Hypertens. (Greenwich). 2010; 12: 869-878.
[108] Bakris GL, Hester A, Dahlof B, Pitt B, Velazquez E, Staikos-Byrne L, Shi V, Jamerson K. ACCOMPLISH Investigators. The diabetes subgroup baseline characteristics of the avoiding cardiovascular events through combination therapy in patients living

with systolic hypertension (ACCOMPLISH) trials. J Cardiometab Syndr. 2008; 3: 229-233.
[109] Litthell HO. Considerations in the treatment of insulin resistance and related disorders with a new sympatholytic agents. J Hypertens. Suppl. 1997; 15: S39-S42.
[110] Kojima M, Dohi Y, Ohashi M, Sato K, Kimura G. Crucial role of kidney function in resistance to antihypertensive therapy in patients with diabetes mellitus. J Hypertens. 2010; 28: 2323-2328.
[111] Czemichow S, Zanchetti A, Tumbull F, Barzi F, Ninomiya T, Kengne AP, Lambers Heerspink HJ, Perkovic V, Huxley R, Arima H, Patel A, Chalmers J, Woodward M, MacMahon S, Neal B; Blood Pressure Lowering Treatment Trialists' Collaboration. The effects of blood pressure reduction and of different blood pressure-lowering regimens on major cardiovascular events according to baseline blood pressure: meta-analysis of randomized trials. J Hypertens. 2011; 29: 4-16.
[112] Perret-Guillaume C, Joly L, Jankowski P, Benetos A. Benefits of the RAS blockade: clinical evidence before the ONTARGET study. J Hypertens. 2009; 279Suppl 2): S53-S57.
[113] Lewin AJ, Weir MR. Antihypertensive efficacy and tolerability of irbesartan/hydrochlorothiazide in hypertensive patients stratified by body mass index and type 2 diabetes mellitus status: a post hoc subgroup analysis of the irbesartan/HCTZ Blood Pressure Reduction in Diverse Patients Populations trial. Clin Ther. 2008; 30: 2354-2365.
[114] Sowers JR, Neutel JM, Saunders E, Bakris GL, Cushman WC, Ferdinand KC, Ofili EO, Weber MA: INCLUSIVE Investigators. J Clin Hypertens (Greenwich). 2006; 8: 470-480.
[115] Grassi G, Mancia G. Implementation of new evidence into hypertension guidelines: the case of the ONTARGET and TRANSCEND trials. J Hypertens. 2009; 27 (Suppl 2); S40-S44.
[116] Sleight P, Redon J, Verdecchia P, Mancia G, Gao P, Fagard R, Schumacher H, Weber M, Bohm M, Williams B, Pogue J, Koon T, Yusuf S; ONTARGET investigators. Prognostic value of blood pressure in patients with high vascular risk in the Ongoing Telmisartan Alone and in combination with Ramipril Global Endopoint Trial study. J Hypertens. 2009; 27: 1360-1369.
[117] Unger T. The ongoing telmisartan alone and in combination with ramipril global endpoint trial program. Am J Cardiol. 2003; 91: 28G-34G.
[118] Kurtz TW. Beyond the classic angiotensin-receptor-blocker profile. Nat Clin Prac Cardiovasc Med. 2008; 5 Suppl 1: S19-S26.
[119] Makita S, Abiko A, Naganuma Y, Moriai Y, Nakamura M. Effects of telmisartan on adiponectin levels and body weight in hypertensive patients with glucose intolerance. Metabolism. 2008; 57: 1473-1478.
[120] Takimoto C, Kumagai H, Osaka M, Sakata K, Onami T, Kamayachi T, Iigaya K, Hayashi K, Saruta T, Itoh H. Candesartan and insulin reduce renal sympathetic nerve activity in hypertensive type 1 diabetic rats. Hypertens Res. 2008; 31: 1941-51.
[121] Ruilpe LM, Segura J. The importance of integrated risk management when treating patients with hypertension: benefits of angiotensin II receptor antagonist therapy. Clin Exp Hypertens. 2008; 30: 397-414.

[122] Scheen AJ. Prevention of type 2 diabetes mellitus through inhibition of the rennin-angiotensin system. Drugs. 2005; 64: 2537-2565.
[123] Weir MR. Effects of renin-angiotensin system inhibition on end-organ protection: can we do better? Clin Ther. 2007; 29: 1803-1824.
[124] Taylor AA, Pool JL. Clinical role of direct renin inhibition in hypertension. Am J Ther. 2011; Feb 10. [Epub ahead of print].
[125] Basile J, Babazadeh S, Lillestol M, Botha J, Yukovic C, Weitzman R. Comparison of aliskiren/hydrochlorothiazide combination therapy with hydrochlorothiazide monotherapy in older patients with stage 2 systolic hypertension: Results of the ACTION study. J Clin Hypertens. (Greenwich). 2011; 13: 162-169.
[126] Basile J, Babazadeh S, Lilestol M, Botha J, Yukovic C, Weltzman R. Comparison of aliskiren/hydrocholorothiazide combination therapy with hydrocholorothiazide monotherapy in older patients with stage 2 systolic hypertension: results of the ACTION study. J Clin Hypertens (Greenwich). 2011; 13: 162-168.
[127] Howard CG, Mullins JJ, Mitchel KD. Direct renin inhibition with aliskiren normalizes blood pressure in Cyp1a1-Ren2 transgenic rats with inducible angiotensin II-dependent malignant hypertension. Am J Med Sci. 2011; Feb 23. [Epub ahead of print].
[128] Gao D, Ning N, Niu X, Wei J, Sun P, Hao G. Aliskiren vs. angiotensin receptor blockers in hypertension: meta-analysis of randomized controlled trials. Am J Hypertens. 2011. Feb 3. [Epub ahead in print].
[129] Persson F, Lewis JB, Lewis EJ, Rossing P, Hollenberg NK, Parving HH. AVOID Study Investigators. Impact of baseline renal function on the efficacy and safety of aliskiren added to losartan in patients with type 2 diabetes and nephropathy. Diabetes Care. 2010; 33: 2304-2309.
[130] Persson F, Rossing P, Reinhard H, Juhi T, Stehouwer CD, Schalkwijk C, Danser AH, Boomsma F, Frandsen E, Parving HH. Optimal antiproteinuric dose of aliskiren in type 2 diabetes mellitus: a randomised crossover trial. Diabetologia. 2010; 53: 1576-1580.
[131] Pitt B. RAAS inhibition/blockade in patients with cardiovascular disease: Implications of recent large scale randomized trials for clinical practice. Heart. 2009; Apr 27. [Epub ahead of print].
[132] Kjeidsen SE, Weber M, Oparil S, Jamerson KA. Combining RAAS and calcium channel blockade: ACCOMPLISH in perspective. Blood Press. 2008; 17: 260-269.
[133] Bramlage P. Fixed-dose combinations of renin-angiotensin blocking agents with calcium channel blockers or hydrochlorothiazide in the treatment of hypertension. Expert Opin Pharmacother. 2009; 10: 1755-1767.
[134] Jemerson K, Weber MA, Bakris GL, Dahlof B, Pitt B, Shi V, Hester A, Gupte J, Gatlin M, Velazquez EJ. ACCOMPLISH Trial Investigators. (Collaborators, 554). Benazepril plus amlodipine or hydrocholorothiazide for hypertension in high-risk patients. N Engl J Med. 2008; 359: 2417-2428.
[135] Bakris GL, Sarafidis PA, Weir MR, Dahlof B, Pitt B, Jamerson K, Velazquez EJ, Staikos-Byrne L, Kelly RY, Shi V, Chiang YT, Weber MA. ACCOMPLISH Trial Investigators (Collaborators, 554). Renal outcomes with different fixed-dose combination therapies in patients with hypertension at high risk for cardiovascular

events (ACCOMPLISH): a pre-specified secondary analysis of a randomized controlled trial. Lancet. 2010; 375: 1173-1181.

[136] Martinez-Martin FJ, Saiz-Satjes M. Add-on manidipine versus amolodipine in diabetic patients with hypertension and microalbuminuria: the MANDHA study. Exprt Rev Cardiovasc Ther. 2008; 6: 1347-1355.

[137] Weiner N, Folker A, Murphy JA, Hung E, Bard M, Perkelcald A, Sowers JR, Bakris GL. Effect of fixed-dose ACE-inhibitor.calcium channel blocker combination therapy vs. ACE-inhibitor monotherapy on arterial compliance in hypertensive patients with type 2 diabetes. Prev Cardiol. 2005; 8: 87-92.

[138] Ruilope LM. Long-term protection in at-risk hypertensive patienrs—a role for nifedipine GITS? Blood Press. 2002; 11: 106-109.

[139] Weycker D, Edelsberg J, Vinncze G, Kjeldsen SE, Jamersson K, Khan ZM, Oster G. Risk of diabetes in real-world setting among patients initiating antihypertensive therapy with valsartan or amlodipine. J Hum Hypertens. 2007; 21: 374-380.

[140] Kuti EL, Baker WL, White CM. The development of new-onset type 2 diabetes associated with choosing a calcium channel blocker compared to a diuretic or beta-blockers. Curr Med Res Opin. 2007; 23: 1239-1244.

[141] Rosen, P.; Ohly, P.; Gleichmann, H. Experimental benefit of moxonidine on glucose metabolism and insulin secretion in the fructose-fed rat. *J. Hypertens..Suppl.* 1997; 15(1): S31-S38.

[142] Sun, Z.; Emsberger, P. Marked insulin resistance in obese spontaneously hypertensive rat adipocytes is ameliorated by in vivo but not in vitro treatment with moxonidine. *J. Pharmacol. Exp. Ther.* 2007; 320(2): 845-852.

[143] Kaaja, R.; Kujala, S.; Manhem, K.; Katzman, P.; Kibarskis, A.; Antikainen, R.; Yliharsila, H.; Erkkola, R.; Tuomilehto, J. Effects of sympatholytic therapy on insulin sensitivity indices in hypertensive postmenopausal women. *Int. J. Clin. Pharmacol. Ther.* 2007; 45(7): 394-401.

[144] Sanjuliani, A.F.; de Abreu, V.G.; Francischetti, E.A. Selective imidazoline agonist moxonidine in obese hypertensive patients. *Int. J. Clin. Prac.* 2006; 60(5): 621-625.

[145] Pater C, Bhatnagar D, Berrou JP, Luszick J, Beckmann K. A novel approach to treatment of hypertension in diabetic patients- a multicenter, double-blind, randomized study comparing the efficacy of combination therapy of Eprosartan versus Ramipril with low-dose Hydrochlorothiazide and Moxonidine on blood pressure levels in patients with hypertension and associated diabetes mellitus type 2-rational and design [ISRCTN5525285]. Curr Controlled Trials in Cardiovas Med. 2004; 5:9. Doi:10.1186/1468-6708-5-0.

[146] Rayner B. Selective imidazoline agonist moxonidine plus the ACE inhibitor ramipril in hypertensive patients with impaired insulin sensitivity: partner in a successful MARRIAGE? Curr Med Res Opin. 2004; 20: 359-367.

[147] Velliquette, R.A.; Kossover, R.; Previs, S.F.; Ernsberger, P. Lipid-lowering actions of imidazoline antihypertensive agents in metabolic syndrome X. Naunyn Schmiedebergs *Arch. Pharmacol.* 2006; 372(4): 300-312.

[148] Vonend, O.; Marsalek, P.; Russ, H.; Wulkow, R.; Oberhauser, V.; Rump, L.C. Moxonidine treatment of hypertensive patients with advanced renal failure. *J. Hypertens.* 2003; 21(9): 1709-1717.

[149] Mukaddam-Daher, S.; Menaouar, A.; El-Ayoubi, R.; Gutkowska, J.; Jankowski, M.; Velliquette, R.A.; Ernsberger, P. Cardiac effects of moxonidine in spontaneously hypertensive obese rats. *Ann. N. Y. Acad. Sci.* 2003; 1009: 244-250.

[150] van Zweiten, P.A. Centrally acting antihypertensive drugs. Present and future. *Clin. Exp. Hypertens.* 1999; 2(5-6): 859-873.

[151] Head, G.A. Central imidazoline- and alpha2-receptors involved in the cardiovascular actions of centrally acting antihypertensive agents. *Ann. N. Y. Acad. Sci.* 1999; 881: 279-286.

[152] Motz, W.; Strauer, B.E. Therapy of hypertensive cardiac hypertrophy and impaired coronary microcirculation. *J. Cardiovasc. Pharmacol.* 1994; 24 Suppl 1: S34-S38.

[153] Ziegler, D.; Haxhiu, M.A.; Kaan, E.C.; Papp, J.G.; Emsberger, P. Pharmacology of moxonidine, a I1-imidazoline receptor agonist. *J. Cardiovasc. Pharmacol.* 1996; 27 Suppl 3: S26-S37.

[154] Sharma, A.M.; Wagner, T.; Marsalek, P. Moxonidine in the treatment of overweight and obese patients with the metabolic syndrome: a postmarketing surveillance study. *J. Hum. Hypertens.* 2004; 18(9): 669-675.

[155] Haenni, A.; Lithell, H. Moxonidine improves insulin sensitivity in insulin-resistant hypertensives. *J. Hypertens. Suppl.* 1999; 17(3): S29-S35.

[156] Elliot WJ, Weir DR, Black HR. Cost-effectiveness of the lower treatment goal (of JNC VI) for diabetic hypertensive patients. Join National Committee on prevention, detection, evaluation, and treatment of high blood pressure. Arch Intern Med. 2000; 160: 1277-1283.

[157] Curb JD, Pressel SL, Cutler JA. Effect of diuretic-based antihypertensive treatment on cardiovascular disease risk in older patients with isolated systolic hypertension. Jama. 1996; 276: 1886-1892.

[158] Borhani NO, Mercuni M, Borhani PA. Final outcome results of the multicenter isradipine diuretics atherosclerosis study (MIDAS). A randomized controlled trial. JAMA. 1996; 276: 785-791.

[159] The ALLHAT Officers and Coordinators for the ALLHAT Collaborative Research Group. Major outcome in high risk hypertensive patients randomized to angiotensin-converting enzyme inhibitor or calcium channel blocker vs. diuretics: the antihypertensive and lipid-lowering treatment to prevent heart attack trial (ALLHAT). JAMA. 2002; 288: 2981-2997.

[160] ALLHAT Collaborative Research Group: Major cardiovascular events in hypertensive patients randomized to doxazosin vs. chlorthalidone: the anti-hypertensive and lipid-lowering treatment to prevent heart attack trial (ALLHAT). JAMA. 2002; 283: 2971-2975.

[161] Lakshman MR, Reda DJ, Materson BJ. Diuretics and beta-blockers do not have adverse effects at 1 year on plasma lipid and lipoprotein profile in men with hypertension. Department of Veterans Affairs Cooperative Study Group on Anti hypertensive Agents. Arch Intern Med. 1998; 159: 551-558.

[162] Weir MR, Moser M. Diuretics and beta-blockers: is there a risk for dyslipidemia? Am Heart J. 2000; 139: 174-183.

[163] Moser M. Lipid abnormality and diuretics. Am Fam Physician. 1989; 40: 213-220.

[164] The Heart Outcome Prevention Evaluation Study Investigators. Effects of an angiotensin-converting enzyme inhibitor, ramipril, on cardiovascular events in high-risk patients. N Engl J Med. 2000; 342: !45-153.
[165] Neal B, McMahon S, Chapman N: for trhe Blood Pressure Lowering Treatment Trialists' Collaboration. Effect of ACE inhibitors, calciyum antagonists, and other blood pressure lowering drugs: results of prospectively designed overviews of randomized trials. Lancet. 2000; 356: 1955-1964.
[166] Gradman AH, Acevedo C. Evolving strategies for the use of combination therapy in hypertension. Curr Hypertens Rep. 2000; 4: 343-349.
[167] Dorsch MP, Gillespie BW, Erickson SR, Bleske BE, Weder AB. Chlorthalidone reduces cardiovascular effects compared with Hydrochlorothiazide. A retrowspective cohort analysis. Hypertension. 2011; 57: 689-694.
[168] Reboldi G, Gentile G, Angeli F, Verdecchia P. Choice of ACE inhibitor combinations in hypertensive patients with type 2 diabetes: update after recent clinical trials. Vasc Health Risk Manag. 2009; 5: 411-427.

14

Diabetic Nephropathy; Clinical Characteristics and Treatment Approaches

Derun Taner Ertugrul, Emre Tutal
and Siren Sezer
Keciören Research Hospital, Department of Internal Medicine
Division of Endocrinology and Metabolism
Baskent University Hospital, Department of Internal Medicine
Division of Nephrology
Turkey

1. Introduction

Diabetes mellitus is a major public health problem and its' prevalance is contuniously rising especially in developed or developing countries. According to World Health Organization (WHO) data the prevalence of diabetes for all age-groups worldwide was estimated to be 2.8% in 2000 and 4.4% in 2030. The total number of people with diabetes is projected to rise from 171 million in 2000 to 366 million in 2030 (1). Despite of improved treatment options for both diabetes mellitus and other associated risk factors, diabetic nephropathy is still a major problem causing increased morbidity and mortality as the increase in total number of diabetic patients finds a reflection in increased prevalence of diabetic patients in end stage renal disease (ESRD) population. There are some studies reporting decreased incidence of diabetic nephropaty in developed countries as a result of better glycemic control and agressive treatment of hypertension with new generation antihypertensives (2). However total number of diabetic nephropathy patients seems to be increasing as a result of increased numbers of diabetic patients and diabetes has become the primary cause of ESRD in the developed countries. Approximately 44% of new patients entering dialysis in the United States are diabetics. In the United States, approximately 20.8 million people, or 7.0% of the population, are estimated to have diabetes, with a growing incidence. Roughly one third of this population, 6.2 million, is estimated to be undiagnosed with type 2 diabetes (3, 4). Similar to these findings prevalence of diabetic nephropahty also increases in in developing countries For example, according to Turkish Society of Nephrology data prevalence of diabetic ESRD patients increased form 7% to 32.5% from 1991 to 2008. A similar trend was also observed for hypertensive nephropathy which raised from 6.3% to 26.8% (5). This hypertensive population is important as according to some previous reports, only one third of essential hypertension patients has normal blood glucose metabolism at diagnosis (6). So it is possible that prevalence of pure diabetic or pure hypertensive nephropathy is lower than predicted but the combination of these two pathological condition is very high in otherwise healthy and ESRD populations.

2. Risk factors

Multiple risk factors for development of diabetic nephropathy were defined. Most important of these seems to be the duration of diabetes mellitus. 20-30% of type I diabetics are supposed to have clinically significant renal involvement (microalbuminuria) after 20 years duration and 15-20% develop ESRD after an additional 10 year (7, 8). These durations are not well defined for type 2 diabetics. 5-25% of these patients might have clinically significant renal failure or even ESRD (1%) at time of diagnosis and approximately 20-30% reach ESRD at 20 years duration (9). The impact of age at time of diabetes diagnosis on development of renal failure is not clear. Among patients with type 2 diabetes, increasing age, along with increasing duration of diabetes was reported to be associated with increased risk for developing albuminuria (10). However some contradicting studies report that, patients who developed diabetes prior to age 20 had a higher risk of progressing to end-stage renal disease (25 versus 5 per 1000 patient years at risk) (11). For type 1 diabetes, the risk of developing ESRD was reported to be very low for patients diagnosed prior to age 5; however at older ages, the relationship of age to progression to ESRD is uncertain (12, 13).

Poor glycemic control is another important risk factor for development of diabetic renal involvement. The Diabetes Control and Complications Trial (DCCT) demonstrated that interventions that improve glycemic control in patients with type 1 diabetes mellitus reduce the risk of development and slow the progression of diabetic microvascular disease, and may also protect against the occurrence of macrovascular disease (14). The United Kingdom Prospective Diabetes Study (UKPDS), a study of over 4000 patients with prolonged follow-up, suggests that strict control also results in a reduced risk of microvascular disease in patients with type 2 diabetes (15).

Hypertension, another important risk factor, is very common in diabetic patients. In fact hypertension is a cause and also a result of diabetic renal disease. Among those with type 1 diabetes, the incidence of hypertension rises from 5% at 10 years, to 33% at 20 years, and 70% at 40 years (16). The blood pressure typically begins to rise within the normal range about three years after the onset of microalbuminuria. Ultimately, the incidence of hypertension is approximately 15 to 25% in all patients with microalbuminuria and 75 to 85% in those with overt diabetic nephropathy (17). On the other hand type 2 diabetic patients have different characteristics. Most of them already have hypertension, even without renal involvement/microalbuminuria at the time of diagnosis (18). Also essential hypertension patients have some glucose metabolism abnormalities including insukin resistance without overt diabetes at time of diagnosis (6).

Obesity and hyperlipidemia might also cause progression of diabetic nephropathy while weight loss and control of hyperlipidemia by using statins might improve renal status (19-22).

Approximately one-half of patients with type 1 diabetes of less than five years duration have an elevated glomerular filtration rate (GFR) that is 25 to 50 percent above normal and this situation was reported to have negative effects on disease progression (23). If GFR is above 150 mL/min risk for developing microalbuminuria significantly increases. In one prospective study, for example, patients with type 1 diabetes and a GFR above 125 mL/min had a risk of developing microalbuminuria within 8 years of approximately 50 percent versus only 5 percent in patients with a lower GFR that was similar to that seen in nondiabetics (23).

Some genetic susceptibilities for developing diabetic renal disease were also reported. Most important of these factors are race, family tendencies and ACE gene polymorphisms (24-28). Considering gene polymorphisms; in patients with type 2 diabetes, the ACE/DD polymorphism was reported to associate with an increased risk for the development of diabetic nephropathy, more severe proteinuria, greater likelihood of progressive renal failure, and mortality on dialysis (26-28).

3. Pathophysiology

Development of diabetic nephropathy depends on different pathogenic processess. Major of these pathyways will be summarized below

a. **Glomerular hyperfiltration:** Studies in experimental animals indicate that dilatation of the afferent (precapillary) glomerular arteriole plays an important role in the hyperfiltration response, by raising both the intraglomerular pressure and renal blood flow (29). Some hormonal factors including insulin-like growth factor I (IGF-1), atrial natriuretic factor and sex hormones were speculated to have effects on hyperfiltration. Most important of these seems to be IGF-1 which induces hyperfiltration, renal vasodilatation and hypertropy in experimental models (30). Increased intracellular sorbitol accumulation, hyperglycemia, glycosylation endproducts and increased sodium reabsorption and tubuloglomerular feedback also has effects on glomerular hyperfiltration
b. **Hyperglycemia and AGEs:** Hyperglycemia is known to have a direct effect on mesangial expansion and injury, a result possibly secondary to increased matrix production or glycosylation of matrix proteins. Glycosylation of tissue proteins also may contribute to the development of diabetic nephropathy. Chronic hyperglycemia causes nonenzymatic glycosylation of free amino acids on circulating or tissue proteins and this process forms reversible early glycosylation products and later irreversible advanced glycosylation end products (AGEs). Circulating AGE levels are increased in particularly diabetics with renal insufficiency, because AGEs are normally excreted in the urine. The net effect is tissue accumulation of AGEs, in part by crosslinking with collagen, which can contribute to the associated renal and microvascular complications (31, 32).
c. **Prorenin:** A recent experimental model has reported a possible pathogenic role for prorenin in the development of diabetic nephropathy in which prolonged prorenin receptor blockade prevented the development of nephropathy without alterin angiotensin II activity (33).
d. **Proinflammatory cytokines and growth factors:** A group of proinflammatory, profibrotic cytokines and growth factors were speculated to have effects on diabetic nephropathy pathogenesis. Most important of these are vascular endothelial growth factor (VEGF), transforming growth factor - beta (TGF-ß). Experimental models reported that VEGF blockade improves albuminuria in diabetic nephropathy (34). Similarly the combination of an anti-TGF-beta antibody and an ACE inhibitor completely normalized proteinuria in experimental diabetic nephropathy models (35).
e. **Proteinuria:** Final result of above mentioned pathogenic factors is proteinuria. Normal protein discharge in urine is lower than 30 mg/day for albumin and 150 mg/day for total protein. Microalbuminuria (30-300 mg/day) is a critical treshold for diabetic nephropathy and after this stage untreated patients usually develop overt proteinuria

(> 300 mg/day microalbuminuria). Proteinuria was reported to induce inflammation, fibrosis, and it is also have direct tubular toxicity which all promote development of diabetic nephropathy

4. Histopathological changes

All components of renal infrastructure can be affected by diabetic nephropathy. Some of these changes are specific for diabetes, some not. Most common and important changes are capillary basal membrane thickening, diffuse glomerulosclerosis and nodular glomerulosclerosis (Kimmelstiel - Wilson nodules). Nodular glomerulosclerosis was described by Kimmelstiel and Wilson in 1936. These nodules are eosinophilic and PAS positive hard masses which are located in the central regions of peripheral glomerular lobules. They appear to be of mesengial origin and when they are pathogomonic for diabetic nephropathy however they are not universal and found only in 10-40% of patients. The diffuse mesengial lesions are more frequent than nodular glomerulosclerosis and present in 50-90% of patients. They include increased mesengial matrix, basala membrane thickening, capillary narrowing, hyalinization and periglomerular fibrosis. Afferent and efferent arteriolar hyalnization is highly specific for diabetic nephropathy, on the other hand only afferent arteriol involvement is a finding of hypertensive nephrosclerosis.

5. Clinical manifestations and natural history

Clinical stages of type 1 diabetes mellitus renal involvement is summarized in Table-1. These stages are also accepted for type 2 diabetic patients however they might not always follow these steps (36). ESRD is not the only major consequence of diabetic nephropathy but patients have increased risk of cardiovascular disease , morbidity and mortality even in the early stages of nephropathy. Microalbuminuria (30-300 mg/day albuminuria) is the first clinical sign of diabetic nephropathy and this situation is highly associated with other complications of diabetes like cardiovascular disease and retinopathy. 24 hour urine or spot urine albumin / creatinine ratios should be used for microalbuminuria follow-up. Overt proteinuria is defined as >300 mg/day albuminuria and at this stage total protei,n loss in urine might exceed 1g/day. 5-7 years after development of overt proteinuria these patients usually develop ESRD.

6. Diagnosis and differential diagnosis

Proteinuria developing in a diabetic patient is an important marker for diabetic nephropathy however in case of atypical presentation renal biopsy might be indicated. A typical diabetic nephropathy presentation is a type 1 diabetes history for at least 10 years, presence of retinopathy, previous microalbuminuria, no macroscopic hematuria and microscopically inactive urinary sediment. Type 2 diabetic patients might not have this kind of a clinic and as previously mentioned 5-25% of these patients might have clinically significant renal failure or even ESRD (1%) at time of diabetes diagnosis (9). In case of atypical presentation a renal biopsy is usually indicated. Possible atypical presentations are as follows; short diabetes duration (> 10 yrs for type 1 diabetics), no previous retinopathy, overt proteinuria without previous microalbuminuria, macroscoic hematuria, red cell or leucocyte casts, presence of systemic manifestations of any other disease that also can involve kidneys like collagen tissue disorders, amyloidosis etc, rapid decline in renal function without significant proteinuria. Long diabetes duration, previous retinopathy and microalbuminuria might not always be present in type 2 diabetics so in these patients presence of glomerulonephritis clinical features or any other systemic disease with possible renal involvement are biopsy indications.

Stage	Duration of diabetes mellitus	GFR and renal perfusion	Urine findings	Serum findings	Clinical findings	Morpho-logical findings
1. Nephro-megaly and hyper-filtration stage	At diagnosis	Increased	Reversible albuminuria	No significant finding	Increased renal size	Glomerular hypertrophy
2. Latent stage	2-5 years	Normal/Incr eased	No significant finding	No significant finding	No significant finding	Increased basal membrane thickness
3. Incident diabetic nephropathy stage	5-15 years	Normal/Incr eased	Microalbumi nuria (30-300 mg/day)	No significant finding	Hypertension	Increased basal membrane thickness and mesengial expansion
4. Overt diabetic nephropathy stage	10-25 years	Decreasing progressively	Overt proteinuria	Increased creatinine	Hypertension and significant nephropathy	Diffuse/nod ular glomeruloscl erosis
5. End stage renal disease stage	15-30 years	Decreased	Overt proteinuria	Uremia	Hypertension and significant nephropathy	Glomeruloscl erosis

Table 1.

Diabetic patients are also prone to some renal diseases or complications which might need to be differentialy diagnosed. Almost every form of glomerular diseases were reported in diabetic nephropathy patients however membranous nephropathy is the most common one. Papillary necrosis, renovascular diseases (arterial or venous), bladder autonomic neuropathy, acute or chronic pyelonephritis, radiocontrast nephropathy and renal tuberculosis should always be kept in mind while evaluating a diabetic patient with renal findings.

7. Treatment and prevention of diabetic nephropathy

Strict glycemic control decreases development of diabetic nephropathy in both type 1 and 2 diabetics. Intensive insulin therapy partially reverse the glomerular hypertrophy and hyperfiltration, delay the development of microalbuminuria, reduce the onset or progression of diabetic nephropathy compared to less intensive therapy, stabilize or decrease protein excretion in patients with microalbuminuria (14, 15, 37, 38). Intensive glycemic not only slow or even prevent development of diabetic nephropathy but also decrease morbidit and mortality ferom other diabetic complications. However the less prominent benefit from strict glycemic control in overt diabetic nephropathy indicates that factors other than hyperglycemia contributes to the glomerular injury. Reducing the intraglomerular pressure with dietary protein restriction or antihypertensive therapy with an angiotensin converting enzyme (ACE) inhibitor or angiotensin receptor blocker (ARB) can minimize progression of or even prevent glomerular disease in the absence of glycemic control. There is now clear evidence that antihypertensive therapy (particularly with RAS blockers) and perhaps protein restriction can reduce the rate of progression in patients with type 1 diabetes and overt nephropathy.

Hypertension increases rate of diabetic nephropathy progression. DCCT and UKPDS trialsdemonstrated that strict blood pressure control decreases microalbuminburia and macroalbuminuria development by 29% and 39% respectively in 6 years follow-up period (14, 15). WHO and JNC advises to keep blood pressure below 130/80 mmHg in diabetic patients. In JNC-VII quideline even a lower level (125/75 mmHg) was proposed for prevention and/or slowing diabetic nephropathy progression (39). ACEI preference in diabetic patients is also recommended in these quidelines. ACEI not only decrease intraglomerular pressure (so decrease proteinuria) by their hemodynamic effects but also decrease glomeruler size and fibrotik process. ACEI were also reported to increase negative charge of basal membrane and so decrease proteinuria. ARBs could also be used alone or in combination with ACEI for increasing nephroprotection (40, 41). Nondihydropyridine class calcium antagonists (NDHCB) are also recommended as a combination with RAS blockers. In BENEDICT trial it was demonstrated that ACEI-NDHCB combination might delay development of microalbuminuria in hypertensive diabetic patients without proteinuria (42). Salt intake should be restricted (< 70 mEq/day) for a beter antirpoteinuric effect as salt seems to blunt effects of both RAS blockers and NDHCB (43, 44). Aldosterone antagonists were also reported to reduce proteinuria when used alone, and to have an additive effect on proteinuria when used in combination with an ACE inhibitor or an ARB in both type 1 and type 2 diabetes (36, 45). Further blood pressure reduction may partially explain the beneficial effect, although an anti-inflammatory mechanism has also been proposed (46). However hyperkalemia in combination treatment ACEI/ARB and aldosterone antagonists) is a significant problem especially in advanced diabetic nephropathy.

Low protein diet decreases hyperfiltration in early stages of diabetic nephropathy and also could slow down GFR loss. However very low protein diets (< 0.6/g/kg/day) could cause malnutrition which is an important mortality risk factor in ESRD population so 0.8 g/kg/day protein diets and essential amino acid supplementations are usually recommended (47).

Hyperlipidemia should also be screened in diabetic patients and must be treated with statins or fibrats if needed. Diabetic patients without hypertension but under simvastatin treatment were reported to have a 25% decrease in microalbuminuria levels (48).

8. Renal replacement treatment in diabetic esrd patients

Diabetic patients usually need renal replacement therapy (RRT) in earlier stages of renal failure. It was reported that nondiabetic patients start receiving RRT when GFR falls below 10 ml/min but on the other hand diabetics need RRT with higher GFR (15-20 ml/min) levels (49). These patients are prone to hypervolemia and lung edema due to accompanying cardiac problems and malnutrition due to proteinuria and dietary restrictions. Diabetic patients developing diuretic resistant edema might need ultrafiltration and start RRT even with higher GFR values.

Patient survival in diabetics on maintenance dialysis is lower than that seen in nondiabetics with end-stage renal failure due to chronic glomerular disease or hypertension (50). As noted in the 2005 USRDS database, only approximately 25 percent of patients with diabetes survived five years after initiation of dialysis and cardiovascular disease is the most common cause of death, accounting for more than one-half of cases (50).

Renal transplantation is a choice of RRT in diabetic ESRD patients however five year survival is clearly lower than other ESRD patients ranging from 75% to 83% (51). Despite of this poor outcome, transplantation still result in decreased extrarenal vascular diseaseand better quality of life compared with either hemodialysis or peritoneal dialysis (51).

Making choice of dialysis modality in diabetic patients is similar with nondiabetic patients. Comorbid conditions, home situation, independence and motivation of the patient, ability to tolerate volume shifts, patients' desire, status of the vasculature and/or abdomen should be evaluated for each patient. The relative effect of hemodialysis and CAPD on survival in diabetic patients is uncertain. Initial reports suggested that CAPD was associated with a better outcome (52). However data from the USRDS case-mix study suggest that mortality may actually be increased in diabetic patients receiving CAPD (53). A subsequent very large study attempted to assess the impact of multiple risk factors, including diabetes, on survival after initiation of either hemodialysis or peritoneal dialysis. Utilizing data from 398,940 patients who initiated dialysis between the years 1995 to 2000 (54). Mortality risk was significantly higher on hemodialysis than PD among younger diabetics with no comorbidity. By comparison, hemodialysis was associated with a lower mortality risk in older diabetics with either no comorbidity or a baseline comorbidity.

9. References

Wild S, Roglic G, Gren A et al. Global prevalence of diabetes. Diabetes Care 2004; 27: 1047-53

Wolf G. New insights into the pathophysiology of diabetic nephropathy: from haemodynamics to molecular pathology. Eur J Clin Invest 2004; 34: 785-96

http://www.usrds.org/adr.htm

American Diabetes Association: Total Prevalence of Diabetes and Pre-diabetes, 2007. Available at http://www.diabetes.org/diabetes-statistics/prevalence.jsp

http://www.tsn.org.tr

Garcia-Puig J, Ruilope LM, Lugue M et al Glucose metabolism in patients with essential hypertension. Am J Med 2006; 119: 318-26

Orchard TJ, Dorman JS, Maser RE, et al. Prevalence of complications in IDDM by sex and duration. Pittsburgh Epidemiology of Diabetes Complications Study II. Diabetes 1990; 39:1116.

Krolewski M, Eggers PW, Warram JH. Magnitude of end-stage renal disease in IDDM: a 35 year follow-up study. Kidney Int 1996; 50:2041.

Adler AI, Stevens RJ, Manley SE, Bilous, RW. Development and progression of nephropathy in type 2 diabetes: The United Kingdom Prospective Diabetes Study (UKPDS 64). Kidney Int 2003; 63:225.

Tapp RJ, Shaw JE, Zimmet PZ, et al. Albuminuria is evident in the early stages of diabetes onset: results from the Australian Diabetes, Obesity, and Lifestyle Study (AusDiab). Am J Kidney Dis 2004; 44:792.

Pavkov Me, Bennett PH, Knowler WC, et al. Effect of youth-onset type 2 diabetes mellitus on incidence of end-stage renal disease and mortality in young and middle-aged Pima Indians. JAMA 2006; 296:421.

Finne P, Reunanen A, Stenman S, et al. Incidence of end-stage renal disease in patients with type 1 diabetes. JAMA 2005; 294:1782.

Svensson M, Nystrom L, Schon S, Dahlquist, G. Age at onset of childhood-onset type 1 diabetes and the development of end-stage renal disease: a nationwide population-based study. Diabetes Care 2006; 29:538.

The Diabetes Control and Complications Trial Research Group. The effect of intensive treatment of diabetes on the development and progression of long-term complications in insulin-dependent diabetes mellitus. N Engl J Med 1993; 329:977.

Intensive blood-glucose control with sulphonylureas or insulin compared with conventional treatment and risk of complications in patients with type 2 diabetes (UKPDS 33). UK Prospective Diabetes Study (UKPDS) Group. Lancet 1998; 352:837.

Epstein M, Sowers JR. Diabetes mellitus and hypertension. Hypertension 1992; 19:403.

Mogensen CE, Hansen KW, Pedersen MM, Christensen, CK. Renal factors influencing blood pressure threshold and choice of treatment for hypertension in IDDM. Diabetes Care 1991; 14 Suppl 4:13.

Hypertension in Diabetes Study (HDS): I. Prevalence of hypertension in newly presenting type 2 diabetic patients and the association with risk factors for cardiovascular and diabetic complications. J Hypertens 1993; 11:309.

Gelber RP, Kurth T, Kausz AT, et al. Association between body mass index and CKD in apparently healthy men. Am J Kidney Dis 2005; 46:871.

Ejerblad E, Fored CM, Lindblad P, et al. Obesity and risk for chronic renal failure. J Am Soc Nephrol 2006; 17:1695.

Morales E, Valero MA, Leon M, et al. Beneficial effects of weight loss in overweight patients with chronic proteinuric nephropathies. Am J Kidney Dis 2003; 41:319.

Zoja C, Corna D, Gagliardini E et al. Adding a statin to a combination of ACE inhibitor and ARB normalizes proteinuria in experimental diabetes, which translates into full renoprotection. Am J Physiol Renal Physiol. 2010 Nov;299(5):F1203-11

Rudberg S, Persson B, Dahlquist G. Increased glomerular filtration rate as a predictor of diabetic nephropathy An 8-year prospective study. Kidney Int 1992; 41:822.

Pettitt DJ, Saad MF, Benneth PH et al. Familial predisposition to renal disease in two generations of Pima Indians with type 2 diabetes mellitus. Diabetologia 33: 438-43, 1990

Earle K, Walker J, Hill C et al. Familial clustering of cardiovascular disease in patients with insulin dependent diabetes and nephropathy. N Eng J Med 7: 2627-35, 1996

Jeffers BW, Estacio RO, Raynolds MV et al. Angiotensin-converting enzyme gene polymorphism in non-insulin dependent diabetes mellitus and its relationship with diabetic nephropathy. Kidney Int 1997; 52:473.

Yoshida H, Kuriyama S, Atsumi Y, et al. Angiotensin I converting enzyme gene polymorphism in non-insulin-dependent diabetes mellitus. Kidney Int 1996; 50:657.

Kuramoto N, Lizuka T, Ito H, et al. Effect of ACE gene on diabetic nephropathy in NIDDM patients with insulin resistance. Am J Kidney Dis 1999; 33:276.

Bank N. Mechanisms of diabetic hyperfiltration. Kidney Int 1991; 40:792.

Hirschberg R, Kopple JD. The growth hormone-insulin-like growth factor I axis and renal glomerular filtration. J Am Soc Nephrol 1992; 2:1417.

Makita Z, Radoff S, Rayfield EJ, et al. Advanced glycosylation end products in patients with diabetic nephropathy. N Engl J Med 1991; 325:836.

Singh AK, Mo W, Dunea G at al. Effect of glycated proteins on the matrix of glomerular epithelial cells. J Am Soc Nephrol 1998; 9:802.

Ichihara A, Suzuki F, Nakagawa T, et al. Prorenin receptor blockade inhibits development of glomerulosclerosis in diabetic angiotensin II type 1a receptor-deficient mice. J Am Soc Nephrol 2006; 17:1950.

Sung SH, Ziyadeh FN, Wang A, et al. Blockade of vascular endothelial growth factor signaling ameliorates diabetic albuminuria in mice. J Am Soc Nephrol 2006; 17:3093.

Benigni A, Zoja C, Corna D et al. Add-on anti-TGF-beta antibody to ACE inhibitor arrests progressive diabetic nephropathy in the rat. J Am Soc Nephrol 2003; 14:1816.

Mogensen CE, Cooper ME. Diabetic renal disease: from recent studies to improved clinical practice. Diabet Med 2004; 21: 4-17

Shichiri M, Kishikawa H, Ohkubo Y et al. Long-term results of the Kumamoto Study on optimal diabetes control in type 2 diabetic patients. Diabetes Care 2000; 23 Suppl 2:B21.

Sustained effect of intensive treatment of type 1 diabetes mellitus on development and progression of diabetic nephropathy: the Epidemiology of Diabetes Interventions and Complications (EDIC) study. JAMA 2003; 290:2159.

Chobanian AV, Bakris GL, Black HR et al. National Heart, Lung and Blood Institute Joint National Committee on Prevention, Detection, Evaluation, and Treatment of High Blood Pressure; National High Blood Pressure Eduv-cation Program Coordinating Committee. Comment in: The Seventh Report of the Joint National Committee on Prevention, Detection, Evaluation and Treatment of Higgh Blood Pressure: JNC 7 report. JAMA 2003; 289: 2560-72

Lewis EJ, Hunsicker LJ, Clarke WR et al. Renoprotective effect of the angiotensin receptor antagonist irbesartan in patients with type 2 diabetes. N Eng J Med 2001; 345: 851-8

Brenner BM, Goper ME, de Zeeuw D et al. RENAAL AStudy Investigators. Effects of losartan on renal and cardiovascular outcomes in patients with type 2 diabetes and nephropathy. N Eng J Med 2001; 345: 861-9

Ruggenenti P, Fassi A, Ilieva AP et al. Preventing microalbuminuria in Type 2 Diabetes. N Eng J Med 2004; 351: 1941-51

Bakris GL, Smith A. Effects of sodium intake on albumin excretion in patients with diabetic nephropathy treated with long-acting calcium antagonists. Ann Intern Med 1996; 125:201.

Bakris GL, Weir MR. Salt intake and reductions in arterial pressure and proteinuria. Is there a direct link?. Am J Hypertens 1996; 9:200S.

Rachmani R, Slavachevsky I, Amit, M, et al. The effect of spironolactone, cilazapril and their combination on albuminuria in patients with hypertension and diabetic nephropathy is independent of blood pressure reduction: a randomized controlled study. Diabet Med 2004; 21:471.

van den Meiracker AH, Baggen RG, Pauli, S, et al. Spironolactone in type 2 diabetic nephropathy: effects on proteinuria, blood pressure and renal function. J Hypertens 2006; 24:2285.

Han SY, Kim CH, Kim HS, et al. Spironolactone prevents diabetic nephropathy through an anti-inflammatory mechanism in type 2 diabetic rats. J Am Soc Nephrol 2006; 17:1362.

Tonolo G, Ciccares M, Brizi P et al. Reduction albumin excretion rate in normotensive microalbuminuric type 2 diabetic patients during long term simvastatin treatment. Diabetes Care 1997; 20: 1891-5

Stein G, Fünfstück R, Schiel R. Diabetes Mellitus and dialysis. Minerva Urol Nefrol 2004; 56: 289-303

United States Renal Data System. Excerpts from the USRDS 2005 annual data report: Atlas of end-stage renal disease in the United States. Am J Kidney Dis 2006; 47(Suppl 1):S1.

Locatelli F, Pozzoni P, Del Vecchio L. Renal replacement therapy in patients with diabetes and end-stage renal disease. J Am Soc Nephrol 2004; 15 Suppl 1:S25.

Wolfe RA, Port FK, Hawthorne VM et al. A comparison of survival among dialytic therapies of choice: In-center hemodialysis versus continuous ambulatory peritoneal dialysis at home. Am J Kidney Dis 1990; 15:433.

Held PJ, Port FK, Turenne MN, et al. Continuous ambulatory peritoneal dialysis and hemodialysis: Comparison of patient mortality with adjustment for comorbid conditions. Kidney Int 1994; 45:1163.

Vonesh EF, Snyder JJ, Foley RN et al. The differential impact of risk factors on mortality in hemodialysis and peritoneal dialysis. Kidney Int 2004; 66:2389.

15

Anemia of Chronic Kidney Disease in Diabetic Patients: Pathophysiologic Insights and Implications of Recent Clinical Trials

Victoria Forte, Miriam Kim, George Steuber, Salma Asad and Samy I. McFarlane
Division of Endocrinology, Department of Medicine, College of Medicine
State University of New York-Downstate Medical Center
Kings County Hospital New York,
USA

1. Introduction

The goals for this chapter are to succinctly describe the definition of anemia, and to describe the pathophysiology and the epidemiology of anemia in diabetic patients with chronic kidney disease. In addition, the cardiovascular risk factors of anemic patients will be explained and a table will be included. A comprehensive visualization will be included which will incorporate the pathophysiology of anemia in chronic kidney disease and the negative impact of anemia on the cardiovascular system. Reasons to treat anemia in this population will be presented. Furthermore, the recent clinical trials on anemia treatment in the diabetic patient with chronic kidney disease will be discussed, including but not limited to the CHOIR, CREATE, ACORD and TREAT trials. Lastly, there will be a summary of the most important points of the chapter. CHOIR (Correction of Hemoglobin and Outcomes in Renal Insufficiency), CREATE (Cardiovascular Risk Reduction by Early Anemia Treatment with Epoetin Beta), ACORD (Anemia Correction in Diabetes) and TREAT (Trial to Reduce Cardiovascular Events with Aranesp Therapy) trials.
With the ongoing pandemic of obesity, diabetes and hypertension, chronic kidney disease is becoming a leading global health problem. Diabetes is currently the most common cause of chronic kidney disease [1]. Patients with diabetes and chronic kidney disease have an increased risk for anemia. Anemia is a risk factor for cardiac dysfunction and is potentially modifiable. Therefore it should be screened for readily in the diabetic population, a particularly vulnerable population, and it should be identified and rectified promptly. However all too often this is not the case.

2. Definition of anemia

According to the National Kidney Foundation Kidney Disease Outcomes Quality Initiative (NKF KDOQI), anemia is defined as hemoglobin levels of less than 13.5g/dL (135 g/L) for men and less than 12.0g/dL (120 g/L) for women [2]. The WHO criteria defines anemia to be less than 13.0g/dL (130 g/L) for men and less than 12.0g/dL for premenopausal women [3].

3. Risk factors for anemia

Patients with diabetes and CKD had the highest risk of anemia (odds ratio 1.73, 95% CI 1.63-1.83) [6,7]. Other risk factors that significantly increase the odds of anemia included lower educational level, diabetes mellitus, hypertension, cardiovascular disease (CVD), and chronic kidney disease (CKD), with risk greatest for patients with diabetes and CKD [6].

Risk Factors For Anemia in CKD patients:
1. Diabetes
2. Chronic Kidney Disease
3. Cardiovascular Disease
4. Hypertension
5. Low Education Levels
6. African American race

4. Ethnicity

African Americans have significantly greater incidences of anemia, with mean hemoglobin being 13.5g/dL for African American vs. 15.3g/dL for white men and 12.5g/dL vs. 14.7g/dL for: African American and White Women respectively [4]. This difference can be due in part to the fact that approximately 30 percent of African Americans carry a 3.7kb deletion in the alpha thalassemia gene. Homozygotes for alpha thalassemia exhibit a mild, microcytic anemia, while even heterozygotes may have a low-normal or mildly decreased hemoglobin. However even when people with alpha thalassemia gene, iron deficiency, renal insufficiency and sickle cell trait are excluded, the difference between the hemoglobin of African Americans and whites still persists, albeit to a lower degree [5]. The cause of this phenomenon still remains to be discovered. In the meantime, it has been debated whether the definition of anemia should be modified for different racial and ethnic groups, although this has not yet been implemented in clinical practice guidelines.

5. Pathophysiology of anemia in diabetics with chronic kidney disease

There are several factors which have been implicated in the development of anemia in CKD which include erythropoietin deficiency, iron deficiency, decreased lifespan of red blood cells, chronic blood loss, secondary hyperparathyroidism, chronic inflammation, oxidative stress, nutritional folate deficiency, uremia and chronic suppression of erythropoesis [6,7].
Diabetes exacerbates many of these factors, leading to a higher degree of anemia in patients with diabetic nephropathy than in patients with kidney disease from other causes.

6. Erythropoietin deficiency

Erythropoietin (EPO) is a glycoprotein hormone that regulates proliferation, differentiation and maturation of red blood cells. EPO is produced by the peritubular capillary cells within the kidney, and this process is mediated by oxygen availability. In normal kidneys, EPO production increases in proportion to the degree of anemia.

Relative deficiency of EPO is the most important cause of anemia in patients with chronic kidney disease. The ability of the kidneys to produce erythropoietin is not impaired in renal disease - the absolute value of EPO can be in the normal or even high, so measuring EPO levels does not aid clinical management. However EPO levels will be inappropriately low relative to the degree of anemia, resulting in a functional EPO deficiency. This is due to the uncoupling of EPO synthesis from hemoglobin concentration so that the protein is no longer upregulated by anemia [8].

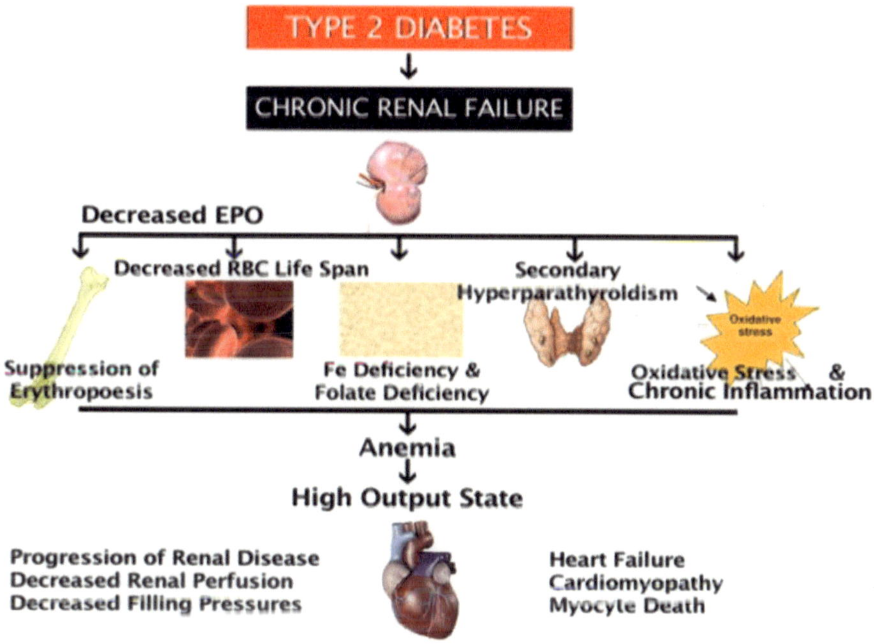

In the diabetic kidney tubulointerstitial dysfunction is observed early in the course of disease [9]. This could cause disruption of the intricate signaling mechanism between the capillaries, interstitial fibroblasts and tubular cells regulating EPO production, thus contributing to the uncoupling of EPO synthesis from hemoglobin levels.

Diabetes also negatively affects hypoxia-inducible factor (HIF), a transcription factor that plays a crucial role in regulating the renal response to hypoxia. HIF regulates the transcriptional activation of many oxygen-sensitive genes, including EPO. Hyperglycemia has been shown to inhibit stabilization of the HIF protein [10].

Autonomic dysfunction has also been suggested as another factor that may contribute to EPO deficiency in diabetic patients. In experimental models, EPO production is impaired when the kidney is denervated [11]. Also, patients with primary disorders of the autonomic nervous system have blunted production of EPO and a high risk of developing anemia [12].

7. Decreased red blood cell lifespan

Patients with renal disease have a 30 to 70 percent reduction in RBC lifespan. The mechanism of this phenomenon has yet to be elucidated satisfactorily. Blood from uremic donors transfused into normal recipients result in normal RBC survival, implying that the uremic environment of patients with chronic kidney disease is the underlying cause of this phenomenon. However advancements in chronic renal replacement therapy does not lead to improvement in RBC survival [13].

The red blood cells of patients with diabetes are metabolically and functionally abnormal. These changes contribute to reduced erythrocyte survival in diabetic patients to a greater degree than in nondiabetic patients with a similar degree of renal impairment [14].

8. Iron deficiency

Uremia causes platelet dysfunction, putting patients with chronic kidney disease at increased risk of bleeding and iron loss. Patients on hemodialysis in particular are prone to losing iron through blood trapping in dialysis machine and repeated phlebotomy.

It has also been shown that patients with chronic kidney disease have impaired absorption of dietary iron. Transferrin is a protein that delivers iron from the gastrointestinal tract and the reticuloendothelial system into the bone marrow to be utilized by maturing erythrocytes. Patients with chronic kidney disease have decreased levels of transferrin, impairing iron mobilization [15].

The overall prevalence of iron deficiency in patients with diabetes is not significantly different from that in the general adult population. However, normal iron indices do not preclude these patients from achieving benefit with iron supplementation. In particular, patients on dialysis are often found to have a functional iron deficiency, in which their iron studies are normal but their anemia improves with parenteral iron supplementation.

9. Chronic inflammation and oxidative stress

Anemia of chronic inflammation is characterized by an impairment of the ability to release iron from the hepatocytes and macrophages of the reticuloendothelial system. Patients with chronic kidney disease exhibit a generalized increase in the inflammatory response due to a variety of factors, including decreased clearance of imflammatory cytokines, volume overload, oxidative stress and their underlying comorbid conditions.

Although decreased GFR and decreased iron stores are major contributing factors to anemia in diabetic patients, EPO deficiency and inflammation are becoming a leading factors in explaining the high prevalence of anemia in diabetics with CKD. These factors lead to anemia and lead to heart failure, cardiomyopathy and myocyte death [16].

10. Epidemiology of anemia in diabetic populations with chronic kidney disease

Anemia occurs earlier, and is more severe in chronic kidney disease related to diabetes than in non-diabetic kidney disease. It often develops when creatinine is within the normal range, and therefore is undiagnosed by primary care physicians. Anemia has a negative impact on patient's quality of life contributing to morbidity, for instance worsening exercise tolerance, lethargy and erectile dysfunction [17]. Furthermore anemia causes hypoxia induced diseases, including angina, cardiac failure and claudication, which are also independently associated with diabetes. Studies have shown that approximately 20 to 30 percent of people with diabetes will be anemic [18]. Unfortunately anemia within the diabetic population anemia is often unrecognized, undetected and untreated in patients with chronic kidney disease [19].

Anemia in diabetic patients although prevalent is often overlooked and undertreated. A cross sectional study comprised of a questionnaire-based interview with 1054 respondents form 6 European countries (Belgium, France, Germany, Greece Italy and the UK) showed that only 32 percent of respondents had been given information about anemia, although 83 percent had heard of anemia. One fifth of those with anemia received no treatment. Although anemia is highly prevalent in those with diabetes, patients are often unaware and undertreated for their anemia [20].

11. Cardiovascular risks of anemic patients with chronic kidney disease

Cardiovascular disease is very common in patients with diabetes and with CKD. There are numerous important interactions between heart disease and renal disease, a term defined as cardiorenal syndrome (CRS). A 2004 report from the National Heart, Lung, and Blood Institute defined CRS as a condition in which therapy to relieve congestive symptoms of heart failure is limited by a decline in renal function as manifested by a reduction in glomerular filtration rate. For instance acute heart failure results in acute kidney injury and chronic heart failure causes progressive chronic kidney disease [21]. This association leads to the vicious circle contributing to premature death [22].

As randomized, placebo-controlled trials have so far been disappointing and unable to show a survival benefit of various treatment strategies, such as lipid-lowering, the risk factor profile seems to be different in CKD compared with the general population. Indeed, seemingly paradoxical associations between traditional risk factors and cardiovascular outcome in patients with advanced CKD have complicated our efforts to identify the real cardiovascular culprits. There are several non-traditional cardiovascular risk factors that are directly linked with CKD such as hyperparathyroidism, hyperphosphatemia, hyperhomocysteinemia and anemia, which are increasingly, recognized as cardiovascular risks [23]. Patients with CKD are more likely to die from cardiovascular events than of end stage renal disease.

12. Cardiovascular risk factors

In a study done involving 69,244 participants in a voluntary screening program and 17,061 participants randomly selected national survey population, CKD was independently associated with MI or stroke [6]. In diabetic patients with CKD the risk of CVD is increased by 20 to 40 percent compared with that in CKD in patients without diabetes [24].

Traditional Risk Factors	Non traditional risk Factors
Diabetes	Chronic inflammation
Dyslipidemia	Anemia
HTN	Oxidative stress
Central obesity	Hyperparathyroidism
Smoking	Hyperhomocysteinemia
Male or postmenopausal female	Endothelial Dysfunction
Family history of MI event	Prothrombotic states

13. Reasons to treat anemia

Type 2 diabetes mellitus and chronic kidney disease frequently coexist, and each disease independently increases the risk of cardiovascular events and end stage renal disease. Intensive treatment of risk factors such as hypertension and elevated LDL reduces cardiovascular morbidity and mortality and slows the progression of the kidney disease [25-27]. Anemia is a risk factor for cardiovascular morbidity and mortality, and is evolving as an attractive target and potentially correctable risk factor [24].

14. Treatment recommendations

All patients with CKD should be screened at least annually for anemia, regardless of stage. Further evaluation of anemia should be initiated in patients with CKD if hemoglobin levels found to be below normal, including iron studies. Erythropoiesis-stimulating agents (ESAs) can be initiated when hemoglobin falls below the target range of 11-12g/dL [16].

ESAs are the mainstay of therapy for anemia of chronic kidney disease. There are currently two agents commercially available, recombinant epoietin alfa (Epogen, Procrit) and darbepoetin alfa (Aranesp). The selection of ESA can be individualized according to clinical circumstances and patient/provider preference.

Patients with serum ferritin, transferrin saturation and/or content of hemoglobin in reticulocytes below target levels should be started on iron supplementation. Patients on hemodialysis should be given parenteral iron therapy as their iron deficiency often fails to correct with oral supplementation.

15. Recent clinical trials

Recommendations regarding the use of erythropoietin and the target hemoglobin are forever changing. In 1994 The FDA first approved a target hemoglobin of 10-11g/dl which was subsequently increased to 10-12g/dl in 1998. The National Kidney Foundation recommended a level of hemoglobin of 11-12g/dl in 2007 [2,6].

In 1998 a study was performed to assess the risks and benefits of normalizing the hematocrit in patients with cardiac disease who were undergoing hemodialysis. There were 1233 patients evaluated in the study, of which 618 were assigned to achieve a hematocrit of 42 percent, and 615 received erythropoietin sufficient to achieve and maintain a hematocrit of 30 percent. After 29 months there were 183 deaths and 19 first nonfatal myocardial infarcts among the patients in the normal hematocrit group and 150 deaths and 14 non-fatal myocardial infarcts among those in the low hematocrit group. The study was prematurely halted due to the higher mortality rate in the normal hematocrit group. The investigators recommended against normalization of hematocrit in patients with clinically evident congestive heart failure or ischemic heart disease who are receiving hemodialysis [28].

In 2006 two other landmark trials were published. The studies were conducted to determine optimal hemoglobin levels in predialysis patients looking at cardiovascular disease outcomes.

The CHOIR (Correction of Hemoglobin and Outcomes in Renal Insufficiency) study was an open-label trial of 1432 patients with CKD. 715 were randomly assigned to receive epoetin alpha to achieve a hemoglobin of 13.5g/dl and 717 were assigned to achieve a level of 11.3g/dl. The endpoint was a composite of death, myocardial infarction, hospitalization for

congestive heart failure, and stroke. There were 222 composite events: 125 in the high hemoglobin group and 97 in the low hemoglobin group. Investigators concluded that the 13.5g/dl target resulted in increased risk, and no improvement in quality of life [29].
The second landmark trial at this time was the CREATE (Cardiovascular Risk Reduction by Early Anemia Treatment with Epoetin Beta) study, which randomly assigned 603 patients with an estimated GFR of 15-35 ml/min and mild to moderate anemia (11-12.5 g/dl) to a target hemoglobin in the normal range (13-15g/dl) or to subnormal values (10.5-11.5g/dl). During the 3 year study complete correction of anemia did not affect the likelihood of a first cardiac death. There was no significant incidence of adverse events between the two groups. Investigators concluded that in patients with CKD, early complete correction of anemia does not reduce the risk of cardiovascular events [30].
The ACORD (Anemia Correction in Diabetes) study, published in 2007, investigated the effect of correcting anemia on heart function in diabetic patients with anemia and early diabetic nephropathy. 172 patients with type 1 or 2 diabetes mellitus, mild to moderate anemia, and stage 1 to 3 chronic kidney disease were randomly assigned to attain a target hemoglobin level of either 13 to 15 g/dL (group 1) or 10.5 to 11.5 g/dL (group 2). The primary end point was change in left ventricular mass index (LVMI), measured by echocardiogram. At study end, hemoglobin levels were 13.5 g/dL in group 1 and 12.1 g/dL in group 2, but no significant differences between study groups were observed in median LVMI after 15 months [31].
In 2009 the TREAT (Trial to Reduce Cardiovascular Events with Aranesp Therapy) trial was conducted to evaluate whether increasing the hemoglobin level with the use of darbepoetin would lower the rate of death, cardiovascular events or end stage renal disease in patients with type 2 diabetes and chronic kidney disease. This was a randomized, double blind placebo controlled trial conducted at 623 sites in 24 countries consisting of 4038 patients. 2012 patients were randomly assigned to receive darbepoetin to achieve a hemoglobin level of approximately 13g/dL, while 2026 patients received placebo, with rescue darbepoetin when the hemoglobin level was less that 9g/dL. Darbepoetin did not reduce the primary end points of death, cardiovascular events or end stage renal disease in patients with diabetes and chronic kidney disease. There was also an increased incident of stroke of 2.1 percent in the darbepoetin arm vs. 1.1 percent in the placebo arm [32].
A subset analysis of TREAT that was published in September 2010 assessed the relationship between responsiveness to darbepoetin, hemoglobin levels achieved, and cardiovascular outcomes in patients with chronic kidney disease and type 2 diabetes. Patients with less than 2 percent change in hemoglobin level after the first two doses of darbepoetin were defined as poor responders. These patients had a lower hemoglobin level at 12 weeks despite receiving higher doses of darbepoetin. They also had higher rates of composite cardiovascular end points or death. The study was unable to determine whether poor response to darbepoetin is a risk factor for adverse outcomes, or whether the risk was augmented by the higher doses of darbepoetin they received [33].

16. Conclusion

Although anemia in chronic kidney disease is often unrecognized and under diagnosed, it is an important predictor of quality of life and contributes to cardiovascular morbidity and mortality in patients with diabetes. Anemia causes hypoxia induced diseases, including angina, cardiac failure and claudication, which are also independently associated with diabetes. Anemia also causes worsening exercise tolerance, lethargy and erectile dysfunction. Anemia, like hypertension and hyperlipidemia is an important modifiable risk factor in patients with chronic kidney disease and diabetes, therefore should be treated as such.

Currently it is recommended to maintain a hemoglobin of 11-12g/dl in patients with chronic kidney disease with correction of nutritional deficiencies and the use of erythropoietin-stimulating agents. Evidence from randomized controlled trials including the CHOIR, CREATE and ACORD studies show that normalization of hemoglobin beyond 12g/dl does not improve outcomes. The TREAT trial showed that using ESAs to increase hemoglobin to a target of 13g/dL increases the risk of stroke. It was also found that patients who had a poor response to ESAs had a higher rate of cardiovascular events.

17. Summary

1. Anemia is pervasive in the diabetic patient with CKD.
2. Anemia occurs earlier, and is more severe in chronic kidney disease related to diabetes than in non-diabetic kidney disease.
3. Reasons for anemia in CKD include EPO deficiency, iron deficiency, decreased lifespan of red blood cells, chronic blood loss, secondary hyperparathyroidism, chronic inflammation, oxidative stress, nutritional folate deficiency, uremia and chronic suppression of erythropoesis.
4. Anemia in diabetic patients although prevalent is often overlooked and undertreated.
5. Cardiovascular disease is very common in patients with diabetes and with CKD.
6. In diabetic patients with CKD the risk of CVD is increased by 20 to 40 percent compared with that in CKD in patients without diabetes.
7. Anemia is a risk factor for cardiovascular morbidity and mortality, and is evolving as an attractive target and potentially correctable risk factor.
8. All patients with CKD should be screened at least annually for anemia, regardless of stage.
9. ESAs are the mainstay of therapy for anemia of chronic kidney disease.
10. Maintaining a hemoglobin of 11-12g/dl is currently recommended.

18. References

[1] Schieppati A, Remuzzi G. Chronic renal diseases as a public health problem; epidemiology, social and economic implications. *Kidney Int Suppl* 98:S7-10, 2005.

[2] KDOQI Clinical Practice Guideline and clinical practice recommendations for anemia in chronic kidney disease: 2007 update of hemoglobin target. *Am J Kidney Dis* 50:471-530, 2007.

[3] World Health Organization (2008). Worldwide prevalence of anaemia 1993–2005. Geneva: *World Health Organization. ISBN 9789241596657.*

[4] Reed, WW; Diehl, LF. Leukopenia, Neutropenia, and Reduced Hemoglobin Levels in Healthy American Blacks *Arch Intern Med* 151:501-505, 1991.

[5] Beutler E, West C. Hematologic differences between African-Americans and whites: the roles of iron deficiency and alpha-thalassemia on hemoglobin levels and mean corpuscular volume. *Blood* 106:740-745, 2005.

[6] McFarlane SI, Chen SC, Whaley-Connell AT et al. Prevalence and associations of anemia of CKD: Kidney Early Evaluation Program (KEEP) and National Health Nutrition Examination Survey(NHANES)1999-2004. *Am J Kidney Dis* 51;S46-55, 2008.
[7] Dharawhat A, Golderberg T, Alam A, Atat Ali, Moore Alexis, McFarlane SI. Cardiovascular disease associated with anemia in diabetic patients with chronic kidney disease. *International Diabetes Monitor* 21:171-178, 2009.
[8] Thomas MC. Anemia in diabetes: marker or mediator of microvascular disease? *Nat Clin Pract Nephrol*. 3:20-30, 2007.
[9] Thomas MC, Burns WC, Cooper ME. Tubular changes in early diabetic nephropathy. *Adv Chronic Kidney Dis* 12:177-186, 2005.
[10] Catrina SB, Okamoto K, Pereira T, Brismar K, Poellinger L. Hyperglycemia regulates hypoxia-inducible factor-1 alpha protein stability and function. *Diabetes* 53:3226-3232, 2004.
[11] Finne PH, Skoglund RW. Erythropoietin production in the rat following splanchnic neurectomy. *J Lab Clin Med* 76:103-106, 1970.
[12] Biaggioni I, Robertson D, Kranz S, Jones M, Haile V. The anemia of primary autonomic failure and its reversal with recombinant erythropoietin. *Ann Intern Med* 121:181-186, 1994.
[13] Ly J, Marticorena R, Donnelly S. Red blood cell survival in chronic renal failure. *Am J Kidney Dis* 44:715-719, 2004.
[14] Manodori AB, Kuypers FA. Altered red cell turnover in diabetic mice. *J Lab Clin Med* 140:161-165, 2002.
[15] Nurko S. Anemia in chronic kidney disease: causes, diagnosis, treatment. *Cleve Clin J Med* 73(3):289-297, 2006.
[16] National Kidney Foundation. KDOQI Clinical Practice Guidelines and Clinical Practice Recommendations for Anemia in Chronic Kidney Disease. *Am J Kidney Dis* 47:S1-S146, 2006.
[17] Valderrabano F. Quality of life benefits of early anaemia treatment. *Nephrol Dial Transplant* 15: 23–28, 2000.
[18] New JP, Aung T, Baker PG et al. The high prevalence of unrecognized anaemia in patients with diabetes and chronic kidney disease: a population-based study. *Diabetic Medicine* 25:564-569, 2008.
[19] Thomas MC, MacIsaac RJ, T salamandris C et al. Unrecognized anemia in patients with diabetes: a cross sectional survey. *Diabetes Care* 26:1164-9, 2003.
[20] Stevens PE, O'Donoghue DJ, Lameire NR. Anaemia in patients with diabetes: unrecognized, undetected and untreated? *Curr Med Res Opin* 19:395-40, 2003.
[21] Ronco C, Haapio M, House AA, Anavekar N, Bellomo R. Cardiorenal syndrome. *J Am Coll Cardiol* 52:1527-39, 2008.
[22] Stenvinkel P, Carrero JJ, Axelsson J, Lindholm B, Heimbürger O, Massy Z. Emerging biomarkers for evaluating cardiovascular risk in the chronic kidney disease patient: how do new pieces fit into the uremic puzzle? *Clin J Am Soc Nephrol* 3:505-21, 2008.
[23] Vlagopoulos PT, Sarnak MJ. Traditional and nontraditional cardiovascular risk factors in chronic kidney disease. *Med Clinic North Americ* 89:587-611, 2005.
[24] Foley R. Cardiac disease in diabetic patients with renal disease. *Acta Diabetol* 39: S9-14, 2002.

[25] Turnbull F, Neal B, Algert C, et al. Effects of different blood pressure-lowering regimens on major cardiovascular events in individuals with and without diabetes mellitus: results of prospectively designed overviews of randomized trials. *Arch Intern Med* 165:1410-1419, 2005.

[26] Baigent C, Keech A, Kearney PM, et al. Efficacy and safety of cholesterol-lowering treatment: prospective meta-analysis of data from 90,056 participants in 14 randomized trials of statins. *Lancet* 366:1267-1278, 2005.

[27] Gaede P, Lund-Andersen H, Parving H-H, Pedersen O. Effect of a multifactorial intervention on mortality in type 2 diabetes. *N Engl J Med* 358:580-591, 2008.

[28] Besarb A, Bolton WK, Browne JK et al. The effects of normal as compared with low hematocrit values in patients with cardiac disease who are receiving hemodialysis and epoetin. *N Engl J Med* 339:584-90, 1998.

[29] Singh AK, Szczech L, Tang KL, et al. Correction of anemia with epoetin alfa in chronic kidney disease. *N Engl J Med* 355:2085-2098, 2006.

[30] Drueke TB, Locatelli F, Clyne N et al. Normalization of hemoglobin level in patients with chronic kidney disease and anemia. *N Engl J M*ed 355:2071-2084, 2006.

[31] Ritz E, Laville M, Bilous RW et al. Target level for hemoglobin correction in patients with diabetes and CKD: primary results of the anemia correction in diabetes (ACORD) study. *Am J Kidney Dis* 49:194-207, 2007.

[32] Pfeffer MA, Burdmann EA, et al. A trial of darbepoetin alfa in type 2 diabetes and chronic kidney disease. *N Engl J Med* 361:2019-2032, 2009.

[33] Hayes C, Alam A, Black-Peart J, McFarlane SI. Mitigating the cardiovascular risk of anemia in patients with type 2 diabetes and CKD: Does darbepoetin help? The TREAT Trial. *Curr Diab Rep*;10(2):87-9

[34] Solomon SD, Uno H, Lewis EF et al. Erythropoietic response and outcomes in kidney disease and type 2 diabetes. *N Engl J Med* 363:1146-1155, 2010.

16

A Diachronic Study of Diabetic Nephropathy in Two Autochthonous Lines of Rats to Understand Diabetic Chronic Complications

Juan Carlos Picena, Silvana Marisa Montenegro, Alberto Enrique D´Ottavio, María Cristina Tarrés and Stella Maris Martínez
National University of Rosario
Argentina

1. Introduction

The worldwide epidemic of Type 2 Diabetes Mellitus, a result of recent deep changes in human lifestyle like sedentary and overly rich nutrition, has dramatic consequences in terms of morbidity, mortality and health care costs (Zimmet *et al.*, 2001). Type 2 Diabetes Mellitus is a complex and multifactorial metabolic disorder which includes distinct nosological entities whose common patterns are hyperglycaemia, resistance to insulin and progressive chronic complications (American Diabetic Association, 2009).
A significant proportion of patients will develop a clinically relevant diabetic nephropathy with glomerulopathy, hyalinization of afferent and efferent arterioles, tubular and interstitial lesions (Fioretto *et al.*, 2008). Nephropathy is a very serious complication in both Type 1 and Type 2 Diabetes Mellitus because patients with diabetic kidney disease are at a higher risk of mortality, mostly from cardiovascular complications, than diabetic patients without diabetic nephropathy (Dronavalli & Barkis, 2008).
In the Western World the incidence of end-stage renal failure associated to the burden of diabetic nephropathy has increased in recent years and represents a failure of current disease control measure with serious public health implications (Stewart *et al*, 2006; Villar & Zaoui, 2010). In Latin America, where incidence of Type 2 Diabetes Mellitus is on the rise and has reached epidemic proportions, people usually have poor disease control with the consequence of very high rates of diabetic nephropathy (Caballero & Tenzer, 2007). A study performed in the Asian Pacific region has also shown that diabetic nephropathy was the most common cause of End-Stage Renal Disease in 9 of the 12 countries surveyed and 6 of the 12 countries had greater than 35% of their dialysis patients age 60 years and older (Lee, 2003). In United States, between 20% and 40% of patients ultimately develop diabetic nephropathy, the most common cause of End-Stage Renal Disease requiring dialysis (Dronavalli & Barkis, 2008). Since 2000, the adjusted rate of prevalent End-Stage Renal Disease cases in the United States population ages 65–74, has increased 25 % with an enormous economic impact on the healthcare systems (United States Renal Data System, 2010). In sum, worldwide incidence of diabetic nephropathy, a frequently silent and unrecognized disease, has increased about a 50% between 1998 and 2008 and is now the leading cause of chronic kidney disease and End-Stage Renal Disease (Unites States Renal

Data System, 2008). These epidemiological findings along with the several pathways which have been implicated in the progression of diabetic nephropathy, such as systemic and glomerular hypertension, metabolic derangements (hyperglycaemia, hyperlipidaemia, hyperinsulinaemia), and oxidative stress among others, indicate the complexity and the magnitude of diabetic nephropathy as a health concern.

Streptozotocin-induced pancreatic injury as well as uninephrectomy have been used for creating both rat and mouse models of Type 1 Diabetes Mellitus which develop renal injury with similarities to human diabetic nephropathy (Tesch & Allen., 2007). Nephropathy is also a complication in rat models of spontaneous Type 2 Diabetes Mellitus as the obese Zucker (fatty) rat, the Goto Kakizaki rat (Janssen *et al.*, 1999) and the hypertensive/NIH-corpulent rat (Nangaku *et al.*, 2005) and in mice models as the BTBR Ob/Ob mutant mice (Hudkins *et al.*, 2010). Either spontaneous or induced, rodent models of diabetes have been extensively used in diabetes research because of their usefulness for understanding the pathogenesis, the complications and the genetic or environmental influences that increase the risks of suffering Type 2 Diabetes Mellitus (Srinivasan & Ramarao, 2007). These models, which depict many clinical features or related phenotypes of the disease, differ among them not only in its metabolic alterations but in their etiopathogenia (Breyer *et al.* 2005; Chatzigeorgiou *et al.*, 2009). Although their use has allowed important advances toward the better understanding of human diabetic nephropathy, it has been recently pointed out that a lack of reliable animal models of diabetic complications still persists (Brosius *et al.*, 2009).

The eSS rat is a spontaneously non-obese diabetic model obtained in Rosario, Argentina, by genetic manipulation, described in detail by Martinez *et al.* (1993). eSS rats evidence a progressive impaired glucose tolerance from 70 days of age onwards with hyperglycaemia and glycosuria worsening with ageing, being these signs much more striking in males (Martínez *et al.*, 1988). Males exhibit insulin resistance and consequent insulin hypersecretion till 12 months of age but the hormone secretion decreases as diabetes progresses in the sequence of events from insulin resistance to overt diabetes (Martínez *et al.*, 1988). This finding is coincident with conspicuous changes in the pancreas of 18 month-old eSS males, such as disruption of islet architecture and areas of pronounced fibrosis (Tarrés *et al.*, 1992; Picena *et al.*, 2007).

During the second year of life, eSS males are known to develop glomerulosclerosis and tubular nephrosis similar to those found in long-term human diabetes (Tarrés *et al.*, 1992; Martínez *et al.*, 1993). Older eSS males also develop bilateral cataracts but not retinopathy (Tarrés *et al.*, 1990; Picena *et al.*, 2005). Hence, the eSS rat was proposed as a model of non-insulin dependent diabetes characterized by complex glucose and lipid disorders (Martínez *et al.*, 1993; Montanaro *et al.*, 2003; Daniele *et al.*, 2010).

eSMT rats (IIMe/Fm eSMT) derived from crossing eSS with ß rats, both parent strains belonging to the IIM stock (Calderari *et al.*, 1991). ß (IIMb/Fm ß) is a line of moderately and spontaneous obese, fertile and hypertriglyceridemic rats (Calderari *et al.*, 1987; Hisano *et al.*, 1994). Upon crossing the F1 to obtain F2, the new colony eSMT was maintained as a closed one, where the full genetic history of each breeding rat is preserved (Tarrés *et al.*, 2000). Young eSMT animals are more robust than eSS and develop higher levels of fasting hyperglycaemia, glycosuria, glucose intolerance, blood triglycerides and total cholesterol (Tarrés *et al.*, 2000; Montenegro *et al.*, 2005). eSMT males of 6 and 9 months show islets with altered shapes and fibrosis, as well as sporadic images of apoptosis and at 12 months of age, islets are reduced in number and size, resembling the histoarchitecture of eSS males during their second year of life (Tarrés *et al.*, 2000). The sexual dimorphism is less evident in eSMT than in eSS diabetic syndrome (Picena, 2007).

The aim of this chapter is to present a wide and diachronic study of renal histopathology in eSS and eSMT rats, two strains which develop hereditary type 2 diabetic syndromes with different expression of the metabolic disorders, in order to characterize morphological changes. The arrival to conclusions could improve our knowledge and understanding of diabetic nephropathy.

2. Material and methods

The study was conducted in highly inbred 139 eSS (males= 71; females= 68) and 122 eSMT (males= 50; females= 72) rats from 3 to 26-30 months of age. Eumetabolic Wistar male rats of 12 (n= 15) and 21 month-old (n=12) were used as controls.

Since the expected life span of the eSS and the eSMT rats in our laboratory ranges from 24-30 months, the morphological studies of diabetic nephropathy covered their entire life span. From 3 months of age onwards, groups of rats from eSS and eSMT strains were euthanized. Previously, glycaemia at 120 min after 10% glucose overload (200 mg/100 g body weight) via stomach tube was assessed. Blood samples were obtained by tail vein puncture. Plasma samples were analysed for glucose by the glucose oxidase enzymatic method using a commercial kit (Wiener Laboratories, Argentina).

Body and kidney weights were registered in every case. Sections of renal tissue were fixed in 10% neutral-buffered formalin for 24 hours, embedded in paraffin, cut into sections of 4 μm thick, stained with hematoxylin-eosin (HE) and Periodic Acid-Schiff (PAS), and examined by light microscopy in a blinded fashion. In each histological specimen, capsular and glomerular diameters of 10 superficial and 10 juxtamedullary nephrons, cut at the vascular pole, were measured through a calibrated Shimadzu ® linear scale, placed in the eyepiece of a light microscopy. Correlations between age and body weights, and age and kidney weights were also performed.

Glomeruli were classified as small when the diameter was lower than 80μm. Mesangial expansion, defined as the thickening mesangium by the deposit of an acidophilic, amorphous, PAS positive matrix substance and by the increase of cellular components, was considered diffuse when the glomerulus was wholly affected, and segmental if it was partially affected. Depending on its severity, it was graded as mild (ME +) or severe (SE ++). Fifty glomeruli per kidney were randomly selected in each animal. Percentages (%) of glomeruli displaying the same degree of injury (small glomeruli, ME+ and SE ++) were obtained per animal. Correlations between age and percentage of small glomeruli, and age and mildly and severely affected glomeruli were calculated. Nodular increases in mesangial matrix as well as the presence of sclerotic or atubular glomeruli and capsular drop were also sought for. Tubulointerstitial and vascular injuries were considered on the basis of tubular dilation and atrophy, interstitial infiltration and fibrosis as well as of intimal thickening and arteriolar hyalinosis, respectively.

eSS rats were maintained in the breeding facilities of our School of Medicine, Rosario University, Rosario, Argentina. Wistar rats came from the animal breeding facilities in the School of Biochemical Science, Rosario University. Breeding conditions were the same for all the animals, including temperature regulation (24°C) and light-darkness cycles as well as the artificial air exchange. In all the cases, the individuals had remained housed since they were 21 days old, in hanging collective cages. All animals were fed on a complete commercial diet, special for laboratory rats, and water was *ad libitum*. These experimental conditions were maintained until the animals were euthanized.

All data are reported as the mean ± standard deviation. Statistical processing was partly carried out with the software SPSS 15, using the parametric and non-parametric methods referred below in the presentation of results.

All experimental procedures presented in this study were previously approved by the Bioethics Commission of School of Medicine, which assures adherence to the standards by the Guide for the Care and Use of Laboratory Animals.

3. Results

Body weights data in the experimental eSS and eSMT animals are seen in Table 1.

Age (months)	Line eSS		Line eSMT		Anova (effect: p)
	Males	Females	Males	Females	
3	266±21 (n=6)	137±14 (n=9)	300±43 (n=11)	207±13 (n=9)	Line:0.015 Sex:0.000 Interaction:0.000
6	342±26 (n=19)	245±43 (n=7)	368±55 (n=5)	284±31 (n=11)	Line:0.016 Sex:0.000 Interaction:0.481
9	362±17 (n=4)	232±14 (n=10	397±61 (n=12)	308±40 (n=6)	Line: 0.004 Sex: 0.000 Interaction: 0.154
12	389±23 (n=14)	252±16 (n= 6)	419±61 (n=6)	338±34 (n=11)	Line:0.002 Sex:0.000 Interaction:0.215
15	399±72 (n=9)	337±15 (n=6)	431±91 (n=5)	370±42 (n=7)	Line:0.051 Sex:0.054 Interaction:0.889
18	402±51 (n=14)	345±36 (n=12)	416±47 (n=8)	350±35 (n=13)	Line:0.440 Sex:0.000 Interaction:0.031
21	357±40 (n=11)	338±26 (n=12)	378±36 (n=8)	348±58 (n=12)	Line:0.063 Sex:0.001 Interaction:0.055
24	282±25 (n=5)	254±52 (n=11)	297±61 (n=4)	319±57 (n=15)	Line:0.087 Sex:0.099 Interaction:0.034
≥ 26		242±26 (n=7)		313±37 (n=4)	Line:0.001

Values expressed as mean ± standard deviation.

Table 1. Body weights (g) in male and female eSS and eSMT rats from 3 to ≥26 months of age.

There was a significant line effect on body weight being eSMT heavier than eSS. A sex-dependent effect was also demonstrated remaining the males heavier than the females.

Table 1 also indicates that body weight increased in male and in female eSS rats till 18 months of age whilst eSMT rats underwent a similar evolution up to 15 months of age. Body weight was significantly correlated with age in both lines (eSS: r=0.171; p=0.050; eSMT: r=0.218; p=0.016). The low values obtained could be owed to the marked declination of body weight in the older animals.

As shown in Table 2, kidney weights increased up to 18 months of age in eSS males and till 15 months of age in eSMT males being always greater in eSMT rats than in eSS rats and in males than in females.

Age (months)	Line eSS		Line eSMT		Anova (effect: p)
	Males	Females	Males	Females	
3	2.30±027	1.25±0.25	2.40±0.22	1.94±0.24	Line:0.005 Sex:0.000 Interaction:0.050
6	2.79±0.32	2.03±0.15	2.84±0.45	2.40±0.19	Line:0.007 Sex::0.000 Interaction:0.022
9	3.55±0.38	2.26±0.16	3.70±0.31	2.55±0.38	Line:0.041 Sex:0.000 Interaction:0.041
12	3.15±0.63	2.63±0.10	4.02±0.94	2.97±0.29	Line: 0.004 Sex: 0.000 Interaction:0.001
15	3.85±0.52	2.75±0.26	4.68±0.36	3.22±0.28	Line:0.952 Sex:0.000 Interaction:0.027
18	4.06±0.57	2.87±0.45	4.39±0.55	3.20±0.44	Line:0.000 Sex:0.000 Interaction:0.026
21	3.68 ± 1.14	2.82±0.35	3.99±0.49	3.17±0.21	Line:0.546 Sex:0.014 Interaction:0.221
24	3.21 ± 1.13	2.78±0.43	3.88±0.46	3.12±0.37	Line:0.546 Sex:0.014 Interaction:0.032
≥ 26		2.67±0.27		3.01±0.10	Line:0.001

Values expressed as mean ± standard deviation

Table 2. Kidney weights (g) in male and female eSS and eSMT rats from 3 to ≥26 months of age

Direct and significant correlations were demonstrated between kidney weight and age in eSS and eSMT lines (eSS: r=0.324; p=0.000; eSMT: r=0.498; p=0.000).

Line and sex effects were shown on glucose tolerance being glycaemia after 120min glucose overload (G120) higher in eSMT rats than in eSS rats and in males than in females. A noticeable worsening of G120 with ageing was also evident (Table 3). eSS males reached the G120 threshold for diagnosis of overt diabetes (G120≥200 mg/dl) from 6 months of age onwards and eSMT males, from 3 months of age. Females displayed similar values later (eSS from 12 months of age and eSMT from 9 m months of age). Wistar rats did not show any significant age-dependent changes remaining normoglycemic until 21 months of age (G120: 109 ± 10 mg/dl).

Age (months)	Line eSS		Line eSMT		Anova (effect: p)
	Males	Females	Males	Females	
3	168±37	124±08	201±75	132±20	Line:0.000 Sex:0.012 Interaction:0.330
6	237±44	179±39	264±41	187±28	Line:0.018 Sex:0.034 Interaction:0.342
9	254±43	188±27	303±34	207±35	Line:0.016 Sex:0.002 Interaction:0.431
12	299±64	201±32	324±43	223±42	Line:0.004 Sex:0.000 Interaction:0.154
15	301±55	222±25	356±44	270±33	Line:0.051 Sex:0.054 Interaction:0.889
18	309±49	226±46	429±27	289±26	Line:0.044 Sex:0.000 Interaction:0.330
21	314±42	235±38	433±52	299±35	Line:0.063 Sex:0.001 Interaction:0.752
24	317±35	240±32	438±64	301±27	Line:0.028 Sex:0.029 Interaction:0.349
≥ 26		242±22		309±46	Line:0.001

Values expressed as mean ± standard deviation

Table 3. Glycaemia after 120min glucose overload (mg/dl) in male and female eSS and eSMT rats from 3 to ≥26 months of age.

Present results indicate that at 3 month of age, when animals are still quite normoglycemic with the exception of eSMT males, kidneys did not show lesions visible under the light microscope and that renal injury became apparent from 6-month-old onward. The most frequent glomerular lesions were ME+ and SE++ diffuse mesangial expansion. Direct and significant correlations were evidenced between the percentage of diffuse mesangial expansion and the age (ME+: eSS ρ= 0.873; p= 0.000. eSMT ρ= 0.689; p= 0.000 and ME++: eSS ρ= 0.832; p= 0.000. eSMT ρ= 0.863; p= 0.000). Nevertheless, an increasing number of small glomeruli (> 80 μm) were also verified in ageing eSS and eSMT individuals (eSS ρ= 0.774; p= 0.000; eSMT ρ= 0.641; p= 0.000). In 12 month-old eSS rats, the glomerular diameter was higher in females (♂: 110 ± 8 μm vs. ♀: 120 ± 6; p<0.01) whilst in eSMT strain these values were not different between sexes (♂:102 ± 9 µm vs. ♀:106 ±11; p>0.05). eSMT females showed similar values of glomerular diameter to those registered in eSS males (eSS ♂: 110 ± 8 µm eSMT vs. eSMT ♀: 106 ±11 ; p>0.05) . Significant correlations between the percentages of small glomeruli, glomeruli with ME+ and with SE++ and age are shown in Figure 1.

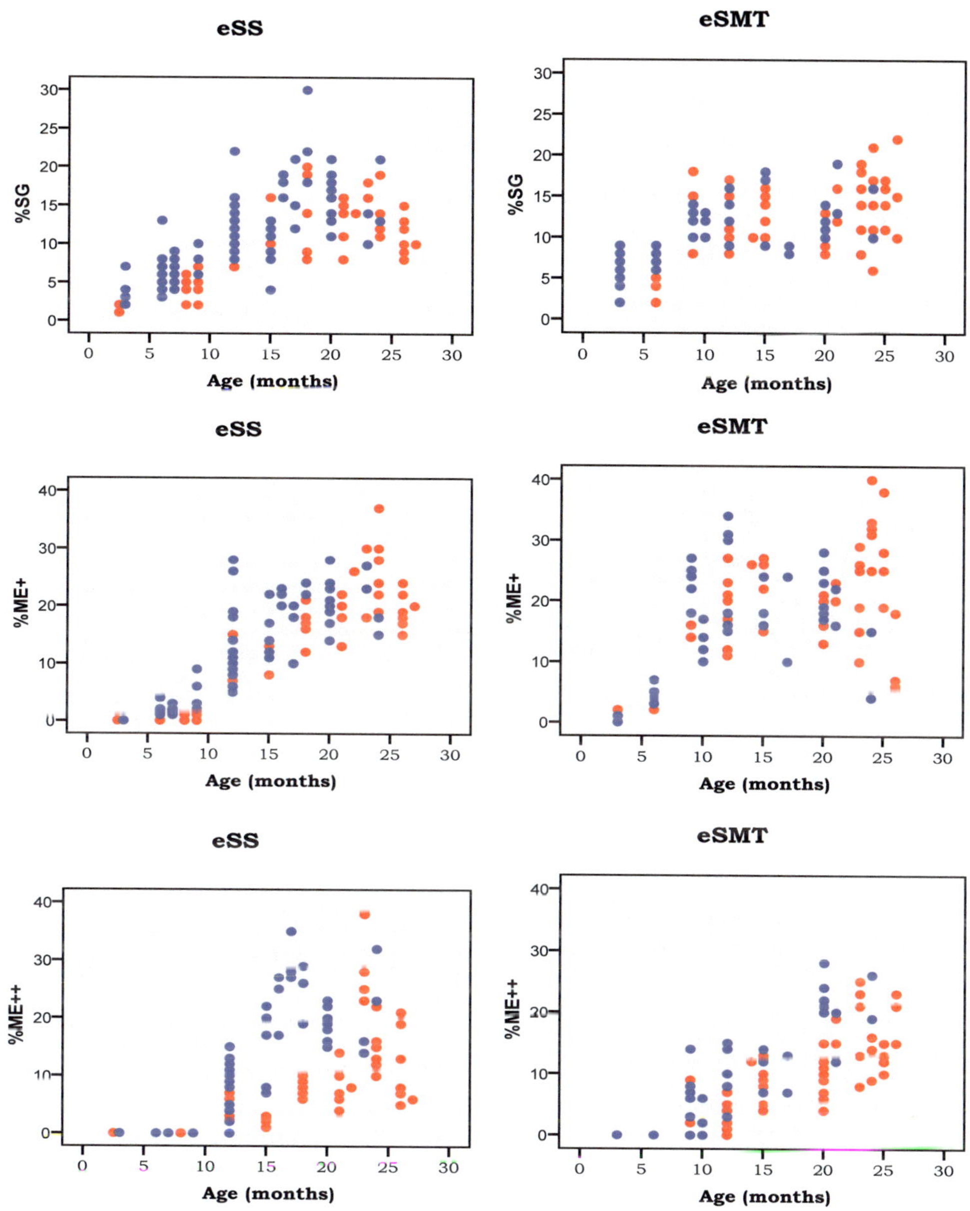

Fig. 1. Correlations between age and percentage of small glomeruli (eSS ρ= 0.774; p= 0.000; eSMT ρ= 0.641; p= 0.000), ME+ (eSS ρ= 0.873; p= 0.000. eSMT ρ= 0.689; p= 0.000), and ME++ (eSS ρ= 0.832; p= 0.000. eSMT ρ= 0.863; p= 0.000) in male (•) and female (•) eSS and eSMT rats.

In both lines, glomerular damage began with thickening of the basement membrane in the peripheral sector of the glomeruli, followed by segmentary or diffuse mesangial expansion due to the deposit of an acidophilic, amorphous, PAS-positive substance in addition to increased cellularity (Fig 2 A and 2 B). Progressively, eSMT y eSS males showed a rising number of small glomeruli (Fig 2 C). While glomerular histology by light microscopy was rather normal in eSS rats younger than 12 months of age, a mild PAS positive thickening of glomerular basement membrane was commonly detected in older males. Mild or severe mesangial expansion was usual in 21 month-old eSS males as well as basement membrane thickening. In eSMT rats, mild thickening of the basement membrane was detected from 6 month-old males onwards, and worsened in older animals.

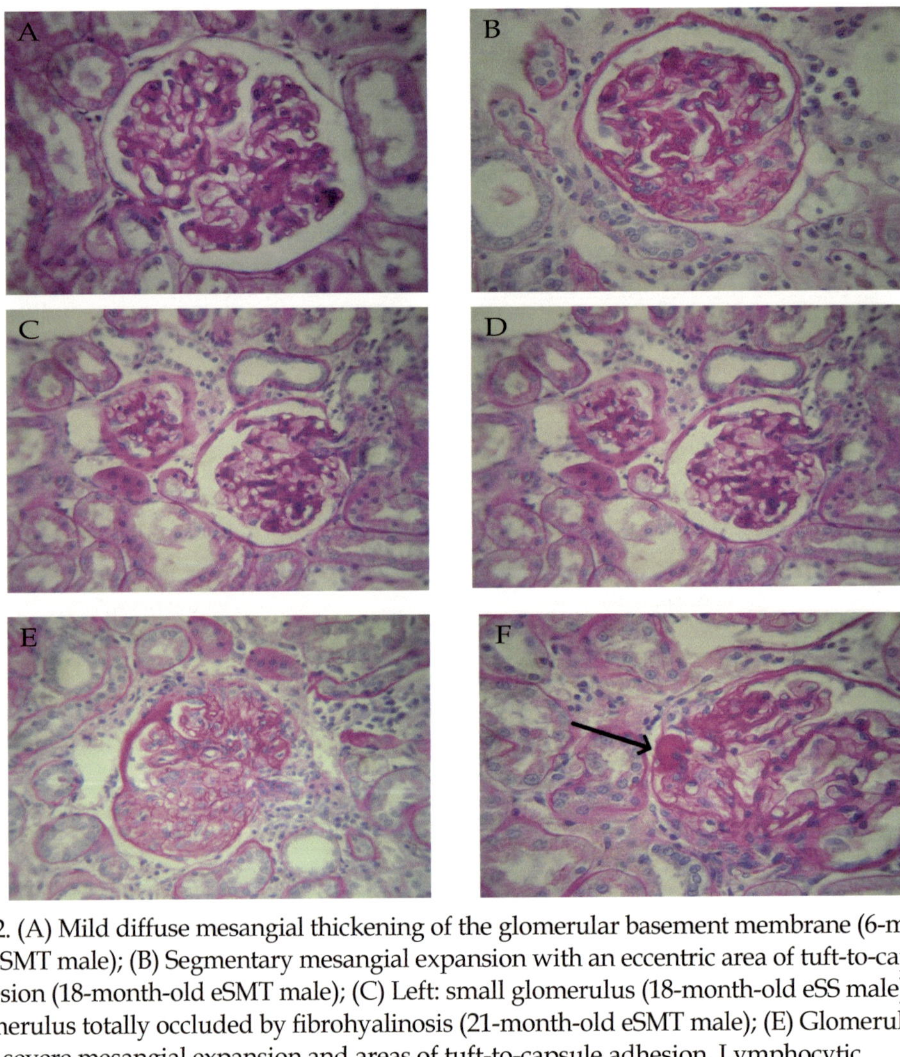

Fig. 2. (A) Mild diffuse mesangial thickening of the glomerular basement membrane (6-month-old eSMT male); (B) Segmentary mesangial expansion with an eccentric area of tuft-to-capsule adhesion (18-month-old eSMT male); (C) Left: small glomerulus (18-month-old eSS male); (D) Glomerulus totally occluded by fibrohyalinosis (21-month-old eSMT male); (E) Glomerulus with severe mesangial expansion and areas of tuft-to-capsule adhesion. Lymphocytic infiltrates near the vascular pole and intertubular interstitium. Atrophic tubules are also observed (24-month-old eSMT male); (F) Arrow: Kimmelstiel-Wilson-like nodular lesion (18-month-old eSMT male). HE and Periodic acid-Schiff (PAS) stain. 300X, except F (400X).

Prominent diffuse or segmentary mesangial expansion and, occasionally, areas of tuft-to-capsule adhesion were evident in the 12- and 18-month-old eSMT males. Severe injury was evidenced by many sclerotic glomeruli totally occluded (Fig 2 D) and a smaller number of atubular glomeruli with tuft adhesions in the older eSMT males (Fig 2 E). Prominent thickening of the peripheral glomerular basement membrane resulted in lobules with an abnormal architecture and a noticeable image of stiffness was observed in 60% of the eSMT rats and in 40% of the eSS after 21 months of age. Glomeruli with capsular drops or fibrin cap were not observed either in eSS or eSMT rats. A Kimmelstiel-Wilson-like nodular lesion was detected only in a 18-month-old eSMT male (Fig 2 F). Sporadically, periglomerular fibrosis was observed in eSMT and eSS females.

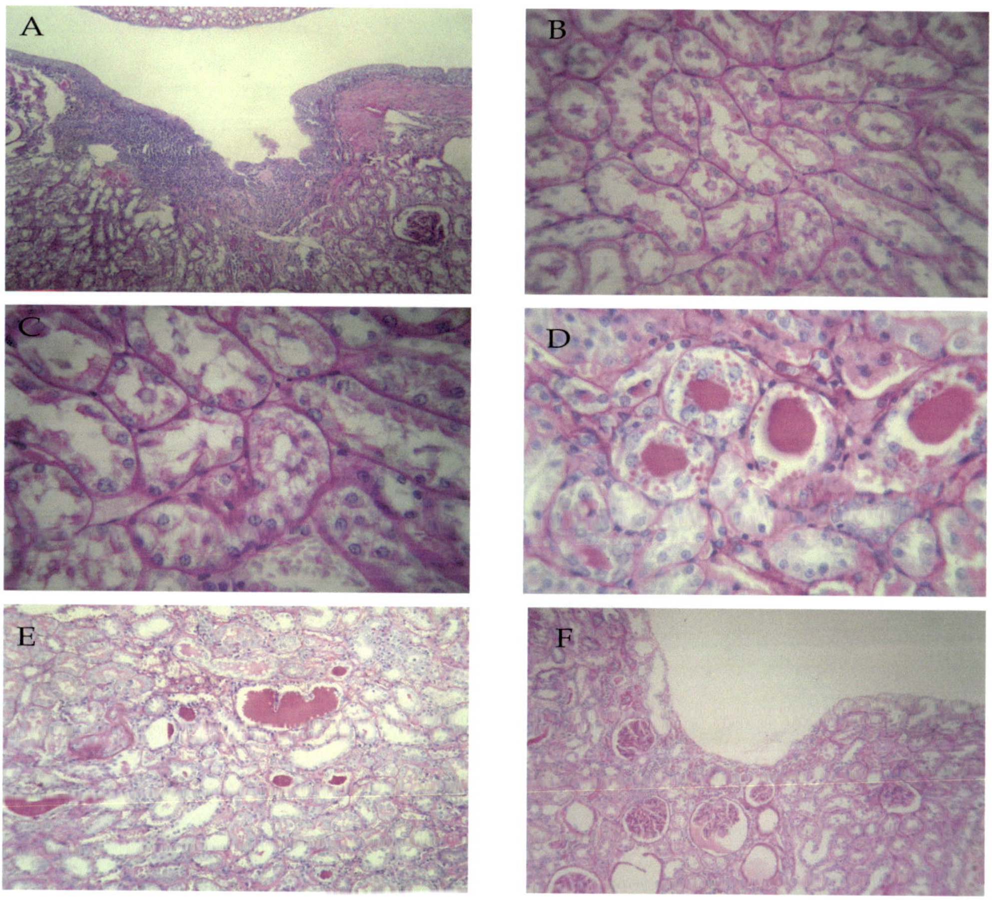

Fig. 3. (A) Intense lymphocytic infiltrate in renal pelvis (18-month-old eSMT female) (40X); (B) Mild tubular lesions (12-month-old eSS female) (300X); (C) Moderate tubular lesions characterized by disgregation of epithelial cells (6-month-old eSMT male) (300X); (D) Group of mildly dilated tubules with lumina containing protein casts (12-month-old eSS male) (300X). (E) Panoramic view of the renal medulla showing different tubular alterations, marked dilatation with protein content (15-month-old eSMT male) (100X); (F) Area of subcapsular retraction due to fibrosis. Parenchymal atrophy and lymphocytic infiltrates (24-month-old eSS male) (40X). HE and Periodic acid-Schiff (PAS) stain.

Areas of arteriolar hyalinosis and thickening of smooth muscle were observed in eSMT males from 9 months, in eSS males and eSMT females from 12 months and in eSS females from 21 month-old.

A few focal interstitial and pyelic mononuclear cell aggregates (Fig 3 A), concomitant with a mild tubular disruption, were apparent in 6-month-old eSS and eSMT males (Fig 3 B and 3 C). Groups of atrophic tubules with their lumina filled by hyaline casts were already noticeable in some 6-month-old eSS and eSMT males, progressing with ageing (Fig 3 D and 3 E). Prominent interstitial fibrosis and tubular atrophy and dilatation with vacuolization and desquamation of tubular cells, were observed in 100% of eSS and eSMT males at 18-24 months of age and older; these features were also detected in some 12-month-old eSS and eSMT females, affecting 80% of 24-month-old individuals. In older animals, subcapsular chronic inflammatory infiltrates, tubular atrophy and fibrosis lead to navel-like retractions of the kidney surface (Fig 3 F).

Renal damage, characterized by diffuse glomerulosclerosis and conspicuous tubular nephrosis, was registered in older eSMT and eSS males. Young eSS females showed the less severe kidney injury.

No changes were observed in glomerular, tubular or interstitial structures of Wistar controls.

4. Discussion and conclusions

Most animal models develop mild renal lesions in early phase diabetes, but not advanced lesions in late phase and even in the best diabetic models, aging is a critical feature in the development of lesions typical of the human DN (Nakagawa, 2009). The relative long-life-span of the eSS and eSMT rats, exceeding their metabolic disturbances, allowed the development of many of the characteristic lesions of diabetic nephropathy. This way, diabetic nephropathy worsened in both lines and sexes during the second year of life. Notwithstanding, results registered in 21-month-old control Wistar males demonstrated that ageing alone was unable to induce either a diabetic syndrome or diabetic renal lesions. It would also be argued that a particularly inherited liability of eSMT line might be an important single factor leading to a more severe renal injury. If so, findings point out that diabetic nephropathy developed as the result of complex interactions between the background genome response, body weight, sex and long-standing metabolic disorders.

Obesity is a very important factor in the beginning and rate of progression of metabolic disturbances and renal chronic complications of type 2 diabetes mellitus, in humans and in experimental models (Price *et al.*, 2002; Nangaku *et al.*, 2005). Even thought eSMT strain is not considered an obese model, these rats are more robust than eSS and this relative overweight has been considered a key factor in the generation of their earlier and more severe hyperglycaemia, hyperlipidaemia and hyperinsulinaemia (Tarrés *et al.*, 2000; Montenegro *et al.*, 2005; Picena *et al.*, 2007). It is important to remark that eSS females, with the lowest body weight, had in turn the minor phenotypic diabetic expression. eSMT females, heavier than eSS females, displayed a more severe diabetic status and showed some glomerular alterations, as reduction in glomerulus's diameter, similar to those found in eSS males.

The degree and duration of hyperglycaemia constitute relevant risk factors regarding the occurrence and severity of renal impairment in people with both Type 1 (Alaveras *et al.*, 1997) and Type 2 Diabetes Mellitus (Ohkubo *et al.*, 1995) as well as in induced diabetic animal models (Kern & Engelman, 1990; Petersen *et al.*, 1988). This way, the greater glucose metabolic disorder in eSS and eSMT males was clearly part of their more severe renal lesions. Several studies have pointed toward an association between sex hormones and the risk of Type 2 Diabetes Mellitus in men and women (Ding *et al.*, 2006). A study in the OLETF rats provided a strong support for this idea by showing that the incidence of Type 2 Diabetes Mellitus was 100% in males and 0% in females (Shi *et al.*, 1994). The higher incidence and severity of nephropathy in Type 2 diabetic male patients and the opposite in women indicate that sex hormones impact in the development and progression of diabetic renal disease by mechanisms yet poorly understood (Maric, 2009). The influence of sex hormones over the eSS diabetic syndrome was studied in rats gonadectomized at 90 days of age (Tarrés *et al.*, 1997). Spayed animals showed higher body weight, early and impaired intolerance to glucose and a decreased number of large pancreatic islets. Despite their lower biomass, castrated males did not evidence impairment in their intolerance to glucose, changes in insulinemia or remarkable modifications in endocrine pancreas histology. Further studies are needed for elucidating the complex interactions between genotype, body weight and sex in the onset of diabetes and the severity of chronic complications in the eSS and eSMT lines.

Transforming growth factor-beta 1 (TGF-beta1) appears to be an important downstream mediator for the development of renal hypertrophy and the accumulation of mesangial extracellular matrix components (Ziyadeh & Wolf, 2008). In the OLETF rats, plasma TGF-beta 1 and vascular TGF-beta type II receptors exist to a greater extent in pre- and early stages of diabetes mellitus when compared with non diabetic rats (Hosomi *et al.*, 2002). Streptozotocin-induced type 2 diabetic rats fed a high fat diet developed a higher proportion of sclerosed glomeruli than type 1 diabetic rats and the expression of CTGF and TGF-beta was significantly increased, despite their lower blood glucose levels and proteinuria (Danda *et al.*, 2005). The connective tissue growth factor (CTGF) is also overexpressed and involving in the pathogenesis of diabetic nephropathy, results from type 2 diabetic ob/ob mice demonstrated that albuminuria strongly correlated with urinary CTGF excretion (Roestenberg *et al.*, 2006). The activated renin-angiotensin system (RAS) has been implicated in the acceleration of diabetic renal disease in type 2 diabetic OLETF rats, as indicated by the long-lasting renoprotective effects of temporary angiotensin II blockage during the prediabetic stage, independent of its effects on glucose metabolism (Nagai *et al.*, 2005). The observation that in the ZDF obese rats reactive oxygen species-associated angiotensinogen enhancement plays an important role in renal damage suggests that reactive oxygen species are partly involved in intrarenal angiotensinogen augmentation, leading to the development of diabetic nephropathy (Kobori *et al.*, 2007).

In summary, mechanisms underlying the development of diabetic nephropathy are extremely complex persisting unclear the nature of the relationship between diabetes and late-onset renal disease. Remain to be clarified whether genetic and environmental factors determining early stages of these disorders are independent from those controlling their progression (Brosius *et al.* 2009; Nobrega, 2009).

The morphological changes in glomeruli of both strains were characterized by basement membrane thickening and diffuse mesangial expansion and, particularly in older eSMT males, by a diffuse or segmental glomerular sclerosis, being exceptional the nodular sclerosis of Kimmelstiel-Wilson. Moreover, it also shows that, even when the principal lesions affected the glomeruli according to the severity of glomerulopathy, the disease extended to the tubulointerstitial compartment. That morphological pattern has been observed in Type 1 diabetic patients (Najafian *et al.*, 2003) and in poorly controlled long-term Type 2 Diabetes Mellitus, ascribed in the Category II of Fioretto et al.'s classification (2008). However, they also suffered from retinopathy, a nonexistent complication in eSS and eSMT rats.

In congruence with Tervaert *et al.* (2010), most of eSS and eSMT animals less than 12-month-old could be classified in Class I (barely evident mesangial lesions) whilst rats exceeding 12 months of age could belong to Class II (diffuse mesangial glomerulosclerosis with moderate to severe expansion of mesangium). It is noteworthy to outline that although the naturally slower progress of the metabolic derangement in eSS males with respect to the eSMT, almost all males over 18 months of age in both lines could be classified as Class IV (advanced glomerulosclerosis). Even though, lesions compatible with Class III (nodular sclerosis or presence of one Kimmelstiel-Wilson nodule at least) were detected in only one 18-month-old eSMT male rat. This single finding makes it exceptional and fits with other spontaneous diabetic murine models (Yuzawa *et al.*, 2008).

It has been reported that nodular glomerulosclerosis is present in diabetic patients with more progressed clinical and pathological features (Jang & Park, 2009). Nevertheless, other authors have sustained that diffuse and nodular sclerosis could be two discrete patterns of glomerulopathy caused by different pathophysiological mechanisms as Kimmelstiel-Wilson lesion correlates with diabetic retinopathy but most of Type 2 diabetic patients without retinopathy develop diffuse mesangial sclerosis (Schwartz *et al.*, 1998). Interestingly, no lesions of retinopathy have ever been detected in either eSS or in eSMT rats (Tarrés *et al.*, 1990; Tarrés *et al.*, 2000; Picena *et al.*, 2005). Moreover, although retinopathy and microalbuminuria are positively associated in Type 1 diabetic patients, the substantial discordances between glomerulopathy and retinopathy reported in Type 2 Diabetes Mellitus (Kanauchi *et al.*, 1998; Boelter *et al.*, 2006) highlights that kidney and retina are distinct organs with diverse underlying pathophysiologic mechanisms (Blum *et al.*, 2011). Further studies on the eSS and eSMT lines rats could be useful for studying the aforesaid differences.

Renal enlargement, particularly perceptible in eSMT males via the increase in kidney weights and diffuse mesangial expansion, evokes early stages of diabetic nephropathy. Notwithstanding, the areas of tubular atrophy detected in some eSS and particularly in the eSMT males at ~6 month, suggest a more advanced phase of diabetic nephropathy. Moreover, progression to macroalbuminuria and uremia already demonstrated in eSS male rats from 6 to 12 months of age in eSS males (Daniele *et al.*, 2000), may be correlated with the increasing loss of glomerular filtration rate accompanying each nephron sclerosis during the progression of diabetic nephropathy. While hyperglycaemia-induced osmotic polyuria has been implied as a relevant role in the onset and evolution of tubulointerstitial injury by causing an early tubular cell injury in the dilated collecting ducts (Wang *et al.*, 2008), careful attention should be paid in the persistent glycosuria detected in eSS and eSMT rats (Martínez *et al.*, 1988, Montenegro *et al.*, 2005). Moreover, the differences found between diabetic rats and Wistar controls as well as between both diabetic lines in superficial and juxtamedullary glomeruli glucidic residues and in convoluted proximal tubules ones could be indicative of alterations in the filtration and in the intracellular tubular processes (Frontini *et al.*, 2008).

As suggested by Murata *et al.*, 2002 in the Otsuka Long-Evans Tokushima Fatty (OLEFT) rats, we guess that the phenomenon of apoptosis could be operating at glomerular level in eSS and eSMT males which displayed a noticeable and increasing number of smaller glomeruli as they get older. Furthermore, apoptosis induced by chronic hyperglycaemia has been related by Picena *et al*, (2007) with the dramatic reduction of the area of the islets of Langerhans described in older eSS males by Gomez Dumm *et al.*, (1989). In diabetic nephropathy, the degree of proteinuria correlates with the progression of glomerulosclerosis and tubulointerstitial fibrosis (Wolf & Ziyadeh, 2007). The early albuminuria from 24-hs collections, the loss of glomerular filtration rate in 6-month-old eSS males and the progression to macroalbuminuria and uremia from 6 to 12 months of age (Daniele *et al.*, 2000), could be due to an increasing number of glomeruli affected associated to the progressive worsening of glucose and lipid disorders, particularly the rising values of hyperglycaemia, triglycerides, non-esterified fatty acids, total cholesterol, and low-density lipoprotein cholesterol with high- density lipoprotein-cholesterol reduced, demonstrated in this strain at 12 month of age (Daniele *et al.*, 2010). Previous studies in humans and animals have also suggested that altered lipid metabolism causes glomerular injury and promotes deterioration of glomerular function (Diamond & Karnovsky, 1987; Kasiske *et al.*, 1988; Maric *et al.*, 2004).

In humans, oxidative stress is linked to multiple chronic diabetic complications (Giacco & Brownlee, 2010). It is increasingly evident that changes in cellular function resulting in oxidative stress play a key role in the development and progression of diabetic nephropathy (Forbes *et al.*, 2008). Moreover, oxidized low density lipoprotein particles and non-esterified fatty acids could damage the mesangial cells and the tubulointerstitial tissue through different pathogenetic mechanisms (Nosadini & Tonolo, 2011). Interestingly, in 12 month-old eSS rats increased basal glycaemia and fructosamine values correlate with those of lipid peroxidation substances and inversely with total antioxidant capacity (Daniele *et al.*, 2007).

In agreement with the data in diabetic patients and in other experimental diabetic models, and taking into account that hyperlipidaemia and oxidative stress have been syndicated as having major roles in the pathogenesis of the diabetic nephropathy (Kume *et al.*, 2008), we suggest that early hyperinsulinemia and lipid disorders, already demonstrated in eSS rats (Montanaro *et al.*, 2003. Daniele *et al.*, 2010) and in eSMT rats (Tarrés MC *et al.*, 2000) as well as the oxidative stress previously verified in eSS male rats (Daniele *et al.*, 2007), are key players in the development of the diabetic nephropathy in eSS and eSMT rats. Though new experiments could be undertaken in eSS and eSMT rats to brighten the genesis and evolution of their nephropathy, we conclude that these two spontaneously diabetic rats closely resemble the advanced human diabetic nephropathy and, simultaneously, have opened valuable opportunities for enhance our understanding about the interactions between glucose and lipid disorders and the pathways towards diabetic nephropathy, a relevant cause of morbidity and mortality in the diabetic population and the leading cause of end-stage renal failure in the Western World.

5. Acknowledgments

The authors are grateful to the School of Medicine, National University of Rosario, for financial support and to Wiener Laboratories for the their invaluable contribution of commercial kits

6. References

Alaveras, AE; Thomas, SM; Sagriotis, A *et al.* (1997). Diabetic Nephropathy: Diagnosis, Prevention, and Treatment: Evaluation of Patients With Diabetic Nephropathy. *Nephrol Dial transplant* 12, Suppl. 2, 71-74, ISSN 0931-0509

American Diabetic Association (ADA) (2009). Diagnosis and Classification of Diabetes Mellitus. *Diabetes Care* 32, Suppl.1, S62-S67, ISSN 0149-5992

Blum, M; Saemann, A & Wolf, G (2011). The eye, the kidney and microcirculation Editorial Comments. *Nephrol Dial Transplant* 26, 1, 4–6, ISSN 0931-0509

Boelter, MC; Gross; JL; Canani LH *et al.* (2006). Proliferative diabetic nephropathy with microalbuminuria in patients with type 2 diabetes. *Braz J Med Biol Res* 39, 8, 1033–1039, ISSN 0100-879X

Breyer, MD; Bottinger, EP; Brosius, FC *et al.* (2005). Mouse models of diabetic nephropathy. *J Am Soc Nephrol* 16, 1, 27–45, ISSN 1046-6673

Brosius, FC; Alpers, CE; Bottinger, EP *et al.* (2009) Mouse models of diabetic nephropathy. *J Am Soc Nephrol* 20, 12, 2503-2512, ISSN 1046-6673

Caballero, AE & Tenzer, P (2007). Building cultural competency for improved diabetes care: Latino Americans and diabetes. *J Fam Pract* 56, 9, S29-S37, ISSN 0094-3509

Calderari, SA; Gonzalez, AC & Gayol, MD (1987). Spontaneous hypertriglyceridemic obesity and hyperglycaemia in an inbred line of rats. *Int J Obes* 11, 6, 571-579, ISSN 0307-0565

Calderari, SA; Font, MT; Garrocq, O *et al.* (1991). The inbred IIM/Fm stock. *Rat News Let* 25, 1, 28-29. ISSN 0309-1848

Chatzigeorgiou, A; Halapas, A; Kalafatakis, K *et al.* (2009). The use of animal models in the study of diabetes mellitus. *In Vivo* 23, 2, 245-258, ISSN 0258-851X

Danda, RS; Habiba, NM; Rincon-Choles, H; Bhandari, BK et al. (2005). Kidney involvement in a nongenetic rat model of type 2 diabetes. *Kidney International 68, 6,* 2562–2571 ISSN 0085-2538

Daniele, S; Arriaga, S; Martínez, SM *et al.* (2000). Onset and evolution of nephropathy in rats with spontaneous diabetes mellitus. *J Physiol Biochem* 56, 1, 45-54, ISSN 1138-7548

Daniele, SM; Picena, JC; Montenegro, SM *et al.* (2007). Hígado graso no alcohólico en ratas machos de una línea con diabetes genética. *Electron J Biomed 7,* 3, 29-39, ISSN 1697-090X

Daniele, SM; Montenegro, SM; Tarrés, MC *et al.* (2010). The eSS rat, a nonobese model of disordered glucose and lipid metabolism and fatty liver. *Diabetol Metabol Syndr* 2, 3, 1-5, ISSN 1758-5996

Diamond, J & Karnovsky, M. (1987) Exacerbation of chronic aminonucleoside nephrosis by dietary cholesterol supplementation. *Kidney Int* 32, 5, 671–678, ISSN 0085-2538

Ding, EL; Song, Y; Malik, VS *et al.* (2006). Sex differences of endogenous sex hormones and risk of type 2 diabetes: a systematic review and metaanalysis. *JAMA* 295, 11, 1288–1299, ISSN 0098748

Dronavalli, S & Barkis GL (2008). Mechanistic Insights into Diuretic-Induced Insulin Resistance. *Hypertension* 52, 6, 1009-1011, ISSN 0194911X

Fioretto, P; Caramori, ML & Mauer, M (2008). The kidney in diabetes: dynamic pathways of injury and repair. The Camillo Golgi Lecture. *Diabetologia* 51, 8, 1347-1355, ISSN 0012-186X

Forbes, JM; Coughlan, MT & Cooper, ME (2008). Oxidative stress as a major culprit in kidney disease in diabetes. *Diabetes* 57, 6, 1446-1154, ISSN 0012-1797

Frontini, AV; Hisano, N & D'Ottavio, AE (2008). La densidad óptica aplicada al estudio lectinhistoquímico de radicales glucídicos néfricos en ratas diabéticas tipo 2. *Electron J Biomed* 6, 1, 36-44, ISSN 1697-090X

Giacco, F & Brownlee, M (2010). Oxidative stress and diabetic complications. *Circ Res* 29, 107, 1058-1070, ISSN 0009-7330

Gomez Dumm, CL; Semino, MC & Gagliardino, JJ (1990). Sequential morphological changes in pancreatic islets of spontaneously diabetic rats. *Pancreas* 5, 5, 533-539, ISSN 0885-3177

Hisano, N; D'Ottavio, AE & Calderari, SA (1994). Female reproductive profile in a fertile genetically obese line of rats. *J Exp Zool* 270, 5, 486-490, ISSN 1932-5223

Hosomi, N; Noma, T; Ohyama H & *et al.* (2002). Vascular proliferation and transforming growth factor-beta expression in pre- and early stage of diabetes mellitus in Otsuka Long-Evans Tokushima fatty rats. *Atherosclerosis* 162, 1, 69-76 ISSN 0021-9150

Hudkins, KL; Pichaiwong, W, *et al.* (2010). Ob/Ob mutant mice model progressive diabetic nephropathy. *J Am Soc Nephrol* 21, 9, 1533-1542, ISSN 1046-6673

Jang, SH & Park, MH (2009). The morphologic patterns of diabetic nephropathy in Koreans. *Korean J Pathol* 43, 1, 36-42, ISSN 1738-1843

Janssen, U; Phillips, AO & Floege, J (1999). Rodent models of nephropathy associated with type II diabetes. *J Nephrol 12*, 3, 159-172, ISSN 1121-8428

Kanauchi, M; Kawano, T; Uyama H *et al.* (1998). Discordance between retinopathy and nephropathy in type 2 diabetes. *Nephron 80, 2, 171–174,* ISSN 0028-2766

Kasiske, B; Cleary, M; O'Donnell, M *et al.* (1988). Mechanisms of glomerular injury in the obese Zucker rat. *Kidney Int* 33, 3, 667–672, ISSN 0085-2538

Kern, TS & Engelman, RL (1990). Arrest of glomerulopathy in diabetic dogs by improved glycaemic control. *Diabetologia 33,* 522-525, ISSN: 0012-186X

Kobori, H; Ozawa, Y; Suzaki, Y; Prieto-Carrasquero, MC (2006). Intratubular angiotensinogen in hypertension and kidney Diseases. *Am J Hypertens* 19, 5, 541–550 ISSN 0895-7061

Kume, S; Uzu, T; Isshiki TK *et al* (2008). Peroxisome proliferator-activated receptors in diabetic nephropathy (Review Article). *PPAR Res 4, 7, 1-11,* ISSN 1687- 4765

Lee, G (2003). End - stage renal disease in the Asian - Pacific region *Semin Nephrol 23, 1,* 107-114, ISSN 0270-9295

Maric, C; Sandberg, K & Hinojosa-Laborde, C (2004). Glomerulosclerosis and tubulo-interstitial fibrosis are attenuated with 17-ß estradiol in the aging Dahl salt-sensitive rat. *J Am Soc Nephrol* 15, 6, 1546-1556, ISSN 1046-6673

Maric, C (2009). Sex, diabetes and the kidneys. *Am J Physiol-Renal Physiol* 296, 4, F680-F688, ISSN 0363-6127

Martínez, SM; Tarrés, MC; Montenegro, SM *et al* (1988). Spontaneous diabetes in eSS rats. *Acta diabetol lat* 25, 4, 303-313, ISSN 0001-5563

Martínez, SM; Tarrés, MC; Picena, JC *et al* (1993). eSS rat, an animal model for the study of spontaneous non-insulin-dependent diabetes, In: *Lessons from Animal Diabetes IV*. E Shafrir, Ed. Smith-Gordon, 75-90, ISBN 1854630075, London, UK

Montanaro, M; Rimoldi, OJ; Igal, RA *et al.* (2003). Hepatic Δ9, Δ6 and Δ5 Desaturations in the Non-Insulin Dependent Diabetic Mellitus eSS Rats. *Lipids* 38, 8, 827-832, ISSN 0024-4201

Montenegro, SM; Tarrés, MC; Picena, JC *et al.* (2005). Conducta alimentaria y perfil glucémico en dos modelos murinos de diabetes genética: eSS y eSMT. *Biomédica* 25, 4, 441-450, ISSN 0120-4157

Murata, I; Takemura, G; Asano, A *et al.* (2002). Apoptotic cell loss following cell proliferation in renal glomeruli of Otsuka Long-Evans Tokushima Fatty rats, a model of type 2 diabetes. *Am J Nephrol* 22, 5-6, 587-595, ISSN 0250-8095

Nagai, Y; Yao, L; Kobori, H *et al.*, (2005). Temporary Angiotensin II blockade at the prediabetic stage attenuates the development of renal injury in Type 2 diabetic rats. *J Am Soc Nephrol* 16, 3, 703–711 ISSN 1046-6673

Najafian, B; Kim, Y; Crosson, JT *et al.* (2003). Atubular glomeruli and glomerulotubular junction abnormalities in diabetic nephopathy. *J Am Soc Nephrol* 14, 4, 908-917, ISSN 1046-6673

Nakagawa, T (2009). A new mouse model resembling human diabetic nephropathy: uncoupling of VEGF with eNOS as a novel pathogenic mechanism. *Clin Nephrol* 71, 2, 103-9, ISSN 0301-0430

Nangaku, M; Izuhara, Y; Usuda, N *et al.* (2005). In a type 2 diabetic nephropathy rat model, the improvement of obesity by a low calorie diet reduces oxidative/carbonyl stress and prevents diabetic nephropathy. *Nephrol Dial. Transplant* 20, 12, 2661-2669, ISSN 0931- 0509

Nobrega, MA; Solberg Woods, LS; Fleming, S; Jacob, HJ (2009). Distinct genetic regulation of progression of diabetes and renal disease in the Goto-Kakizaki rat. *Physiol Genomics* 39: 38–46 ISSN 1531-2267

Nosadini, R & Tonolo, G. (2011). Role of oxidized low density lipoproteins and free fatty acids in the pathogenesis of glomerulopathy and tubulointerstitial lesions in type 2 diabetes. *Nutr Metab Cardiovasc Dis* 21, 2, 79-85, ISSN 0939-4753

Ohkubo, Y; Kishikawa, H; Araki, E *et al.* (1995). Intensive insulin therapy prevents the progression of diabetic microvascular complications in Japanese patients with non-insulin-dependent diabetes mellitus: a randomized prospective 6-year study. *Diabetes Res Clin Pract* 28, 2, 103-117, ISSN 0168-8227

Petersen, J; Ross, J & Rabkin, R (1988). Effect of insulin therapy on established diabetic nephropathy in rats. *Diabetes* 37, 10, 1346-1350, ISSN 0012-1797

Picena, JC; Daniele, SM; Tarrés, MC *et al.* (2005). An animal model fits for studying divergences among diabetic microvascular complications. *Electron J Biomed* 3, 2, 39-43, ISSN 1697-090X

Picena, JC; Montenegro, SM; Tarrés, MC *et al.* (2007). Modificaciones dinámicas en los islotes de Langerhans de dos líneas de ratas espontáneamente diabéticas: eSS y eSMT. *Medicina (B Aires)* 67, 4, 331-340, ISSN 0025-7680

Price, DA; Lansang, MC; Osey, SY *et al.* (2002). Type 2 diabetes, obesity and the renal response to blocking the renin system with irbesartan. *Diabetic Med* 19, 10, 858-861, ISSN 0742-3071

Roestenberg, P; van Nieuwenhoven, FA; Joles, JA; Trischberger, C *et al*, (2006). Temporal expression profile and distribution pattern indicate a role of connective tissue growth factor (CTGF/CCN-2) in diabetic nephropathy in mice. *Am J Physiol Renal Physiol 290, 6,* F1344-1354 ISSN 1522-1466

Schwartz, MM; Lewis, EJ; Leonard-Martin, T *et al.* (1998). Renal pathology patterns in type II diabetes mellitus: relationship with retinopathy. The Collaborative Study Group. *Nephrol Dial. Transplant.* 13, 10, 2547-2552, ISSN 0931- 0509

Shi, K; Mizuno, A; Sano, T *et al.* (1994). Sexual difference in the incidence of diabetes mellitus in Otsuka-Long-Evans-Tokushima-Fatty rats: effects of castration and sex hormone replacement on its incidence. *Metabolism* 43, 10, 1214–1220, ISSN 0026-0495

SPSS (2006). IBM SPSS Statistics, 15.0.1 version, SPSS Inc, New York, USA

Srinivasan, K & Ramarao, P (2007). Animal models in type 2 diabetes research: an overview. *Indian J Med Res* 125, 3, 451-472, ISSN 0971-5916

Stewart, JH; McCredie, MR; Williams, SM *et al.* (2006). The enigma of hypertensive ESRD: observations on incidence and trends in 18 European, Canadian, and Asian-Pacific populations, 1998 to 2002. *Am J Kidney Dis* 48, 2, 183-191, ISSN 0272-6386

Tarrés, MC; Martínez, SM; Montenegro, SM *et al.* (1990). Relación entre dieta, biomasa y expresión de la diabetes en la rata eSS. *Medicina (Buenos Aires)* 50, 3, 235-243, ISSN 0025-7680

Tarrés, MC; Martínez, SM; Montenegro, SM *et al.* (1992). The eSS rat: A new model of non-insulin-dependent human diabetes. *Am J Pathol* 141, 3, 761-763, ISSN 0002-9440

Tarrés, MC; Martínez, SM; Montenegro, SM *et al.* (1997). Influence of gonadectomy in eSS diabetic rats. *J Physiol Biochem* 53, 2, 211-216, ISSN 1138-7548

Tarrés, MC; Montenegro, S; Martínez, SM *et al.* (2000). The eSMT rat: a murine model of type 2 human diabetes. Chapter: Animal models in the study of human diseases, In: *Animal Research and Welfare. A Partnership. Proceedings of the International Joint Meeting between 12th ICLAS General Assembly & Conference and the 7th Felasa Symposium.* Laboratory Animals Ltd., 93-94, ISBN: 0-901334-13-8. London, UK

Tervaert, TW; Mooyaart, AL; Amann, K *et al.* (2010) Pathologic classification of diabetic nephropathy. *J Am Soc Nephrol* 21, 4, 556-563, ISSN 1046-6673

Tesch, GH & Allen, TJ (2007). Rodent models of streptozotocin-induced diabetic nephropathy. *Nephrology* (Carlton) 12, 3, 261-266, ISSN1320-5358

U.S Renal Data System (USRDS) (2008). Annual Data Report: Atlas of Chronic Kidney Disease and End-Stage Renal Disease in the United States, National Institutes of Health, National Institute of Diabetes and Digestive and Kidney Diseases. Bethesda, MD. 2, Précis, 29-33

U.S Renal Data System (USRDS) (2010). Annual Data Report: Atlas of Chronic Kidney Disease and End-Stage Renal Disease in the United States, National Institutes of Health, National Institute of Diabetes and Digestive and Kidney Diseases, Bethesda, MD. 2, Précis, 209-222

Villar, E & Zaoui, P (2010). Diabetes and chronic kidney disease: Lessons from renal epidemiology. *Nephrol Ther* 6, 7, 585-590, ISSN 1769-7255

Wang, S; Mitu, GM & Hirschberg, R (2008). Osmotic polyuria: an overlooked mechanism in diabetic nephropathy. *Nephrol Dial Transplant* 23, 7, 2167-2172, ISSN 0931- 0509

Wolf, G & Ziyadeh, FN (2007). Cellular and molecular mechanisms of proteinuria in diabetic nephropathy. *Nephron Physiol* 106, 2, 26-31, ISSN 1660-2137

Yuzawa, Y; Niki, I, Kosugi, T *et al.* (2008). Overexpression of Calmodulin in Pancreatic β Cells Induces Diabetic Nephropathy. *J Am Soc Nephrol* 19, 9. 1701-1711, ISSN 1046-6673

Ziyadeh, FN & Wolf, G (2008). Pathogenesis of the podocytopathy and proteinuria in diabetic glomerulopathy. *Curr Diabetes Rev* 4, 1, 39-45 ISSN 1573-3998

Zimmet, P; Alberti, KGM & Shaw, J (2001). Global and societal implications of the diabetic epidemic. *Nature* 414, 12, 782-787, ISSN 0028-0836

Part 4

Diverse Organ Involvement/Dysfunction in Diabetes

17

Pathogenic Features of Insulin Resistance and Critical Organ Damage in the Liver, Muscle and Lung

Kei Nakajima[1], Toshitaka Muneyuki[2], Masafumi Siato[1] and Masafumi Kakei[2]
[1]*Division of Clinical Nutrition, Department of Medical Dietetics Faculty of Pharmaceutical Sciences Josai University, Sakado*
[2]*First Department of Comprehensive Medicine, Saitama Medical Center Jichi Medical University School of Medicine, Omiya Japan*

1. Introduction

1.1 Overall pathogenic features of insulin resistance

Over the last two decades, type 2 diabetes and metabolic syndrome (MetS) have been increasing worldwide in concert with an increasing obesity pandemic [Grundy, 2005; Kopelman, 2007; Dixon, 2010]. In particular, abdominal obesity predisposes to development of type 2 diabetes and MetS through the pathogenic feature of insulin resistance, mostly accompanied by hyperinsulinemia to compensate for impairment of insulin action, especially in the early stage of these diseases [Bartnik, 2007]. In addition to genetic background, generally unfavorable lifestyles, such as smoking, infrequent exercise, sedentary working, overeating, and unbalanced nutrition provoke insulin resistance and cause progress in cooperation with obesity [Grundy, 2005; Kopelman, 2007; Bartnik, 2007; American Diabetes Association, 2010]. Once excess abdominal obesity is present, numerous cytokines, chemokines, and free fatty acids (FFA) are secreted from hypertrophic visceral fat as well as trunk subcutaneous fat, leading to deterioration of such pathogenicity [Capeau, 2008; Meshkani, 2009; Gustafson, 2010]. Type 2 diabetes and MetS have emerged as major public health problems as comorbid conditions not only with microvascular disease but also with macrovascular disease [Grundy, 2005; Kopelman, 2007; Dixon, 2010; Bartnik, 2007; American Diabetes Association, 2010]. Because insulin resistance and resultant hyperinsulinemia are a pivotal pathophysiology, these etiologies simultaneously contribute to hypertension, dyslipidemia (increased triglycerides and decreased high-density lipoprotein cholesterol), and hyperuricemia in a complex manner, in addition to causing abnormal glucose metabolism [Grundy, 2005; Kopelman, 2007; Dixon, 2010; Bartnik, 2007; American Diabetes Association, 2010].

Currently, insulin resistance is not limited to traditional insulin-sensitive tissues and organs such as skeletal muscle; it also affects other critical organs such as the kidney [Kubo, 1999; Chen, 2003; Guarnieri, 2010] or possibly the lung [Kaparianos, 2008; Klein, 2010; Fimognari, 2010], which are involved in the development of cardiovascular diseases and impaired quality of life. In addition, glucose and FFA as fundamental energy substrates are closely related to each other; this relationship was originally conceptualized as the "glucose-fatty acid cycle" by Randle et al. half a century ago [Randle, 1963]. Therefore, clinicians in different fields, including cardiology, lipidology, and hepatology, and clinical scientists should be aware of the pathophysiology of insulin resistance, extending far beyond the narrow range of clinical diabetology, for the prevention, care and improvement of critical diseases comprising microvascular and macrovascular diseases, and organ damage.

1.2 Effect of hyperinsulinemia

It is unknown whether the insulin resistance exerts similar effects in all tissues and organs. Hyperinsulinemia per se has substantial effects on many tissues and organs because in addition to precise regulation of glucose metabolism, insulin has pleiotropic actions. These actions are mostly anabolic properties, leading to storage of lipids and glucose substrates, and increased protein synthesis and cell proliferation and growth, which are activated via the MAP kinase pathway [Meshkani, 2009; Godsland, 2009]. However, these often result in adverse outcomes such as vascular endothelial thickening, polycystic ovary syndrome, and provoking latent cancers as well as acanthosis nigricans, a skin lesion characterized by thickened and hyperpigmented plaques around the neck [Harwood, 2007; Higgins, 2008]. Furthermore, insulin has been shown to have antinatriuretic actions (Na^+ reabsorption by the kidney and circulating volume retention) and enhanced sympathetic nervous system activation, eventually resulting in elevated blood pressure, which is one of the components of MetS. Notably, chronic hyperinsulinemia in turn deteriorates insulin resistance in tissues originally sensitive to insulin because the insulin receptor is downregulated by a feedback mechanism or is degraded along with insulin [Capeau, 2008].

1.3 Progression of insulin resistance

As shown in **Figure 1** [Laakso, 2003], the amount of circulating insulin, i.e., hyperinsulinemia, normal insulinemia, or hypoinsulinemia, can interfere with the effects of insulin resistance in the progression of type 2 diabetes and MetS, with varying degrees of glucose toxicity and/or lipotoxicity. However, insulin resistance will continue to progress unless the individual improves an unhealthy life style and abdominal obesity, regardless of an irreversible and progressive decline in insulin secretion.

Type 2 diabetes has a strong genetic component [American Diabetes Association, 2010]. Of note, the prevalence of impaired glucose tolerance is high in many Asian countries [Sharma, 2010]. Therefore, a strong gene-environmental interaction may be one of the causes for the rapidly increasing rate of diabetes, especially in Asians, who are now becoming accustomed to an unhealthy lifestyle [Sharma, 2010]. Among the Asian peoples, particularly the Japanese, they show a lower insulin secretory capacity after glucose loading, suggesting a smaller potential for pancreatic beta cell function than in Western people [Kaku, 2010]. Furthermore, most Asians also have a genetic background of the "thrifty gene", including specific polymorphisms of peroxisome proliferator-activated receptor (PPAR), beta 3-adrenagic receptor, and ucp- 1 [Hara, 2000; Kahara, 2002].

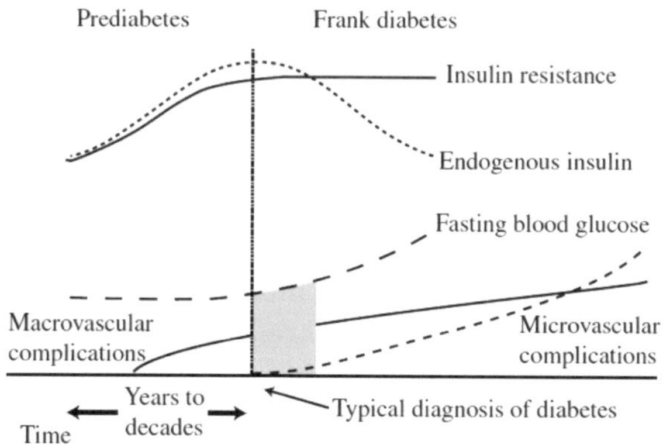

Fig. 1. Insulin resistance, impaired insulin secretion, and fasting glucose in relation to micro- and macrovascular diseases (Laakso, 2003).

Worldwide, it is unknown which factor factors occur first, insulin resistance or insulin deficiency. People with type 2 diabetes probably have both conditions in varying degrees. In this chapter, we discuss the pathophysiology of insulin resistance and organ damage (liver, muscle, and lung) particularly in the stages of hyperinsulinemia with mild glycemia, where restrict more stringent glucose control soon after diagonosis of diabetes is important for the so called "legacy effect" long-term legacy effect that is known as long-term reduction of myocardial infarction and all-cause mortality in intensive treatment cohort as compared to the standard arm after further 10-years follow up UKPDS [Chalmers, 2008; Murray, 2010].

1.4 Common mechanisms of multiple organ damage in relation to insulin resistance

Common mechanisms of organ damage that relate to insulin resistance appear to be dyslipidemia, abnormal glucose metabolism, subtle inflammation, oxidative status, low blood flow systemically as well as locally because of reduced nitric oxide (NO) synthesis, and hypertension, most of which enhance the renin-angiotensin-aldosterone system (RAAS) and Rho/Rho kinase signaling, which attenuate microvessel function in many organs [Capeau, 2008; Meshkani, 2009; Gustafson,2010; Lastra, 2010; Choi, 2010]. Several animal and cellular studies have shown that activation of the RAAS as well as Rho/Rho kinase signaling is associated with impaired insulin signaling and insulin resistance in most organs, including the liver, muscle, and kidney [Choi, 2010; Lastra, 2006].

Regarding abnormal glucose metabolism, euglycemia or mild hyperglycemia with resultant hyperinsulinemia is observed in the early stage of type 2 diabetes, whereas reduced insulin secretion and chronic hyperglycemia with lasting insulin resistance is still observed in advanced stages [Bartnik, 2007; American Diabetes Association, 2010]. Specific mechanisms according to organs (liver, muscle, and lung) are described in the following sections. The effects of insulin on cell metabolism are mediated by binding of insulin to its receptor on the cell surface, leading to phosphorylation of tyrosine residues, followed by the activation of phosphatidylinositol 3-kinase (PI 3-kinase) [Liu, 2010; Tatoń, 2010; Tarantino, 2010]. The main receptor is insulin receptor substrate (IRS), which has four isoforms (IRS1-4). Many organs and tissues have both IRS-1 and IRS-2 with different actions [Tatoń, 2010; Tarantino, 2010]. IRS-3 is mainly involved in adipocytes and IRS-4 is involved in the kidney/thalamus. Insulin resistance appears to occur at the receptor level by the inhibition of receptor tyrosine kinase activity, although a relatively reduced number of insulin receptors on the cell surface may also affect insulin resistance. Because a comprehensive description of insulin resistance in all organs is beyond the scope of this review, we will highlight major organ damage (liver and muscle) as well as the emerging field of the lung.

2. Insulin resistance and liver and skeletal muscle

It is now commonly accepted that in addition to critical immune functions such as natural killer cells and digestive function such as formation of bile acid as well as actions of detoxification, the liver plays a central role in regulating systemic metabolism, including protein, carbohydrate, and lipid metabolism, all of which are under close control by a series of hormones secreted from various organs [Tarantino, 2010]. Of these hormones, in particular, circulating insulin substantially interferes with these hepatic functions and systemic metabolism [Capeau …] 2008; Meshkani, 2009; Gustafson, 2010; Lastra, 2010; Choi, 2010; Liu, 2010; Tatoń, 2010; Tarantino, 2010; Samuel, 2010].
Originally, simple steatosis, i.e., fatty liver, was thought to remain benign throughout life. However, currently, fatty liver or so called non-alcoholic fatty liver disease (NAFLD) and its worsened condition, non-alcoholic steatohepatitis (NASH), have been emerging as one of the conditions that cause critical organ damage in the general population, mostly accompanied by type 2 diabetes and MetS [Capeau, 2008; Meshkani, 2009; Liu, 2010]. Similar to other lifestyle-related diseases, most people with NAFLD remain untreated with few or no symptoms until a blood test or abdominal ultrasound are conducted in the clinical setting. Generally, serum hepatic enzymes, especially alanine aminotransferase, are often elevated beyond the normal range [Schindhelm, 2006; Chang, 2007; Ghouri, 2010]. However, these hepatic enzymes occasionally remain within the normal ranges [Chang, 2007] and are overlooked until an abdominal ultrasound test is performed. Importantly, NASH may occasionally progress to cirrhosis (10-15%) and rarely to hepatic cancer after several decades [Estep, 2010]. NAFLD generally follows the presence of abdominal hypertrophic fat cells in clinical practice. Plausible main causes are direct influx via the portal vein of FFA (long chain FFA), glycerol, and proinflammatory cytokines comprising tumor necrosis factor (TNF)-α, interleukin (IL)-6, and IL-1 from visceral and upper body fat, which follow insulin resistance at visceral fat tissues by activating hormone sensitive lipase and adipose tissue triacylglycerol lipase [Capeau, 2008; Meshkani, 2009; Gustafson, 2010; Nakajima, 2010].

2.1 FFA metabolism in hepatic cells

Chronically elevated fatty acids can impair the function of pancreatic β-cells [Bollheimer, 1998]. In addition, elevated fatty acids enter hepatic cells via fatty acid transporter protein CD 36 and fatty-acid-binding protein [Makowski, 2004], providing a major amount of FFA, which are converted into triglycerides (TG) and secreted by the liver in the form of very low density lipoprotein (VLDL). FFAs from lipolysis of adipose fat account for approximately 60% of the total FFA in the liver [Donnelly, 2005]. In contrast, chylomicron, an exogenous triglyceride-rich lipoprotein synthesized from the diet in the intestine, enters the circulation via the thoracic duct after being absorbed into the lymph duct, and eventually is taken up through remnant receptors by the liver, and this accounts for 15% of the total FFA in the liver. The rest of the FFAs are those newly synthesized by the liver. Therefore, theoretically, a substantial improvement of NAFLD and NASH would not occur until body fat is substantially reduced. FFA has lipotoxic effects and exerts hepatic injury, whereas TG formation, which may be less toxic, is protective in hepatic cells [Capeau, 2008; Tarantino, 2010; Cnop, 2001]. These FFAs do not develop significant metabolic disturbances as long as they are successfully oxidized in well-functioning mitochondria in target tissues. Consistently, in the early stage of NAFLD, fat accumulation in the form of TG with intact β-oxidation is considered to be rather benign and is called the "first hit" stage. However, excess β-oxidation increases reactive oxygen species (ROS), and this is considered to provoke the so called "second hit" process to NASH [Gentile, 2008; Tessari, 2009]. Insufficient action of superoxide dismutase, which neutralizes superoxide free radicals, may contribute to increased ROS in the cytosol [Faraci, 2004; Miao, 2009]. Increased ROS in turn activates the immune system and hepatocytes and stellate cells, followed by increased collagen synthesis and transforming growth factor secretion, resulting in development and progression of hepatic fibrosis [Gressner, 2008; Matsuzaki, 2009].

2.2 FFA metabolites and impairment of insulin signaling

Excess long-chain fatty acyl CoAs, diacylglycerol (DAG), and FFA metabolites cause IRS-1 serine phosphorylation via protein kinase C (PKC), thereby inhibiting the PI 3-kinase pathway [Shulman, 2000]. In this situation, inhibition of FOXO1 via Akt does not occur, resulting in increased glyconeogenesis and reduced glycogen synthesis [Sharma, 2010], because glucose enters the liver through glucose transporter GLUT2, which is always present at the cell membrane, independent of insulin action. TNF-α inhibits insulin signal transduction by activating Jun kinase and IKKβ, which cause serine phosphorylation of IRS [Gustafson, 2010; Shulman, 2000; Popa, 2007].

With regard to glucose metabolism, the liver appears to play a pivotal role because liver IRS knockout mice show systemic insulin resistance, whereas muscle IRS knockout mice do not have insulin resistance, regardless of increased fat mass and circulating fatty acids [Brüning, 1998; Kim, 2000]. Nevertheless, controversy still remains because extra-hepatic IRS2 dependent mechanisms may be involved in the regulation of glucose homeostasis [Simmgen, 2006].

Under most conditions, hepatic insulin resistance and peripheral insulin resistance progress in parallel, although the clinical relevance and mechanisms have not been fully elucidated. Under conditions of hepatic insulin resistance, glucogenolysis and gluconeogenesis are stimulated because of decreased suppression by insulin, resulting in hyperglycemia, especially in the fasted state, and the storage of glycogen in the liver is reduced.

The liver has both IRS-1 and IRS-2 with different actions [Capeau, 2008; Meshkani, 2009, Tatoń, 2010; Morino, 2006] Kubota et al. showed that IRS-2 mainly functions during fasting and immediately after refeeding, and IRS-1 functions primarily after refeeding [Kubota, 2008]. Furthermore, liver-specific IRS-2-knockout mice display insulin resistance during fasting but not after refeeding. Therefore, IRS-2 may be involved in the fasting state via limitation of hepatic glucose production by controlling phosphoenolpyruvate carboxykinase and glucose 6-phoshatase [Capeau, 2008; Haeusler, 2008]. Thus, insufficient amount of hepatic IRS-2 during fasting due to insulin resistance may result in abnormal glucose metabolism with postprandial hyperglycemia [Kubota, 2008].

2.3 Insulin resistance and abnormal lipogenesis

There is a paradoxical mechanism in the lipogenic metabolism of hepatocytes in subjects with insulin resistance. Although the mechanism has not been fully elucidated yet, de-novo lipogenesis is activated by sterol regulatory element- binding protein (SREBP)-1c, which is insulin sensitive and is enhanced by elevated insulin [Eberlé, 2004; Ferré, 2007]. Alternatively, such lipogenesis is partially explained as a result of endoplasmic reticulum stress, activating the cleavage of SREBP-1c [Ferré, 2007; Ferré, 2010].

The three SREBP isoforms, SREBP-1a, SREBP-1c and SREBP-2, have different roles in lipid synthesis. Animal studies using transgenic and knockout mice suggest that SREBP-1c is involved in FFA synthesis and glucose metabolism, whereas SREBP-2 is relatively specific to cholesterol synthesis [Eberlé, 2004; Ferré, 2007; Ferré, 2010]. The SREBP-1c isoform appears to be mainly regulated at the transcriptional level by insulin. Indeed, SREBP-1c knockout mice are likely to have high plasma glucose during a carbohydrate feeding period [Liang, 2002], suggesting that SREBP-1c expression is involved in the pathophysiology of type 2 diabetes and MetS. Although extensive studies have been limited to animal studies, liver X receptor, which is a nuclear hormone receptor highly expressed in the liver and it responds to oxysterol, enhances fatty acid synthesis by activating SREBP-1c, which in turn activates lipogenesis as well as VLDL assembly and secretion [Liang, 2002; Okazaki, 2010]. Therefore, there is a complicated relationship between glucose metabolism and lipid metabolism, which includes many transcriptional factors

The liver can store extra fat that should be originally accumulated in adipose tissue or skeletal muscle. However, such fat accumulation eventually aggravates organ function. Ectopic fat deposition, especially as triglycerides, in the liver may be a rough hallmark of insulin resistance, particularly in adipose tissue. However, organ damage does not occur yet, although impaired insulin signaling is imminent. Excess fat accumulation and their metabolites may provoke a second stage. Therefore, NAFLD and NASH may be more severe clinical conditions than simple obesity regardless of the visceral or subcutaneous type. Tarantino et al. [Tarantino, 2010] suggested that hepatocytes are the last type of cell to store fat when other cell types are full with fat. Therefore, lifestyle intervention and possible treatments should be initiated at simple steatosis instead of overt steatohepatitis.

2.4 Possibility of pharmacological treatment

Recently, it has been shown that a relatively long time (1-2 years) of treatment with vitamin E and thiazolidinediones improves NAFLD and NASH [Aithal, 2008; Duvnjak, 2009; Sanyal, 2010; Musso, 2010], suggesting that anti-oxidative agents and PPAR-γ agonists may improve the pathophysiology of the liver as well as clinical variables in patients with NASH and NAFLD. PPAR-γ, which belongs to the nuclear hormone receptor family, is mainly expressed in adipose tissues [Anghel, 2007] and exerts substantial actions such as adipocyte differentiation and fibroblast differentiation into mature adipocyte types [Anghel, 2007; Mandrup, 1997]. Therefore, improvement of NASH and NAFLD may be predominantly caused through improvement of the etiology in the visceral tissue or upper subcutaneous fat, although the precise underlying mechanism is unknown. Considering the discrepancy between the site of PPAR-γ expression and that of the pharmacological effects, the plausible mechanism is that thiazolidinediones restore fat accumulation from the liver or muscle into adipose tissues and confine it in adipose tissue at the long term expense of adipose cells [Samuel, 2010]. Mayerson et al. [1997] showed that treatment with rosiglitazone results in a significant reduction of hepatic triglyceride content along with successful suppression of adipocyte lipolysis. Unexpectedly, there is also increased intramyocellular fat as triglycerides accompanied by improved insulin sensitivity in muscle. This suggests that intramyocellular fat alone is unlikely to reflect insulin resistance, similar to triglyceride accumulation in the liver and the "first hit" stage in the second hit theory of NASH.

Such apparent improvement in insulin resistance often results in adverse outcomes, such as an increase in the amount of adipose cells by differentiation of adipose cells, eventually leading to weight gain and systematic edema [Duvnjak, 2009; Sanyal, 2010], which in turn loads the heart and aggravates latent heart failure. Long-term treatment of thiazolidinediones, in which pioglitazone may be better than rosiglitazone in terms of less side effects [Tang, 2006; Tzoulaki, 2009], can result in intolerance for some people with diabetes because of these adverse effects, regardless of whether they provoke heart failure. Likewise, the safety and efficacy of long-term treatment with vitamin E has not been established yet in the clinical setting. Metformin (biguanide), an insulin-sensitizer, is considered as the first choice for type 2 diabetes because it has fewer side effects and a mild lipid-lowering property. However, the outcomes of clinical trials are conflicting [Duvnjak, 2009]. Therefore, it is not recommended to treat NAFLD patients with metformin unless they have abnormal glucose metabolism.

In contrast, 3-hydroxy-3-methyglutaryl-coenzyme A (HMG-CoA) reductase inhibitors (statins) do not seem to be an effective treatment for NASH, with conflicting outcomes [Nelson, 2009; Kimura, 2010]. Statins are used in clinical practice to improve lipid metabolism, particularly low density lipoprotein-cholesterol. In addition, they have a pleiotropic effect including anti-inflammatory actions [Davignon, 2004] in which proinflammatory cytokines, such as C-reactive protein (CRP) and TNF-α, are substantially reduced by the use of statins. Notably, although CRP and TNF-α are related to insulin resistance and metabolic abnormalities, statins are unlikely to improve the histology of NALD and NASH. This finding might be related to the fact that statins are associated with deterioration of glucose metabolism [Sattar, 2010; Koh, 2010]; however, further in depth studies are required.

2.5 Liver cirrhosis and Insulin resistance

Liver cirrhosis causes hepatic insulin resistance, resulting in hyperinsulinemia and diabetes because of both decreased insulin clearance and increased secretion of insulin from the pancreas [Petrides, 1994; Hickman, 2007; Garcia-Compean, 2009]. A substantial amount of patients with cirrhosis have glucose intolerance (~96%) and a relatively small amount of them may have overt diabetes (~30%) [Hickman, 2007; Garcia-Compean, 2009]. In patients with liver cirrhosis, particularly in the decompensated stage, substantial hyperglycemia as well as hypoglycemia occur as a result of a lack of glucose control because of lack glucose uptake in the postprandial state and glucose secretion by the liver in the fasting state. Such diabetes and abnormal glucose metabolism, which develop as a complication of cirrhosis, are known as "hepatogenous diabetes" [Garcia-Compean, 2009] and they worsen the clinical outcomes of patients along with malnutrition associated with advanced cirrhosis. Hepatitis C virus (HCV) and hemochromatosis are known to frequently accompany diabetes and insulin resistance [Hickman, 2007; Garcia-Compean, 2009]. Although underlying mechanisms between HCV infection and insulin resistance are not clearly known, HCV induces insulin resistance primarily because of TNF-α overproduction, regardless of obesity and hepatic fibrosis stage [Kawaguchi, 2010].

2.6 Skeletal muscle and insulin resistance

Skeletal muscle is a large organ that consumes a variety of nutrients including glucose, lipids, and proteins. After a meal, approximately one third of absorbed glucose is taken up by the liver and the rest is mainly taken up by the skeletal muscle [Abdul-Ghani, 2010]. Therefore, skeletal muscle can substantially interfere with systemic glucose metabolism and alter peripheral insulin sensitivity as well as hepatic insulin sensitivity [Samuel, 2010; Turcotte, 2008]. Therefore, the pathogenic features of skeletal muscle need to be considered in relation to the liver and adipocytes. In liver and muscle, there are many common mechanisms of lipid and glucose metabolism. Ectopic fat accumulation in skeletal muscle is often observed in patients with type 2 diabetes and MetS. Such fat deposition is considered to be the cause of insulin resistance [Tarantino, 2010; Samuel, 2010; Abdul-Ghani, 2010]. However, while the amount of intramyocellular lipids can be used as a marker of insulin resistance in general, similar to the liver, these neutral triglycerides themselves are not thought to be harmful [Abdul-Ghani, 2010; Eckarde, 2011]. In addition, storage of carbohydrates as glycogen in muscle is impaired in people with insulin resistance [Samuel, 2010].

FFA metabolism and increased fatty acid metabolites such as long-chain acyl CoA, DAG, and ceramide, are likely to play a pivotal role in the development of insulin resistance in skeletal muscle [Samuel, 2010]. Accumulated DAG has a high affinity for PKC, which in turn cause a reduction of tyrosine phosphorylation of IRS-1, followed by reduced glucose uptake via GLUT4. A plausible reason why lipid intermediates accumulate in muscle cells is because of an unbalance between a higher rate of FFA uptake and a lower rate of FFA disposal, which is primarily performed by β–oxidation in the mitochondria. High circulating FFA may result from adipocyte lipolysis because of insulin resistance in adipose tissue. Because higher circulating FFA are correlated with a higher uptake of FFA by muscle, consequent high FFA in muscle may be related to insulin resistance in adipose tissue.

Muscle oxidation capacity is reduced in patients with type 2 diabetes and obesity, leading to increasing oxidative stress in skeletal muscle [Abdul-Ghani, 2010; Turcotte, 2008; Eckardt, 2011; Tsutsui, 2011]. Increased oxidative stress, such as ROS, in the muscle deteriorates exercise capacity [Tsutsui, 2011], resulting in muscle weakness and disuse muscle atrophy.

It is well known that favorable modulation of mitochondrial oxidative capacity in skeletal muscle by exercise training improves the oxidation of fatty acids, leading to effective insulin downstream signaling. It has been suggested that insulin resistance of muscle in the elderly may contribute to the development of sarcopenia [Volpi, 2004; Boirie, 2001], an unintended loss of muscle mass, strength, and function. In fact, when glucose is ingested with a regular meal, it is likely that increased insulin has a negative effect on muscle protein synthesis, particularly in older individuals [Volpi, 2004], suggesting that increasing muscle protein synthesis via insulin may be impaired in the elderly. It is unknown whether this negative effect is also observed in patients with type 2 diabetes; studies in relation to insulin effects on skeletal muscle are required to prevent "diabetes disability" in the elderly and people with insulin resistance.

Adiponectin, a hormone secreted by normal-sized adipocytes, stimulates AMPK activation, fatty-acid oxidation, glucose uptake, and lactate production in skeletal muscle [Yamauchi, 2002]. Adipocyte-myocyte crosstalk is an important modulator in the development of skeletal muscle insulin resistance [Havekes, 2010]. Accumulating evidence suggests that not only adipose cells but also skeletal muscle synthesize and secrete specific cytokines called "myokines" that modify metabolic crosstalk between organ systems. A substantial amount of IL-6 is released from skeletal muscle during and after exercise, i.e., contracting skeletal muscle, which is correlated with increases in AMPK activity in many tissues [Pedersen,

2007]. A slight to mild increase in serum IL-6 levels is often observed in obese people and individuals with type 2 diabetes, whereas a greater increase in IL-6 levels after exercise is considered as a facilitator of increased fuel metabolism, leading to adipocyte lipolysis and fat oxidation. Therefore, under certain conditions, IL-6 and other muscle-derived cytokines may play a role in preventing metabolic abnormalities such as type 2 diabetes [Pedersen, 2007] and damage to skeletal muscle.

3. The lung and insulin resistance

Complications of diabetes affect many tissues and organs, resulting in retinopathy, nephropathy, neuropathy, cardiovascular diseases, peripheral vascular diseases, stroke, and periodontal pathologies. Diabetes as well as MetS and hypertension, which are associated with insulin resistance and hyperinsulinemia, contribute to these complications and organ damage/failure. We discuss here impaired lung function in relation to the pathogenic features of insulin resistance.

Impaired lung function and lung diseases have been rarely discussed in terms of metabolic abnormalities. Although the diabetic lung was topically discussed in early human studies [Kaparianos, 2008; Klein, 2010], there have been limited investigations for metabolic abnormalities and impaired lungs.

With regard to respiratory function, respiratory diseases are generally divided into obstructive or restrictive lung diseases. To date, chronic obstructive pulmonary disease (COPD) is a leading cause of mortality in many countries and is increasing mainly because of the expanding number of smokers as well as the advancing age of the population. The association of COPD with all-cause mortality and cardiovascular events has been intensively studied in numerous prospective and cross-sectional studies [Fimognari, 2010; Rabe, 2007]. Molecular and cellular studies have explored the detailed mechanisms of COPD, which are considered to be related to local inflammation in the lung and systemic inflammation as assessed by elevated CRP and TNF-α levels [Fimognari, 2010; Rabe, 2007]. Although elevated CRP levels have been considered to be related to insulin resistance [Ndumele, 2006; Lu, 2010], metabolic abnormalities including type 2 diabetes and MetS have not been found to be involved in the etiology of COPD or an obstructive spirometric pattern [Fimognari, 2010]. Accumulating evidence is now questioning the association between the pathogenic features of insulin resistance and COPD because of elevated plasma adiponectin and the absence of either dyslipidemia, at least quantitatively [Basili, 1999], or insulin resistance [Fimognari, 2010] in COPD patients.

3.1 Restrictive lung disease and metabolic abnormalities

In recent years, some studies have addressed the association between low vital capacity, i.e., restrictive lung disease (RLD), and fatal and critical diseases. However, the magnitude of the increased mortality risk for RLD, e.g., the hazard ratio, appears to be comparable with that of mild-to-moderate COPD [Mannino, 2003a, 2003b; Purdue, 2007]. Although the etiology and cause of RLD are unknown, the prevalence of RLP is similar to that of COPD; it is approximately half to equal that in COPD or obstructive lung disease in some studies [Mannino, 2003a, 2003b; Purdue, 2007; Ford, 2004, Guerra, 2010].

In addition to earlier studies on the diabetic lung [Kaparianos, 2008], relatively recent cross-sectional studies and prospective studies, which investigated the relationship between

restrictive lung disease and cardiometabolic risks, have yielded almost uniform outcomes. They found that the restrictive pattern is associated with MetS (insulin resistance, dyslipidemia), type 2 diabetes, and inflammatory markers, especially CRP [Fimognari, 2010; Ford, 2004; Nakajima, 2008; Lin, 2006; Fimognari, 2007; Lee, 2008; Yeh, 2008; Chance, 2008].
Fimognari et al. [2007] revealed an association between RP and MetS in older persons in terms of insulin resistance. They observed that insulin resistance was much higher in the restriction group than that in the obstruction group and normal controls. Intriguingly, type 1 diabetes has been reported to be predominantly associated with features of RP [Schnack, 1996; Makkar, 2000; Boulbou, 2003]. Generally, type 1 diabetes is not accompanied by insulin resistance. Therefore, the results suggest a possible link between endocrine disorders, i.e., insufficient insulin action and impaired pulmonary function.

3.2 Determination of RLD in the clinical setting

Pulmonary function testing is often used and recommended for the assessment and management of impaired pulmonary function. However, spirometer-diagnosed COPD and RLD in such large studies could be equivocal because of controversy regarding the definitions and limitations in each facility. Furthermore, RLD may involve characteristics that reflect a restrictive pattern, some of which are caused by extrapulmonary impairment. This restrictive pattern includes various etiologies including classical RLDs such as interstitial lung diseases, respiratory muscle weakness, congestive heart failure, pneumonia, restrictive thoracic cage and, possibly, severe obesity. Theoretically, the determination of RLD should be assessed based on the reduction of total lung capacity (TLC) instead of a decline in vital capacity or forced vital capacity (FVC). According to the American Thoracic Society and the European Respiratory Society (ATS/ERS) task force [Pellegrino, 2005], a restrictive ventilatory defect is characterized by a reduction in TLC below the 5th percentile of the predicted value and a normal forced expiratory volume in 1 second (FEV_1)/vital capacity (VC). Therefore, it is not possible to accurately diagnose RLD using only an ordinary spirometer. However, measuring TLC is unfeasible in large studies as it is time consuming, expensive, and requires special facilities and trained technicians. It has been reported that a slightly increased FEV_1/FVC is often caused by submaximal inspiratory or expiratory efforts, or peripheral air flow obstruction [Pellegrino, 2005]. In our previous study, we showed that a stricter restrictive pattern was substitutively defined as a combination of low FVC assessed by lower limits of normal and relatively high FEV_1/FVC ($\geq$ 85%) [Nakajima, 2008].
Despite these limitations in the assessment of RLD, RLD and COPD have been associated with mortality and fatal incidents from cardiovascular disease [Mannino, 2003a, 2003b; Purdue, 2007; Hozawa, 2006, Guerra, 2010], but there is a lack of adequate understanding of the underlying mechanisms. Mannino et al. [2003b] reported that moderate and severe COPD were associated with an increased mortality risk in current and former smokers, but not in people who never smoked. In contrast, RLD was associated with an increased risk of mortality to a similar extent in all three smoking categories (current, former, and never smoked), suggesting that the mortality risk of COPD is mostly dependent on smoking status, whereas that of restrictive pattern is not. Likewise, in white people who have never smoked, the incidence of stroke is significantly increased along with reduced FVC, but not FEV_1/FVC [Hozawa, 2006]. Similar trends have also been recognized in other studies [Mannino, 2003a; Purdue, 2007] Therefore, factors other than smoking appear to deteriorate the fundamental pathogenesis of RLD.

3.3 Relation of RLD to cardiometabolic risks

Our laboratory and other investigators [Nakajima, 2008; Lee, 2008; Yeh, 2008, Klein, 2010] have reported that the mean FVC in persons with MetS or diabetes is reduced by approximately 6.0% compared with those without the diseases. In three studies [Nakajima, 2008; Lee, 2008; Yeh, 2008], the mean predicted FVC in persons with metabolic abnormalities, MetS, or diabetes (88-97%) ranges within the normal limit but it is higher in patients with a specific RLD, e.g., nonspecific interstitial pneumonia (59-83%) [Martinez, 2006]. The clinical relevance of a 6-7% decline in FVC within the normal range is unclear. Additional tests such as the 6-minute walk test and ventilation function test (carbon monoxide diffusion capacity) may give additional information on the features of the metabolic disorder-related restrictive lung pattern.

Regarding plausible underlying mechanisms between RLD and metabolic abnormalities, central obesity, particularly visceral fat and fatty liver diseases such as NAFLD, may physically impede the descent of the diaphragm, leading primarily to restrictive respiration impairment. However, a significant association between the restrictive pattern and type 2 diabetes and MetS remains, even after statistical adjustment for body mass index (BMI) and after stratification by BMI [Ford, 2004; Nakajima, 2008; Lin, 2006; Fimognari, 2007; Nakajima, 2010]. This suggests that for a given BMI, individuals with cardiometabolic abnormalities have a lower vital capacity than those without cardiometabolic abnormalities. Therefore, metabolic abnormalities and, possibly in part, mechanical limitation, may contribute to the development and progression of the restrictive pattern.

With regard to the cause of RLD, some prospective studies appear to suggest that restrictive patients are expected to develop metabolic abnormalities such as diabetes compared with subjects with normal spirometry. In the NHANES study [Ford, 2004], non-diabetes subjects with a restrictive pattern had an increased risk of developing diabetes in the follow-up. In the ARIC study [Yeh, 2008], low pulmonary function, defined as low forced vital capacity and low FEV_1, predicted the new onset of diabetes.

Metabolic abnormalities may cause impaired lung function. For example, insulin resistance may reduce the uptake of glucose by respiratory muscle, resulting in respiratory muscle weakness and poor ventilatory performance [Fimognari, 2010]. Nevertheless, regarding the cause-effect relationship, it has not been established which occurs first, the restrictive pattern or metabolic abnormalities. Alternatively other factor such as insulin resistance might cause both simultaneously.

3.4 Possible underlying mechanisms

Given that insulin resistance and related etiologies are the main cause of the restrictive lung, a plausible explanation for this is that several malignant cytokines, such as IL-6, CRP, TNF-α, and PAI-1, as well as decreased levels of adiponectin, which originate mostly from visceral and trunk subcutaneous adipocytes [Capeau, 2008; Meshkani, 2009; Gustafson,2010; Nakajima, 2010; Wannamethee, 2010], hyperglycemia, nonenzymatic glycosylation [Kaparianos, 2008; Chance, 2008], and diabetes-related growth hormones, such as insulin-like growth factor-I, insulin-like growth factor binding proteins, and transforming growth factor-β [Ezzat, 2008; Pilewski, 2005], may be related to histopathological alterations and functional abnormality because of oxidative and inflammatory processes. These molecules and resultant hyperinsulinemia, as well as ectopic fat deposition, leukocyte-endothelial cell adhesion, extracellular matrix deposition, fibroblast proliferation, pulmonary capillary leak, pulmonary microangiopathy, and thickening of alveolar epithelia, may all converge into decreased lung compliance and diffusing capacity. Postmortem studies support the notion that the lung is a target organ for diabetic microangiopathy [Kaparianos, 2008; Klein, 2010]. Insulin resistance and resultant hyperinsulinemia may result in diastolic dysfunction of the lung via respiratory muscle weakness and functional failure by a similar pathology of skeletal muscle. Notably, lung-derived surfactant protein (SP)-A is associated with altered glucose tolerance and insulin resistance [Fernández-Real, 2008]. Fernández-Real (2008) found that SP-A levels in the blood were significantly higher among patients with glucose intolerance and type 2 diabetes than in those with normal glucose tolerance, even after adjustment for BMI, age, and smoking status. Additionally, SP-D, a lung-derived innate immune protein, is also associated with inflammation and metabolic abnormalities including insulin sensitivity [Fernández-Real, 2010]. Indeed, in the obese type 2 diabetes animal model, many qualitatively similar changes as in type 1 diabetes develop with extensive lipid deposition, altered alveolar type-2 cell ultrastructure and surfactant protein expression patterns [Foster, 2010]. Foster et al. (2010) recently reported in their study using obese diabetic rats that numerous lipid droplets were visible within alveolar interstitium, lipofibroblasts, and macrophages, particularly in subpleural regions, and that triglyceride content was higher not only in the liver but also in the lung. These findings suggest a definite relationship between metabolic abnormalities relating to insulin resistance and impairment of the lung. Potential histopathological features in the diabetic or metabolic abnormal lung are presented in **Figure 2**.

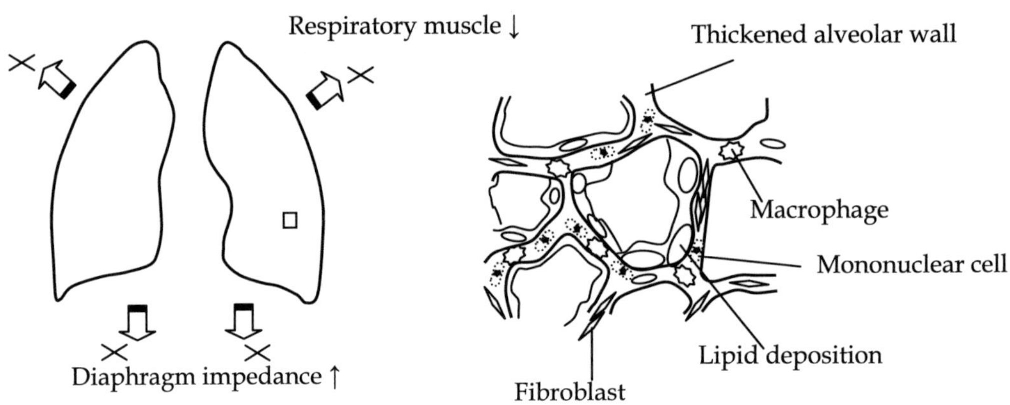

Fig. 2. A. Diastolic dysfunction of lung due to reduced respiratory muscle and increased diaphragm impedance. B. Histopathological features of alveolar space referring to Foster et al., 2010 and Klein et al., 2010. Lipid droplets are present in alveolar interstitium. Alveolar-capillary membrane is thickened with fibrotic changes.

3.5 Possible treatment for impaired lungs

The use of statins has been frequently discussed for patients with COPD [Fimognari, 2010; Dobler, 2009; Young, 2009], but their effect is unknown in RLD [Keddissi, 2007]. Statins prevent the decline in FEV_1 and FVC, irrespective of obstructive or restrictive disease

[Keddissi, 2007]. Considering that statins have a pleiotropic effect, this lung-protective effect may be because of the pleiotropic effect, including anti-inflammatory, anti-oxidant, anti-thrombogenic, and vascular function-restoring actions [Davignon, 2004]. Therefore, the mechanism underlying the association between metabolic disorders and RLD might be, at least in part, similar to that between cardiometabolic risk and cardiovascular disease. In addition, statin use is associated with slower rates of lung function decline in the elderly. These findings suggest a possible treatment for patients with impaired lung function and this possibility should be investigated further. However, lifestyle intervention is critical beyond any medications because insulin resistance and related etiologies develop and progress according to an unfavorable lifestyle.

3.6 Clinical perspective with respect to impaired lung function

Both types of impaired lung function, obstructive and restrictive lung disease, have been associated with an increased risk for high mortality and critical pathophysiology such as cardiovascular diseases probably because of chronic inflammation and oxidative stress. However, there is likely to be a difference in the underlying mechanism between obstructive and restrictive lung disease in terms of metabolic abnormalities.

Metabolic abnormalities, especially insulin resistance, and restrictive lung/reduced vital capacity belong to apparently unrelated fields. If there is a real association between insulin resistance and restrictive lung, it would be of substantial clinical interest and important for preventing possible synergic effects on the development and progression of fatal diseases. Although restrictive lung has been confirmed to be associated with increased mortality, particularly from diabetes, in recent studies [Fimognari, 2010, Guerra, 2010], it is unclear whether the restrictive pattern associated with metabolic abnormalities is a direct cause of mortality. Alternatively, RLD or the restrictive pattern might represent complications of longitudinal diabetes such as the three major complications of diabetes, because reduced lung volume and alveolar perfusion are correlated with extrapulmonary microangiopathy [Schnack, 1996]. Once RLD occurs in such patients, it may in turn worsen diabetes and metabolic abnormalities, resulting in aggravation of the pathogenesis. Intervention of the restrictive pattern by pulmonary rehabilitation or medication would clarify the cause-effect relationship between the restrictive pattern or RLD and cardiometabolic risks.

Further prospective as well as cross-sectional studies and clinical trials that address both fields are required to consider the potential importance of the subclinical restrictive pattern compared with obstructive lung, and to elucidate the complicated relationships between them.

4. Conclusion

Insulin resistance plays pivotal roles in all organs and tissues including the kidney and skin lesions. Ectopic fat deposition in the liver, muscle, and lung may be an initial hallmark of peripheral insulin resistance, particularly adipose tissue, which predominantly accumulates surplus energy as fat. If such conditions continue without proper treatment or intervention, second stages comprising oxidative stress, inflammation, and degeneration can occur and worsen organ function, along with impairment of insulin downsignaling in the cells of the target organ. Although some candidates have been considered for pharmacotherapy, these drugs may transiently improve the pathophysiology by redistribution of fat and change the direction of surplus lipids and carbohydrates, i.e., push back accumulated fat to original adipose tissues. Because of controversial clinical data concerning pharmacological therapies

as well as the cost and unknown adverse reactions, lifestyle interventions seem to be the only fundamental treatment for insulin resistance-related organ damage.
Further animal and human studies considering systemic organ damage and abnormal metabolism are required to explore the underlying complicated mechanisms and effective treatment and medications.

5. References

Abdul-Ghani MA, DeFronzo RA. Pathogenesis of insulin resistance in skeletal muscle. J Biomed Biotechnol. 2010;2010:476279.

Aithal GP, Thomas JA, Kaye PV, Lawson A, Ryder SD, Spendlove I, Austin AS, Freeman JG, Morgan L, Webber J. Randomized, placebo-controlled trial of pioglitazone in nondiabetic subjects with nonalcoholic steatohepatitis. Gastroenterology. 2008 ;135(4):1176-84.

American Diabetes Association Diagnosis and Classification of Diabetes Mellitus Diabetes Care, Vol 33 2010

Anghel SI, Wahli W. Fat poetry: a kingdom for PPAR gamma. Cell Res. 2007 ;17(6):486-511.

Bartnik M, Norhammar A, Rydén L. Hyperglycaemia and cardiovascular disease. J Intern Med. 2007 ;262(2):145-56.

Basili S, Ferroni P, Vieri M, Cardelli P, Ceci F, Paradiso M, Labbadia G, Gazzaniga PP, Cordova C, Alessandri C. Lipoprotein(a) serum levels in patients affected by chronic obstructive pulmonary disease. Atherosclerosis. 1999 Dec;147(2):249-52.

Boirie Y, Gachon P, Cordat N, Ritz P, Beaufrère B. Differential insulin sensitivities of glucose, amino acid, and albumin metabolism in elderly men and women. J Clin Endocrinol Metab. 2001 Feb;86(2):638-44.

Bollheimer LC, Skelly RH, Chester MW, McGarry JD, Rhodes CJ. Chronic exposure to free fatty acid reduces pancreatic beta cell insulin content by increasing basal insulin secretion that is not compensated for by a corresponding increase in proinsulin biosynthesis translation. J Clin Invest. 1998 1;101(5):1094-101.

Boulbou MS, Gourgoulianis KI, Klisiaris VK, Tsikrikas TS, Stathakis NE, Molyvdas PA. Diabetes mellitus and lung function. Med Princ Pract. 2003 Apr-Jun;12(2):87-91.

Brüning JC, Michael MD, Winnay JN, Hayashi T, Hörsch D, Accili D, Goodyear LJ, Kahn CR. A muscle-specific insulin receptor knockout exhibits features of the metabolic syndrome of NIDDM without altering glucose tolerance. Mol Cell. 1998 ;2(5):559-69.

Capeau J. Insulin resistance and steatosis in humans. Diabetes Metab. 2008 Dec;34(6 Pt 2):649-57.

Chalmers J, Cooper ME. UKPDS and the legacy effect. N Engl J Med. 2008 9;359(15):1618-20.

Chance WW, Rhee C, Yilmaz C, et al. 2008. Diminished alveolar microvascular reserves in type 2 diabetes reflect systemic microangiopathy. Diabetes Care 31: 1596-60

Chang Y, Ryu S, Sung E, Jang Y. Higher concentrations of alanine aminotransferase within the reference interval predict nonalcoholic fatty liver disease. Clin Chem. 2007 ;53(4):686-92

Chen J, Muntner P, Hamm LL, Fonseca V, Batuman V, Whelton PK, He J. Insulin resistance and risk of chronic kidney disease in nondiabetic US adults. J Am Soc Nephrol. 2003 Feb;14(2):469-77.

Choi K, Kim YB. Molecular mechanism of insulin resistance in obesity and type 2 diabetes. Korean J Intern Med. 2010 ;25(2):119-29.

Cnop M, Hannaert JC, Hoorens A, Eizirik DL, Pipeleers DG. Inverse relationship between cytotoxicity of free fatty acids in pancreatic islet cells and cellular triglyceride accumulation. Diabetes. 2001 ;50(8):1771-7.

Foster DJ, Ravikumar P, Bellotto DJ, Unger RH, Hsia CC. Fatty Diabetic Lung: Altered Alveolar Structure and Surfactant Protein Expression Am J Physiol Lung Cell Mol Physiol 2010

Davignon J. Beneficial cardiovascular pleiotropic effects of statins. Circulation. 2004 Jun 15;109(23 Suppl 1):III39-43.

Dixon JB. The effect of obesity on health outcomes. Mol Cell Endocrinol. 2010 Mar 25;316(2):104-8

Dobler CC, Wong KK, Marks GB. Associations between statins and COPD: a systematic review. BMC Pulm Med. 2009 Jul 12;9:32.

Donnelly KL, Smith CI, Schwarzenberg SJ, Jessurun J, Boldt MD, Parks EJ. Sources of fatty acids stored in liver and secreted via lipoproteins in patients with nonalcoholic fatty liver disease. J Clin Invest. 2005 ;115(5):1343-51.

Duvnjak M, Tomasic V, Gomercic M, Smircic Duvnjak L, Barsic N, Lerotic I. Therapy of nonalcoholic fatty liver disease: current status. J Physiol Pharmacol. 2009 Dec;60 Suppl 7:57-66.

Eberlé D, Hegarty B, Bossard P, Ferré P, Foufelle F. SREBP transcription factors: master regulators of lipid homeostasis. Biochimie. 2004 ;86(11):839-48.

Eckardt K, Taube A, Eckel J. Obesity-associated insulin resistance in skeletal muscle: Role of lipid accumulation and physical inactivity. Rev Endocr Metab Disord. 2011 Feb 19.

Estep JM, Birerdinc A, Younossi Z. Non-invasive diagnostic tests for non-alcoholic fatty liver disease. Curr Mol Med. 2010 ;10(2):166-72.

Ezzat VA, Duncan ER, Wheatcroft SB, Kearney MT. 2008. The role of IGF-I and its binding proteins in the development of type 2 diabetes and cardiovascular disease. *Diabetes Obes Metab* 10: 198-211.

Faraci FM, Didion SP. Vascular protection: superoxide dismutase isoforms in the vessel wall. Arterioscler Thromb Vasc Biol. 2004 ;24(8):1367-73.

Fernández-Real JM, Chico B, Shiratori M, Nara Y, Takahashi H, Ricart W. Circulating surfactant protein A (SP-A), a marker of lung injury, is associated with insulin resistance. Diabetes Care. 2008 May;31(5):958-63.

Fernández-Real JM, Valdés S, Manco M, Chico B, Botas P, Campo A, Casamitjana R, Delgado E, Salvador J, Fruhbeck G, Mingrone G, Ricart W. Surfactant protein d, a marker of lung innate immunity, is positively associated with insulin sensitivity. Diabetes Care. 2010 Apr;33(4):847-53.

Ferré P, Foufelle F. Hepatic steatosis: a role for de novo lipogenesis and the transcription factor SREBP-1c. Diabetes Obes Metab. 2010 ;12 Suppl 2:83-92

Ferré P, Foufelle F. SREBP-1c transcription factor and lipid homeostasis: clinical perspective. Horm Res. 2007;68(2):72-82.

Fimognari FL, Pasqualetti P, Moro L, et al. 2007. The association between metabolic syndrome and restrictive ventilatory dysfunction in older persons. J Gerontol A Biol Sci Med Sci 62: 760-65.

Fimognari FL, Scarlata S, Antonelli-Incalzi R. Why are people with "poor lung function" at increased atherothrombotic risk? A critical review with potential therapeutic indications. Curr Vasc Pharmacol. 2010 Jul;8(4):573-86.

Ford ES, Mannino DM. 2004. Prospective association between lung function and the incidence of diabetes: findings from the National Health and Nutrition Examination Survey Epidemiologic Follow-up Study. Diabetes Care 27: 2966-70.

Garcia-Compean D, Jaquez-Quintana JO, Gonzalez-Gonzalez JA, Maldonado-Garza H. Liver cirrhosis and diabetes: risk factors, pathophysiology, clinical implications and management. World J Gastroenterol. 2009 Jan 21;15(3):280-8.

Gentile CL, Pagliassotti MJ. The role of fatty acids in the development and progression of nonalcoholic fatty liver disease. J Nutr Biochem. 2008 ;19(9):567-76.

Ghouri N, Preiss D, Sattar N. Liver enzymes, nonalcoholic fatty liver disease, and incident cardiovascular disease: a narrative review and clinical perspective of prospective data. Hepatology. 2010 ;52(3):1156-61.

Godsland IF. Insulin resistance and hyperinsulinaemia in the development and progression of cancer. Clin Sci (Lond). 2009 23;118(5):315-32.

Gressner OA, Gressner AM. Connective tissue growth factor: a fibrogenic master switch in fibrotic liver diseases. Liver Int. 2008 ;28(8):1065-79

Grundy SM, Cleeman JI, Daniels SR, Donato KA, Eckel RH, Franklin BA, Gordon DJ, Krauss RM, Savage PJ, Smith SC Jr, Spertus JA, Costa F; American Heart Association; National Heart, Lung, and Blood Institute.Diagnosis and management of the metabolic syndrome: an American Heart Association/National Heart, Lung, and Blood Institute Scientific Statement. Circulation. 2005 Oct 25;112(17):2735-52.

Guarnieri G, Zanetti M, Vinci P, Cattin MR, Pirulli A, Barazzoni R. Metabolic syndrome and chronic kidney disease. J Ren Nutr. 2010 Sep;20(5 Suppl):S19-23.

Guerra S, Sherrill DL, Venker C, Ceccato CM, Halonen M, Martinez FD. Morbidity and mortality associated with the restrictive spirometric pattern: a longitudinal study. Thorax. 2010 Jun;65(6):499-504

Gustafson B. Adipose tissue, inflammation and atherosclerosis. J Atheroscler Thromb. 2010 Apr 30;17(4):332-41.

Haeusler RA, Accili D. The double life of Irs. Cell Metab. 2008 ;8(1):7-9.

Hara K, Okada T, Tobe K, Yasuda K, The Pro12Ala polymorphism in PPAR gamma2 may confer resistance to type 2 diabetes. Biochem Biophys Res Commun. 2000 Apr 29;271(1):212-6.

Harwood K, Vuguin P, DiMartino-Nardi J. Current approaches to the diagnosis and treatment of polycystic ovarian syndrome in youth. Horm Res. 2007;68(5):209-17.

Havekes B, Sauerwein HP. Adipocyte-myocyte crosstalk in skeletal muscle insulin resistance; is there a role for thyroid hormone? Curr Opin Clin Nutr Metab Care. 2010 Nov;13(6):641-6.

Hickman IJ, Macdonald GA. Impact of diabetes on the severity of liver disease. Am J Med. 2007 Oct;120(10):829-34.

Higgins SP, Freemark M, Prose NS. Acanthosis nigricans: a practical approach to evaluation and management. Dermatol Online J. 2008 15;14(9):2.

Hozawa A, Billings JL, Shahar E, Ohira T, Rosamond WD, Folsom AR. 2006. Lung function and ischemic stroke incidence: the Atherosclerosis Risk in Communities study. Chest 130: 1642-49

Kahara T, Takamura T, Hayakawa T, Nagai Y, Prediction of exercise-mediated changes in metabolic markers by gene polymorphism. Diabetes Res Clin Pract. 2002 Aug;57(2):105-10.

Kaku K. Pathophysiology of Type 2 Diabetes and Its Treatment Policy. JMAJ 53(1): 41–46, 2010

Kaparianos A, Argyropoulou E, Sampsonas F, Karkoulias K, Tsiamita M, Spiropoulos K. Pulmonary complications in diabetes mellitus. Chron Respir Dis. 2008;5(2):101-8.

Kawaguchi T, Sata M. Importance of hepatitis C virus-associated insulin resistance: therapeutic strategies for insulin sensitization. World J Gastroenterol. 2010 28;16(16):1943-52.

Keddissi JI, Younis WG, Chbeir EA, Daher NN, Dernaika TA, Kinasewitz GT. 2007. The use of statins and lung function in current and former smokers. *Chest* 132: 1764-71.

Kim JK, Michael MD, Previs SF, Peroni OD, Mauvais-Jarvis F, Neschen S, Kahn BB, Kahn CR, Shulman GI. Redistribution of substrates to adipose tissue promotes obesity in mice with selective insulin resistance in muscle. J Clin Invest. 2000 ;105(12):1791-7.

Kimura Y, Hyogo H, Yamagishi S, Takeuchi M, Ishitobi T, Nabeshima Y, Arihiro K, Chayama K. Atorvastatin decreases serum levels of advanced glycation endproducts (AGEs) in nonalcoholic steatohepatitis (NASH) patients with dyslipidemia: clinical usefulness of AGEs as a biomarker for the attenuation of NASH. J Gastroenterol. 2010 ;45(7):750-7.

Klein OL, Krishnan JA, Glick S, Smith LJ. Systematic review of the association between lung function and Type 2 diabetes mellitus. Diabet Med. 2010 Sep;27(9):977-87.

Koh KK, Quon MJ, Han SH, Lee Y, Kim SJ, Shin EK. Atorvastatin causes insulin resistance and increases ambient glycemia in hypercholesterolemic patients. J Am Coll Cardiol. 2010 23;55(12):1209-16.

Kopelman P. Health risks associated with overweight and obesity. Obes Rev. 2007 Mar;8 Suppl 1:13-7.

Kubo M, Kiyohara Y, Kato I, Iwamoto H, Nakayama K, Hirakata H, Fujishima M. Effect of hyperinsulinemia on renal function in a general Japanese population: the Hisayama study. Kidney Int. 1999 Jun;55(6):2450-6.

Kubota N, Kubota T, Itoh S, Kumagai H, Kozono H, Takamoto I, Mineyama T, Ogata H, Tokuyama K, Ohsugi M, Sasako T, Moroi M, Sugi K, Kakuta S, Iwakura Y, Noda T, Ohnishi S, Nagai R, Tobe K, Terauchi Y, Ueki K, Kadowaki T. Dynamic functional relay between insulin receptor substrate 1 and 2 in hepatic insulin signaling during fasting and feeding. Cell Metab. 2008 ;8(1):49-64.

Laakso M and J. Kuusisto J. Understanding patient needs Diabetology for cardiologists (2003) 5 (Supplement B), B5–B13

Lastra G, Dhuper S, Johnson MS, Sowers JR. Salt, aldosterone, and insulin resistance: impact on the cardiovascular system. Nat Rev Cardiol. 2010 ;7(10):577-84.

Lastra G, Manrique C, McFarlane SI, Sowers JR. Cardiometabolic syndrome and chronic kidney disease. Curr Diab Rep. 2006 ;6(3):207-12

Lee HM, Le TV, Lopez VA, Wong ND. 2008. The association of C-reactive protein to reduced forced vital capacity in a non-smoking U.S. population with metabolic syndrome and diabetes. Diabetes Care 2008 Oct;31(10):2000-2

Liang G, Yang J, Horton JD, Hammer RE, Goldstein JL, Brown MS. Diminished hepatic response to fasting/refeeding and liver X receptor agonists in mice with selective deficiency of sterol regulatory element-binding protein-1c. J Biol Chem. 2002 15;277(11):9520-8.

Lin WY, Yao CA, Wang HC, Huang KC. 2006. Impaired lung function is associated with obesity and metabolic syndrome in adults. Obesity (Silver Spring) 14: 1654-61.

Liu Q, Bengmark S, Qu S. The role of hepatic fat accumulation in pathogenesis of non-alcoholic fatty liver disease (NAFLD). Lipids Health Dis. 2010 28;9:42.

Lu B, Yang Y, Yang Z, Feng X, Wang X, Zhang Z, Hu R. Insulin resistance in Chinese patients with type 2 diabetes is associated with C-reactive protein independent of abdominal obesity. Cardiovasc Diabetol. 2010 Dec 19;9:92.

Makkar P, Gandhi M, Agrawal RP, Sabir M, Kothari RP. Ventilatory pulmonary function tests in type 1 diabetes mellitus. J Assoc Physicians India. 2000 Oct;48(10):962-6.

Makowski L, Hotamisligil GS. Fatty acid binding proteins--the evolutionary crossroads of inflammatory and metabolic responses. J Nutr. 2004 ;134(9):2464S-2468S.

Mandrup S, Lane MD. Regulating adipogenesis. J Biol Chem. 1997 28;272(9):5367-70.

Mannino DM, Aguayo SM, Petty TL, Redd SC. 2003. Low lung function and incident lung cancer in the United States: data from the First National Health and Nutrition Examination Survey follow-up. *Arch Intern Med* 163: 1475-80.

Mannino DM, Buist AS, Petty TL, Enright PL, Redd SC. 2003. Lung function and mortality in the United States: data from the First National Health and Nutrition Examination Survey follow up study. *Thorax* 58(5): 388-93.

Martinez FJ, Flaherty K. 2006. Pulmonary function testing in idiopathic interstitial pneumonias. *Proc Am Thorac Soc* 3: 315-21

Matsuzaki K. Modulation of TGF-beta signaling during progression of chronic liver diseases. Front Biosci. 2009 1;14:2923-34

Mayerson AB, Hundal RS, Dufour S, Lebon V, Befroy D, Cline GW, Enocksson S, Inzucchi SE, Shulman GI, Petersen KF. The effects of rosiglitazone on insulin sensitivity, lipolysis, and hepatic and skeletal muscle triglyceride content in patients with type 2 diabetes. Diabetes. 2002 ;51(3):797-802.

Meshkani R, Adeli K. Hepatic insulin resistance, metabolic syndrome and cardiovascular disease. Clin Biochem. 2009 Sep;42(13-14):1331-46.

Miao L, St Clair DK. Regulation of superoxide dismutase genes: implications in disease. Free Radic Biol Med. 2009 15;47(4):344-56.

Morino K, Petersen KF, Shulman GI. Molecular mechanisms of insulin resistance in humans and their potential links with mitochondrial dysfunction. Diabetes. 2006 ;55 Suppl 2:S9-S15.

Murray P, Chune GW, Raghavan VA. Legacy effects from DCCT and UKPDS: what they mean and implications for future diabetes trials. Curr Atheroscler Rep. 2010 ;12(6):432-9.

Musso G, Gambino R, Cassader M, Pagano G A meta-analysis of randomized trials for the treatment of nonalcoholic fatty liver disease. Hepatology. 2010 ;52(1):79-104.

Nakajima K, Ebata M, Saito M. The relationship between low vital capacity and impaired glucose metabolism in men. Diabet Med. 2010 Dec;27(12):1460-1.

Nakajima K, Kubouchi Y, Muneyuki T, Ebata M, Eguchi S, Munakata H. A possible association between suspected restrictive pattern as assessed by ordinary pulmonary function test and the metabolic syndrome. Chest. 2008 Oct;134(4):712-8. Epub 2008 Jul 14.

Nakajima K. Pharmacotherapy of mixed dyslipidemia in the metabolic syndrome. Curr Clin Pharmacol. 2010 1;5(2):133-9.

Ndumele CE, Pradhan AD, Ridker PM. Interrelationships between inflammation, C-reactive protein, and insulin resistance. J Cardiometab Syndr. 2006 Summer;1(3):190-6.

Nelson A, Torres DM, Morgan AE, Fincke C, Harrison SA. A pilot study using simvastatin in the treatment of nonalcoholic steatohepatitis: A randomized placebo-controlled trial. J Clin Gastroenterol. 2009 -;43(10):990-4

Okazaki H, Goldstein JL, Brown MS, Liang G. LXR-SREBP-1c-phospholipid transfer protein axis controls very low density lipoprotein (VLDL) particle size. J Biol Chem. 2010 26;285(9):6801-10.

Pedersen BK. IL-6 signalling in exercise and disease. Biochem Soc Trans. 2007 Nov;35(Pt 5):1295-7.

Pellegrino R, Viegi G, Brusasco V, et al. 2005. Interpretative strategies for lung function tests. *Eur Respir J* 26: 948-68.
Petrides AS, Vogt C, Schulze-Berge D, Matthews D, Strohmeyer G. Pathogenesis of glucose intolerance and diabetes mellitus in cirrhosis. Hepatology. 1994 ;19(3):616-27.
Pilewski JM, Liu L, Henry AC, Knauer AV, Feghali-Bostwick CA. 2005. Insulin-like growth factor binding proteins 3 and 5 are overexpressed in idiopathic pulmonary fibrosis and contribute to extracellular matrix deposition. *Am J Pathol* 166: 399-407.
Popa C, Netea MG, van Riel PL, van der Meer JW, Stalenhoef AF. The role of TNF-alpha in chronic inflammatory conditions, intermediary metabolism, and cardiovascular risk. J Lipid Res. 2007 ;48(4):751-62.
Purdue MP, Gold L, Järvholm B, Alavanja MC, Ward MH, Vermeulen R. 2007. Impaired lung function and lung cancer incidence in a cohort of Swedish construction workers. *Thorax* 62: 51-6.
Rabe KF, Beghé B, Luppi F, Fabbri LM. 2007. Update in chronic obstructive pulmonary disease 2006. *Am J Respir Crit Care Med* 175: 1222-32.
Randle PJ, Garland PB, Hales CN, Newsholme EA.The glucose fatty-acid cycle. Its role in insulin sensitivity and the metabolic disturbances of diabetes mellitus. Lancet. 1963 Apr 13;1(7285):785-9.
Samuel VT, Petersen KF, Shulman GI. Lipid-induced insulin resistance: unravelling the mechanism. Lancet. 2010 26;375(9733):2267-77.
Sanyal AJ, Chalasani N, Kowdley KV, McCullough A, Diehl AM, Bass NM, Neuschwander-Tetri BA, Lavine JE, Tonascia J, Unalp A, Van Natta M, Clark J, Brunt EM, Kleiner DE, Hoofnagle JH, Robuck PR; NASH CRN. Pioglitazone, vitamin E, or placebo for nonalcoholic steatohepatitis. N Engl J Med. 2010 6;362(18):1675-85.
Sattar N, Preiss D, Murray HM, Welsh P, Buckley BM, de Craen AJ, Seshasai SR, McMurray JJ, Freeman DJ, et al. Statins and risk of incident diabetes: a collaborative meta-analysis of randomised statin trials. Lancet. 2010 27;375(9716):735-42.
Schindhelm RK, Diamant M, Dekker JM, Tushuizen ME, Teerlink T, Heine RJ. Alanine aminotransferase as a marker of non-alcoholic fatty liver disease in relation to type 2 diabetes mellitus and cardiovascular disease. Diabetes Metab Res Rev. 2006 - ;22(6):437-43.
Schnack C, Festa A, Schwarzmaier-D'Assié A, Haber P, Schernthaner G. Pulmonary dysfunction in type 1 diabetes in relation to metabolic long-term control and to incipient diabetic nephropathy Nephron. 1996;74(2):395-400
Sharma V, Kumar V. Diabetes in Asia. Lancet. 2010 Mar 20;375(9719):982.
Shulman GI. Cellular mechanisms of insulin resistance. J Clin Invest. 2000 ,106(2):171-6
Simmgen M, Knauf C, Lopez M, Choudhury AI, Charalambous M, Cantley J, Bedford DC, Claret M, Iglesias MA, Heffron H, Cani PD, Vidal-Puig A, Burcelin R, Withers DJ. Liver-specific deletion of insulin receptor substrate 2 does not impair hepatic glucose and lipid metabolism in mice. Diabetologia. 2006 ;49(3):552-61.
Sykiotis GP, Papavassiliou AG. Serine phosphorylation of insulin receptor substrate-1: a novel target for the reversal of insulin resistance. Mol Endocrinol. 2001 ;15(11):1864-9
Tang WH. Do thiazolidinediones cause heart failure? A critical review. Cleve Clin J Med. 2006 ;73(4):390-7.
Tarantino G, Savastano S, Colao A. Hepatic steatosis, low-grade chronic inflammation and hormone/growth factor/adipokine imbalance. World J Gastroenterol. 2010 Oct 14;16(38):4773-83.

Tatoń J, Czech A, Piatkiewicz P. Insulin as the main regulator of cellular glucose utilization--aetiological aspects of insulin resistance. Endokrynol Pol. 2010 -;61(4):388-94.

Tessari P, Coracina A, Cosma A, Tiengo A. Hepatic lipid metabolism and non-alcoholic fatty liver disease. Nutr Metab Cardiovasc Dis. 2009 ;19(4):291-302.

Tsutsui H, Kinugawa S, Matsushima S, Yokota T. Oxidative stress in cardiac and skeletal muscle dysfunction associated with diabetes mellitus. J Clin Biochem Nutr. 2011 Jan;48(1):68-71.

Turcotte LP, Fisher JS. Skeletal muscle insulin resistance: roles of fatty acid metabolism and exercise. Phys Ther. 2008 Nov;88(11):1279-96.

Tzoulaki I, Molokhia M, Curcin V, Little MP, Millett CJ, Ng A, Hughes RI, Khunti K, Wilkins MR, Majeed A, Elliott P. Risk of cardiovascular disease and all cause mortality among patients with type 2 diabetes prescribed oral antidiabetes drugs: retrospective cohort study using UK general practice research database. BMJ. 2009 3;339:b4731.

Volpi E, Nazemi R, Fujita S. Muscle tissue changes with aging. Curr Opin Clin Nutr Metab Care. 2004 Jul;7(4):405-10.

Wannamethee SG, Shaper AG, Rumley A, Sattar N, Whincup PH, Thomas MC, Lowe GD. Lung function and risk of type 2 diabetes and fatal and nonfatal major coronary heart disease events: possible associations with inflammation. Diabetes Care. 2010 Sep;33(9):1990-6.

Yamauchi T, Kamon J, Minokoshi Y, Ito Y, Waki H, Uchida S, Yamashita S, Noda M, Kita S, Ueki K, Eto K, Akanuma Y, Froguel P, Foufelle F, Ferre P, Carling D, Kimura S, Nagai R, Kahn BB, Kadowaki T. Adiponectin stimulates glucose utilization and fatty-acid oxidation by activating AMP-activated protein kinase. Nat Med. 2002 Nov;8(11):1288-95.

Yeh HC, Punjabi NM, Wang NY, et al. 2008. Cross-sectional and prospective study of lung function in adults with type 2 diabetes: the Atherosclerosis Risk in Communities (ARIC) study. Diabetes Care 31: 741-46.

Young RP, Hopkins R, Eaton TE. Pharmacological actions of statins: potential utility in COPD. Eur Respir Rev. 2009 Dec 1;18(114):222-32.

18

Implications of Type II Diabetes Mellitus on Gastrointestinal Cancers

Diana H. Yu and M. Mazen Jamal
Section of Gastroenterology, Long Beach Veterans Affairs (VA) Healthcare System
Long Beach, California
Department of Medicine, University of California Irvine College of Medicine
Irvine, California
United States of America

1. Introduction

The rapid growth of the prevalence of Type II Diabetes Mellitus (DM) and its complications among adults has become a major public health problem that is approaching epidemic proportions worldwide. The world prevalence of diabetes among adults is estimated to be 285 million in 2010, and this number is projected to reach 439 million by 2030 (Shaw et al., 2010). While the pathogenesis of hyperglycemia in Type I DM is secondary to lack of insulin due to islet destruction, the hyperglycemia in Type II DM results from complex genetic interactions, the expression of which is modified by environmental factors such as increased age, reduced physical activity and obesity (Inzucchi & Sherwin, 2007). The over-production of insulin and the influence of hyperinsulinemia in enhancing free or bioavailable concentrations of insulin-like growth factor-1 (IGF-1) have been postulated to increase carcinogenesis through a tyrosine kinase growth factor cascade in enhancing tumor cell proliferation (Campbell et al., 2010; Giovannucci, 1995; McKeown-Eyssen, 1994; Moore, 1998).

Type II DM has been demonstrated by numerous epidemiologic studies to be associated with increased risk of many gastrointestinal cancers: esophageal adenocarcinoma, colorectal cancer, pancreatic cancer, biliary tract cancers (primary gallbladder carcinoma, extrahepatic/intrahepatic cholangiocarcinoma) and hepatocellular carcinoma. This review focuses on the expanding body of clinical evidence that supports the association between Type II DM and the increased risk of gastrointestinal cancers. Implications of Type II DM on each respective gastrointestinal cancer are divided into proposed etiology and pathophysiology, and review of epidemiologic studies to support the suggestion that Type II DM independently increase the risk of gastrointestinal cancers.

2. Implication of Type II DM on esophageal adenocarcinoma

2.1 Etiology and pathophysiology

One of the postulated mechanisms to explain the association between Type II DM and esophageal adenocarcinoma is that the metabolic changes associated with DM and adiposity, such as hyperinsulinemia, establishes a hormonal environment which promotes the development of nascent tumors (Calle & Kaaks, 2004; Neale et al., 2009).

Insulin is the hormone integral to the 'metabolic hormonal hypothesis,' proposed by Calle and colleagues. Insulin activates the insulin receptor, and consequently the intracellular signaling cascades with mitogenic and anti-apoptotic effects. Insulin also promotes synthesis and activity of insulin-like growth factor-1 (IGF-1), a peptide hormone with similar structure of insulin, which regulates cellular proliferation in response to available energy and reserves (Calle & Kaaks, 2004). *In vitro* studies have clearly established that both insulin and IGF-1 act as growth factors that promote cell proliferation and inhibit apoptosis (Ish-Shalom et al., 1997; Khandwala, 2000; Lawlor & Alessi, 2001; Le Roith, 2000; Prisco et al., 1999).

As hyperinsulinemia is positively associated with the risk of esophageal adenocarcinoma, association with type II DM, "a proxy for pre-existing hyperinsulinemia," was observed independently of other obesity-related factors by Neale and colleagues (Neale et al., 2009).

2.2 Epidemiologic studies

In a large population-based case-control study in Australia, Neale and colleagues observed consistently higher risks of esophageal adenocarcinoma among those with diabetes within each category of Body Mass Index (Neale et al., 2009). People with diabetes who were also obese were at a 3.5 fold higher risk of esophageal adenocarcinoma than those with neither risk factor (Odds Ratio (OR) 3.55, 95% Confidence Interval (CI) 1.87-6.76). Esophageal adenocarcinoma risks were somewhat lower in those with either obesity or diabetes alone (Obesity: OR 2.67, 95% CI 1.8-3.96; Diabetes: OR 1.86, 95% CI 0.65-5.31).

Hemminki and colleagues also conducted a large population-based study of 125,126 in Sweden, which assessed cancer risks in patients who were hospitalized for Type II DM. For the entire follow-up period (All: 1 year or 5 years), the risk for esophageal cancer was significant in Type II diabetic patients. Standardized incidence ratio (SIR) for esophageal cancer was 2.19 (95% CI 1.83-2.59). The association between number of hospitalizations and esophageal cancer was also observed (Hemminki et al., 2010).

The case-control study by Neale and colleagues is consistent in demonstrating that Type II diabetic patients have about two-fold increased risk of esophageal adenocarcinoma. Hemminki et al. also supported the finding that Type II DM is associated with about two-fold increased risk of esophageal cancer overall; however, no distinction was made between adenocarcinoma and squamous cell carcinoma.

3. Implication of Type II DM on colorectal cancer

3.1 Etiology and pathophysiology

Obesity, reduced physical activity and abdominal distribution of adiposity, which are determinants of the metabolic syndrome, have been implicated in increased risk of colorectal cancer (Giovannucci, 2007; Glade, 1999). Hyperglycemia and hyperinsulinemia, which are the underlying metabolic defects of the metabolic syndrome and are especially pronounced during the early state of Type II DM, have been proposed as mediators for association between metabolic syndrome and colorectal cancer (Campbell et al., 2010; Giovannucci, 1995; McKeown-Eyssen, 1994).

Chronic hyperinsulinemia of Type II DM leads to insulin resistance as a metabolic adaptation to increased circulating levels of free fatty acids released from adipocytes. Increased free fatty acids leads to reduced capacity of livers, muscle and other tissues to absorb, store and metabolize glucose (Bergman & Ader, 2000). In addition to free fatty acids, adipocytes also release endocrine signaling factors, adiponectin and leptin, which play a role in regulation of insulin sensitivity in liver, muscle and other tissues (Havel, 2002). Furthermore, insulin positive feedback influences levels of leptin, a mitogenic adipocytokine, which has been demonstrated to be associated with cancers of the colon, breast and prostate (Stattin et al., 2003; Tessitore et al., 2000).

3.2 Epidemiologic studies

A 2005 meta-analysis of epidemiologic studies reported that DM was associated with a moderate increased risk of CRC overall, with almost identical associations when men and women were analyzed separately (Larsson et al., 2005). Analysis of 15 studies (six case-control and nine cohort studies), with 2,593,935 participants, showed that diabetes was associated with an increased risk of colorectal cancer when compared to non-diabetic controls (Pooled RR of colorectal cancer incidence = 1.3, 95% CI 1.20-1.40), without heterogeneity between studies. In a Singapore Chinese Health Study of diabetic cohort, with distinct body type and lifestyle profiles from those of Western population, Type II DM was also statistically significantly associated with colorectal cancer risk in both men (RR = 1.5, 95% CI = 1.2-2.1) and women (RR = 1.4, 95% CI = 1.0-1.9) (Seow et al., 2006) [Table 1].

More recent studies, however, consistently demonstrate stronger associations for men than for women (Inoue et al., 2006; Kuriki et al., 2007; Limburg et al., 2006; Seow et al, 2006;) [Table 1]. Many studies which examine the association between Type II DM and CRC published since the 2005 meta-analysis by Larsson, analyze statistics in men and women separately in the same study, which suggest that the association among women is not as significant relative to men.

A more recent large, prospective cohort-study by Campbell et al. demonstrated the association between Type II DM and CRC among men (RR 1.24, 95% CI 1.08-1.44), but not among women (RR 1.01, 95% CI 0.82-1.23) (Campbell et al., 2010). Limburg and colleagues have also supported a statistically significant relationship between Type II DM and CRC (especially proximal colon CRC vs. distal CRC) in men, but not statistically significant in women. Over 19,158 person-years of follow-up, 51 incident CRC cases were identified within the type 2 DM cohort of 1,975, while only 36.8 cases were expected based on data from the general population (Standardized Incidence Ratio (SIR) = 1.39, 95% CI 1.03-1.82). In men, Type II DM was associated with increased overall (SIR = 1.67, 95% CI 1.16-2.33) and proximal (SIR = 1.96, 95% CI 1.16 3.10) CRC risks, with statistically not significant increase in distal CRC risk. Conversely, in women, Type II DM was not a risk factor for overall, proximal or distal CRC (SIR = 1.03, 95% CI 0.60-1.66; SIR = 1.17, 95% CI 0.58-2.09; and SIR = 0.74, 95% CI 0.24-1.72, respectively) (Limburg et al., 2006) [Table 1].

Large population-based case-control studies conducted by Ren et al. in China, and by Kuriki et al. and Inoue et al. in Japan, established that association between Type II DM and CRC is statistically significant in both men and women; however, Type II DM women showed less pronounced risk for CRC compared to Type II men (Inoue et al., 2006; Kuriki et al., 2007: Ren et al., 2009). Kuriki and colleagues studied the associations between Type II DM and multi-site cancer risks in a case-control study of 11,672 cancer cases (5341 men, 6331 women) and 47,768 cancer-free controls. Adjusted for confounding factors such as age, BMI, alcohol, smoking, physical exercise, bowel movement, family history of CRC, family history of DM, vegetable intake and dietary restriction, past/present history of diabetes was associated with increased CRC risk for both men and women (OR=1.3, 95% CI 1.0-1.65, OR=1.13, 95% CI 0.72-1.76, respectively) (Kuriki et al., 2007). A more significant association between Type II DM and CRC was observed by Ren and colleagues in their population-based case-control study conducted in China (SIR = 1.82, 95% CI 1.23-2.4 in Type II DM men, SIR = 1.36, 95% CI 0.85-1.88 in Type II DM women) (Ren et al., 2009). Inoue and colleagues have observed moderately increased risk of colon CA in diabetic men (HR 1.36, 95% CI 1.0-1.85) and rectal CA in diabetic women (HR 1.65, 95% CI 0.8-3.39), without statistically significant increase of colon CA in diabetic women and rectal CA in diabetic men.

Study	Control	Case	Adjusted Risk for Colorectal Cancer	Adjustment
Seow et al.	Non-Diabetic (Cases of CRC) 55,851 (546)	Diabetic (Cases of CRC) 5,469 (90)	RR = 1.5 (95% CI 1.2-1.8)	Age, Sex, Dialect group, Education, Body Mass Index, Smoking, Alcohol, Familial Hx of CRC, Physical activity
Inoue et al.	Non-Diabetic † (Cases of Colon CA) 43,451 (445)	Diabetic † (Cases of Colon CA) 3,097 (46)	HR = 1.36 (95% CI 1.0-1.85)	Age, Study area, Hx of cerebrovascular disease, Hx of ischemic heart disease, Smoking, Alcohol, Body Mass Index, Physical activity, Vegetable intake, Coffee intake
	Non-Diabetic ‡ (Cases of Colon CA) 49,652 (293)	Diabetic ‡ (Cases of Colon CA) 1,571 (10)	HR = 0.83 (95% CI 0.42-1.61)	
	Non-Diabetic † (Cases of Rectal CA) 43,451 (228)	Diabetic † (Cases of Rectal CA) 3,097 (15)	HR = 0.8 (95% CI 0.47-1.36)	
	Non-Diabetic ‡ (Cases of Rectal CA) 49,652 (145)	Diabetic ‡ (Cases of Rectal CA) 1,571 (8)	HR = 1.65 (95% CI 0.8-3.39)	
Limburg et al.	Non-Diabetic † (EI of CRC) Not Specified (20.4)*	Diabetic † (OI of CRC) 997 (34)	SIR = 1.67** (95% CI 1.16-2.33)	
	Non-Diabetic ‡ (EI of CRC) Not Specified (16.4)*	Diabetic ‡ (OI of CRC) 978 (17)	SIR = 1.03** (95% CI 0.6-1.66)	
Kuriki et al.	Without CRC† (Case of DM) 13,254 (945)	With CRC† (Case of DM) 686 (76)	OR = 1.3 (95% CI 1.0-1.68)	Age, Body Mass Index, Alcohol, Smoking, Physical exercise, Bowel movement, Family Hx of CRC, Family Hx of DM, Vegetable intake, Dietary restriction
	Without CRC‡ (Case of DM) 32,789 (780)	With CRC‡ (Case of DM) 527 (22)	OR = 1.13 (95% CI 0.72-1.76)	
Ren et al.	Non-Diabetic † (EI of CRC) Not Specified (20.3)*	Diabetic † (OI of CRC) 3,792 (37)	SIR = 1.82** (95% CI 1.23-2.4)	
	Non-Diabetic ‡ (EI of CRC) Not Specified (19.8)*	Diabetic ‡ (OI of CRC) 4146 (27)	SIR = 1.36** (95% CI 0.85-1.88)	

RR = Risk Ratio, HR = Hazard Ratio, SIR = Standardized Incidence Ratio, OR = Odds Ratio
DM = Diabetes Mellitus, CRC = Colorectal Cancer, Hx = History, EI = Expected Incidence, OI = Observed Incidence

† Men ‡ Women

* Number of EI calculated according to age & gender-specific incidence rate of general population

** Calculated as ratio of Observed Incidence cases to Expected Incidence cases

Table 1. Type II DM and Colorectal CA

These studies, taken as a whole, suggest Type II DM is associated with a moderately increased risk of CRC overall, with more recent studies consistently demonstrating stronger associations for men than for women.

4. Implication of Type II DM on pancreatic cancer

4.1 Etiology and pathophysiology

The precise etiology of pancreatic cancer remains unclear. Several environmental factors have been implicated, but evidence of a causative role exists only for tobacco use.

Many epidemiologic studies have reported a positive association between DM and pancreatic cancer risk, with concern that diabetes may be a consequence, rather than a cause (Noy & Bilezikian, 1994). However, other studies have demonstrated an association between elevated plasma glucose, insulin and C-peptide levels - characteristics of long-standing DM – with increased risk for pancreatic cancer (Batty et al., 2004; Gapstur et al., 2000; Jee, et al., 2005; Michaud, et al., 2007; Stattin, et al., 2007).

Some studies have demonstrated an increased incidence of pancreatic cancer among patients with chronic pancreatitis or history of DM (Batty et al., 2009; Genkinger et al., 2009; Hildalgo, 2010; Landi, 2009; Lowenfels & Maisonneuve, 2006). Though less conclusive, there is also evidence that chronic cirrhosis, high-cholesterol diet and previous cholecystectomy are associated with an increased incidence of pancreatic cancer (Batty et al., 2009; Genkinger et al., 2009; Hildalgo, 2010; Landi, 2009; Lowenfels & Maisonneuve, 2006).

Considerable number of recent epidemiologic studies suggests that DM may be a predisposing factor in pancreatic carcinogenesis (Gapstur et al., 2000).

4.2 Epidemiologic studies

A meta-analysis conducted by Everhart et al. has shown that a history of diabetes for greater than or equal to 5 years increases the incidence of pancreatic cancer by twofold (Everhart & Wright, 1995). Among 20 studies included in meta-analysis, 18 demonstrated a positive association between preexisting diabetes and the occurrence of pancreatic cancer. The pooled Relative Risk (RR) of 20 epidemiologic studies for those diabetes was diagnosed at least 1 year prior to either diagnosis of pancreatic cancer or mortality was 2.1 with 95% CI of 1.6-2.8. In an analysis requiring a 5-year duration of diabetes resulted in similar results, with RR of 2.0 (95% CI 1.2-3.2) in 11 epidemiologic studies [Table 2].

In a hospital based case-control study, Bonelli et al. have demonstrated that the risk of pancreatic cancer was increased by 6.2 fold in patients with diabetes, which necessitated insulin therapy for greater than 5 years (Bonelli et al., 2003). Jamal and colleagues further supported these findings with their large population-based case-control study of 1,172,496 patients, by demonstrating that occurrence of pancreatic cancer was increased by threefold in DM patients compared to controls (frequency of pancreatic cancer in DM subjects 0.9% compared to control subjects 0.3% with OR:3.22, 95% CI: 3.03-3.42) (Jamal et al., 2009) [Table 2].

A more recent three large case-control studies conducted by Li and colleagues have shown that diabetes is associated with 1.8 fold risk of pancreatic cancer (95% CI: 1.5-2.1), adjusted for age, sex, race, education, smoking, alcohol consumption and Body Mass Index (BMI). Risk estimates decreased with increasing years with diabetes. Among diabetics, risk was higher in insulin users vs. non-users (OR: 2.2, 95%CI 1.6-3.7). Insulin use of >10 years was associated with reduced risk of pancreatic cancer (OR: 0.5 95% CI: 0.3-0.9). Lastly, Hispanic/Latino-American men and Asian-Americans had higher risks of diabetes-associated pancreatic cancer when compared to Caucasian-Americans and African-Americans, but the differences were not statistically significant (Li et al., 2011) [Table 2].

Study	Control	Case	Adjusted Risk for Pancreatic Cancer	Adjustment
Jamal et al.	Non-Diabetic (% with pancreatic CA) 836,283 (0.3)	Diabetic (% with pancreatic CA) 278,761 (0.9)	OR = 3.22 (95% CI 3.03-3.42)	Smoking, Obesity, Pancreatitis and other Pancreatic disorders
Li et al.†	Without Pancreatic CA (% with DM) 5113 (11)	With Pancreatic CA (% with DM) 2192 (20.4)	OR = 1.8 (95% CI 1.5-2.1)	Age, Sex, Race, Education, Smoking, Alcohol, Body Mass Index, Study site
Gapstur et al.‡	Non-Diabetic (No. of pancreatic CA mortality) 16,158 (30)	Diabetic (No. of pancreatic CA mortality) 2,578 (23)	RR = 2.15 (95% CI 1.22-3.8)	Age, Race, Categories of postload plasma glucose [ ], Smoking, Body Mass Index
Everhart et al.¶	NA	NA	DM (1yr)* RR= 2.1 (95% CI 1.6-2.8) DM (5yr)** RR= 2.0 (95% CI 1.2-3.2)	Age (Each epidemiologic study included in Meta-analysis with own variables)
Calle et al.	Non-Diabetic (No. of pancreatic CA mortality) 1,035,758 (2953)	Diabetic (No. of pancreatic CA Mortality) 53,828 (249)	RR = 1.48 (95% CI 1.3-1.68)	Age, Race, Smoking, Family Hx of pancreatic CA, Body Mass Index, Education

OR = Odds Ratio, RR = Risk Ratio, CI = Confidence Interval, CA = Cancer, NA = Non- applicable, Hx = History, DM = Diabetes Mellitus, [ ] = Concentration, No. = Number, yr = year

† Data pooled from 3 case-control studies (M.D. Anderson Cancer Center Study, University of California San Francisco Bay Area Study, National Cancer Institute Study)

‡ Non-diabetic designated to participants with postload plasma glucose [ ] ≤ 119mg/dL (6.6mmol/L). Diabetic designated to participants with postload plasma glucose [ ] ≥ 200mg/dL (11.1mmol/L)

Meta-analysis: Pooled RR of 20 epidemiologic studies* 11 epidemiologic studies **

Table 2. Type II DM and Pancreatic CA

Gapstur and colleagues have also demonstrated a positive association between post-load plasma glucose level and risk of pancreatic cancer mortality. Risk was 2.2 fold higher (RR

2.15 CI 1.22-3.8, p 0.01) for participants whose post load plasma glucose level was at least 200mg/dL at baseline compared to those with less or equal to 119mg/dL, adjusted for age, race, cigarette smoking status and BMI. This association was independent of other known and suspected pancreatic cancer risk factors such as age, race, cigaretts smoking and BMI (Gapstur et al., 2000) [Table 2].

Lastly, Calle et al. have also concluded from their study, after 12 years of follow-up in 1,089,586 men and women, that a history of self-reported diabetes was associated with increased pancreatic cancer mortality RR = 1.48 (95% CI 1.3-1.68) [Table 2]. This association was similar in men RR = 1.49 (95% CI 1.25-1.77) and women RR = 1.51 (95% CI 1.24-1.85). (Calle et al., 1998) [Table 2].

These studies, taken as a whole, suggest Type II DM is independently associated with about two-fold increased risk in pancreatic cancer. This finding is consistent throughout all studies which adjusted for tobacco use, which remains to be the only environmental factor that plays a causative role in the risk of pancreatic cancer.

5. Implication of Type II DM on biliary tract cancer (primary carcinoma of gallbladder and extrahepatic/intrahepatic cholangiocarcinoma)

5.1 Etiology and pathophysiology

Type II DM is associated with insulin resistance, compensatory hyperinsulinemia and up-regulated level of insulin-like growth factors (IGFs). Cai and colleagues have recently demonstrated that IGFs may stimulate cholangiocyte growth through cellular proliferation and inhibition of apoptosis (Cai et al., 2008). Furthermore, the integral role IGFs may play in the carcinogenesis of cholangiocytes is supported by *in vitro* and *in vivo* studies (Alvaro et al., 2006).

The etiology of primary gall bladder carcinoma is not well understood. However, several factors have been postulated to place patients at a greater risk. These risk factors include gallstone disease, obesity, female sex, tobacco use and an anomalous pancreaticobiliary ductal union (Jones, 1990; Strom et al., 1995). Some international population-based studies have also shown that diabetes is independently associated with a higher risk of gallstones, which is one of the major risk factors for primary carcinoma of the gallbladder (Festi et al., 2008; Shebl et al., 2010).

In a recent study by Biddinger and colleagues, the mechanistic link between the well-documented association between gallstones and the metabolic syndrome has been proposed (Biddinger et al., 2008). Their study using the LIRKO mouse model (mice with isolated hepatic insulin resistance created by liver-specific disruption of the insulin receptor), showed that hepatic insulin resistance leads to increased biliary cholesterol secretion and cholesterol gallstone formation, both of which are features of the human metabolic syndrome (Attili et al., 1997; Bennion & Grundy, 1975; Shaffer & Small, 1977). These effects are due to disinhibition of the forkhead transcrtiption factor (FoxO1), which drives the expression of the biliary cholesterol transporters (Abcg5 and Abcg8), in addition to the enzymes of gluconeogenesis (Biddinger et al., 2008).

5.2 Epidemiologic studies

In a large population-based case-control study conducted among 1,172,496 American Veterans, Jamal and colleagues have found that Type II DM was associated with an increased

risk of gallbladder cancer. The risk of gallbladder (OR 2.2, 95%CI 1.56-3) cancer was increased by two-fold in diabetic patients when compared to controls (Jamal et al., 2009) [Table 3]. A case-control study using a large United Kingdom primary care database, Grainge et al. also demonstrated that the relative risk of gallbladder cancer in diabetic patients compared to non-diabetic controls was 1.43 (95% CI: 0.81-2.52) (Grainge et al., 2009) [Table 3].
A similar analysis was performed by investigators, Shebl and colleagues in a population-based case-control study of 627 biliary tract cancers, 1037 biliary tract stones, and 959 controls in Shanghai, China. Independent of BMI, diabetes was associated with significantly increased risks of gallbladder cancer and biliary stones, OR 2.6 (95% CI 1.5-4.7) and 2.0 (95% CI 1.2-3.3), respectively. Furthermore, about 60% of the effect of diabetes on biliary tract cancer was mediated in part by gallstones and 17% by high-density lipoprotein (HDL). However, no significant association was found with extrahepatic biliary cancer and cancer of Ampulla of Vater. (Shebl et al., 2010) [Table 3].

Study	Control	Case	Adjusted OR for Biliary Tract Cancer	Adjustment
Jamal et al.†‡	Non-Diabetic (% with Gallbladder CA) 836,283 (0)	Diabetic (% with Gallbladder CA) 278,761 (0.03)	OR = 2.2 (95% CI 1.56-3.0)	Gallstone disease, Smoking, Obesity
	Non-Diabetic (% with Extrahepatic Biliary CA) 836,283 (0.02)	Diabetic (% with Extrahepatic Biliary CA) 278,761 (0.1)	OR = 2.1 (95% CI 1.61-2.53)	
Grainge et al.†‡	Without Gallbladder CA (% DM) 5760 (5.9)	With Gallbladder CA (% DM) 5760 (8.7)	OR = 1.43 (95% CI 0.81-2.52)	Sex, Age
	Without Cholangiocarcinoma (% DM) 5760 (5.9)	With Cholangiocarcinoma (% DM) 372 (9.4)	OR = 1.48 (95% CI 1.0-2.17)	
Shebl et al.†	Without Gallbladder CA (% DM) 902 (7.54)	With Gallbladder CA (% DM) 367 (13.9)	OR = 2.63 (95% CI 1.47-4.68)	Age, Sex, Education, Diabetes duration, Body Mass Index, Waist-to-hip ratio, Aspirin use
Welzel et al.‡	Without ECC (% DM) 102,782 (22.1)	With ECC (% DM) 549 (30.1)	OR = 1.5 (95% CI 1.3-1.8)	Age, Sex, Race, Geographic location
	Without ICC (% DM) 102,782 (22.1)	With ICC (% DM) 535 (33.1)	OR = 1.8 (95% CI 1.5-2.1)	
Tao et al.‡	Without ECC (% DM) 380 (9.5)	With ECC (% DM) 129 (18.6)	OR = 3.2 (95% CI 1.7-5.9)	Age, Sex, DM, Cholelithiasis, Hx of Cholecystectomy
	Without ICC (% DM) 380 (9.5)	With ICC (% DM) 6.1 (4.9)	NA	

OR = Odds Ratio, CI = Confidence Interval, CA = Cancer, NA = Non-applicable
Hx = History, DM = Diabetes Mellitus, ECC = Extrahepatic Cholangiocarcinoma
ICC = Intrahepatic Cholangiocarcinoma
† Gallbladder CA
‡ Extrahepatic and/or Intrahepatic Cholangiocarcinoma

Table 3. Type II DM and Biliary Tract CA

However, several other studies have shown that there is significant association between Type II DM and bile duct cancers. Jamal et al. in the same large population-based case-control study, described above, showed that extrahepatic biliary cancer was increased by two-fold in diabetic patients (OR 2.1, 95% 1.61-2.53) (Jamal et al., 2009). Grainge and colleagues, in their large UK study, described above, also support the finding of increased risk of cholangiocarcinoma in diabetic patients compared to non-diabetic controls (RR = 1.48, 95% CI: 1.0-2.17) (Grainge et al., 2009) [Table 3].
Welzel et al. further demonstrated that Type II DM was significantly more common among both Extrahepatic Cholangiocarcinoma (ECC) and Intrahepatic Cholangiocarcinoma (ICC). The study examined the prevalence of following risk factors for both ECC and ICC in patients age 65 years and older with diagnosis of ECC or ICC using the SEER (Surveillance, Epidemiology, and End Results) database in the United States: Biliary cirrhosis, cholelithiasis, choledocholithiasis, cholecystitis, cholecystectomy, alcoholic liver disease, liver cirrhosis, Type II DM, thyrotoxicosis and chronic pancreatitis. Prevalence of Type II DM was significantly higher in patients with ECC compared to those without ECC (OR = 1.5, 95% CI 1.3-1.8). Similar result was found in patients with ICC compared to those without ICC (OR = 1.8, 95% CI 1.5-2.1) [Table 3].
A similar study was conducted by investigators in China by Tao and colleagues, who also supported Welzel's findings that Type II DM had a positive association with ECC (OR = 3.2, 95% CI 1.7-5.9), adjusted for age, gender, history of cholelithiasis and cholecystectomy. However, in this Chinese population-based study, an inverse association between Type II DM and ICC were reported (increased DM cases among patients with ICC than those without ICC) (Tao et al., 2009) [Table 3].

6. Implication of Type II DM on hepatocellular carcinoma

6.1 Etiology and pathophysiology

The main etiology of hepatocellular carcinoma (HCC) is chronic infection with hepatitis B and hepatitis C viruses. However, there are other important factors that contribute to the international burden of HCC. Among these are obesity, diabetes, non-alcoholic steatohepatitis (NASH) and dietary exposures (Blonski et al, 2010). Diabetes is a part of the metabolic syndrome that is characterized by insulin resistance and is thought to predispose to nonalcoholic fatty liver disease (NAFLD), including its more severe form, nonalcoholic steatohepatitis (NASH) (El-Serag, et al., 2006). Diabetes has also been identified as an independent factor for disease progression and for more advanced liver disease in patients with NAFLD.
HCC as a complication of diabetes-associated NASH has been described (Di Bisceglie et al., 1998; El-Serag et al., 2001) and diabetes has been found to be prevalent in patients with HCC and cryptogenic cirrhosis (Marchesini et al., 1999; Matteoni et al., 1999). However, the pathophysiology underlying the increased risk of chronic nonalcoholic liver disease and HCC with diabetes is uncertain. Proposed pathyphysiology involves increased insulin resistance in NAFLD patients compared with control subjects (Marchesini et al., 1999). Insulin resistance facilitates peripheral lipolysis, decreases mitochondrial beta-oxidation of fatty acids and increases accumulation of free fatty acids in the liver, which can lead to NAFLD (Chitturi & Farrell, 2001; Pessayre et al., 2001). Recent studies have shown that

HCC can result as a consequence of DM-related NASH (Cotrim et al., 2000; Shimada et al., 2002; Zen et al., 2001).

6.2 Epidemiologic studies

In a large retrospective cohort study of veteran patient populations (DM cohort: 173,643. Control: 650,620), El-Serag and colleagues have shown that the incidence of chronic nonalcoholic fatty liver disease (NAFLD) was significantly higher among patients with diabetes compared to control patients (Incidence rate: 18.13 vs. 9.55 per 10,000 person-years, respectively). Corresponding results were obtained for higher rates of HCC among diabetic patients compared to non-diabetic patients (incidence rate: 2.39 vs. 0.87 per 10,000 person-years, respectively), supporting previously published studies with positive association between Type II DM and HCC (El-Serag et al., 2004).

Furthermore, in a recent systematic review of 13 case-control studies, 11 supported an association between diabetes and the development of HCC. Among the 13 case-control studies, subjects with diabetes were found to have a two-fold increase in the risk of HCC. This association was also appreciated amongst 12 cohort studies evaluated (El-Serag et al., 2006).

7. Conclusion

Type II Diabetes Mellitus and its complications is a growing public health problem worldwide. Increased morbidity and mortality associated with various gastrointestinal cancers as one of the complications of Type II DM holds strong public health and clinical relevance. There is a growing body of evidence suggesting that Type II DM and its metabolic defects (hyperinsulinemia and hyperglycemia) are associated with increased risk of various gastrointestinal cancers. Although further studies are required to definitively validate this association, the current understanding between Type II DM and gastrointestinal cancers warrants attention for its potential implications in the clinical practice of diabetic management and novel targeted cancer therapy.

8. References

Alvaro, D. & Barbaro, B. et al. (2006). Estrogens and insulin-like growth factor I modulate neoplastic cell growth in human cholangiocarcinoma. *Am J Pathol*, Vol.169, No.3 (September 2006), pp. 877-888.

Attili, A.F. & Capocaccia, R. et al. (1997). Factors associated with gallstone disease in the MICOL experience. Multicenter Italian Study on Epidemiology of Cholelithiasis. *Hepatology*, Vol.26, No.4 (October 1997), pp. 809-818.

Batty, G.D.; Kivimaki, M.; Morrison, D.; Huxley, R.; Smith, G.D.; Clarke, R.; Marmot, M.G. & Shipley, M.J. (2009). Risk factors for pancreatic cancer mortality: extended follow-up of the original Whitehall study. *Cancer Epidemiol Biomarkers Prev*, Vol.18, No.2 (February 2009), pp. 673-675.

Batty, G.D.; Shipley, M.J.; Marmot, M. & Smith, G.D. (2004). Diabetes status and post-load plasma glucose concentration in relation to site-specific cancer mortality: findings from the original Whitehall study. *Cancer Causes Control*, Vol. 15, No. 9 (November 2004), pp. 873-881.

Bennion, L.J. & Grundy, S.M. (1975). Effects of obesity and caloric intake on biliary lipid metabolism in man. J *Clin Invest,* Vol. 56, No.4 (October 1975), pp. 996-1011.

Bergman, R.N. & Ader, M. (2000). Free fatty acids and pathogenesis of type 2 diabetes mellitus. *Trends Endocrinol Metab,* Vol. 11, No.9 (November 2000), pp. 351-356.

Biddinger, S.B. & Hass, J.T. et al. (2008). Hepatic insulin resistance directly promotes formation of cholesterol gallstones. *Nat Med,* Vol.14, No.7 (July 2008), pp. 778-782.

Blonski, W.; Kotlyar, D.S. & Forde, K.A. (2010). Non-viral causes of hepatocellular carcinoma. *World J of Gastroenterology,* Vol.16, No.29 (August 2010), pp. 3603-3615.

Bonelli, L.; Aste, H.; Hovo, P.; Cavallini, G.; Felder, M.; Gusmaroli, R.; Morandini, E.; Ravelli, P.; Briglia, R.; Lombardo, L.; De Micheli, A. & Pugliese, V. (2003). Exocrine pancreatic cancer, cigarette smoking, and diabetes mellitus: a case-control study in northern Italy. *Pancreas,* Vol.27, No.2 (August 2003), pp. 143-149.

Cai, H.H.; Sun, Y.M.; Bai, J.F.; Shi, Y.; Zhao, H.L. & Miao, Y. (2008). Relationship between the GH-IGFs axis and the proliferation of bile duct cancer cell line QBC939 in vitro. *Hepatobiliary Pancreat Dis Int,* Vol. 7, No.1 (February 2008), pp. 76-81.

Calle, E.E. & Kaaks, R. (2004). Overweight, obesity and cancer: epidemiological evidence and proposed mechanisms. *Nat Rev Cancer,* Vol.4, No.8 (August 2004), pp. 579-591.

Calle, E.E.; Murphy, T.K.; Rodriguez, C.; Thun, M.J. & Heath C.W.Jr. (1998). Diabetes mellitus and pancreatic cancer mortality in a prospective cohort of United States adults. *Cancer Causes Control,* Vol. 9, No. 4. (August 1998), pp. 403-410.

Campbell, P.T.; Deka, A.; Jacobs, E.J.; Newton, C.C.; Hildebrand, J.S.; McCullough, M.L.; Limburd, P.J. & Gapstur, S.M. (2010). Prospective study reveals associations between colorectal cancer and type 2 diabetes mellitus or insulin use in men. *Gastroenterology,* Vol.139, No.4 (October 2010), pp. 1138-1146.

Chitturi, S. & Farrell, G. (2001). Etiopathogenesis of nonalcoholic steatohepatitis. *Sem Liver Dis,* Vol.21, No.1 (2001), pp. 27-41.

Cotrim, H.P.; Parana, R.; Braga, E. & Lyra, L. (2000). Nonalcoholic steatohepatitis and hepatocellular carcinoma: natural history? *Am J Gastroenterol,* Vol.95, No.10 (October 2000), pp. 3018-3019.

Di Bisceglie, A.M.; Carithers, R.L. Jr. & Gores, G.L. (1998). Hepatocellular carcinoma. *Hepatology,* Vol.28, No.4 (October 1998), pp. 1161-1165.

El-Serag, H.B.; Hampel, H. & Javadi, F. (2006). The association between diabetes and hepatocellular carcinoma: a systematic review of epidemiologic evidence. *Clin Gastroenterol Hepatol,* Vol.4, No.3 (March 2006), pp. 369-380.

El-Serag, H.B.; Richardson, P.A. & Everhart, J.E. (2001). The role of diabetes in hepatocellular carcinoma: a case-control study among United States veterans. *Am J Gastroenterol,* Vol.96, No.8 (August 2001), pp. 2462-2467.

El-Serag, H.B.; Tran, T. & Everhart, J.E. (2004). Diabetes increases the risk of chronic liver disease and hepatocellular carcinoma. *Gastroenterology,* Vol.126, No.2 (February 2004), pp. 460-468.

Everhart, J. & Wright, D. (1995). Diabetes Mellitus as a risk factor for pancreatic cancer. A meta-analysis. *JAMA,* Vol.273, No.20 (May 1995), pp. 1605-1609.

Festi, D. & Dormi, A. et al. (2008). Incidence of gallstone disease in Italy: results from a multi-center, population-based Italian study. *World J Gastroenterology,* Vol.14, No.34. (September 2008), pp. 5282-5289.

Gapstur, S.M.; Gann, P.H.; Lowe, W.; Liu, K.; Colangelo, L. & Dyer, A. (2000). Abnormal glucose metabolism and pancreatic cancer mortality. *JAMA*, Vol. 283, No. 19 (May 2000), pp. 2552-2558.

Genkinger, J.M. & Spiegelman, D. et al. (2009). Alcohol intake and pancreatic cancer risk: A pooled analysis of fourteen cohort studies. *Cancer Epidemiol Biokmarker Prev*, Vol.18, No.3 (March 2009), pp. 765-776.

Glade, M.J. (1999). Food, nutrition, physical activity, and the prevention of cancer: a global perspective. American Institute for Cancer Research/World Cancer Research Fund, American Institute for Cancer Research, 1997. *Nutrition*, Vol.15, No.6, (June 1999), pp 523-526.

Grainge, M.J.; West, J.; Solaymani-Dodaran, M.; Aithal, G.P. & Card, T.R. (2009). The antecedents of biliary cancer: a primary care case-control study in the United Kingdom. *Brit J Cancer*, Vol.100, No.1 (January 2009), pp. 178-180.

Giovannucci, E. (1995). Insulin and colon cancer. *Cancer Causes* Control, (March 1995), Vol.6, pp. 164-179.

Giovannucci, E. (2007). Metabolic syndrome, hyperinsulinemia, and colon cancer: a review. *Am J Clin Nutr*, Vol. 86, No.3, (September 2007), pp. s836-42.

Havel, P.J. Control of energy homeostasis and insulin action by adipocyte hormone: leptin, acylation stimulating protein, and adiponectin. *Curr Opin Lipidol*, Vol. 13, No.1 (February 2002), pp. 51-59.

Hemminki, K.; Li, X.; Sundquist, J. & Sundquist K. (2010). Risk of Cancer Following Hospitalization for Type 2 Diabetes. *The Oncologist*, Vol. 15, No. 6 (May 2010), pp. 548-555.

Hidalgo, M. (2010). Pancreatic Cancer. *New Engl J Med*, Vol.362, No.17 (April 2010), pp. 1605-1617.

Inoue, M.; Iwasaki, M.; Otani, T.; Sasazuki, S.; Noda, M. & Tsugane, S. (2006). Diabetes mellitus and the risk of cancer: results from a large-scale population-based cohort study in Japan. *Arch Intern Med*, Vol.166, No.17 (September 2006), pp. 1872-1877.

Inzucchi, S.E & Sherwin R.S. (2007). Chapter 248: Type 2 Diabetes Mellitus, In: *Cecil Medicine, 23rd Edition*. Goldman, L. & Ausiello, D. (Ed.), pp. 1748-1760, Saunders Elsevier, ISBN: 978-1-4160-2805-5, Philadelphia, Pennsylvania, USA.

Ish-Shalom, D. & Christoffersen, C.T. et al. (1997). Mitogenic properties of insulin and insulin analogues mediated by the insulin receptor. *Diabetologia*, Vol. 40, No. Suppl2 (July 1997), pp. 25-31.

Jamal, M.M.; Yoon, E.J.; Vega, K.J.; Hashemzadeh, M. & Chang, K.J. (2009). Diabetes mellitus as a risk factor for gastrointestinal cancer among American veterans. *World J Gastroenterol*, Vol.15, No.42. (November 2009), pp. 5274-5278.

Jee, S.H.; Ohrr, H.; Sull, J.W.; Yun, J.E.; Ji, M. & Samet, J.M. (2005). Fasting serum glucose level and cancer risk in Korean men and women. *JAMA*, Vol. 293, No. 2 (January 2005), pp. 194-202.

Jones, R.S. (1990). Carcinoma of the gallbladder. *Surg Clin North Am*, Vol.70, No.6. (December 1990), pp. 1419-1428.

Khandwala, H.M.; McCutcheon, I.E.; Flyvbjerg, A. & Friend, K.E. (2000). The effects of insulin-like growth factors on tumorigenesis and neoplastic growth. *Endocr Rev*, Vol.21, No.3 (June 2000), pp. 215-244.

Kuriki, K.; Hirose, K. & Tajima, K. (2007). Diabetes and cancer risk for all and specific sites among Japanese men and women. *Eur J Cancer Prev,* Vol.16, No.1 (February 2007), pp. 83-89.

Landi, S. (2009). Genetic predisposition and environmental risk factors to pancreatic cancer: a review of the literature. *Mutat Res,* Vol.681, No.2-3 (March-June 2009), pp. 299-307.

Larsson, S.C.; Orsini, N. & Wolk, A. (2005). Diabetes Mellitus and risk of colorectal cancer: a meta-analysis. *J Natl Cancer Inst,* Vol.97, No.22 (November 2005), pp. 1679-1687.

Lawlor, M.A. & Alessi, D.R. (2001). PKB/Akt: a key mediator of cell proliferation, survival and insulin responses? *J Cell Sci,* Vol. 114, No.16 (August 2001), pp. 2903-2910.

Le Roith, D. (2000). Regulation of proliferation and apoptosis by the insulin-like growth factor I receptor. *Growth Horm IGF Res,* Vol. 10, Suppl A. (April 2000), pp. S12-13.

Li, D.; Tang, H.; Hassan, M.M.; Holly, E.A.; Bracci, P.M. & Silverman, D.T. (2011). Diabetes and risk of pancreatic cancer: a pooled analysis of three large case-control studies. *Cancer Causes Control,* Vol.22, No.2 (February 2011), pp. 189-197.

Limburg, P.J. & Vierkant, R.A. et al. (2006). Clinically confirmed type 2 diabetes mellitus and colorectal cancer risk: a population-based, retrospective cohort study. *Am J Gastroenterol,* Vol.101, No.8 (August 2006), pp. 1872-1879.

Lowenfels, A.B. & Maisonneuve, P. (2006). Epidemiology and risk factors for pancreatic cancer. *Best Pract Res Clin Gastroenterol,* Vol.20, No.2 (April 2006), pp. 197-209.

Marchesini, G.; Brizi, M.; Morselli-Labate, A.M.; Bianchi, G.; Bugianesi, E.; McCullough, A.; Forlani, G. & Melachionda, N. (1999). Association of nonalcoholic fatty liver disease with insulin resistance. *Am J Med,* Vol. 107, No.5 (November 1999), pp. 450-455.

Matteoni, C.; Younossi, Z.; Gramlich, T.; Bopari, B.; Liu, Y. & McCullough, A. (1999). Nonalcoholic fatty liver disease: a spectrum of clinical and pathological severity. *Gastroenterol,* Vol. 116, No.6 (June 1999), pp. 1413-1419.

McKeown-Eyssen, G (1994). Epidemiology of colorectal cancer revisited: are serum triglycerides and/or plasma glucose associated with risk? *Cancer Epidemiol Biomarkers* Prev, Vol.3, No.8 (December 1994), pp. 687-695.

Michaud, D.S. & Wolpin, B. et al. (2007). Prediagnostic plasma C-peptide and pancreatic cancer risk in men and women. *Cancer Epidemiol Biomarkers Prev,* Vol. 16, No. 10 (October 2007), pp. 2101-2109.

Moore, M.A.; Park, C.B. & Tsuda, H. (1998). Implications of the hyperinsulinemia-diabetes cancer link of for preventive efforts. *Eur J Cancer Prev,* Vol.7, No.2 (April 1998), pp. 89-107.

Neale, R.E.; Doecke, J.D.; Pandeya, N.; Sadhegi, S.; Green, A.C.; Webb, P.M. & Whiteman, D.C. (2009). Does type 2 diabetes influence the risk of oesophageal adenocarcinoma? *Brit J of* Cancer, Vol.100, No.5, (March 2009), pp. 795-798.

Noy, A. & Bilezikian, J.P. (1994). Clinical review 63: Diabetes and pancreatic cancer: clues to the early diagnosis of pancreatic malignancy. *J Clin Endocrinol Metab,* Vol. 79, No. 5 (November 1994), pp. 1223-1231.

Pessayre, D.; Berson, A.; Formenty, B. & Mansouri, A. (2001). Mitochondria in steatohepatitis. *Sem Liver Dis,* Vol.21, No.1 (2001), pp. 57-69.

Prisco, M.; Romano, G.; Peruzzi, F.; Valentinis, B. & Baserga, R. (1999). Insulin and IGF-I receptors signaling in protection from apoptosis. *Horm Metab Res,* Vol. 31, No.2-3 (February-March 1999), pp. 80-89.

Ren, X. & Zhang, X. et al. (2009). Type 2 diabetes mellitus associated with increased risk for colorectal cancer: evidence from an international ecological study and population-based risk analysis in China. *Public Health,* Vol.123, No.8 (August 2009), pp. 540-544.

Seow, A.; Yuan, J.M.; Koh, W.P.; Lee, H.P. & Yu, M.C. (2006). Diabetes mellitus and risk of colorectal cancer in the Singapore Chinese Health Study. *J Natl Cancer Inst,* Vol.98, No.2 (January 2006), pp. 135-138.

Shaffer, E.A. & Small, D.M. (1977). Biliary lipid secretion in cholesterol gallstone disease. The effect of cholecystectomy and obesity. *J Clin Invest,* Vol.59, No.5 (May 1977), pp. 828-840.

Shaib, Y.H. & El-Serag, H.B. et al. (2007). Risk factors for intrahepatic and extrahepatic cholangiocarcinoma: a hospital-based case-control study. *Am J Gastroenterol,* Vol.102, No.5 (May 2007), pp. 1016-1021.

Shaw, J.E.; Sicree, R.A. & Zimmet, P.Z. (2010). Global estimates of the prevalence of diabetes for 2010 and 2030. *Diabetes Res Clin Pract,* Vol.87, No.1 (January 2010), pp. 4-14.

Shebl, F.M. & Andreotti, G. et al. (2010). Diabetes in relation to biliary tract cancer and stones: a population-based study in Shanghai, China. *Brit J Cancer,* Vol. 103, No.1 (June 2010), pp. 115-119.

Shimada, M.; Hashimoto, E.; Taniai, M.; Hasegawa, K.; Okuda, H.; Yayashi, N.; Takasaki, K. & Lugwig, J. (2002). Hepatocellular carcinoma in patients with non-alcoholic steatohepatitis. *J Hepatol ,* Vol.37, No.1 (July 2002), pp. 154-160.

Stattin, P. & Bjor, O. et al. (2007). Prospective study of hyperglycemia and cancer risk. *Diabetes Care,* Vol. 30, No. 3 (March 2007), pp. 561-567.

Stattin, P.; Palmqvist, R.; Soderberg, S.; Biessy, C.; Ardnor, B.; Hallmans, G.; Kaaks, R. & Olsson, T. (2003). Plasma leptin and colorectal cancer risk: a prospective study in Northern Sweden. *Oncol Rep,* Vol.10, No.6 (November-December 2003), pp. 2015-2021.

Strom, B.L.; Soloway, R.D.; Rios-Dalenz, J.L.; Rodriguez-Martinez, H.A.; West, S.L.; Kinman, J.L.; Polansky, M. & Berlin, J.A. (1995). Risk factors for gallbladder cancer. An international collaborative case-control study. *Cancer,* Vol.76, No.10 (November 1995), pp. 1747-1756.

Tao, L.Y. & He, X.D. et al. (2010). Risk factors for intrahepatic and extrahepatic cholangiocarcinoma: a case-control study in China. *Liver Int,* Vol.30, No.2 (February 2010), pp. 215-221.

Tessitore, L.; Vizio, B.; Jenkins, O.; De Stefano, I.; Ritossa, C.; Argiles, J.M.; Benedetto, C. & Mussa, A. (2000). Leptin expression in colorectal and breast cancer patients. *Int J Mol Med,* Vol.5, No.4 (April 2000), pp. 421-426.

Welzel, T.M. & Graubard, B.I. et al. (2007). Risk factors for intrahepatic and extrahepatic cholangiocarcinoma in the United States: a population-based case-control study. *Clin Gastroenterol Hepatol,* Vol.5, No.10 (October 2007), pp. 1221-1228.

Zen, Y.; Katayanagi, K.; Tsuneyama, K.; Harada, K.; Araki, I. & Nakanuma, Y. (2001). Hepatocellular carcinoma arising in non-alcoholic steatohepatitis. *Pathol Int,* Vol.51, No.2 (February 2001), pp. 127-131.

19

Prevention for Micro- and Macro-Vascular Complications in Diabetic Patients

Kyuzi Kamoi
University of Niigata Prefecture
Japan

1. Introduction

One of the goals in long-term cares for patients with diabetes mellitus (DM) is to prevent the development of micro-and macro- vascular complications (The International Diabetes Federation, 2011). To achieve this purpose, an adequate control of blood pressure (BP) as well as a good glycaemic control is crucial (The International Diabetes Federation, 2011). The American Diabetes Association recommended that the BP goal should be lowered to 130/80 mmHg in the daytime of clinic setting (The American Diabetes Association, 2002-2011).

However, in 4733 patients with type 2 DM at high risk for cardiovascular events followed the mean of 4.7 years, targeting a systolic casual/clinic BP (CBP) in the daytime of less than 120 mmHg as compared with less than 140 mmHg, did not reduce the rate of a composite outcome of fatal and nonfatal major cardiovascular events (ACCORD Study Group, 2010). Further, in 16,893 patient-years of follow up at 862 sites in 14 countries, a tight control of systolic CBP in the daytime among patients with DM and cardiovascular disease to achieve systolic CBP in the daytime of less than 130 mmHg and diastolic CBP of less than 85 mmHg was not associated with improved cardiovascular outcomes compared with usual control (Cooper-DeHoff et al, 2010). At present, the reasons of difference are not clear.

Recently, a discrepancy between screening BP by CBP measurment and ambulatory BP by ambulatory blood pressure monitaring (ABPM) has been noted. It has also been shown that in patients with essential hypertension, home BP (HBP) measurement in the morning has a stronger predictive power for mortality than CBP measurements in the daytime (Aihara et al, 1998, Ohkubo et al, 1998, Imai et al, 1999). Accordingly, the difference of results (ACCORD Study Group, 2010, Cooper-DeHoff et al, 2010) may be due to be not evaluated BP in the midnight or in the morning by ABPM or HBP measurements.

To evaluate the usefulness of HBP measurement in the morning in patients with DM, we examined whether BP elevations at the awakening-up in the morning detected by HBP were more predictive than those in the daytime detected by CBP for micro- and macro- vascular complications in patients with type 1 or 2 DM, as observed in patients with essential hypertension (Aihara et al, 1998, Ohkubo et al, 1998, Imai et al, 1999).

Our cross-sectional studies have demonstrated that HBP measurements at the awakning-up in the morning offer stronger predictive power for micro- and macro-vascular complications in patients with type 1 and 2 DM than CBP measurements in the daytime (Kamoi et al, 2002-2003). Further, a study examined which of HBP at the awakning-up in the morning or CBP in the daytime provides the stronger predictive power for outcomes by comparing cumulative events between hypertensive and normotensive patients over 6 years in a prospective and longitudinal study of patients with type 2 DM (Kamoi et al, 2010).

2. Research design and methods

2.1 Subjects

2.1.1 A cross-sectional study

In a cross-sectional study, 10 years ago we studied on 53 Japanese patients with type 1 DM who visited our clinics regularly (Kamoi et al, 2003). The diagnosis of type 1 DM was based on the World Health Organization (WHO) criteria (AlbertiK et al, 1998). Numbers of female patients were twice of male patients. The age was 23 to 81 year old and the duration was 2 to 47 years (Table 1). Of 53 patients, 38 (72%) were treated by multiple daily insulin injections and remaining (28%) by subcutaneous continuous insulin infusion therapy for DM. Twenty two patients (42%) were treated with anti-hypertensive drugs at the beginning of the study (Table 2). Also, we studied on 170 Japanese patients with type 2 DM. They visited our clinic regularly (Kamoi et al, 2002). The diagnosis of type 2 DM was based on the WHO criteria (AlbertiK et al, 1998). The clinical characteriscs are shown in the Table 3. Ratio of numbers in female and male patients was similar. The mean age was middle and the mean BMI was within normal range (Table 3). Of 170 patients, 153 (90%) were treated with oral hypoglycaemic drugs and/or insulin regimens for DM, whereas 80 (47%) were treated with anti-hypertensive drugs at the beginning of the study (Table 4).

2.1.2 A longitudinal study

In a longitudinal study, subjects comprised 400 Japanese patients with type 2 DM enrolled between 1999 and 2005 including the patients participated in the cross-sectional study (Kamoi et al, 2010). After a detailed baseline examination (Table 5), subjects were followed up for all-cause mortality and morbidity.

All participants visited our clinic regularly and were observed until February 28, 2007. Mean survey duration of all patients was 42 ± 20 months (range, 3–72 months). Type 2 DM was diagnosed according to WHO criteria (AlbertiK et al, 1998). No significant difference in the number of patients was noted between females and males. Mean subjects were also middle ages. The mean BMI was within normal range (Table 5). At the beginning of the study, 329 patients (82%) were receiving treatment with oral hypoglycaemic drugs and/or insulin regimens for DM and 196 patients (49%) were receiving treatment with various anti-hypertensive drugs (angiotensin-converting enzyme inhibitors, angiotensin receptor blockers, calcium channel blocker, and others) for hypertension (Table 6). For ethical reasons, patients were treated with various anti-hypertensive, anti-diabetic, anti-dyslipidemia, and/or anti-hypercoagulation agents during the course of the study by the patients' own doctors as a part of a continuing standard of medical care.

All patients were fully informed about the purposes and the procedures for study and provided oral consent at enrolment.

	CH group			CN group			
	MH group	MN group	Total	MHgroup	MNgroup	Total	All subjects
Number	6	11	17	8	28	36	53
Age (years)	68 ± 13‡	53 ± 7	58 ± 12	54 ± 15	51 ± 16	52 ± 17	54 ± 15
Sex (female/male)	5/1	8/3	13/4	4/4	19/9	23/13	36/17
BMI (kg/m²)	22 ± 2	23 ± 1	23 ± 2	22 ± 2	22 ± 3	22 ± 3	22 ± 3
Disease duration (yr)	19 ± 11	17 ± 11	18 ± 11	23 ± 12	15 ± 9	17 ± 10	17 ± 10
Blood pressure (mmHg)							
SBP							
Clinic	154 ± 11	160 ± 18	152 ± 9*	120 ± 8	118 ± 11	118 ± 10	129 ± 19
Morning	144 ± 10‡	122 ± 9*	123 ± 14*	151 ± 197‡*	121 ± 13	121 ± 21	124 ± 20
DBP							
Clinic	103 ± 25‡	85 ± 8	91 ± 17†	75 ± 15	71 ± 9	73 ± 11	78 ± 16
Morning	81 ± 11*	74 ± 8*	76 ± 10*	82 ± 10‡*	69 ± 8	72 ± 10	73 ± 10*
HbA1c (JDS%)	6.9 ± 1.2	6.9 ± 0.9	6.9 ± 1.0	7.6 ± 1.3	7.0 ± 0.9	7.2 ± 1.0	7.0 ± 0.9
TG (mg/dl)	65 ± 36	99 ± 47	87 ± 46	116 ± 54	92 ± 34	97 ± 43	94 ± 44
T-CH (mg/dl)	210 ± 30	204 ± 38	206 ± 34	202 ± 20	198 ± 33	199 ± 30	201 ± 32
LDL (mg/dl)	112 ± 27	110 ± 26	111 ± 26	112 ± 20	102 ± 26	105 ± 25	107 ± 25
HDL (mg/dl)	84 ± 8	73 ± 14	77 ± 13	71 ± 16	74 ± 21	73 ± 20	75 ± 18
Serum Cr (mg/dl)	0.9 ± 0.2‡	0.7 ± 0.1	0.7 ± 0.2	1.0 ± 0.6‡	0.7 ± 0.2	0.8 ± 0.3	0.8 ± 0.3
UERA (μg/mg Cr)	107±112‡	6.9±3.7	42±79	324±567‡	7.1±6.9	7.8±287	66±240

Data are means ± SD. The systolic BP (SBP) and the diastolic BP (DBP) levels in all patients were measured at the clinic in the daytime and at the home at the awakening-up in the morning, resepectively. CH; clinic hypertension, CN; clinic normotension, MH; morning hypertension, MN; morning normotension, Cr; creatinine, UERA; urinary excretion rate of albumin. **P<0.01 versus patients with CN; ‡P<0.01 versus patients with MN; and †P<0.01 versus patients measured at the clinic in the daytime.

Table 1. Characteristics of patients with type 1 diabetes mellitus in a cross-sectional study

2.2 Method

2.2.1 Blood pressure

2.2.1.1 CBP

CBP levels were measured once in clinical setting of a daytime during each clinic visit. HBP was also measured once each morning, in the sitting position within 10 min after awakening, for every day. For the CBP levels in the daytime, when patients with DM had clinic systolic BP 130 mmHg and/or clinic diastolic BP 85 mmHg, we classified these patients as having clinic hypertension (CH) by the criteria of the WHO and International Society of Hypertension guide lines (Guide lines Subcommittee, 1999).

	CH group			CN group				
	MH group (n=6)	MN group (n=11)	Total (n=17)	MH group (n=8)	MN group (n=26)	Total (n=36)	All subjects (n=53)	Odds ratio (95% CI)
Medical events								
Nephropathy	4	0	4	7	0	7	11	1.3 (0.3 to 5.1)
Microalbuminuria	3	0	3	5	0	5	8	1.3 (0.3 to 6.4)
Clinical albuminuria	1	0	1	2	0	2	3	1.1 (0.1 to 12.6)
Retinopathy	1	4	5	4	4	8	13	1.5 (0.5 to 5.4)
Non-proliferative	0	3	3	0	2	2	5	3.0 (0.5 to 19.7)
Preproliferative	0	1	1	1	1	2	3	1.1 (0.1 to 12.6)
Proliferative	1	0	1	3	1	4	5	0.5 (0.1 to 4.9)
Medical treatment								
Therapy for hypertension								
Oral drugs	5	4	9	6	7	13	22	2.0 (0.6 to 6.4)
Therapy for diabetes mellitus								
MDI	4	8	12	7	19	26	38	0.9 (0.3 to 3.3)
CSII	2	3	5	1	9	10	15	1.0 (0.3 to 3.9)

Data are number. Odds ratio for CH and CN groups was calculated. MDI; multiple daily insulin injections, CSII; subcutaneous continuous insulin infusion, CI; confidence interval.

Table 2. Prevalence of micro- and macro- vascular events and medical treatment in patients shown in the table 1

2.2.1.2 HBP

When the HBP levels at the awakening-up in the morning were systolic HBP 130 mmHg and/or diastolic HBP 85 mmHg, we classified these patients as having morning hypertension (MH). When these values were 130 mmHg of systolic BP and 85 mmHg of diastolic BP, we classified these patients as having clinic normotension (CN) or morning normotension (MN), respectively.

All subjects were divided into two groups: with CH or MH and without CH or MH. Finally, we examined whether CBP in the daytime and HBP at the awakening-up in the morning is more predictive of these events.

2.2.2 Micro- and macro- vascular complications

The microvascular complications detected in this study were nephropathy and retinopathy. Occurrence of nephropathy was evaluated each three months in the clinic setting from beginning of the study based on urinary excretion rate of albumin (UERA), whereas occurrence of retinopathy was evaluated at least once each 6 months during the study. The macrovascular complications defined were coronary heart disease (CHD) and cerebrovascular disease (CVD) assessed by clinical situation. Prevalence of these events was confirmed by medical history at the beginning of the study.

	CH group			CN group			
	MH group	MN group	Total	MH group	MN group	Total	All subjects
Number	74	57	131	23	16	39	170
Age (years)	67 ± 8	64 ± 8	66 ± 9	71 ± 9†	63 ± 9	68 ± 10	66 ± 9
Sex (female/male)	47/27	24/33	74/57	7/16	9/7	16/23	90/80
BMI (kg/m²)	24 ± 3†	23 ± 2	23 ± 3*	23 ± 3†	22 ± 3	22 ± 3	23 ± 3
Blood pressure (mmHg)							
SBP							
Clinic	167 ± 18†	158 ± 14	163 ± 17*	124 ± 12†	117 ± 9	121 ± 11	153 ± 26
Morning	163 ± 19†	127 ± 7†	147 ± 24‡	166 ± 17†‡	116 ± 10	146 ± 29‡	147 ± 25‡
DBP							
Clinic	97 ± 14†	93 ± 9	95 ± 12*	75 ± 8	73 ± 9	74 ± 9	90 ± 14
Morning	88 ± 11†‡	75 ± 8‡	83 ± 12‡	88 ± 15†‡	69 ± 10	80 ± 16‡	82 ± 13‡
Laboratory variables							
HbA1c (JDS%)	6.5 ± 0.9	6.5 ± 0.9	6.5 ± 0.9	6.7 ± 1.0	6.4 ± 0.7	6.6 ± 0.9	6.5 ± 0.9
TG (mg/dl)	153 ± 77	40 ± 92	148 ± 83	138 ± 74	109 ± 46	126 ± 65	143 ± 80
T-CH (mg/dl)	198 ± 32	96 ± 31	197 ± 3	182 ± 44	204 ± 24	191 ± 38	196 ± 33
LDL (mg/dl)	109 ± 32	01 ± 31	106 ± 31	92 ± 34	122 ± 21	105 ± 33	106 ± 32
HDL (mg/dl)	61 ± 16	66 ± 18	63 ± 17	57 ± 24	59 ± 10	58 ± 20	62 ± 18
Serum Cr (mg/dl)	0.8 ± 0.2	0.8 ± 0.2	0.8 ± 0.2*	1.1 ± 0.4†	0.7 ± 0.2	1.0 ± 0.4	0.9 ± 0.3
UERA (μg/mg Cr)	212±524†	11±8*	125±405*	1,113±2,449†	7.5±5.0	660±1,943	248±1,013

Data are means ± SD. The systolic BP (SBP) and the diastolic BP (DBP) levels in all patients were measured at the clinic in the daytime and at the home at the awakening-up in the morning, resepectively. CH; clinic hypertension, CN; clinic normotension, MH; morning hypertension, MN; morning normotension, Cr; creatinine, UERA; urinary excretion rate of albumin. **P<0.01 versus patients with CN ;‡P<0.01 versus patients with MN ; and †P<0.01 versus patients measured at the clinic in the daytime.

Table 3. Characteristics of patients with type 2 diabetes mellitus in a cross-sectional study

2.2.3 Glycaemic control and other variables

Glycaemic control was evaluated by HbA1c values (JDS: normal range 4.5–5.7%) (Kasezawa et al, 1987). Other variables, including serum concentrations of electrolytes and lipids, were also measured (Kamoi et al, 2002). Albumin concentration in random spot urine was measured by the latex agglutinination photometric immunoassay method (Kamoi et al, 2002).

2.2.4 Analytical methods

2.2.4.1 CBP

CBP level was measured by patient's self at the clinic in the daytime in the left arm after a 5-min rest in a sitting position using an automatic device based on the cuff-oscillometric method (FT-200; Parama-Tech, Fukuoka, Japan).

	CH group			CN group				
	MH group (n=74)	MN group (n=57)	Total (n=131)	MH group (n=23)	MN group (n=16)	Total (n=39)	All subjects (n=170)	Odds ratio (95% CI)
Medical events								
Nephropathy	69†	0	39	91†	0	54	43	0.6 (0.3 to 1.1)
Microalbuminuria	67†	0	32	52†	0	31	32	1.0 (0.5 to 2.3)
Clinical albuminuria	12†	0	7	39†	0	24	10	0.2 (0.1 to 0.7)*
Retinopathy	32†	18	28	33†	6	24	26	1.3 (0.5 to 2.9)
Non-proliferative	18	9	15	4	0	3	12	6.4 (0.8 to 50)
Preproliferative	9†	2	6	13	0	8	7	0.8 (0.2 to 3.1)
Proliferative	5	8	7	17†	6	13	8	0.5 (0.2 to 1.6)
CHD	8	11	9	35†	0	20	11	0.5 (0.2 to 1.3)
CVD	23	11	18	35†	0	21	18	0.8 (0.3 to 1.9)
Medical treatment								
Therapy for hypertension								
Oral drugs	61†	15	48	70†	6	44	47	1.2 (0.6 to 2.5)
Therapy for diabetes mellitus								
Oral drugs or insulin	91	86	89	100	88	95	90	0.2 (0.0 to 1.5)

Data are %. The prevalence is a percent ratio of patient with MH, MN, CH, CN, or all patients. Odds ratio for CH and CN groups was calculated. *P<0.01 versus patients with CN, †P<0.01 versus patients with MN. CI: confidence interval.

Table 4. Prevalence of micro- and macro- vascular events and medical treatment in patients shown in the table 3

2.2.4.2 HBP

HBP level was measured at the home in the morning within 10 min after awakening, by a patient's self or a family member, in the left arm in a sitting position. Semiautomatic devices based on the cuff-oscillometric principles that generate a digital display of both systolic BP and diastolic BP were used. All devices met the criteria set by the Association for the Advancement of Medical Instrumentation. A standard arm cuff was used to measure both CBP and HBP levels.

2.2.4.3 Variable parameters

Venous samples were collected during each clinic visit and were analysed for HbA1c levels and concentrations of total cholesterol (TC), low densty lipoprotein cholesterol (LDL), high densty lipoprotein chesterol (HDL), triglyceride (TG), and creatinine without fasting. Microalbuminuria and clinical albuminuria were defined as UERA 30 and 300 μg/mg creatinine, respectively (The American Diabetes Association, 2002).

Variable	MH	MN	CN	CH
n (%)	286 (72*)	114 (28*)	283 (71*)	117 (29*)
Age (years)	66±9†	61±10	65±9	64±10
Sex (F/M)	136/150	52/62	140/143	48/69
Duration (years)	14.1±8.5†	11.2±7.5	13.8±8.2	12.1±8.6
BMI (kg/m²)	24±3†	23±4	24±3†	23±3
Blood pressure (mmHg)				
Systolic				
Morning	151±19†	117±8**	146±22†	130±20**
Clinic	148±22†	132±20	155±17†	117±9
Diastolic				
Morning	84±11†**	73±10**	82±12†**	77±13**
Clinic	87±16†	78±13	90±14†	71±9
Laboratory variables				
HbA1c (%)	6.7±1.1	6.5±0.8	6.7±1.1	6.6±1.0
TG (mg/dl)	155±122	138±84	154±117	140±100
T-C (mg/dl)	199±33	197±30	198±32	198±32
LDL-C (mg/dl)	109±30	112±27	108±28†	115±31
HDL-C (mg/dl)	60±19	59±17	60±18	60±20
Serum Cr (mg/dl)	0.8±0.3†	0.7±0.2	0.8±0.3	0.8±0.3
UERA (μ g/mg Cr)	206±646†	26±113	141±369	187±854

Data represent mean ± SD. Morning and clinic blood pressures were measured at the home at the wakening up in the morning and at the clinic in the daytime, respectively. CH; clinic hypertension, CN; clinic normotension, MH; morning hypertension, MN; morning normotension, Cr; creatinine, UERA; urinary excretion rate of albumin. For comparisons of UERA, unpaired *t* test with Welch's correction was used. †P<0.05 versus patients with normotension; **P<0.01 versus patients measured at the clinic in the daytime.

Table 5. Baseline characteristics of patients with type 2 diabetes mellitus on the basis of HBP measurement in a longitudinal study

Variable	MH	MN	Odds ratio (95% CI)	CN	CH	Odds ratio (95% CI)
Medical events (%)						
Microvascular complications	271 (68*)	36 (9.0*)	38 (20 to 75)†	235 (59*)	72 (18*)	3.0 (1.9 to 5.0)†
Nephropathy	157 (39*)	14(3.5*)	8.7 (4.7 to 15.9)†	133 (33*)	38 (10*)	1.8 (1.1 to 2.7)†
Microalbuminuria	121	13	6.3 (3.4 to 11.6)†	105	29	1.7 (1.0 to 2.8)†
Clinical albuminuria	36	1	16.3 (2.0 to 120)†	28	9	1.3 (0.6 to 2.8)
Retinopathy	114 (29*)	22 (5.5*)	2.8 (1.6 to 4.7)†	102 (26*)	34 (8.5*)	1.3 (0.8 to 2.1)
Non-proliferative	66	15	2.0 (0.7 to 3.6)†	61	20	1.3 (0.7 to 2.2)
Pre-proliferative	14	0	12.1 (0.7 to 206)†	11	3	1.3 (0.7 to 2.2)
Proliferative	34	7	2.1 (0.9 to 4.8)†	30	11	1.0 (0.5 to 2.3)
Macrovascular complications	100 (25*)	10 (2.5*)	5.6 (2.8 to 11.1)†	78 (20*)	32 (8.1*)	1.0 (0.6 to 1.6)
Coronary heart disease	36 (9.0*)	4 (1.0*)	4.0 (2.0 to 11.4)†	28 (7.0*)	12 (3.0*)	1.0 (0.5 to 2.0)
Cerebrovascular disease	64 (16*)	6 (1.5*)	5.1 (2.2 to 12.2)†	50 (13*)	20 (5.0*)	1.0 (0.6 to 1.8)
Medical treatment (%)						
Therapy for hypertension	173 (43*)	23 (5.8*)	6.1 (3.6 to 10.1)†	125 (40*)	71 (10*)	2.6 (1.7 to 4.2)†
Therapy for diabetes mellitus						
Oral drugs/or insulin	240 (60*)	89 (22*)	1.5 (0.9 to 2.5)	225 (56*)	104 (26*)	0.5 (0.3 to 0.9)
Therapy for dyslipidemia	71 (18*)	17 (4.3*)	1.9 (1.1 to 3.4)†	71 (18*)	17 (4.3*)	3.5 (1.9 to 6.4)†
Therapy for hypercoagulation	56 (14*)	4 (1.0*)	6.7 (2.4 to 11)†	44 (11*)	6 (1.5*)	3.4 (1.4 to 8.3)†
Therapy for others	4 (1.0*)	3 (0.8*)	0.5 (0.1 to 2.4)	3 (0.8*)	4 (1.0*)	0.3 (0.07 to 1.4)

Data represent means ± SD. Morning and clinic blood pressures were measured at the home at the awkening-up in the morning and in the clinic in the daytime, respectively. *Numbers in parentheses represent a percentage ratio of patients in each type for all subjects. CI: confidence interval. †$P<0.05$ versus patients with normotension; **$P<0.01$ versus patients measured at the clinic.

Table 6. Prevalence of micro- and macro- vascular events and medical treatment in patients shown in the table 5

2.3 Statistical analysis

2.3.1 Baseline

All values are presented as means ± SD. Mean values were compared using chi square test or un-paired Student's *t* test. To compare the prevalence of micro- and macro-vascular complications in groups with and without the hypertension, Yates 'continuity corrected x2 test with two-tailed P value was performed and odds ratios were calculated; if prevalence of the events was 0.5 was added to all values before calculating the odds ratio and 95% CIs were provided. Multiple logistic analyses were used to determine the contribution of the variables to the events. Correlation between HBP and CBP levels was calculated. In addition, receiver operating characteristic (ROC) curves for HBP and CBP with various end points were used to examine whether HBP levels in the morning and CBP levels in the daytime behave differently in allowing ascertainment of the true risk or whether the 130/85 mmHg cut points are better for HBP levels in the morning than for CBP levels in the daytime.

	Multivariate-adjusted odds ratio	95% CI
Age (years)	1.03	0.97–1.10
Sex (female/male)	0.85	0.29–2.45
BMI (kg/m^2)	1.29†	1.08–1.55
HbA_{1c} (%)	0.84	0.49–1.45
Clinic blood pressure		
SBP (mmHg)	1.00	0.97–1.04
DBP (mmHg)	0.93†	0.89–0.98
Morning blood pressure		
SBP (mmHg)	1.07‡	1.04–1.10
DBP (mmHg)	1.02	0.97–1.07
Triglycerides (mg/dl)	1.00	0.99–1.01
Total cholesterol (mg/dl)	0.98	0.96–1.01
LDL cholesterol (mg/dl)	1.03*	1.00–1.06
HDL cholesterol (mg/dl)	1.02	0.99–1.06
Serum creatinine (mg/dl)	43.2*	1.53–1,225
Anti-hypertensive drugs	5.90*	1.27–9.49
Anti-diabetic drugs	4.89	0.86–27.7

Odds ratio for continuous variables represent a difference of 1 SD. $^*P < 0.05$; $^†P < 0.01$; $^‡P < 0.001$.

Table 7. Multivariate-adjusted odds ratios and 95%CIs of risk factors for nephropathy in patients with type 1 diabetes

2.3.2 Endpoints and outcome measures

Differences in outcomes for each endpoint of death, and new or worsened micro- and macro- vascular complications between hypertensive and normotensive patients on the basis of HBP levels in the morning or CBP levels in the daytime were assessed using survival curves calculated according to Kaplan-Meier methods, then compared by a hazard ratio using the log-rank test. Within the survey time previously defined, a time until censoring or death (or occurrence of the event) was calculated for each endpoint.

2.3.3 Risk factor assessment for outcomes

In a longitudinal study, risk factors related to outcomes determined statistically by a log-rank test were assessed using hazard ratios by Cox proportional hazards model. For outcomes of microvascular complications, risk factors were determined in new, worsened, or improved events. Omnibus tests were used to determine the appropriateness of Cox proportional hazards modelling. Confounding factors used in this analysis were variables with MH in the morning or CH in the daytime at baseline and additional therapy for each disease. The analysis was based on the first event of each participant, thereby, allowing each participant to enter once in the Cox proportional hazard models.

These analyses were performed using the GraphPad Prisms of software (version 3.02-5.01; GraphPad Soft-ware, San Diego, CA, USA), the Statistical Package for the Biosciences (SPBS;

Winesteem Institute of Community Medicine, Tokyo, Japan) and the Dr. SPSSII for Windows (SPSS Japan, Tokyo, Japan). A two-tailed value of P< 0.05 was considered statistically significant.

	Multivariate-adjusted odds ratio	95% CI
Age (years)	1.03	0.97–1.10
Sex (female/male)	0.85	0.29–2.45
BMI (kg/m²)	1.29†	1.08–1.55
HbA_{1c} (%)	0.84	0.49–1.45
Clinic blood pressure		
SBP (mmHg)	1.00	0.97–1.04
DBP (mmHg)	0.93†	0.89–0.98
Morning blood pressure		
SBP (mmHg)	1.07‡	1.04–1.10
DBP (mmHg)	1.02	0.97–1.07
Triglycerides (mg/dl)	1.00	0.99–1.01
Total cholesterol (mg/dl)	0.98	0.96–1.01
LDL cholesterol (mg/dl)	1.03*	1.00–1.06
HDL cholesterol (mg/dl)	1.02	0.99–1.06
Serum creatinine (mg/dl)	43.2*	1.53–1,225
Anti-hypertensive drugs	5.90*	1.27–9.49
Anti-diabetic drugs	4.89	0.86–27.7

Odds ratio for continuous variables represent a difference of 1 SD. *$P < 0.05$; †$P < 0.01$; ‡$P < 0.001$.

Table 8. Multivariate-adjusted odds ratios and 95%CIs of risk factors for nephropathy in patients with type 2 diabetes

3. Results

3.1 In a cross-sectional study

3.1.1 A type 1 diabetes mellitus

As shown in the figure 1, in type 1 diabetic groups with both CH and CN, the kinds of anti-hypertensive medicines administered after taking breakfast in the groups with MH were greater than in the groups with MN. There were no significant differences in the prevalence of nephropathy and retinopathy between the two groups with CH and CN. In contrast, the prevalence of nephropathy with 8 microalbuminuria and 3 clinical albuminuria in the patients with MH was significantly higher than those with MN (Table 2). The prevalence of proliferative retinopathy in the patients with MH was significantly higher than that in those with MN, although there was no significant difference in all types of retinopathy between two groups. There was no occurrence of CHD or CVD in the two groups. Specifically, systolic MH made a significant (r = 0.66, P = 0.001) contribution to the occurrence of nephropathy by multiple regression analysis, whereas the difference is not related to age, sex, duration of diabetes, BMI, HbA1c, and serum lipid concentrations or use of different methods of insulin therapy and anti-hypertensive drugs. Meanwhile, the duration of diabetes had a significant (r = 0.4, P = 0.001) contribution to the occurrence of retinopathy (Table 7). No relationships between systolic HBP and diastolic HBP, and systolic CBP and diastolic CBP measurements were observed (morning systolic HBP = 0.28, systolic CBP = 0.07, P = 0.06 and diastolic HBP = 0.25, diastolic CBP = 0.14, P = 0.005). The area under the ROC curve (AUC) of morning systolic HBP (0.99 ± 0.01) was significantly higher (P < 0.001) than that of systolic CBP (0.49 ± 0.10) in nephropathy (Figure 2). There was no statistical difference in AUC between them in other events. In nephropathy, sensitivities of 130 mmHg threshold in morning and clinic systolic BP were 1.0 (95% CI 1.0–1.0) and 0.55 (0.23–0.83), respectively, whereas those of 85 mmHg threshold in morning and clinic diastolic BP were 0.64 (0.31-0.89) and 0.55 (0.23–0.83), respectively. Specificities of 130 mmHg threshold in morning and clinic systolic BP were 0.95 (0.84–0.99) and 0.48 (0.32–0.64) (Figure 3), respectively, whereas those of 85 mmHg threshold in morning and clinic diastolic BP were 0.14 (0.05–0.29) and 0.29 (0.16–0.45), respectively.

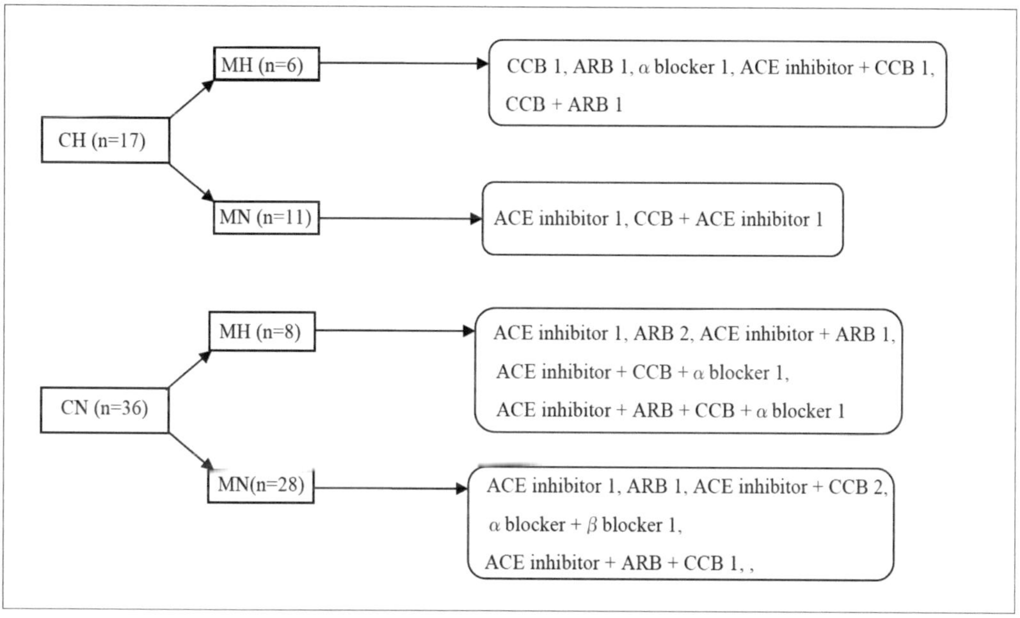

Fig. 1. Various kinds of anti-hypertensive medicines in each group with CH or CN and MH or MN in patients with type 1 diabetes mellitus in a cross-sectional study. These anti-hypertensive medicines were administered after taking a breakfast. CH; clinic hypertension, CN; clinic normotension,MH; morning hypertension, MN; morning normotension, ARB; angiotensin II receptor blocker, CCB; calcium channel blocker , ACE inhibitor; angiotensin converting enzyme inhibitor.

3.1.2 A type 2 diabetes mellitus

As shown in the figure 4, in the type 2 diabetic groups with both CH and CN, the kinds of anti-hypertensive medicines administered after taking breakfast in the groups with MH were also greater than in the groups with MN as those in patients with type 1 diabetes (Table 4). Comparing the characteristics of patients with and without CH, the following trends were noted. The prevalence of CH was four times higher than CN. BMI in CH patients was slightly higher than in CN patients. In contrast, serum creatinine concentration and UERA in CH patients were significantly lower than in CN patients (Table 3). No significant differences in other variables were noted between the two groups (Tabel 4). A total of 48% of CH patients were being treated with anti- hypertensive drugs, compared with 44% of CN patients (Tabel 4).

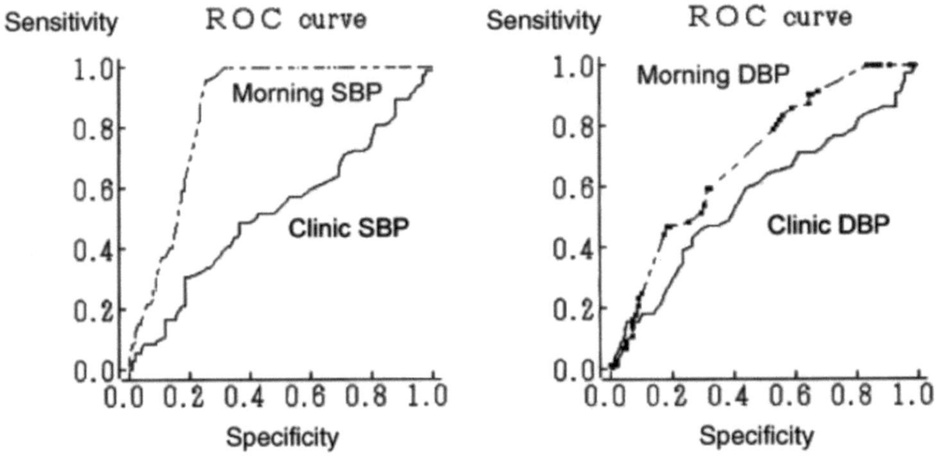

Fig. 2. ROC analysis in nephropathy in patients with type 1 and 2 diabetes mellitus.

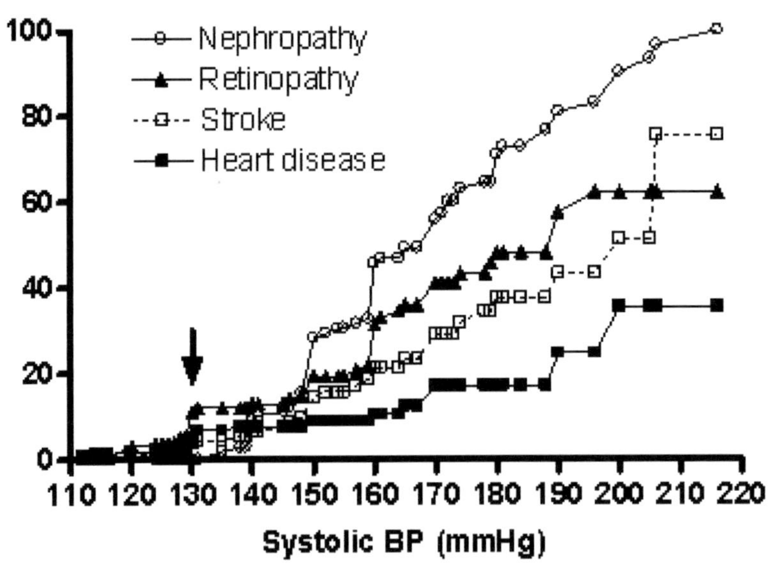

Fig. 3. Threshold of systolic HBP at the wakening-up for prevalence of micro- and macro-vascular events in patients with type 1 and 2 diabetes mellitus. The vertical arrow indicated the value of threshold of systolic HBP.

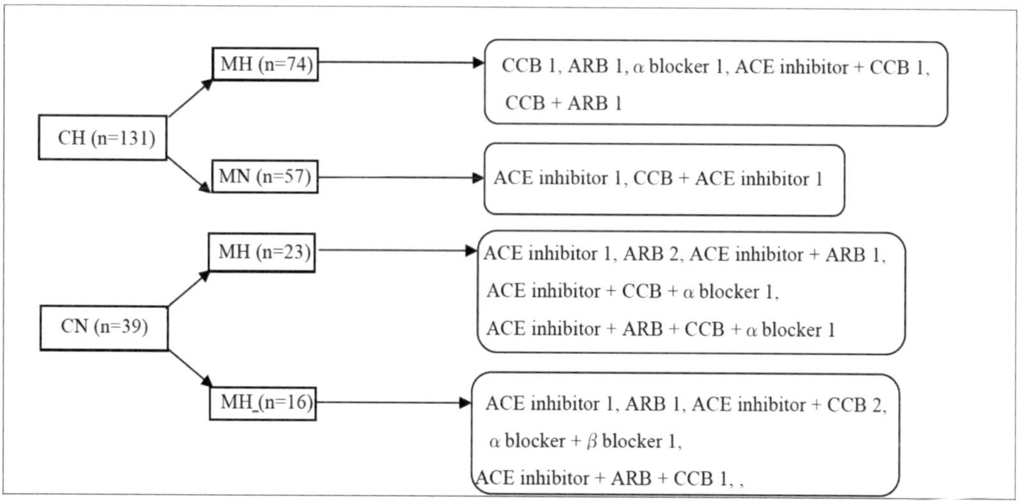

Fig. 4. Various kinds of anti-hypertensive medicines in each group with CH or CN and MH or MN in patients with type 2 diabetes mellitus in a cross-sectional study. CH; clinic hypertension, CN; clinic normotension, MH; morning hypertension, MN; morning normotension, ARB; angiotensin II receptor blocker, CCB; calcium channel blocker , ACE inhibitor; angiotensin converting enzyme inhibitor

When we compared the prevalence of diabetic complications in the two groups, there were no significant differences in the prevalence of nephropathy, retinopathy, CHD, and CVD between the two groups. However, the prevalence of clinical albuminuria in CH patients was lower than in CN patients (Table 2).

The CH patients were further divided into two groups: with and without MH (Table 3). BMI in MH patients was slightly higher than in MN patients. Systolic BP, diastolic BP, and UAER in MH patients were significantly higher than those in MN patients. There were no significant differences in other variables between the two groups. Nephropathy was observed in 69% of MH patients, whereas there was no nephropathy in MN patients. The prevalences of retinopathy and CVD in MH patients were also significantly higher than in MN patients (Table 4). The prevalence of treatment with anti- hypertensive drugs was higher in MH than in MN (Table 4).

The CN patients were also divided into two groups: with and without MH (Table 3). The means of age, BMI, systolic HBP, and diastolic HBP in MH patients were significantly higher than those in MN patients. Serum creatinine concentration and UAER were also higher in MH than in MN. No significant differences in other variables were shown between the two groups. However, the prevalence of nephropathy in MH patients was high (91%), whereas no nephropathy was observed in MN patients. The prevalences of retinopathy, CHD, and CVD in MH patients were also higher than in MN patients. More MH patients than MN patients were being treated with anti- hypertensive drugs (Table 4).

Comparing the characteristics of the two patient groups with and without MH, the following trends were noted (Table 3). The means of age, sex, HbA1c levels, and lipid concentrations were not different between the two groups. However, systolic BP and diastolic BP, based on HBP in the morning, in MH patients were significantly higher than in MN patients. Serum creatinine concentration and UAER were also higher in MH patients

(Table 3). The prevalences of treatment with anti-hypertensive and anti-diabetic drugs were 3 and 1.5 times higher, respectively, in MH patients compared with MN patients (Table 4). The prevalence of nephropathy in MH patients was 75%, whereas no nephropathy was noted in MN patients. The prevalence of retinopathy in MH patients was twice that found in MN patients, although there was no difference in the prevalences of non-proliferative and proliferative retinopathies between the two groups (Table 4). The prevalences of CHD and CVD in MH patients were four and six times higher, respectively, than in MN patients.

Specifically, the prevalence of nephropathy in all subjects was highly associated ($P < 0.001$) with systolic MH, but not with age, sex, HbA1c, serum lipid concentrations without LDL, and use of anti-diabetic drugs by multiple logistic analysis. However, prevalence of nephropathy was associated with BMI, LDL concentration, serum creatinine concentration, and use of anti-hypertensive drugs and was negatively associated with diastolic CBP (Table 8).

The relationships between systolic HBP and diastolic HBP in morning and clinic measurements were described by regression equations of morning systolic HBP = 0.23 systolic CBP + 111 and morning diastolic HBP = 0.26 diastolic CBP + 58, respectively. The correlations were poor (morning versus clinic systolic BP, $r = 0.05$, $P = 0.004$; morning versus clinic diastolic BP, $r = 0.09$, $P = 0.0001$). In comparison of ROC curves for HBP and CBP with the events, the areas under ROC curves of morning systolic HBP (0.86 ± 0.39) and morning diastolic HBP (0.70 ± 0.52) were significantly higher ($P < 0.001$ and $P = 0.035$, respectively) than those of systolic CBP (0.52 ± 0.60) and diastolic CBP (0.57 ± 0.59) in nephropathy, indicating that HBP has a higher predictive value than CBP (Figure 2). In contrast, there were no statistical differences between them in other events. In nephropathy (Figure 2), sensitivities of the 130 mmHg threshold in morning and clinic systolic BP were 1.00 (1.00–1.00 95% CI) and 0.18 (0.10–0.29), respectively, whereas those of the 85 mmHg threshold in morning and clinic diastolic BP were 0.49 (0.37–0.61) and 0.43 (0.31–0.55), respectively. Specificities of the 130 mmHg threshold in morning and clinic systolic BP were 0.68 (0.58–0.77) and 0.85 (0.76–0.91) (Figure 3), respectively, whereas those of the 85 mmHg threshold in morning and clinic diastolic BP were 0.75 (0.65–0.83) and 0.73 (0.64–0.82), respectively.

3.2 In a longitudinal study

3.2.1 Baseline characteristics of patients

In the patients with a type 2 DM, baseline characteristics of patients classified as hypertensive or normotensive on the basis of HBP and CBP are shown in Tables 5, respectively. Based on HBP, prevalence of MH was double that of MN. Mean age, duration of disease, BMI, systolic BP and diastolic BP in both HBP and CBP, serum creatinine concentration and UAER were also significantly higher with MH than with MN (Table 5). In MH patients, morning diastolic HBP was significantly lower than diastolic CBP. In MN patients, morning systolic and diastolic HBP were significantly lower than systolic and diastolic CBP, respectively. No significant differences were noted in other laboratory variables between the two groups. Prevalence of microvascular complications was significantly great higher with MH than with MN, and prevalence of nephropathy was about 9-fold higher with MH than with MN (Table 6), although there was no dialysis. Prevalence of macrovascular complications was also significantly higher with MH than with MN. Most patients showing MH received anti-hypertensive and anti-diabetic drugs. The prevalence of patients receiving anti-hypertensive drugs was 6-fold higher for MH than for MN. The prevalence of patients receiving anti-diabetic drugs appeared 1.5-fold higher with MH than with MN, although no significant difference was evident. Prevalences of using anti-dyslipidemia and anti-hypercoagulation agents were also significantly higher with MH than with MN (Table 6), but prevalences were lower than those for anti-hypertensive and anti-diabetic drugs.

On the basis of CBP, most characteristics of CH and CN patients at baseline were similar to those of MH and MN patients, respectively (Table 5). However, no significant differences in mean age, duration of disease, serum creatinine concentration or UAER or in prevalences of retinopathy and macrovascular complications were noted between these patients. Meanwhile, mean LDL was significantly lower with CH than with CN. In patients with CN, morning systolic and diastolic HBP were significantly higher than systolic and diastolic CBP, respectively (Table 5).

3.2.2 Endpoints and outcome measures

Nine cumulative events (2.3%) of death were observed for 6 years (Figure 6). They were with sustained MH, whereas none occurred in patients with sustained MN (Table 9). The hazard ratio was significantly (5-fold) higher with sustained MH than with sustained MN.

	Patient Status on the Basis of HBP Measurement (n = 400)				Patient Status on the Basis of CBP Measurement (n = 400)			
Outcome	Hypertension (n=286)	Normotension (n = 114)	Hazard Ratio (95% CI)	P	Hypertension (n=283)	Normotension (n = 117)	Hazard Ratio (95% CI)	P
Primary outcome								
Death	9	0	4.87 (1.23–19.3)	0.02*	6	3	0.62 (0.13–2.87)	0.54
Secondary outcome								
Microvascular complications	55	17	2.06 (1.25–3.38)	0.01*	50	22	0.89 (0.53–1.51)	0.67
Macrovascular complications	20	1	3.85 (1.56–9.47)	0.01*	20	1	3.11 (1.16–8.30)	0.02*

Characteristics of patients at baseline on the basis of HBP and CBP measurement are shown in Tables 1 and 2, respectively. The 400 patients in each group were classified as having hypertension or normotension according to values of blood pressure measured at home or in the clinic at the start of this study, respectively. Differences in outcomes for new or worsened events of each endpoint between sustained hypertensive patients and sustained normotensive patients in each group were assessed using survival curves from the Kaplan-Meier method and comparisons were analyzed using hazard ratios by the log-rank test.
*Significant difference between hypertensive and normotensive patients.

Table 9. Primary and secondary outcomes in a longitudinal study.

On the causes of death, 3, 3, 2 and 1 patients in the MH group were due to cancer with brain, breast or pancreas, CVD, CHD and unknown cause, respectively. while 3, 1, 1 and 1 patients in the CH group were due to cancer with brain, breast or pancreas, CVD, CHD and unknown cause, respectively, and 2 and 1 patients in the CN group were due to CVD and CHD, respectively (Kamoi et al, 2010). As shown in figure 7, new or worsened events of microvascular complications were observed in 72 patients (18%) included 36 with retinopathy and 59 with nephropathy, while improved events of microvascular complications were shown in 102 patients (25.5%) included 27 with retinopathy and 79 with nephropathy. New or worsened events of macrovascular complications were shown in 21 patients (5.3%) included 8 patients with myocardial infarction, 3 with heart failure, 1 with atrial fibrillation, 7 with cerebral infarction and 2 with cerebral bleeding. These new or worsened cumulative events were also significantly higher with sustained MH than with sustained MN, whereas no significant difference was seen between sustained CH and CN.

In terms of macrovascular complications, cumulative events also occurred significantly with sustained CH (Table 9).

On the outcome of each group with normotension, white coat hypertension, masked hypertension or sustained hypertension, we were not able to survey their outcomes with statistics as a cohort study, because that each number participated in this study was small.

3.2.3 Risk factor assessment for outcomes

In terms of death, macrovascular complications at baseline represented a significant risk factor for patients with sustained MH, as determined by a Cox proportional hazard model that was significantly (P<0.001) appropriate according to Omnibus tests. Serum creatinine and UAER at baseline levels also represented significant confounding factors. However, as hazard ratios for these parameters were 0.01 and 1.00, respectively, these represented negative or small associated risk (Table 10).

In terms of microvascular complications, MH at baseline on the basis of HBP was a significant risk factor related to new, worsened or improved events of events according to a Cox proportional hazard model that was significantly (P<0.001) appropriate by Omnibus tests. Additional therapies for hypertension and DM also represented significantly confounding factors, but displayed negative associations with this outcome (Table 10).

In terms of macrovascular complications, HbA1c and presence of micro- and macro-vascular complications at baseline in patients with sustained MH were significantly associated with this outcome, as determined by a Cox proportional hazard model that was significantly (P<0.001) appropriate by Omnibus tests. Additional therapy for hypertension represented a negative confounding factor significantly (Table 4). In patients with sustained CH on the basis of CBP, a Cox proportional hazard model was found to be significantly (P<0.001) appropriate by Omnibus tests, and additional therapies for hypercoagulation and others represented a significant confounding factor (P=0.025; Hazard ratio 5.71). No other significant risk factors were identified other than serum TG level at baseline (P=0.025), for which the hazard ratio was 1.00. Additional therapy for hypertension also represented significantly confounding factors, but displayed negative associations with this outcome (P=0.001; Hazard ratio 0.10) (data not shown in the table).

4. Discussion

4.1 Blood pressure (BP)

Over the past 100 years, BP has been measured in the clinic of daytime, which has been called casual or clinic BP (CBP). As hypertension research and treatment methodologies have substantially advanced since the development of CBP, the gold standard of BP measurement for practice and research has been CBP (Imai et al, 2004). Namely, an evaluation for BP is based on the value of CBP. However, an alternative to the CBP was proposed soon after the introduction of BP measurements. Recent studies show that a discrepancy between CBP and ABPM has been noted. It has also been shown that in patients with essential hypertension, HBP measurement in the morning has a stronger predictive power for mortality than CBP measurements in the daytime (Aihara et al, 1998, Ohkubo et al, 1998, Imai et al, 1999). Further, BP measurements by using ABPM or HBP revealed that there is a white hypertension that BP by CBP in the daytime is high, whereas

BP byHBP in the daytime is normal or a masked hypertension that BP in the daytime is normal but BP in the night or in the morning is high in peoples (Pickering, 1992), whch has worsend outcomes for complications in patients, is paied attention to many researchers.

Variable	Death		Microvascular Events		Macrovascular Events	
	Hazard Ratio	P	Hazard Ratio	P	Hazard Ratio	P
Baseline						
Age (years)	1.22	0.13	1.00	0.21	1.10	0.20
Sex	5.61	0.28	1.02	0.86	2.59	0.24
Duration (years)	1.12	0.10	0.99	0.94	0.94	0.11
BMI (kg/m^2)	0.97	0.84	1.00	0.85	1.16	0.10
Blood pressure (mmHg)						
Morning hypertension	0.01	0.95	2.10	0.01*	4.16	0.25
Clinic hypertension	0.11	0.15	0.87	0.27	4.22	0.08
Laboratory variables						
HbA1c (%)	0.73	0.68	1.07	0.22	1.90	0.01*
Triglycerides (mg/dl)	1.00	0.79	1.00	0.95	1.00	0.28
Total cholesterol (mg/dl)	1.01	0.71	1.00	0.83	1.01	0.38
LDL-cholesterol (mg/dl)	1.00	0.91	1.00	0.84	0.99	0.63
HDL-cholesterol (mg/dl)	1.07	0.28	1.00	0.64	1.03	0.10
Serum creatinine (mg/dl)	0.01	0.01*	0.90	0.69	0.53	0.58
Urinary albumin excretion (mg/g creatinine)	1.00	0.03*	1.00	0.98	1.00	0.72
Medical events						
Microvascular complications	0.24	0.78	1.07	0.16	1.67	0.04*
Macrovascular complications	46.0	0.02*	1.08	0.57	3.87	0.01*
Medical treatment						
Therapy for hypertension						
Baseline	0.01	0.07	0.96	0.71	0.99	0.98
Additional	1.18	0.93	0.39	0.01*	0.02	0.01*
Therapy for diabetes mellitus						
Baseline	0.82	0.81	1.04	0.54	1.21	0.50
Additional	0.04	0.07	0.38	0.01*	1.21	0.46
Therapy for dyslipidemia						
Baseline	0.19	0.35	1.14	0.35	0.36	0.19
Additional	0.01	0.99	1.09	0.84	0.01	0.98
Therapy for hypercoagulation and others						
Baseline	26.3	0.21	1.05	0.79	4.43	0.07
Additional	0.01	0.99	0.38	0.07	0.77	0.86

macro- vascular

Each outcome of death, and new, worsened or improved micro- and new or worsened macrovascular events was determined in patients with sustained morning hypertension on the basis of home blood pressure (HBP), which was determined by the log-rank test. Confounding factors were variables at baseline and additional therapy for each disease. Associated risk factors among the confounding factors were assessed using hazard ratio by Cox proportional hazards modeling.
*P value was significant for each risk factor.

Table 10. Risk factors for each outcome of events in patients with sustained morning hypertension on the basis of HBP

4.1.1 Method for blood pressure

4.1.1.1 Clinic Blood Pressure (CBP)

In 1896, Riva-Rocci developed an indirect arm-cuff method for the BP measurement, and in 1905, Korotkoff introduced the use of auscultation. Since then, the method for BP measurement with sphygmomanometers has remained essentially unchanged for 100 years. Nowadays, the oscillometric method takes the plase of sphygmomanometers for having a favorable environment.

4.1.1.2 Home Blood Pressure (HBP)

4.1.1.2.1 ABPM by automated BP measurements

However, alternative methods to the CBP are proposed as HBP. To evaluate the HBP, many methods have developed in the world. One of the methods is ABPM. There are many reports on the results using ABPM for several decades (Imai et al, 2004). Clinically, Sokolow M and his colleagues developed the initial semiautomatic ABPM device in 1962. It consisted of a BP cuff that was manually inflated by the subject and of a tape recorder on which the Korotkoff sounds were recorded. Now, ABPM provides automated measurements of arterial BP for 24 hours or longer. Most modern ABPM monitors use the oscillometric technique. The monitors are programmed to take readings at desired intervals, usually every 15 to 30 minutes, throughout the day and night. At the end of recording, the readings are downloaded onto a computer.
ABPM demonstrated the variability of BP during the daytime and its relatively poor correlation with CBP and first showed that ABPM correlates more closely than CBP with damage to heart and arteries caused by hypertension. They also provided that ABPM improves the ability to predict risk. Nowadays, ABPM is reliable and quiet, and can be programmed to be fully automatic and be worn with little discomfort. Rrecordings by ABPM demonstrate the well-known diurnal pattern of BP, with the higher pressures in the afternoon, with the lower readings in the evening, with the nadir during sleep, and the well-reported early morning surge starting. The BP measurement by ABPM showed there is a white coat hypertension or a masked hypertension (Pickering, 1992). Thus, the ABPM provides BP information in relation to time.

4.1.1.2.2 HBP by self-BP measurement

Another method is self-BP measurement. In 1940, Ayman and Goldshine first reported the concept of "self-BP measurement" and demonstrated an apparent difference between the CBP and the self measured BP. Initially, self-measurement was done using the auscultation method. In the 1970s, an electric device based on the microphone method was marketed, but not widely distributed because of high price, mechanical difficulties, and the issue of auscultation gap. Explosive distribution of HBP measurement devices since the 1980s is mediated by the development of devices based on the cuffoscillometric principle. The basic algorithm of the principle has been improved by procedures to correctly approximate the characteristic changes during phase I and phase V Korotkoff sounds owing to electronic development. Recently, the accuracy of the automatic device is determined by comparison with the auscultation method and no other standard method is currently available for this purpose. At present, three types of electrical devices for HBP measurements are commercially available: the arm-cuff device, the wrist-cuff device, and the finger-cuff device. Ten million such electrical devices are produced each year in the Far East (including

Japan, Korea, Taiwan and China), which represents 85% of the world production. Of those, 35% are wrist-cuff devices. Finger-cuff devices commanded a considerable portion of the market share owing to their convenience and ease-of-use. Nowdays, manufacturers have decreased production of finger-cuff devices owing to technical problems and extensively increased production of wrist-cuff devices. In Japan, wrist-cuff devices possess 30% of the market share. Wrist-cuff devices are much easier to handle and more portable, but include serious shortcomings (Imai et al., 2004). The reference level for BP measurement is the right atrium. When the measurement site is 10 cm below (above) the right atrium, systolic BP and diastolic BP are measured 7 mmHg higher (lower) than those at the level of the right atrium. Even after appropriate correction of the hydrostatic pressure, another issue remains concerning the anatomy of the wrist. At the wrist, the radial and ulnar arteries are surrounded by the radial bone, the ulnar bone and several long tendons, including the palmaris longus tendon. Therefore, even a sufficient amount of cuff pressure over the arterial area does not necessarily occlude these arteries completely. As a result, wrist-cuff devices sometime provide erroneous readings, especially for systolic BP. Therefore, arm-cuff devices based on the cuff-oscillometric method are recommended for HBP measurement (Imai et al, 2004), which is recommended by guidline of many societies for hypertension (the European Society of Hypertension and the European Society of Cardiology, 2007, the American Heart Association, American Society of Hypertension and Preventive Nurses Association, 2008, the Japanese Society of Hypertension , 2009).

4.1.1.1.3 Differences between ABPM by automated-BP measurement and HBP by self-BP measurement

It is very important to know the characteristcs of the difference between ABPM and HBP. ABPM is measured under several psychological and physiological conditions by automated BP measuremnt, while HBP is measured under relatively stable conditions by self-BP measurment. Although both ABPM and HBP are able to evaluate BP in the night time, an estimation of BP in the short-time by HBP is inadequate. Meanwhile, an estimation of BP in the long-time for more than 24 hours including the drug effect by ABPM is inadequate and occasionally insufficient due to regression to the mean, and reproducibility owing to measure BP under psychological and physiological conditions by ABPM is poor (Imai et al, 2004). Further, the costs for ABPM by automated BP measurement including devices are higher than those for HBP by self-BP measurement. However, we confirmed that ABPM is sometimes better to check the accuracy of HBP measurement method.

4.1.2 Variation

4.1.2.1 Variation of BP by HBP in healthy subjects

There is no difference in BP by HBP using Omron device between left and right arms for a day and for one month. Further, there is no difference in BP using left arm- cuff by HBP between summer and winter.

4.1.2.2 Variation of BP by HBP in diabetic patients

As mentioned in above, the variation of BP by HBP at the awakening-up using wrist-cuff in a diabetic patient is sometimes higher than that using arm-cuff. In diabetic patients, BP by HBP at the wakening-up is also increased sometimes by stress for a month. In them, more than 10% of day-by-day coefficient variation (CV) in HBP at the wakening-up for a month leads to have more occurences of complications with micro- and macro-vascular disturbences than less than 10% of CV (Figure 5) as shown in a diabetic patient who had acute myocardial infarction. These findings were demonstrated by Ohasma study (Imai et al, 2004). Short-term BP variability is a risk factor for cardiovascular diseases (Imai et al, 2004). Although short-term information is available from ABPM, the information on day-by-day variability is obtained only with home BP measurements. The Ohasama study demonstrated that day-by-day variability reflects the risk of cardiovascular diseases. Thus, home BP measurements can now replace ABPM (Imai et al , 2004).

4.1.3 Threshold

Subjects from the Ohasama population aged 40 years and over were followed up for an average of 10.6 years. In the study, when the relationship between BP level and stroke incidence being analyzed by a Cox regression model was adjusted for age, sex, and drug treatment, the study suggested that there is higher predictability of HBP when compared with CBP. The linear regression analysis deduced that 140/90 mmHg for CBP corresponds to 125/80 mmHg for HBP, suggesting that the normative value of HBP is less than 125/80 mmHg (Imai et al, 2004)

In our study, we used thresholds of once HBP value at the awakening-up in the morning and those of CBP in the daytime as <130/85 mmHg value based on the criteria of CH owing to the 1999 WHO-International Society of Hypertension guidelines (Guide lines Subcommittee, 1999). This studies showed the threshold of 130 mmHg of systolic BP at the awakening-up in the morning for micro- and macro-vasclualr complications is significant (Figure 3), while diastolic BP of HBP at the wakening-up is persistently referred to assement the BP for the complications.

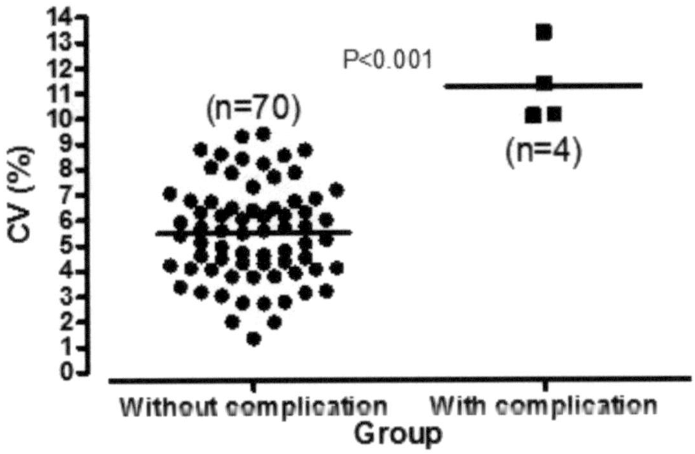

Fig. 5. Relationship between variations of BP by HBP measured at the awakening-up in the morning and vascular comlications in diabetic patients in comparison with those of less than 10% and more than 10% of CV for a month. In diabetic patients, the mean of more than of 10% for CV has demonstrated that there were more complications than that of less than 10% for CV.

Recently, all guidelines recommended a threshold for HBP by 5-10 mmHg is lower than for CBP (Mancia et al, 2007, Pickering et al, 2008, Ogihara et al, 2009). The guidelines indicated that the target HBP goal for treatment is <130–135/85 mmHg in the morning (Mancia et al, 2007) and <135/85 mmHg or <130/80 mmHg in the morning in high-risk patients (Pickering et al, 2008). The Japanese Society of Hypertension defined the threshold of controlled BP is < 135 /85 mmHg of HBP in the morning (Ogihara et al,2009).

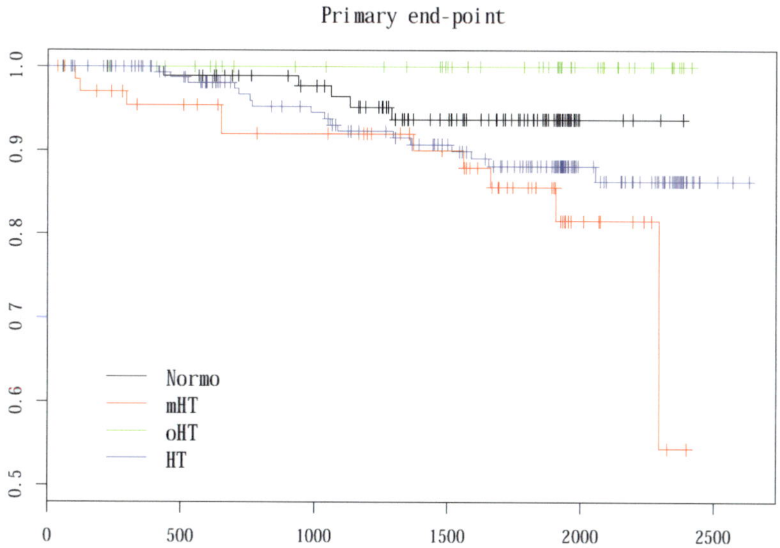

Fig. 6. Event-free survival curve of primary endpoints in patients with type 2 diabetes in a longitudinal study. Normo; MN and CN, mHT; MH, oHT; CH, HT; MH and CH

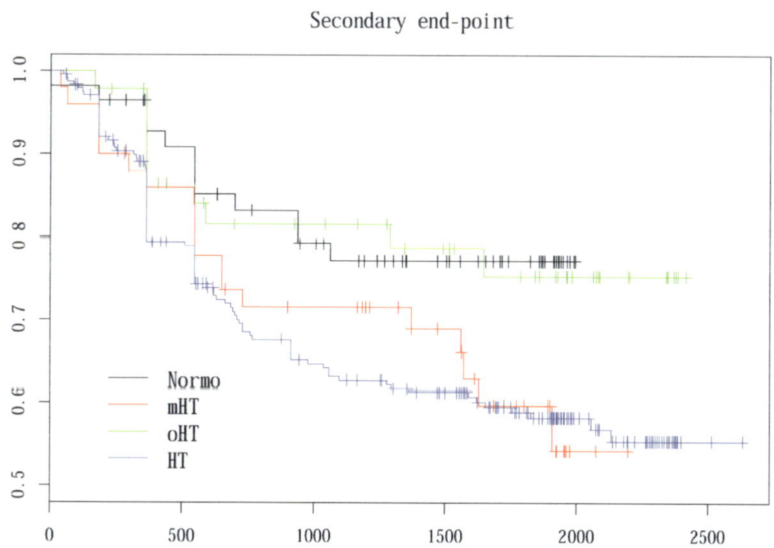

Fig. 7. Event-free survival curve of secondary endpoints in patients with type 2 diabetes in a longitudinal study. Normo; MN and CN, mHT; MH, oHT; CH, HT; MH and CH

4.2 In a cross-sectional study

4.2.1 In a type 1 diabetes mellitus

As shown in the figure 1, in the type 1 diabetic groups with CH or CN, the anti-hypertensive medicines in the groups with MH were larger number than in the groups with MN. The prevalence of nephropathy in the patients with MH was significantly higher than in those without MH, even though they had CN (Table 2). In contrast, the occurrence was not observed in those without MH, even though they had CH. Specifically, nephropathy, including clinical albuminuria, was observed in patients with systolic MH but not in patients without MH. Analysis by ROC curves also indicates that home BP in the morning has a stronger predictive power than clinic BP, especially in nephropathy (Figure 2). The cut point of 130-mmHg morning systolic BP has higher sensitivity and higher specificity than that of clinic systolic BP (Figure 3). This finding indicates that nephropathy in type 1 diabetic patients may be strongly related to morning home BP rather than clinic BP (Kamoi et al, 2003). The reason may be explained by several factors, such as white coat hypertension, nondipper hypertension, and morning surge. Particularly, an increase in nocturnal BP, as detected by ABPM, in type 1 diabetes is related to the development of microalbuminuria (Moore et al, 1992, Lurbe et al, 2003). These phenomena are thought to be caused by many neuroendocrine and hematological factors, especially autonomic neuropathy (Spallone et al, 1993, Lafferty et al, 2000, Torbjornsdotter et al, 2001). Although we did not measure 24-h ambulatory BP, the greater range in the relation of morning home BP and clinic BP may be partially explained by true and white coat hypertension, reverse-dipping hypertension, and the effects of treatment with anti- hypertensive drugs. In contrast, the prevalence of retinopathy in type 1 diabetic patients did not relate to BP, including morning home BP, although the degree of retinopathy was strengthened by MH. The duration of diabetes contributed to retinopathy significantly. They support the hypothesis that sustained long-term hyperglycaemia is the strongest predictor for developing retinopathy and that high morning home BP accelerates retinopathy as well as nephropathy.

4.2.2 In a type 2 diabetes mellitus

In the type 2 diabetic patients who were regularly treated with diet and exercise or medications for hyperglycaemia and hypertension, we found that one half of CH patients had MN, whereas two thirds of CN patients had MH. The prevalences of nephropathy, retinopathy, CHD, and CVD in patients with MH were significantly higher than in patients without MH, even though they had CN. In contrast, the prevalence of these vascular disturbances was significantly lower in patients without MH than in patients with MH, even though they had CH. Specifically, nephropathy, including clinical albuminuria, was observed in patients with systolic MH but not in any patients without MH. The difference is not related to age, sex, BMI, HbA1c, serum lipid concentrations, or use of anti-diabetic and anti-hypertensive drugs. The finding in the present cross-sectional study indicates that micro- and macro- vascular complications of type 2 diabetic patients may be strongly related to HBP in the morning rather than CBP.

The reason for the underlying relation of high HBP in the morning rather than high CBP to the vascular complications is not clearly determined by this study. However, several possibilities are postulated. First, type 2 diabetic patients have high prevalence of increased CBP but normal HBP in the morning (white coat hypertension) (Burgess et al, 1991, Puig et al, 1995). White coat hypertension seems to be a low risk for vascular complications

(Pickering, 1996, Nielson et al, 1997). Second, O'Brien et al (O'Brien et al, 1988) and Imai et al (Imai et al, 1990) reported that nocturnal decline in BP in patients with essential hypertension is often diminished (non-dipper hypertension) and sometimes inverts to become a nocturnal elevation (inverted dipper hypertension). Non-dipper hypertension, particularly inverted dipper hypertension, accelerates vascular disturbances (Shimada et al, 1990, Okubo et al, 1997), including microalbuminuria (Opsahl et al, 1988). Many studies have reported that type 2 diabetic patients have non-dipper hypertension (Forgari et al, 1994, Spalone et al, 1993, Farmer et al, 1998, Sturrock et al, 2000, White, 2001, Aronson, 2001). Therefore, it seems that blunted nocturnal and/or inverted dipper hypertension may cause micro- and macro- vascular complications in type 2 diabetic patients. Third, a morning surge in BP may be related to these events. A number of reports indicate that the early morning surge in BP acts as a trigger for vascular events (White, 2001, Aronson, 2001). Most diabetic patients have the morning surge (Aronson, 2001). These phenomena in diabetic patients are considered to be caused by many neuroendocrine and haematological factors, including autonomic neuropathy, which may result in glomerular hyperfiltration, hypercoagulability, and hypofibrinolysis, promoting micro- and macro- vascular disturbances. In fact, a high prevalence of these phenomena was observed in MH but not in MN. In addition, the severity of MH in CN patients tended to be greater than in CH patients. Moreover, the relation of MBP and CBP levels was a greater range, indicating true and white coat hypertension, and MBP level in some patients was higher than the corresponding CBP level, indicating that reverse dipping hypertension might occur, although we did not measure 24-h ambulatory BP. It is hypothesized that treatment with anti- hypertensive drugs reduced daytime BP but did not restore blunted nocturnal hypertension, did not decrease nocturnal hypertension, and could not attenuate the morning surge in BP (Spalone et al, 1993, Imai et al, 1999). The greater range in relation of MBP and CBP, and the negative association between events of nephropathy and clinic DBP may be partially explained by the effect of treatment with anti- hypertensive drugs, as hypothesized above.

Analysis by ROC curves also indicates that HBP has a stronger predictive power than CBP, especially in nephropathy. The cut points of 130/85 mmHg have higher sensitivity in morning measurement than in clinic measurement (Figure 2), although specificity in the cut point of 130 mmHg SBP in the morning measurement was lower than in the clinic measurement. Accordingly, measurement of HBP in the morning is a useful method of determining these phenomena, as indicated by the Ohasama study (Imai et al, 1990-2004, Okubo et al, 1995-1998), and high HBP levels at the awakening-up in the morning in type 2 diabetic patients may be related to micro and macro vascular complications of diabetes.

All findings indicate that high BP levels at the awakening-up in the morning, obtained by means of self-measurement in type 2 diabetic patients, should be treated as hypertension.

4.3 In a longitudinal study

4.3.1 General

We analysed the influence of HBP at the awakening-up in the morning and of CBP in the daytime on outcomes of events including death, microvascular complications as nephropathy and retinopathy, and macrovascular complications as CHD and CVD for data obtained over 6 years in a prospective, longitudinal study of type 2 diabetic patients. To clarify which of HBP or CBP provides the stronger predictive power for the outcomes, the

400 patients were classified as with or without hypertension based on HBP and CBP measurements at baseline, because that although the cross-sectional studies have demonstrated that HBP measurements at the awakening-up in the morning offer stronger predictive power for micro- and macro-vascular complications in patients with type 1 and 2 DM than CBP measurements in the daytime (Kamoi et al, 2002-2003) and the MH may be caused by micro- and macro-vascular complications.

All subjects were Japanese patients with type 2 diabetes. Subject characteristics were broadly similar to those described previously (Kamoi et al, 2002), except that patients with CH showed a higher prevalence of nephropathy than patients with CN.

Recently, all guidelines recommended a threshold for HBP by 5-10 mmHg lower than for CBP (Mancia et al, 2007, Pickering et al, 2008, Ogihara et al, 2009) as mention. In this study, the use of the same thresholds based on the criteria of CH owing to the 1999 WHO-International Society of Hypertension guidelines (WHO, 1999) for both methods resulted to MN patients with higher threshold and more severe MH patients selected with HBP. Nevertheless, the cumulative event of death was observed in sustained MH patients, but not in sustained MN patients. United Kingdom Prospective Diabetes Study (UKPDS) reported that the cumulative incidence of death was 12.4 % (597 of 4801 patients with type 2 diabetes) for ten years (Adler et al, 2000). In the study, the incidence was 2.3 % for 6 years. Although the reason is unclear why the incidence in this study is lower than in UKPDS, the hazard ratio was significantly (5-fold) higher in sustained MH patients than in sustained MN patients, while no significant difference was seen between sustained CH and CN patients. In addition, cumulative events of new or worsened microvascular complications were significantly (2-fold) higher in sustained MH patients than in sustained MN patients, while no significant difference was seen between sustained CH and CN patients. The incidence of the events is about 50% higher in the MH patients as compared to the MN patients (19.2% vs. 14.9%), while the hazard ratio indicates that the risk of an event in the MH patients is about twice as high as the risk of an event in the MN patients. This may be explained by that the follow-up time in the MH patients is much shorter than the follow-up time in the MN patients. Furthermore, UKPDS reported that the cumulative incidence of CHD was 12.5 % (600 of 4801 patients with type 2 diabetes) for ten years. In the study, the incidence was 5.3 % for 6 years. Also, although the reason is unclear why the incidence in this study is lower than in UKPDS (Adler et al, 2000), cumulative events of new or worsened macrovascular complications were significantly higher in sustained MH patients than in sustained MN patients, and significantly higher in sustained CH patients than in sustained CN patients.

The present results indicate that cumulative events of death and new or worsened micro- and macro- vascular complications are more strongly related to sustain MH, although sustained CH is also related to them,

In terms of death among sustained MH patients, the finding that presence of macrovascular complications at baseline was a significant risk factor indicates that sustained MH may be a trigger for death among patients with macrovascular complications. In the event of new or worsened microvascular complications, the fact that MH at baseline was the only associated risk factor indicates that sustained MH also represents a strong contributor to new or worsened microvascular complications. The finding that additional therapy for hypertension suppressed occurrence of new or worsened microvascular complications supports this view. In the event of new or worsened macrovascular complications, the identification of glycaemic control and presence of micro- and macro- vascular complications at baseline among patients with sustained MH as associated risk factors indicates that sustained MH, as along with glycaemic control and presence of micro- and macro-vascular complications (American Diabetes Association, 2009), is important risk factor. It is supported this view that age, sex, serum creatinine, LDL and proteinuria were not risk factors. Moreover, additional therapy for hypertension improved or prevented the macrovascular events, supporting this idea. Meanwhile, the finding that sustained CH was related to the macrovascular events is consistent with the findings of a previous report (Aldler et al, 2000). Accordingly, not only sustained CH but also sustained MH is related to the new or worsened macrovascular events.

All findings indicated that events of death and new or worsened micro- and macro-vascular complications in type 2 diabetic patients are strongly related to sustained MH, irrespective of sustained CH as demonstrated in a cross-sectional study (Kamoi et al, 2002-2003) and in the Ohasama study (Okubo et al, 1998), and support the view that the available evidence suggests that HBP has strong prognostic value, which appears to be superior to that of the conventional CBP measurements. The reasons of differencnt results by studies of ACCORD and Cooper-DeHoff et al may be obtained by evaluation of BP by HBP measurement at the wakening-up.

4.3.2 Limitations of this study

In a longitudinal study, this study was that the numbers of patients participating and events occurring over the 6 years of the study were heterogeneous and small, so we were unable to survey outcomes and compare differences among baseline groups of patients with MH, MN, CH and CN as a cohort study. Further, there were no evening measurements as well as 24 hours BP monitoring to compare them. Instead, we classified the 400 patients into patients with or without hypertension based on HBP and CBP measurements and compared differences in cumulative events between sustained hypertensive and normotensive patients in each group. These patients' classifications obviously overlapped. Accordingly, the censoring date depends on whether HT and NT are defined according to CBP or HBP and the same censoring time was not used in the 2 analyses. Furthermore, for ethical reasons, most patients received treatment with various anti-hypertensive agents and other medications during follow-up. Therefore, we were unable to examine outcomes without changing treatments from baseline over the 6 years of the study and whether these drugs would thus have influenced the outcomes of events in this study. At baseline 49% of the subjects received anti- hypertensive treatment. Anti-hypertensive drugs are most likely prescribed on the basis of CBP. Therefore, somebody argues that it is not appropriate to classify patients taking anti- hypertensive drugs and having a normal BP as normotension, and the untreated CBP in most of these patients may be probably in the hypertensive range. This may introduce a bias in the comparison between CBP and HBP.

Particularly, it is clinically more informative to evaluate the prognostic value of both white coat hypertension and masked hypertension based on CBP and HBP among subjects with diabetes. However, we were not able to survey their outcomes with statistics as a cohort study, because that each number participated in this study was small.

Someone may indicate that the prognostic values of CBP and HBP should be assessed as not only categorical data, but also continuous variables. The analysis using continuous variables may give more significant meaning, but in this study, BP as continuous variables showed high fluctuation and the numbers participated were small. Accordingly, as the analysis with statistics is complex, we did not examine it in this study.

By meta-analysis, compared with clinic BP monitoring alone, systolic BP at daytime by home BP monitoring has the potential to overcome therapeutic inertia and lead to a small but significant reduction in systolic and diastolic BP. Hypertension control with home BP monitoring can be enhanced further when accompanied by plans to monitor and treat elevated BP, although there is not a systematic review on the morning BP by home BP measurement (Agarwal et al, 2011).

4.3.3 A mechanism undering awakening-up hypertension related to vascular complications in patients with diabetes mellitus

As shown in Figure 8, when subjects had awakening-up from sleeping, their parasympathic activity changed to sympathic activity. Such changes at the awakening-up have most increase in activiation of renin-angiotenin-aldosteron-vasopressin system, coaglulation system and oxidant stress, and most decreases in activation of plasminogen activator inhibitor and fibilinolytic system. The alterations have companied with most conctriction of blood vessel owing to most decreased endothelial function in the day (Figure 9) (Otto et al, 2004). In the states, hypertension may lead to have a vascular injury, resulting in vascular disturbances. Most patients with diabetes have hypertension when we used measurement of BP by HBP at the awkening-up as well as CBP in the daytime.

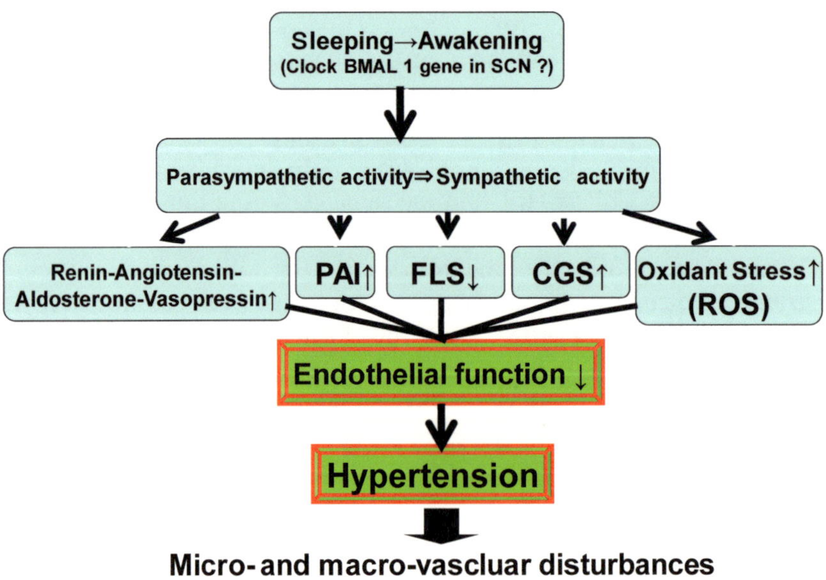

Fig. 8. Scheme of mechanism underling awakening-up hypertension related vascular disturbences in diabetic patients. BMAL ; Brain-Muscle-Arnt-Like-protein, SCN ; supra optic nucleus, PAI; plasminogen activator inhibitor, FLS ; fibilinolytic system, CGS; coaglulation system

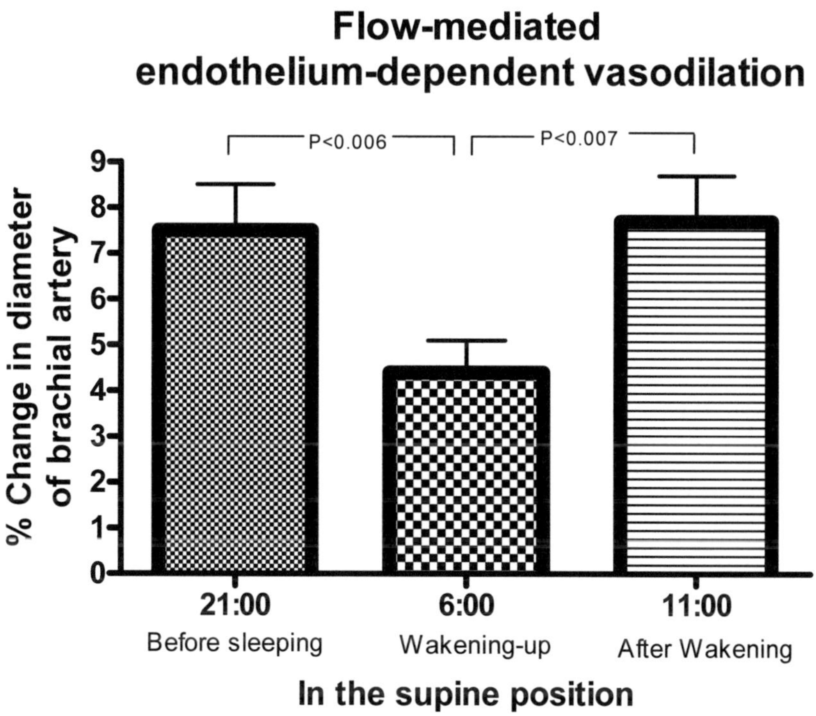

Fig. 9. Change in diameter of brachial artery at the awakening-up, after the wakening and before sleeping in the supine postion of healthy subjects by evaluation using flow-mediated echogram.

4.3.4 A reason why we measure BP at the wakening-up by HBP

There were more occurrences of CVD and CHD in the morning and in the evening in Japanese peoples in 1994 (Sato et al, 1994). However, the reason was unclear. Also, Stergiou GS et al in 2002 showed that the incidences of vascular complications in patients with hypertension at the awakening-up in Siesta were greater number than those in patients with normotension at the awakening-up (Stergious et al, 2002) (Figure 10). Our previous studies demonstrated that secretions of hormones related to BP in the upright position are higher than in the recumbent position (Kamoi et al, 1988). These findings indicated that the differences may be related to the difference of parasymapthic- and sympathic-nerves activities. Further, the increased hormones have decresded immediately after bias by various factors including own or other helps. In fact, HBP at the morning has been decreased immediately after awakening-up and second or third measurement of HBP is more decreased than first measurement of BP. Therefore, we chosed first HBP measurement once at the awakening up except another points of BP in a day, although someone thinks that the once mesurment may be strict, because that many reseachers have a mean of BP for several mesuremnts of BP becasuse that most patients desire to pass urine after awakening. When they are unbearable to pass it, I recommend once measurement of BP after passing the urine. Most patients have awakening-up in the eary morning, but some patients who have worked in midnight have awakening-up in the late morning. Therefore, I recommend patients to measure BP at awakening-up in the day. The method is simple and accurate to assess HBP.

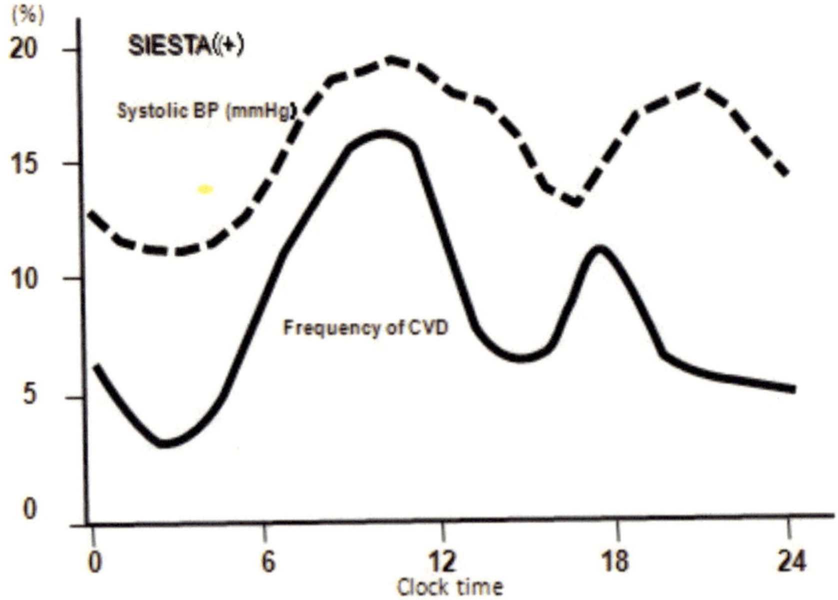

Fig. 10. Relationship between systolic blood pressure at the awkening-up in Siesta of Greece and cerebral vascular diseases (CVD).

4.3.5 An usefulness of BP by HBP in the disaster

First, Kario et al observed that there were more occurences CVD or CHD in patients with MH, which increased after several days after Hanshin-Awaji earthquake using ABPM in 1994 (Kario et al, 2002). The mechanism may be due to activity of sympathic nerve, which was supported by administration of α blockers. They proposed if peoples have the MH by HBP or ABPM, α blockers administration into the peoples have been recommended, which needs few weeks post the disaster. To evaluate MH in the morning, BP must be measured by a device of measurements HBP or ABPM. However, in Japan, nowadays, peoples in the public refuge houses have BP measurement in the daytime, but not upon awakening in the morning.

Our expérices in the 2004 Mid-Niigata Prefecture Earthquake in 2004 (Kamoi et al, 2006) are same as Kario et al. The patients measured HBP in the awkening-up in his own house showed an increased HBP within a few weeks afer earthquake and the patients suppressed HBP in the awalening-up by taking anti-hypertensive medicines for MH before the earthquake had no vascular complications (Figure 12), whereas peoples without measured HBP had many CHD, CVD or dialysis during 6 months after the earthquake (Kamoi et al, 2006). These findings suggest that it is important to control MH as we11 as CH during a disaster to prevent vascular complications, particularly such as nephrophaty. However, our study showed only one-third of patients measured their HBP within three months after the shock. Although the reasons why they did not measure their HBP were not clarified by the study, it is known that some patients lost their HBP measurement equipment, some had their equipment destroyed, and some suffered from anxiety, in particular sleep disturbance, as result of the devastation caused by the strong earthquake. In the public refuge houses, all patients have BP measurements in the daytime as the report by Kario et al, but not upon awakening in the morning. Therefore, we recommend strongly that there is need to develop a procedure of BP measurement upon awakening in the morning during a disaster in the public refuge houses as well as in their homes and to educate individuals about appropriate adaptation mechanisms following a disaster such as taking special care of themselves during the initial three months following a disaster. Appropriate information about morning hypertension should be provided to all affected people using all possible means, including the mass media, to decrease the potential for adverse consequences.

4.3.6 Treatment methods for awakening-up hypertension, by HBP in patients with diabetes melitus

First, restriction of salt ingestion in diabetic patients is necessary to have better BP by HBP at the awakening-up as patients with hypertension in the daytime. As hyperglycaemia causes increased urinary excretion of glucose via convoluted tubule, reabsorption of sodium cloride from the convoluted tubule into blood is increased. Hence, volume expansion in the blood and activation of sympathic nerve occure in them. They lead to occure MH in the morning as CH in the daytime. Therefore, restriction of salt ingestion (less than 7.0 g/day) is usefull to control MH

Second, howeve, the treatment is not effective in most diabetic patients. Some patients have MN in the admission of hospital, but have MH in their homes. Probably, the sympathic activity of them may increase in the daily life, which shows the MH at the awakening-up but CN in the daytime as masked hypertension. Further, some patients have orthostatic hypotension by nerve disturbenes, which shows that BP are hypotension by CBP in the daytime, whereas they are MH by HBP at the awakening-up in the morning. In such patients, switched bedtime adminstration of α blockers is effective (Figure 11) (Kamoi et al, 2006).

Third, when the patients have CH in the daytime and MH at the awakening-up, administration of long active anti-hypertensive medicines after taking breakfast as a conventinal method for hypertension is usfull. Sometimes, such adminstraton is not effective in the patients with MH. In that case, switched bedtime administration is effective (Kamoi et al, 2006) In the world, many studies by researchers on administration methods of them are proceeding.

Fourth, we meet many patients who had albeit such treatments, the therapy had no effective for MH. In such diabetic patients, clock time disturbed may be accompanied (Figure 8). As it is difficult to treat such patients, the treatment methods remain to be not resolved completely.

Any way, controlling high BP at the wakening-up by using various methods prevents for micro- and macro- vascluar complications.

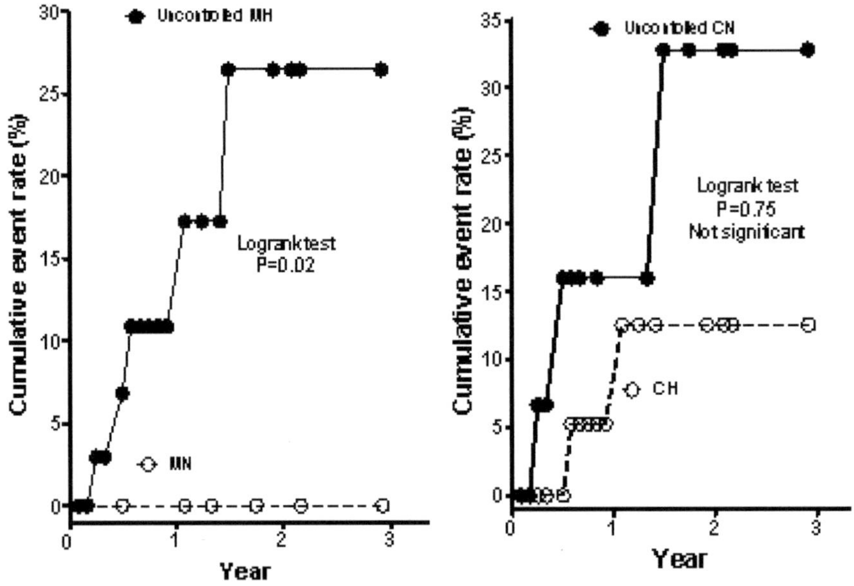

Fig. 11. Effect of α blocker administration at bedtime in type 2 diabetic patients on nephropathy. The patients were treated with doxosine received at bedtime for 3 years for MH.

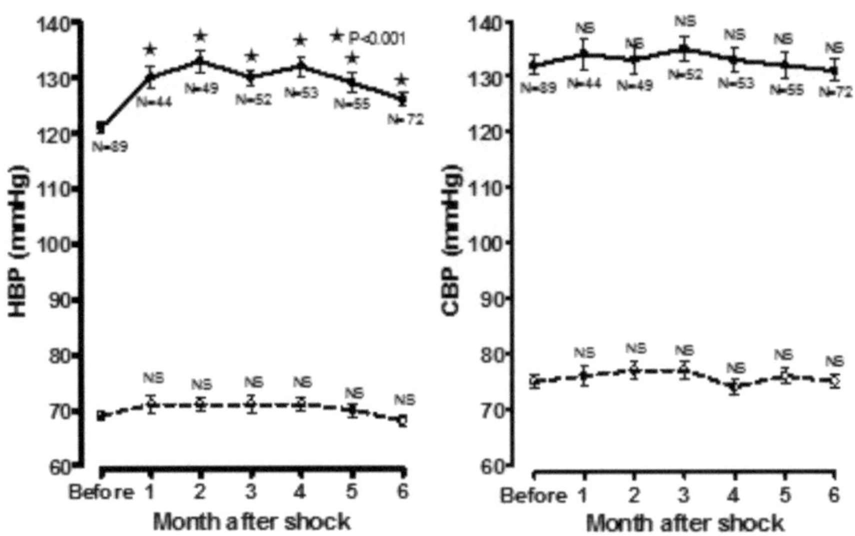

Fig. 12. Effect of earthquake (magnitude 7.0) on HBP and CBP at the awakening-up in type 2 diabetic patients for 6 months. Increased BP at the awakening-up in the morning owing to devastation by earthquake continued for several months, whereas CBP was not changed, eventhough the patient had received anti-hypertensive medicines before occuring earthquake.

5. Conclusion

In conclusion, elevations of blood pressure on self-measurement at the awakening-up in the morning as well as clinical blood pressure measurement in the daytime in type 1 and 2 diabetic patients are strongly related to microvascular complications, especially nephropathy, and the control of morning hypertension may prevent to have a development of micro- and macro-vascular complications in patients with diabetes mellitus.

6. Acknowledgment

We thank Emeritus Professor Yutaka Imai, MD (Tohoku University Graduate School of Medicine and Pharmaceutical Science) for helpful comments.

7. References

ACCORD Study Group.; Cushman, W.C., Evans, G.W., Byington, R.P., Goff, D.C. Jr, Grimm, R.H. Jr, Cutler, J.A., Simons-Morton, D.G., Basile, J.N., Corson, M.A., Probstfield, J.L., Katz, L., Peterson, K.A., Friedewald, W.T., Buse, J.B., Bigger, J.T., Gerstein, H.C. & Ismail-Beigi, F. (2010). Effects of intensive blood-pressure control in type 2 diabetes mellitus. *N Engl J Med* Vol 362, No. 17, (Apr 2010), pp 1575-1585, ISSN: 00284793.

Adler, A.I. ; Stratton, I.M., Neil, H.A., Yudkin, J.S., Matthews, D.R., Cull, C.A., Wright, A.D., Turner, R.C. & Holman, R.R. (2000). Association of systolic blood pressure with macrovascular and microvascular complications of type 2 diabetes (UKPDS 36): prospective observational study. *BMJ* Vol 321, No.7258, (Aug 2000), pp 412-419, ISSN: 17592151

Agarwal, R. ; Bills, J.E., Hecht, T.J. & Light, R.P. (2010). Role of home blood pressure monitoring in overcoming therapeutic inertia and improving hypertension control: a systematic review and meta-analysis. *Hypertension* Vol 57, No. 1, (Jan 2011), pp 29-38, ISSN: 0194911X

Aihara, A. ; Imai, Y., Sekino, M., Kato, J., Ito, S., Ohkubo, T.,Tsuji, I., Satoh, H., Hisamichi, S. & Nagai, K. (1998). Discrepancy between screening blood pressure and ambulatory blood pressure: acommunity based study in Ohasama. *Hypertens Res* Vol 21, No. 2, (Jun 1998), pp127–136, ISSN: 09169636.

Alberti, K. G. & Zimmet, P. Z. (1998). Definition, diagnosis and classification of diabetes mellitus and its complications. Part1. Diagnosis and classification of diabetes mellitus provisional report of a WHO consultation. *Diabet Med* Vol 15, No. 7, (Jul 1998), pp 539–553, ISSN: 07423071

American Diabetes Association. (2002). Summary of revisions for the 2002. Clinical practice recommendations. *Diabetes Care* Vol 25 (Suppl. 1), No. 1, (Jan 2002), pp S3, ISSN: 01495992

American Diabetes Association. (2002). Clinic practice recommendations 2002: diabetic nephropathy. *Diabetes Care* Vol 25 (Suppl.1), No. 1 (Jan 2002), pp S85–S89, ISSN: 01495992

American Diabetes Association. (2009). Clinical practice recommendations 2009, Standards of medical care-2009. *Diabetes Care* Vol 32 (Suppl 1), No. 1 (Jan 2009), pp S13-S61, ISSN: 01495992.

American Diabetes Association. (2011). Summary of revisions for the 2011. Clinical practice recommendations. *Diabetes Care* Vol 34 (Suppl 1), No. 1, (Jan 2011), pp S3, ISSN: 01495992

Aronson, D. (2001). Impaired modulation of circadian rhythms in patients with diabetes mellitus: a risk factor for cardiac thrombotic events? *Chronobiol Int* Vol 18, No. 1, (Jan 2001), pp109–121, ISSN: 07420528

Burgess, E.; Mather, K., Ross, S. & Josefsberg, Z. (1991). Offce hypertension in type2 (non-insulin-dependent) diabetic patients. *Diabetologia* Vol 34, No. 9, (Sep 1991), pp 684–685, ISSN: 0012186X

Cooper-DeHoff, R.M. ; Gong, Y., Handberg, E.M., Bavry, A.A., Denardo, S.J., Bakris, G.L. & Pepine, C.J. (2010).Tight blood pressure control and cardiovascular outcomes among hypertensive patients with diabetes and coronary artery disease. *JAMA* Vol 304, No. 1, (Jul 2010), pp 61-68, ISSN: 00987484

1999 Guide lines Subcommittee. (1999). World Health Organization-International Society of Hypertension guide lines for the management of hypertension. *J Hypertens* Vol 17, No.2, (Feb 1999), pp 151–183, ISSN: 02636352

Farmer, C. K.; Goldsmith, D. J., Quin, J. D., Dallyn, P., Cox, J., Kingswood, J. C. & Sharpstone, P. F. (1998). Progression of diabetic nephropathy--is diurnal blood pressure rhythm as important as absolute blood pressure level? *Nephrol Dial Transplant* Vol 13, No.3, (Mar 1998), pp 635–639, ISSN: 09310509

Fogari, R.; Zoppi, A., Malamani, G. D., Lazzari, P., Albonico, B. & Corradi, L. (1994). Urinary albumin excretion and nocturnal blood pressure in hypertensive patients with type II diabetes mellitus. *Am J Hypertens* Vol 7, No. 7, (Sep 1994), pp 808–813, ISSN: 08957061

Imai, Y.; Abe, K., Munakata, M., Sakuma, H., Hashimoto, J., Imai, K., Sekino, H.& Yoshinaga, K. (1990). Circadian blood pressure variation under different pathophysiological conditions. *J Hypertens* Vol 8 (Suppl 6), No. 7, (Dec 1990), pp125–132, ISSN: 0263652

Imai, Y. ; Nishiyama, A., Sekino, M., Aihara, A., Kikuya, M., Ohkubo, T., Matsubara, M., Hozawa, A.,Tsuji, I., Ito, S., Satoh, H., Nagai, K. & Hisamichi, S. (1999). Characteristics of blood pressure measured at home in the morning and in the evening: the Ohasama study. *J Hypertens* Vol 17, No. 7, (Jul 1999), pp 889–898, ISSN: 02636352

Imai, Y.; Ohkubo, T.,Tsuji, I., Satoshi, H. & Hisamichi, S. (1999). Clinical signifcance of nocturnal blood pressure monitoring. *Clin Exp Hypertens* Vol 21, No.5-6, (Jul-Aug 1999), pp 717–727, ISSN: 10641963

Imai,Y.; Ohkubo, T., Tsuji, I., Hozawa, A., Nagai, K., Kikuya, M., Aihara, A., Sekino, M., Michimata, M.,Matsubara, M., Ito, S., Satoh, H. & Hisamichi, S. (1999). Relationships among blood pressures obtained using different measurement methods in the general population of Ohasama, Japan. *Hypertens Res* Vol 22, No. 2, (Feb 1999), pp 261–272, 1SSN: 09182918

Imai, Y.; Ohkubo, T., Kikuya, M. & Hashimoto, J. (2004). Practical aspect of monitoring hypertension based on selfmeasured blood pressure at home. *Internal Medicine* Vol 43, No. 9, (Sep 2004), pp 771–778, ISSN: 09182918

Kamoi, K.; Sato, F., Arai, O., Ishibashi, M. & Yamaji, T. (1988). Effects of plasma volume and osmolality on secretion of atrial natriuretic peptide and vasopressin in man. *Acta Endocrinol (Copenh)* Vol 118, No. 1, (May 1988), pp 51-58. ISSN: 00015598

Kamoi, K. ; Miyakoshi, M., Soda, S., Kaneko, S. & Nakagawa, O. (2002). Usefulness of home blood pressure measurement in the morning in type 2 diabetic patients. *Diabetes Care* Vol 25, No.12, (Dec 2002), pp 2218-2223, ISSN: 01495992

Kamoi, K.; Imamura, S. & Kobayashi, T. (2003). Usefulness of home blood pressure measurement in the morning in type 1 diabetic patients. *Diabetes Care* Vol 26, No.8, (Aug 2003), pp 2473-2475, ISSN: 01495992

Kamoi, K. & Ikarashi, T. (2005).The bedtime administration of doxazosin controls morning hypertension and albuminuria in patients with type-2 diabetes: evaluation using home-based blood pressure measurements. *Clin Exp Hypertens* Vol 27, No. 4, (May 2005), pp 369-376, ISSN: 10641963

Kamoi, K.; Tanaka, M., Ikarashi, T. & Miyakoshi, M.(2006). Effect of the 2004 Mid-Niigata Prefecture earthquake on home blood pressure measurement in the morning in type 2 diabetic patients. *Clin Exp Hypertens* Vol 28, No. 8, (Nov 2006), pp 719-729, ISSN: 10641963

Kamoi, K.; Ito, T., Miyakoshi, M. & Minagawa, S. (2010). Usefulness of home blood pressure measurement in the morning in patients with type 2 diabetes: long-term results of a prospective longitudinal study. *Clin Exp Hypertens* Vol 32, No. 3, (May 2010), pp 184-192, ISSN: 10641963

Kasezawa, N.; Shinzato, M., Maruyama, N., Urata, T., Kobayashi, S., Shimamune, Y., Sekino, C., Sakai, Y., Katagiru, T., Izu, K., Aai, O., Kaneko, K. & Kamoi, K. (1987). Development of rapid automated simultaneous measurements of stable and labile glycosylated hemoglobins and fetal hemoglobin by high performance liquid chromatography and studies on the clinical evaluation. *Rinsho Byori* Vol 35, No. 2, (Feb 1987), pp 203-210, ISSN: 00471860

Mancia, G. ; De Backer, G., Dominiczak, A., Cifkova, R., Fagard, R., Germano, G., Grassi, G., Heagerty, A.M., Kjeldsen, S.E., Laurent, S., Narkiewicz, K., Ruilope, L., Rynkiewicz, A., Schmieder, R.E., Boudier, H.A., Zanchetti, A., Vahanian, A., Camm, J., De Caterina, R., Dean, V., Dickstein, K., Filippatos, G., Funck-Brentano, C., Hellemans, I., Kristensen, S.D., McGregor, K., Sechtem, U., Silber, S., Tendera, M., Widimsky, P., Zamorano, J.L., Erdine, S., Kiowski, W., Agabiti-Rosei, E., Ambrosioni, E., Lindholm, L.H., Viigimaa, M., Adamopoulos, S., Agabiti-Rosei, E., Ambrosioni, E., Bertomeu, V., Clement, D., Erdine, S., Farsang, C., Gaita, D., Lip, G., Mallion, J.M., Manolis, A.J., Nilsson, P.M., O'Brien, E., Ponikowski, P., Redon, J., Ruschitzka, F., Tamargo, J., van Zwieten, P., Waeber, B. & Williams, B. (2007). Management of Arterial Hypertension of the European Society of Hypertension; European Society of Cardiology. 2007 Guidelines for the Management of Arterial Hypertension: The Task Force for the Management of Arterial Hypertension of the European Society of Hypertension (ESH) and of the European Society of Cardiology (ESC). *J Hypertens* Vol 25, No 6, (Jun 2007), pp 1105-1187, ISSN: 02636352

Moore, W. V.; Donaldson, D.L., Chonko, A.M.,Ideus,P. & Wiegmaon,T.B. (1992). Ambulatory blood pressure in type I diabetes mellitus: comparison to presence of incipient nephropathy in adolescents and young adults. *Diabetes* Vol 41, No 9, (Sep 1992), pp1035–1041, ISSN: 00121797

Lafferty,A.R.;Werther,G.A. &Clarke,C.F. (2000). Ambulatory blood pressure, microalbuminuria, and autonomic neuropathy in adolescents with type 1 diabetes. *Diabetes Care* Vol 23, No. 4, (Apr 1992), pp 533–538, ISSN: 01495992

Lurbe, E.; Redon,J.,Kesani,A.,Pascual,J.M.,Tacons,J.,Alvarez,J. & Batlle,D. (2002). Increase in nocturnal blood pressure and progression to microalbuminuria in type 1 diabetes. *N Eengl J Med* Vol 347, No. 11, (Sep 2002), pp797–805, ISSN: 00284793

Nielson, F. S. ; Gaede, P., Vedel, P., Pederson, O. & Parving, H. H. (1997). White coat hypertension in NIDDM patients with and without incipient and overt diabetic nephropathy. *Diabetes Care* Vol 20, No.5, (May 1997) , pp 859–863, ISSN: 01495992

O'Brien, E. ; Sheridan, J. & O'Mallely, K. (1988). Dipper and non-dippers (Letter). *The Lancet* Vol 2, No. 8687, (Aug 1988), pp397-405, ISSN: 01406736

Ogihara, T. ; Kikuchi, K., Matsuoka, H., Fujita, T., Higaki, J., Horiuchi, M., Imai, Y., Imaizumi, T., Ito, S., Iwao, H., Kario, K., Kawano, Y., Kim-Mitsuyama, S., Kimura, G., Matsubara, H., Matsuura, H., Naruse, M., Saito, I., Shimada, K., Shimamoto, K., Suzuki, H., Takishita, S., Tanahashi, N., Tsuchihashi, T., Uchiyama, M., Ueda, S., Ueshima, H., Umemura, S., Ishimitsu, T., Rakugi, H. & on behalf of The Japanese Society of Hypertension Committee. (2009). The Japanese Society of Hypertension Guidelines for the Management of Hypertension (JSH 2009). *Hypertens Res* Vol 32, No.1, (Jan 2009), pp 3-107, ISSN: 09169636

Ohkubo, Y.; Kishikawa, H., Araki, E., Miyata, T., Isami, S., Motoyoshi, S., Kojima, Y., Furuyoshi, N. & Shichiri, M. (1995). Intensive insulin therapy prevents the progression of diabetic microvascular complications in Japanese patients with non-insulin-dependent diabetes mellitus: a randomized prospective 6-year study. *Diabetes Res Clin Pract* Vol 28, No. 2, (Feb 1995), pp 103-117, ISSN: 01688227

Ohkubo,T.; Imai, Y.,Tsuji, I., Nagai, K., Watanabe, N., Minami, N., Kato, J., Kikuchi, N., Nishiyama, A., Aihara, A., Sekino, M., Sato, H. & Hisamichi, S. (1997). Relationship between nocturnal decline in blood pressure and mortality: the Ohasama Study. *Am J Hypertens* Vol 10, No 11, (Nov 1997), pp 1201-1207, ISSN: 08957061

Ohkubo,T.; Imai, Y., Tsuji, I., Nagai, K., Kato, J., Kikuchi, N., Nishiyama, A., Aihara, A., Sekino, M. Kikuya, M., Ito, S., Satoh, H. & Hisamichi, S. (1998). Home blood pressure measurement has a stronger predictive power for mortality than does screening blood pressure measurement: a population-based observationin Ohasama, Japan. *J Hypertens* Vol 16, No. 7, (Jul 1998), pp 971-975, ISSN: 02636352

Opsahl, J, A. ; Abraham, P. A., Halstension, C. E.& Keane, W. F. (1988). Correlation of offce and ambulatory blood pressure measurements with urinary albumin and N-acetyl-beta-D-glucos aminidase excretion in essential hypertension.*Am J Hypertens* Vol 1, No. Pt 3, (Jul 1988), pp 1175–1205, ISSN: 08957061

Otto, M.E. ; Svatikova, A., Barretto, R.B., Santos, S., Hoffmann, M., Khandheria, B. & Somers, V. (2004). Early morning attenuation of endothelial function in healthy humans. *Circulation* Vol 109, No. 21, (Jun 2004), pp 2507-2510, ISSN: 00097322

Pickering, T.G. (1992). Ambulatory blood pressure monitoring: An historical perspective. *Clin Cardiol* Vol 15 , No. Suppl I, (Oct 1992), pp II 3- II 5, ISSN: 07414218

Pickering, T. G. (1996). White coat hypertension. *Curr Opin Nephrol Hypertens* Vol 5, No. 2, (Mar 1996), pp 192–198, ISSN: 10624821

Pickering, T.G. ; Miller, N. H., Ogedegbe, G., Krakoff, L. R., Artinian, N.T. & Goff, D. (2008). American Heart Association; American Society of Hypertension; Preventive Cardiovascular Nurses Association. Call to action on use and reimbursement for home blood pressure monitoring: a joint scientific statement from the American Heart Association, American Society of Hypertension, and Preventive Cardiovascular Nurses Association. *Hypertension* Vol 52, No.1, (Jan 2008), pp 10-29, ISSN: 0194911X

Puig, J. G. ; Ruilope, L.M. & Ortega, R. (1995). Antihypertensive treatment effcacy in type II diabetes mellitus: dissociation between causal and 24 hour ambulatory blood pressure. *Hypertension* Vol 26, No.Pt 2 (Dec 1995), pp 1093–1099, ISSN: 0194911X

Sato, T.; Hayashi S. & Toyoshima, H. (1994). *Coronary* Vol 11, No. 3, (Mar 1994), pp189-195, ISSN: 09103031

Shimada, K. ; Kawamoto, A., Matsubayashi, K. & Ozawa, T. (1990). Silent cerebrovascular disease in the elderly: correlation with ambulatory pressure. *Hypertension* Vol 16, No. 6, (Dec 1990), pp 692–699, ISSN: 0194911X

Spallone, V. ; Bernardi, L., Ricordi, L., Solda, P., Maiello, M. R., Calciati, A., Gambardella, S., Fratino, P.& Menzinger, G. (1993). Relationship between the circadian rhythms of blood pressure and sympathovagal balance in diabetic autonomic neuropathy. *Diabetes* Vol 42, No.12, (Dec 1993), pp 1745–1752, ISSN: 00121797

Staessen, J.A. ; Beilin, L., Parati, G., Waeber, B. & White, W. (1999). Task force IV: Clinical use of ambulatory blood pressure monitoring. Participants of the 1999 Consensus Conference on Ambulatory Blood Pressure Monitoring. *Blood Press Monit* Vol 4, No. 6, (Dec 1999), pp 319-331, ISSN:.13595237

Stergiou, G.S. ; Vemmos, K.N., Pliarchopoulou, K.M., Synetos, A.G., Roussias, L.G. & Mountokalakis, T.D. (2002). Parallel morning and evening surge in stroke onset, blood pressure, and physical activity. *Stroke* Vol 33, No. 6, (Jun 2002), pp 1480-1486, ISSN: 00392499

Stergiou, G.S. ; Kalogeropoulos, P.G.& Baibas, N.M. (2007). Prognostic value of home blood pressure measurement. *Blood Press Monit* Vol 12, No. 6, (Jun 2007), pp 391-392, ISSN: 13595237.

Sturrock, N. D. , George, E., Pound, N., Sturrock, N. D., George, E., Pound, N., Stevenson, J., Peck G, M. & Sowter, H. (2000). Non-dipping circadian blood pressure and renal impairment are associated with increased mortality in diabetes mellitus. *Diabet Med* Vol 17, No.5, (May 2000), pp 360–364, ISSN: 07423071

The Diabetes Control and Complications Trial Research Group. (1993). The effect of intensive treatment of diabetes on the development and progression of long-term complications in insulin-dependent diabetes mellitus. *N Engl J Med* Vol 329, No.14, (Set 1993), pp 977-986, ISSN: 00284793.

The International Diabetes Federation. http://www.idf.org/

Torbjornsdotter,T.B.; Jaremko, G.A. & Berg,U.B. (2001). Ambulatory blood pressure and heart rate in relation to kidney structure and metabolic control in adolescents with type I diabetes. *Diabetologia* Vol 44, No. 7, (Jul 2001), pp 865–873,ISSN: 0012186X

White, W. B. (2001). Cardiovascular risk and therapeutic intervention for the early morning surge in blood pressure and heart rate. *Blood Press Monit* Vol 6, No. 2, (Apr 2001), pp 63–72, ISSN: 13595237

Part 5

Aspects of the Treatment of Type 2 Diabetes

20

Emerging Challenge of Type 2 Diabetes: Prospects of Medicinal Plants

Rokeya Begum[1], Mosihuzzaman M[2], Azad Khan AK[1,2],
Nilufar Nahar[3] and Ali Liaquat[1,2]
[1]Bangladesh Institute of Research and Rehabilitation in Diabetes, Endocrine and Metabolic Disorder (BIRDEM);
[2]Bangladesh Institute of health sciences (BIHS);
[3]Dept of Chemistry, University of Dhaka
Bangladesh

1. Introduction

Diabetes mellitus, a complex metabolic disorder is an increasing concern, worldwide in terms of health. The disorder affects more than 100 million people worldwide and by 2030 it is predicted to affect 366 million. Type 2 diabetes, the commonest form of the disease globally, has now reached epidemic proportions in most parts of the world; rapidly developing countries are the forefront of this epidemic (WHO, 2006). This explosive increase in the prevalence of diabetes and the consequences of its complications and associated disorders represent the greatest health care challenge the world facing today.

It has been stated that, in the 'epidemics' of diabetes the developing world will suffer the most, with a predicted 170% increase in cases that will mainly affect the 45-64 years age group; by contrast, the diabetic population in developed countries will increase by only 40%, and particularly among those aged >65 years (King et. al, 1998). Diabetes is an expensive disease, both to manage and because the associated morbidity and premature death impact so heavily on work and productivity; the massive increase among people of working age in the developing world will put a huge strain on the already overstretched health care resources in these countries.

Type 2 diabetes is a complex disease. It is characterized by the combination of several interacting mechanisms like disturbances in insulin secretion, insulin action, glucose production and glucose uptake. Defect in one or more of these mechanisms due to either environmental and/or genetic factors, can lead to a dysregulated glucose homeostasis depicted by hyperglycemia, the cardinal finding of diabetes. The long-term consequences of hyperglycemia are severe including eye, heart, kidney and nerve damage. There is evidence that hyperglycemia is the primary cause of microvascular complications i.e retinopathy, neuropathy and nephropathy (ADA, 2003). Hyperglycemia also plays a vital role in the premature and accelerated development of macrovascular complications such as cardiovascular and peripheral vascular diseases. Incidence of coronary heart disease is much more common than in non-diabetic people, and up to 75% of patients die from cardiovascular causes. Life expectancy for middle-aged patients is shortened by 5-10 years,

as compared with the general population (ADA, 2001; Katsilambros et al., 1991; Stamler et al., 1993).
Treatment of Type 2 diabetes is complicated by several factors inherent to the disease process. Diet and exercise play very important roles for diabetes management (Tuomilehto et al., 2001; Knowler et al., 2002). Oral hypoglycemic agents and/or insulin are being used to treat type 2 diabetes, all of which act through one of the pathways important in diabetes pathophysiology. However, even with these therapies diabetes remains an exceedingly difficult disease to control. No single agent has so far been unequivocally accepted to be 'the drug' in the management of diabetes. There is, therefore, an urgent need to develop new medications or strategies to counter the huge increase in cases expected in the future.

2. Prospects of medicinal plants in the management of type 2 diabetes

Plants have been used for the treatment of diabetes for centuries. However, their scientific evaluation has not constituted a substantial area of front-line pharmacological research in diabetes. A limited number of these plant species have been studied and validated for their hypoglycemic activities using diabetic animal models and in clinical studies using human subjects. Recently interest in plants has been increased particularly due to the relative lack of progress in the development of proper and save antidiabetic agents. Better understanding of the etipathogenesis of diabetic syndrome has paved the way for a more targeted use of plant materials in a modern pharmacological sense. In the perspective of the multiplicity of the pharmacological approaches against type 2 diabetes it is evident that plants provide interesting possibilities in these area because they contain thousands of compounds of which some may be useful as antidiabetic agents by themselves. Morever, the plant compound may form the basis for further manipulate to develop proper antidiabetic agents. Therefore, search for improved drug(s) against diabetes has remained a major goal among the biomedical researchers. Since approach of the scientists for synthesis of the conventional drugs has not yet brought expected results, many of them, in recent years, are focusing their attention on natural compounds to find, at least a lead if not a compound, of such antidiabetic agents.

2.1 Management of Type 2 diabetes with traditional systems of medicine

Traditional medicines are a fundamental aspect of basic health care needs globally. Over 64% of world's population (ca. 4.4 bn) use plants, in either crude or extract form as a primary health care source (Farnsworth, et al., 1985). A number of plants used as herbal drugs for diabetes therapy has been described in Ayurveda, Unani and other indigenous systems of medicine. Most of these traditional medicines are prepared from herbs, spices and plants, which do not form part of normal diet (Day & Bailey, 1986; Bailey & Day 1989). However, several common components of the diet are traditionally recommended for regular consumption, and some are additionally taken as infusions, decoctions or alcoholic extracts.
Plant materials have formed the basis for the treatment of diabetes in traditional medicines systems for thousands of years. These medicines for the treatment of diabetes mellitus are probably based mainly on treatment of its obvious symptoms. In ancient Ayurvedic medical texts such as the Charaka Samhita (Ca 2500 B.C.) and Sushruta Samhita (Ca 1000 B.C.)

glycosuria was recognized as a symptom of diabetes (Nagarajan et al., 1982) whereas etiopathogenesis, clinical features and complications of diabetes have been described in another Ayurvedic medical text as Rogovinischaya (12thCentury A.D). The Ayurvedic way of diabetes management include: advice for active life style, control over diet and different formulations for the treatment of diabetic complications. Sixty formulations of herbal and herbo-mineral origin under different categories like powder, paste, decoctions, etc. have been used in Ayurveda for diabetes management. Many mineral preparations (Bhasma) are also recommended.

2.2 Plant materials and diabetes: Present scenario

World's Ethnobotanical information about medicinal plants reports that almost 800 plants are used in the control of diabetes mellitus (Ajgaoonkar, 1979, Alarcon- Aguilara et al., 1998). More than 400 plants world-wide have been documented for the treatment of diabetes and majority await proper scientific and medical evaluation (Day & Bailey, 1986). Over the last three decades, several comprehensive reviews (Oliver-Bever et al., 1979; Bailey, 1989; Ivorra et al., 1989; Subbulakshmi and Naik, 2001; Grover et al., 2002; Srinivasa, 2007) and extensive surveys (Marles & Farnsworth, 1995; Simmonds & Howes, 2006) have been published highlighting the fact that higher plants are of use in the treatment of diabetes, providing discussion on botany, phytochemistry, pharmacology and, in some cases, toxicology of the botanical agents. The extensive survey by Marles and Farnsworth (1995) reported that more than 1200 species of plants (in 725 genera and 183 families) are in use, and Simmonds and Howes (2006) mentioned that 656 plant species (in 437 genera and 11 families) have been used to treat diabetes and/or been investigated for antidiabetic activity. Recently a database of antidiabetic plants have been published (Singh et al., 2007) which contains information of medicinal plants having antihyperglycemic or antidiabetic activity. It includes 238 plants species and 123 Indian industries, which are using them.

There are very large and widely distributed families of antidiabetic plants, so the large number of species reported to have been used traditionally or experimentally for the treatment of diabetes may be coincidental. The most frequently cited families are Fabaceae, Asteraceae, Lamiaceae, Liliaceae, Poaceae and Euphorbiaceae (Marles & Farnsworth, 1995). The phylogenetic distance between even this select group of families is a strong indication of the varied nature of the active constituents.

2.3 Reported hypoglycemic plant compounds

Cumulative research over the last few decades have already indicated some promising results that plants may serve as a source of antidiabetic compounds (Day, 1995). In many instances the chemical constituent(s) in the plant responsible for the biological activity has been isolated and identified, and some information is also available concerning the mechanism of action. A wide range of plant- derived principles belonging to different compounds have demonstrated bioactivity against hyperglycemia (Bailey & Day, 1989; Ivorra et al., 1988; Ivorra et al., 1989; Bressler et al., 1969; Day, 1990; Marles & Farnsworth, 1995). Hypoglycemic Natural Products of different classes are presented in Table 1.

The wide variety of chemical classes indicate that a variety of mechanisms must be involved in the lowering of the blood glucose levels. Some of these compounds may have therapeutic potential, while others may produce hypoglycemia, as side effects of their toxicity that is also another important concern.

Chemical class	Number active
Alkaloids	38
Carbohydrates	66
Coumarins	1
Cyanogenic glycosides	1
Favonoids	7
Glycopeptides	20
Inorganic salts	3
Iridoids	4
Lipids	6
Peptides and amines	15
Phenolics (simple)	4
Phenolpropanoid	1
Steroids	7
Stilbenes	1
Sulfur compounds	2
Terpenoids	17
Vitamins	2
Xanthenes	2

Table 1. Hypoglycemic Natural Products

2.4 Research work on antidiabetic plant materials done by the Dhaka group

Collaborative studies between the Biomedical Research group of BIRDEM and the Department of Chemistry, University of Dhaka, Bangladesh are conducted on antidiabetic plant materials following a standardized approach (Ali et al., 1993). Bangladesh and neighboring countries have a rich tradition in indigenous herbal medicine, therefore, in search of a new agent, considerable attention has been given on research with antidiabetic plant materials. Although screening of plant materials for hypoglycemic activities are abundantly found in literature, in-depth studies on the mechanism of action of these products are relatively lacking. In this design, a single plant material is tested in three models (nondiabetic, Type 1 and Type 2) of rats in three prandial states (fasting, simultaneously with oral glucose load, and 30 min before oral glucose load). Analysis of the results of these nine series of experiments helps not only to screen the hypoglycemic effects of the plant material, but also to postulate on their possible mechanism of action in target tissue(s). This, in turn, enables the investigator to conduct further in-depth studies on specific target tissue(s).

During the last twenty years 82 plants from Bangladesh, India, Pakistan, Nepal, Sri-lanka, China and Cameroon have been screened following the above approach. Some of them have shown promising results. From the results it was evident that screening of plant materials for hypoglycemic effects is not a straightforward task. The materials are active in particular model(s) and in particular prandial state(s) but may be inactive in other models and other prandial states. For example, bulb of a plant *Stephania hernandifolia,* used as antidiabetic remedy by the local people and traditional healers of Eastern Himalayan Belt, India, showed significant hyperglycemic activity in nondiabetic rats, no significant activity in Type 2 model rats and significant hypoglycemic activity in Type 1 model rats (Mosihuzzaman et al., 1994). The plants which showed promising results on screening, may be summarized into the groups as shown in Table 2 on the basis of their probable mechanism of action they have been classified into the following groups.

It is evident that, even the 9 series of experiments, as followed by us, are not fully exhaustive as other options are readily conceivable. Moreover, experiments have been done only after oral administration. A plant material may well be active when administered through other routes.

Possible mechanism of action	Name of the plant material
1. Enhance or promote insulin secretion	
Momordica charantia (Ali et al., 1993)	*Costus speciosus* (Mosihuzzaman et al., 1994)
Coccinia indica (Nahar et al., 2000 & Rokeya et al., 2003)	*Premna integrifolia Linn* (Alamgir et al., 2000)
Spirulina platensis (Rokeya et al., 1999)	*Bridelia ndellensis* (Soheng et al., 2005)
Nephrolepsis tuberosa (Mosihuzzaman et al., 1994)	*Swetenia mahagoni* (Rokeya et al., 2005)
Pterospermum semisagittum (Khan et al., 2003)	
2. Inhibition of glucose absorption	
Trigonella foenum graceum (Ali et al., 1995 & Hannan et al., 2003)	*Syzgium cumini* (Rokeya et al., 1999)
Plantago ovata (Rokeya et al., 1999)	*Musa paradisiaca* (Rokeya et al., 2000)
Allium cepa (Rokeya et al., 1999)	*Pterospermum acerifolium* (Mamun et al., 2001)
Allium sativum (Rokeya et al., 1999 & Retal et al., 1999 & 2000)	*Costus Specious* (Mosihuzzaman et al., 1994)
Allium Wallicha	*Spirulina platensis* (Rokeya et al., 1999)
Asparagus racemosus (Hannan et al., 2007)	*Crateava Religiosa*
Ocimum sanctum (Alamgir et al., 2000)	*Mangifera indica* (Bhowmik et al., 2009)
Ipomoea aquatica (Sokeng et al., 2007)	*Tamarindus indicus*
3. Action on the peripheral tissues	
Coccinia indica (Nahar et al., 2000)	*Nephrolepsis tuberosa* (Mosihuzzaman et al., 1994)
Costus speciosus (Mosihuzzaman et al., 1994)	
4. Mixed activity	
Hemidesmus indicus (Murshed et al., 2005)	*Gymnema sylvestre* (Rokeya et al., 2000)
Caesalpinia bonducella (Chakrabarti et al., 2003)	*Ocimum sanctum* (Alamgir et al., 2001)
Allium sativum (Rokeya et al., 2000)	
5. Prevention of islet damage or possibility of β-cell regeneration	
Gymnema sylvestre (Rokeya et al., 1999)	*Stephania hernandifolia* (Mosihuzzaman et al., 1994)
6. Improving insulin sensitivity	
Gymnema sylvestre (Ali et al., 2005)	

Table 2. Anidiabetic plant materials reported by the Dhaka Group

2.4.1 Studies on the antidiabetic effect and mechanism of action of *Nyctanthes Arbortristis Linn.*

This is one example of screening methodology followed by mechanistic study. *Nyctanthes arbortristis* Linn (Seoli) is a shrub (a C_3 plant; Rao & Kodandaramaiah, 1982) cultivated as a garden plant throughout Bangladesh and in the Sub-Himalayan region. In Ayurvedic and Unani medicine the leaves of this plant is used extensively for the treatment of various ailments (Singh et al., 1995; Chopra et al., 1956; Srivastava et al., 1990). In Ayurvedic system of medicine the seeds are being used for throat and eye diseases, skin infections, intestinal worm infection, leprosy, etc (RB Singh & Jindal, 1985). To the best of our knowledge there is no published report on the antidiabetic properties of this plant. As a routine screening programme this plant has been undertaken for studying the effect on serum glucose level of nondiabetic and diabetic rat models. Ripe seeds and fresh leaves of *N arbortristis* were collected from Dhaka, Bangladesh. The plant was identified at Bangladesh National Herbarium and a voucher specimen (DACB-35121) was deposited.

2.4.1.1 Materials & methods

Aquous extract of seed and 2% ethanol extract of leaf were used for the study at a dose of 1.25 g/kg bw. Male Long-Evans rats bred at BIRDEM Animal House, weighing between 180-200 gm were used to carry out the experiment. All the experiments were carried out following the International Guidelines for handling of laboratory Animals (Derrell, 1966). Type 1 and Type 2 diabetes were produced with *intraperitoneal* injection of Streptozotocin using conventional methods and following the procedure standardized in BIRDEM. Acute experiments were done in normal, Type 1 and Type 2 diabetic model rats at different prandial states. Blood samples were collected by cutting the tail tip under mild ether anesthesia. The glucose levels in the serum samples in duplicate were estimated by GOD-PAP method (Boehringer Mannheim GMBH). Statistical analyses were performed by using one- way ANOVA.

2.4.1.2 Results

Screening result for hypoglycemic activity of aqueous extract of seed and 2% ethanol extract of leaf in nondiabetic rats showed no effect in the fasting or postprandial state when fed simultaneously with glucose load. Ethanol extract of *arbortristis* seed significantly ($p<0.05$) opposed the rise of serum glucose at 60min when the extract was fed 30 minutes before glucose load in nondiabetic rats (data not shown).

Aquous seed and leaf extract did not show any hypoglycemic activity in Type 1 rats in fasting and 30 minutes before the glucose load state (Table 3). When administered simultaneously with glucose, leaf extract showed significant anti-hyperglycemic effect at 75min ($p<0.05$).

Nyctanthes arbortristis seed extract significantly lowered fasting blood glucose levels in Type 2 diabetic rats at 120min ($p<0.05$) and also showed significant anti-hyperglycemic effect at 75min ($p<0.01$) when fed simultaneously with glucose (Table 4).

Aquous extract of seed was effective in lowering serum glucose level of nondiabetic rats only in postprandial states when fed 30 min before glucose load indicating more of a systemic action. These also include the possibility of inhibition of gastric emptying (Lembcke, 1987) and also the involvement of gut hormones (Creutzfeld, 1979). Seed extract also showed significant effect in Type 2 rats at the fasting and in postprandial states when fed simultaneously with glucose load. This extract might contain some hypoglycemic

Group	Serum glucose level mmol/l		
Fasting	**0 min**	**60 min**	**120 min**
Water control (n = 6)	22.10 ± 2.91	22.02 ± 2.53	20.29 ± 1.33
Insulin control (n = 6)	20.33 ± 0.99	3.60 ± .57***	2.35 ± 0.12***
N arbortristis ripe seed (n = 7)	22.72 ± 2.53	22.37 ± 2.74	21.11 ± 2.49
N arbortristis leaf (n = 7)	21.87 ± 2.20	20.92 ± 2.26	22.29 ± 3.02
Simultaneously with glucose load	**0 min**	**30 min**	**75 min**
Water control (n = 6)	22.25 ± 1.86	34.19 ± 1.31	32.03 ± 0.75
Insulin control (n = 6)	22.52 ± 0.47	22.10 ± 0.66***	11.40 ± 1.15***
N arbortristis ripe seed (n = 10)	24.45 ± 1.20	32.50 ± 1.16	27.11 ± 2.30
N arbortristis leaf (n = 8)	22.33 ± 0.82	30.56 ± 1.08	25.91 ± 2.79*
30 min before glucose load	**0 min**	**60 min**	**105 min**
Water control (n = 5)	22.16± 4.64	30.35±3.34	26.65±2.82
Insulin control (n = 6)	21.38±3.18	9.47± 4.12***	5.21±1.97 ***
N. arbortristis ripe seed (n = 7)	19.63 ± 3.25	27.68 ± 2.98	24.35 ± 2.77
N arbortristis leaf (n = 6)	19.47±6.07	27.32±3.82	27.21± 4.03

Values are mean ± SE; n = number of rats; *p<0.05, **p<0.01, ***p<0.001 compared to control rat.

Table 3. Effect of aqueous extract of *Nyctanthes arbortristis* seeds and 2% ethanol extract of leaves on serum glucose levels of Type 1 diabetic models rats in different prandial states.

Group	Serum glucose level mmol/l		
Fasting	**0 min**	**60 min**	**120 min**
Water control (n = 6)	8.48 ± 0.47	8.36 ± 0.33	7.85 ± 0.22
Glibenclamide control (n = 6)	8.36 ± 0.25	7.25 ± 0.32*	6.750 ± 0.24 **
N arbortristis seed (n = 7)	7.21 ± 0.18	8.83 ± 0.10	6.99 ± 0.14*
N arbortristis leaf (n = 7)	6.90 ± 0.24	7.77 ± 0.08	7.49 ± 0.13
Simultaneously with glucose load	**0 min**	**30 min**	**75 min**
Water control (n = 6)	8.08 ± 0.99	17.06± 0.49	15.89± 0.54
Glibenclamide control (n=6)	8.28 ± 0.78	19.19± 1.42	16.97± 1.16
N arbortristis seed (n = 8)	8.32 ± 0.92	15.43 ± 1.09	9.01 ± 0.05**
N arbortristis leaf (n = 7)	7.12±0.85	15.42± 1.39	16.22 ± 0.96
30 min before glucose load	**0 min**	**60 min**	**105 min**
Water control (n = 6)	9.21 ± 0.50	18.57 ± 1.61	17.63 ± 0.95
Glibenclamide control (n = 7)	8.99 ± 0.47	16.78 ± 1.94	15.03± 1.68
N arbortristis seed (n = 5)	9.43 ± 0.28	19.50 ± 1.79	19.01± 1.74
N arbortristis leaf(n = 6)	9.76 ± 0.81	17.64± 1.74	19.36± 1.62

Values are mean ± SE; n = number of rats; *p<0.05, **p<0.01, ***p<0.001 compared to control rat.

Table 4. Effect of aqueous extract of *Nyctanthes arbortristis* seeds and 2% ethanol extract of leaves on fasting serum glucose levels of Type 2 diabetic models rats in different prandial states.

principles, which act probably by stimulation of insulin secretion from β-cells of islets or acting either at the gut level or at the peripheral tissues. Analysis of the nature of the action of the 2% ethanol extract of leaf in Type 1 model (no effect in fasting state and 30min before glucose load, but significant effect when fed simultaneously with glucose load) indicates its probable effect at the glycogen synthesis level, since glycogenesis (enhanced by feeding) is the predominant mechanism at fed state in contrast to the gluconeogenesis which is characteristically activated at fasting state in diabetic animals (Felig & Bergman, 1990).
The results of the oral acute hypoglycemic effects on normal and Type 2 diabetic rats at fasting and postprandial conditions suggested that blood glucose lowering effect of the seed extract of *N arbortristis* is probably due to enhanced insulin-releasing activity.

2.4.1.3 Studies on the mechanism of insulin secretion

The effect of the ethanol (PE080) and chloroform (PE081) extracts of seed were also evaluated on insulin secretion together with exploration of their mechanism of action together with exploration of their mechanism of action in isolated perfused rat pancreas and BRIN-BD11 insulin secreting cell (Rokeya et al., 2006).
Experimental procedure: To study the effects of the extracts on insulin secretion Long-Evans rats were anesthetized with sodium pentobarbital solution and the pancreas was isolated and perfused through mesenteric and celiac vessels of whole pancreas at 37^{0}C according to the Method of Giroix et al. (1983). Both the extracts were dissolved at a dose of 0.1mg/ml in Krebs-Ringer bicarbonate buffer containing 2.8 mM or 11.1 mM D glucose. The perfusate was continuously gassed with a mixture of O2:CO (95:50). After 20 min equilibration period the composition of the perfusate was changed every ten min with plant extracts and other reagents. The effluent was collected at 1 minute interval from the portal vein. Effluent samples were frozen and stored at -20^{0}C for insulin assay.
Clonal BRIN-BD11 cells (McClenaghan et al., 1996) were also used to evaluate the action of ethanol and chloroform extracts on insulin secretion. Cell viability was evaluated by modified neutral assay (this part of wrk was done in the Diabetes Research Group, University of Ulster, UK).
For perfusion studies and studies with BRIN-BD11 cells insulin was measured by ELISA and by radioimmunoassay respectively. Results are presented as mean±SD for a given number of observations(n). Data from each set of observations were compared using unpaired Student's t-test and Mann-Whitney U test where appropriate (SPSS for Windows). One-way ANOVA was performed and comparisons to the control group was made using Dunnet's test to preserve overall error rate of 5%. Differences were considered significant if $p<0.05$.

Results

Fig. 1 shows that PE080 stimulated insulin secretion in isolated perfused rat pancreas which caused a significant increase in insulin release during 10 minute perfusion with almost a 6-fold increase above basal level (Insulin, M±SD ng/ml; 0.204±0.02 basal *vs* 1.22±0.12 PE080, Peak value; $p<0.001$). PE081 did not evoke a significant increase on insulin secretion.
It is establised that studies using insulinotropic antagonists can define the possible mechanism of action in enhancing insulin secretion and confirm absence of insulin leakage by more lysis of cells. Therefore, in our experiment one such inhibitor utilized was diazoxide, an ATP-sensitive K+ chanel opener. Fig 2 shows that diazoxide (300µM) inhibited the insulin enhancing effects of PE080 in the perfused panceaes (Insulin M±SD, ng/ml;

1.22±0.12 PE080 *vs* 0.42±0.05 PE080 + diazoxide; p<0.01) indicating the involvement of the extract in the stimulus-secretion coupling pathway at the closure of K+-ATP channels (Henquin, 1992).

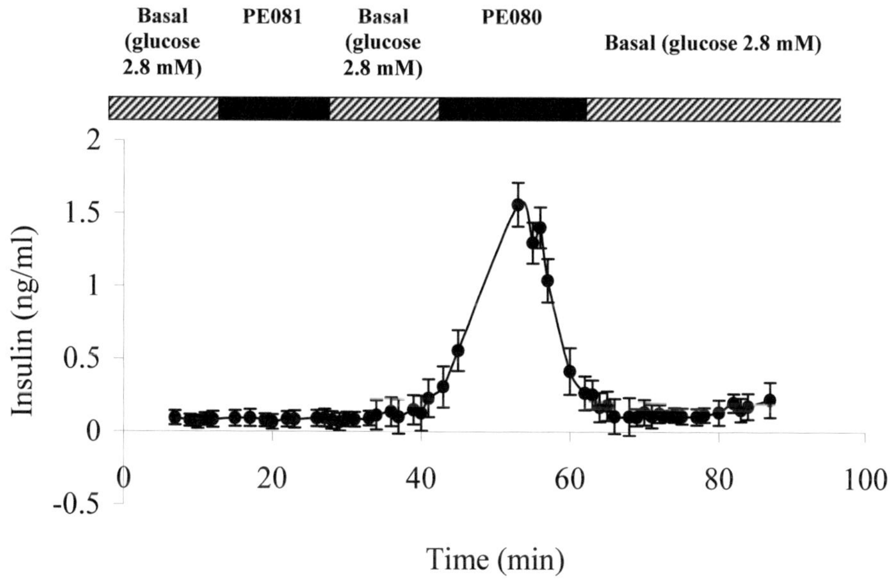

Fig. 1. Effects of PE081 and PE080 on insulin secretion from perfused rat pancreas in basal state. Insulin released in presence of PE080

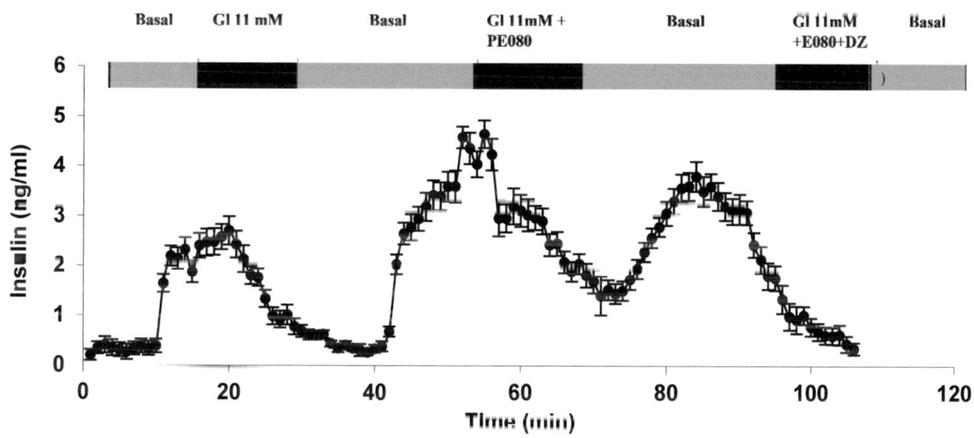

Fig. 2. Insulin release in glucose stimulated state and in presence of diazoxide.

The insulinotropic effects and cellular detrimental effects of PE080 and PE081 with two concentrations of each (50 gμ/ml and 100 μg/ml) were evaluated in BRIN-BD11 cell line. It was found that, in this cell line (Table 5) PE080 stimulated insulin release in both the concentrations (50 and 100 μg/ml) compared to control (5.6 mM glucose). The Table 5 shows that the higher concentration did not affect cell viability. PE081 in 100μg/ml concentration stimulated insulin release which was also not associated with a significant reduction in cell viability.

These findings revealed that PE080 and PE081 exert stimulatory effects on insulin secretion from the β-cells mediated through a physiological insulinotropic pathway. *In vivo* studies also indicate that aquous extract of *Nyctanthes arbortristis* seeds decreased serum glucose in Type 2 diabetic model rats. The identification of active principle(s) from seeds of *Nyctanthes arbortristis* PE080 and PE081 may provide interesting possibilities against diabetes.

Group	**Cell viability (%)**	**Insulin (ng/ml)**
5.6 mM glucose	98.58±5.19	1.45±0.087
PE081 (50 μg/ml)	96.70±4.81	1.46±0.23
PE081 (100 μg/ml	92.02±3.87**	2.29±0.41***
PE080 (50 μg/ml)	96.39±4.07	2.26±0.25***
PE080 (100 μg/ml)	93.30±5.15	3.36±0.60***
t/p value		
5.6 mM gl vs PE081 (50 μg/ml)	0.75/0.465	0.032/0.975
5.6 mM gl vs PE081 (100 μg/ml)	2.86/0.012	7.044/0.001
5.6 mM gl vs PE080 (50 μg/ml)	0.94/0.364	10.39/0.001
5.6 mM gl vs PE080 (100 μg/ml)	2.041/0.061	10.87/0.001

Table 5. Effects of different concentrations of PE081 and PE080 of on BRIN-BD11 cell viability and insulin secretion.

2.4.2 Studies on the retardation of glucose absorption in the gut

The retardation of carbohydrate digestion and absorption in the gut is now a potential therapeutic approach for the management of diabetes mellitus. The intestinal disaccharidase enzymes (α-glucosidase) are involved in the digestion and absorption of carbohydrate and inhibition of these enzymes by the agents may slow this process and thus leads to a slower and less pronounced rise in postprandial blood glucose levels. It has been confirmed that some plant fractions i.e hot water extract extract of *T foenumgraecum* *P. ovata* and ethanol extracts of *O sanctum, A racemosus, M indica (Bhowmik 2009), T indica* (not published) significantly inhibited the absorption of glucose during perfusion of gut with glucose solution, a mechanism postulated before through *in vivo* experiments. *T foenumgraecum* (Hannan, et.al., 2003 & 2007a) , *P. ovata* (Hannan, et.al., 2006a) *O sanctum* (Hannan, et.al., 2006b) and *A racemosus*, (Hannan, et.al., 2007b) increased unabsorbed sucrose content throughout gut when administered with sucrose and also inhibitited intestinal disaccharidase enzyme activity, which reveals that the retardation of carbohydrate absorption is related to the inhibition of gut enzyme activity. However, they did not increase GI tract motility (by Barium meal studies) which suggests that inhibition of glucose absorption is not related to enhance peristaltic movement of gut.

2.4.3 Discussion

It is utmost important to compile information regarding the toxicity of all medicinal plants as plant extracts may exert different types of toxicities like hepatic, renal, cardiac, hematological and other toxicities through their inherent properties. Therefore, antidiabetic plants which show hypo-/antihyperglycemic properties in animal models or in humans should be tested for their possible toxicities. If found to have some degree of toxicity, the risks can be weighed against the benefits and decisions can be made regarding their continued availability. The plant materials which have been mentioned here, a few of them were studied with a longer durationin in streptozotocin induced diabetic model rats (Chakrabarti et al 2005; Bandara et al 2010) and also inType 2 diabetic subjects (Bandara et al 2019). After chronic oral feeding their serum alanine amino transferase (ALT) and serum creatinine levels have been determined as a marker of liver and kidney toxicities. Chronic consumption of these plant materials did not indicate any adverse effect on liver and kidney functions of Type 2 rats or Type 2 patients as serum ALT and creatinine levels remained unchanged throughout study period. It should be kept in mind that the inherent properties of the plants are not the sole source of plant related hepatic, renal, cardiac, hematological or other disorders. There may be some other factors like i) plant material and drug interactions, ii)mistakes in dosage and identification and iii) presence of adulterants etc. All these issues of concern should be taken into account to eliminate toxicity and ensure the safety of not only the antidiabetic but all medicinal plant products.

2.4.4 Practical guidelines regarding usefulness

To study the traditionally used plant materials is not only a scientific but also a social responsibility. Whether liked or not a large number of people, particularly in the developing countries, are still dependent on plants. It is important to screen their efficacy and it may also be helpful if the best timing, dose and the method of administration of these materials can be suggested. It is also important to warn people against injudicious dependence on plants for the management of diabetes. Although, the modern treatment for diabetes has not reached perfection, it has become possible to control the disorder and lead a normal and productive life. So, a clinician must be aware that the well-being of the patient is not scarified merely due to a psychological preference to use plant materials. If diabetes of a patient is not under control after using plant materials, the clinician should not hesitate to use the modern drugs against diabetes.

3. Conclusions

Prevalence of diabetes mellitus is increasing and it causes substantial morbidity and mortality through macro- and microvascular complication, especially in developing countries where adequate treatment is often unavailable. Since almost 90% of the people in rural areas of developing countries still rely on traditional medicines for their primary health care and scientific investigations of traditional medicines have led to the discovery of 122 compounds obtained from only 94 species of plants which are used as drugs worldwide (Fabricant & Farnsworth, 2001) therefore, the development of new antidiabetic drug(s) from traditionally used plants seems to be probable. From the existing evidence it appears that plants have got a vast potential to provide source materials for antidiabetic agents. However, this potential has remained largely unexplored. A rationally designed interdisciplinary research program i.e. involvement of scientists from diverse disciplines of biomedical sciences, may also lead to the development of scientifically tested indigenous, remedies for diabetes through sustainable and cost-effective use of medicinal plant resources.

4. Acknowledgments

We gratefully acknowledge the active advice and support of the Department of Medical Cell Biology, Uppsala Univesity, Sweden (group led by Prof Bo Hellman and Prof Erik Gylfe) and the Dept of Chemistry, Mahidol University, Bangkok (group led by Prof Vichai Reutrakul) during these studies. We also express our sincere thanks to International Program in the Chemical Sciences (IPICS), Uppsala University, Sweden, International Foundation for Sciences (IFS), Stockholm, Sweden, Asian Netwirk of research on antidiabetic plant materials (ANRAP) Dhaka, Bangladesh, Diabetic Association of Bangladesh, Ministry of Science and Information and Communication Technology, Bangladesh, University Grant Commission and Dhaka University, Bangladesh for their financial and logistic support in all our studies.

5. References

Ajgaonkar, S.S. (1979). Herbal drugs in the treatment of diabetes. *Int Diabetes Fed Bull,* Vol. 24, pp. 10-17.

Alamgir, M.; Rokeya, B.; Chowdhury, N.S. and Choudhury, M.S.K (2001). Antihyperglycemic effect of aqueous extract of Ocimum sanctum Linn (Labiateae) in type 2 diabetic model rats. *Diab Res,* Vol.36, pp. 019-027

Alamgir, M.; Rokeya, B.; Hannan, J.M.A. & Choudhuri, M.S.K. (2001). The effect of *Premna integrifolia* Linn. (Verbenaceae) on blood glucose in streptozotocin induced type 1 and type 2 diabetc rats. *Pharmazie,* Vol. 56, pp. 903-904.

Alarcon-Aguilara, F.J.; Roman-Ramos, R.; Perez-Gutierrez, S.; Aguliar-Contreras, A.; Contreras-Weber, C.C. & Flores-Saenz, J.L. (1998). Study of the hypoglycemic effect of plants used as antidiabetics, *F Ethnopharmacol ,* Vol. 61. pp.101-110.

Ali, L.; Azad Khan, A.K.; Hassan, Z.; Mosihuzzaman, M.; Nahar, N.; Nasreen, T.; Nur-e-Alam, M.; Parveen, M.; Rokeya, B. (1995). Characterization of the hypoglycemic effects of Trigonella foenum graecum seed extracts on normal and diabetic model rats. *Planta Medica,* Vol. 61, pp. 358-360.

Ali, L.; Chowdhury, N.; Rokeya, B.; Chaudhury, H.S.; Hannan, J.M.A.; Khaleque, J.; Akhter, M.; Hassan, Q.; Murshed, S.; Nahar, N.; Azad Khan, A.K.; Mosihuzzaman, M. (2005). Antidiabetic effects of plant extract PE052 on type 1 diabetic model rats. *Diabetologia;Suppl 1* pp. *763:* A

American Diabetes Association. (2003). Standards of medical care for patients with diabetes mellitus. *Diabetes care,* Vol. 26, No. 1, pp. S33-S50.

American Diabetes Association. Mortality. (2001). In: American Diabetes Association, eds. Diabetes Vital Statistics. Alexandria, VA: American Diabetes Association; pp. 77-85.

Bandara, T.; Rokeya, B.; Khan, S.; Ali, L.; Ekanayake, S.; Balasubramanium, K. (2009). Effects of Gymnema lactiferum leaves on, glycemic and lipidemic status in type 2 diabetes subjects. *Bangladesh J Pharmacol,* Vol. 4, pp.92-98.

Bandara, T.; Rokeya, B.; Ekanayake, S.; Ali, L.; Raddy, E.; Balasubramanium, K. (2010). Effects of Gymnema lactiferum leaf on serum glucose and cholesterol levels of Streptozotocin induced diabetic rats. *Int J Boil Chem Sci,* Vol. 9, pp.815-819.

Bailey, C.J. & Day, C. (1989). Traditional plant medicines as treatments for diabetes. *Diabetes Care,* Vol.12, pp.553-64.

Bhowmik, A., Liakot, A. K.; Akhter, M. & Rokeya, B. (2009). Study on Antidiabetes effects of mango (*Mangifera indica*) stem-barks and leaves on Nondiabetic and Diabetic model rats. *Bangladesh J Pharmacol (BDPS)*, Vol. 4, No. 2, pp. 110-114.

Bressler, R.; Correndor, C. & Brendel, K. (1969). Hypoglycin and hypoglycin-like compounds. *Pharmacol Revs,* Vol. 21, pp.105-30.

Chakrabarti, S.; Biswas, T.K.; Rokeya, B.; Ali, L.; Mosihuzzaman, M.; Nahar, N.; Azad Khan, A.K. & Mukherjee, B.P. (2003) Advanced studies on the hypoglycemic effect of *Caesalpinia bonducella* F. in type I and II diabetes in Long Evans rats. *J of Ethnopharmacology,* Vol. 84, pp. 41-46.

Chakrabarti S., Biswas T. K., Seal T., Rokeya B., Ali L., Azad Khan AK, Nahar N. , Mosihuzzaman M. and Mukherjee B.: Antidiabetic activity of Caesalpinia bonducella F. in chronic type 2 diabetic model in Long Evans rats and evaluation of insulin secretagogue property of its fractions on isolated islets. *J Ethnopharmacology* 2005, *97:* p-117-122.

Chopra, R.N.; Nayar, S.L. & Chopra, I.C. (1956). Glossary of Indian Medicinal Plants. *CSIR,* New Delhi, pp. 177.

Creutzfeld, W. (1979). The incretion concept today. *Diabetologia,* Vol.16, pp.75-85.

Day, C. (1995). Hypoglycemic plant compounds Pract. *Diabetes,* Vol. 12, pp. 245-96.

Day, C.; & Bailey, C.J. (1986). Hypoglycemic agents from traditional plant treatments for diabetes. *Int Indus Biotechnol,* Vol. 8, pp. 5-8.

Derrell, C. (1996). Guide for the care and use of laboratory animals. Istitute of Laboratory Animal Resources. *National Academy Press,* Washington DC, USA.

Fabricant, D.S. & Farnsworth, N. (2001). R.The Value of Plants Used in Traditional Medicine for Drug DiscoveryEnviron *Health* Perspect 109(suppl 1):69 - 75.

Famsworth, N. R.; Akerele, O.; Bingel, A. S.; Soejarto, D. D. & Guo, Z.G.(1985). Medicinal plants in therapy. *Bull. WHO,* Vol. 63, pp. 965-981.

Felig, P. & Bergman, M. (1990). In Diabetes Mellitus: Theory and Practice. 2nd Edition (ed. H.Rifkin and D. Jr. Portc), pp. 51-60.

Giroix, M.H.; Portha, B.; Kergoat, M.; Bailbe, D. & Picon, L. (1983). Glucose insensitivity and amino-acid hypersensitivity of insulin release in rats with non-insulin-dependent diabetes: a study with the perfused pancreas. *Diabetes.* Vol. 32, pp. 445-51.

Grover,J.K.; Yadav, S.; & Vats, V. (2002). Medicinal plants of India with anti-diabetic potential. *J Ethnopharmacol,* Vol. 81, pp. 81-100.

Hannan, J.M.A.; Ali, L.; Rokeya, B.; Khaleque, J.; Akhter, M.; Flatt, P.R. & Abdel-Wahab, Y.H (2007a). Soluble dietary fibre fraction of Trigonella foenum graecum (fenugreek) seed improves glucose homeostasis in animal models of type 1 and type 2 diabetes by delaying carbohydrate digestion and absorption, and enhancing insulin action. *Br J Nutr,* Vol. 97, No. 3, pp. 514-21

Hannan, J.M.A.; Marenah, L.; Ali, L.; Rokeya, B.; Flatt PR & Wahab YHA (*2007b*): Insulin secretory actions of extracts of *Asparagus racemosus* root in perfused pancreas, isolated islets and clonal pancreatic beta-cells. *J Endocrinology; 192:* 159-68.

Hannan, J.M.A.; Marenah, L.; Ali, L.; Rokeya, B.; Flatt, P.R. & Wahab, Y.H.A (2006). *Ocimum sanctum* leaf extracts stimulated insulin secretion from perfused pancreas, isolated islets and clonal pancreatic beta-cells. *J Endocrinology,* 189 (No 1): 127-136.

Hannan, J.M.A.; Rokeya, B.; Faruque, O.; Nahar, N.; Mosihuzzaman, M. & Ali, L. (2003). Effect of Soluble Dietary Fibre fraction of *Trigonella foenum-graecum* on glycemic, insulinemic, lipidemic and platelet aggregation status of Type 2 diabetic model rats. *J Ethnopharmacology*, Vol. 88, pp. 73-77.

Henquin, J.C.; Debuyser, A.; Drews, G. & Plant, T.D. (1992). Regulation of K^+ permeability and membrane potential in insulin-secretory cells. In: Flatt PP (ed) Nutrient regulation of insulin secretion. Porland, London, pp. 173-192.

Ivorra, M.D., D, Ocon, M.P.; Paya, M. & Villar, A. (1988). Anti hyperglycemic and insulin - releasing effects of β-sitosterol-3-b-Dglucoside and its aglycon, β-sitosterol. *Arch Int Pharmaodyn Therap*, Vol. 296, pp. 224-31.

Ivorra, M.D.; Paya, M.; Villar, A. (1989). A review of natural products and plants as potential antidiabetic drugs , *J Ethnopharmacol*, Vol. 27, pp. 243-75.

Katsilambros, N.; Hatzakis, A.; Perdicaris, G.; Pefanis, A. & Touloumi, G. (1991). Total and cause-specific mortality in a population based cohort in Greece. *Diabetes Metab,* Vol. 17, pp. 410-14.

Khan, S.H.; Mosihuzzaman, M.; Nahar, N.; Rashid, M.A.; Rokeya, B.; Ali, L. & Azad Khan, A.K. (2003). Three Megastigmane Glycosides from the leaves of *Perospermum semisagittatum*. *Pharmaceutical Biology,* Vol. 41, pp. 512-515.

King, H.; Aubert, R.E. & Herman, W.H. (1998). Global burden of diabetes, 1995-2025: prevalence, numerical estimates, and projections. *Diabetes Care*, Vol. 21, pp. 1414-31.

King, *H.*; Aubert, R.E. & Herman, W.H. *(*1998). Global burden of diabetes, 1995-2025: prevalence, numerical estimates and projections. *Diabetes Care,* Vol. 21, pp. 1414-31.

Knowler, W.C.; Barrett-Connor, E. Fowler, S.E.; Hamman, R.F.; Lachin, J.M.; Walker, E.A. & Nathan, D.M. (2002). Reduction in the incidence of type 2 diabetes with lifestyle intervention or metformin. *N. Engl. J. Med,* Vol. 346, pp. 393–403. [PMC free article] [PubMed]

Lembcke, B. (1987). Control of absorption: delaying absorption as a therapeutic principle. In: Structure and Function of the Small Intestine (edited by W. F. cospary). *Excerpta Medica, Amsterdam,* pp. 263-280.

Mamun, M.I.R.; Rokeya, B.; Chowdhury, N.S.; Muniruzzaman, M.; Nahar, N.; Ahmed, M.U.; Mosihuzzaman, M.; Ali, L., Azad Khan, A.K. & Khan, S.H. (2001). Anti-hyperglycemic effect of *Pterospermum acerifolium* Willd. And *Pterospermum semisagittatum* Ham. *Diab Res*, Vol. 35, pp.163-170.

Marles, R.J. & Farnsworth, N.R. (1995). Antidiabetic plants and their active constituents. *Phytomedicine,* Vol. 2, No. 2, pp. 137-189.

McClenaghan, N.H.; Barnett, C.R.; Ah-Sing, E.; Abdel-Wahab, Y.H.A.; O'Harte, F.P.M.; Yoon, T.W.; Swanston-Flatt, S.K. & Flatt, P.R. (1996). Characterization of a novel glucose responsive insulin-secreting cell line, BRIN-BD11, produced by electrofusion, *Diabetes,* Vol. 45, pp. 1132-140.

Mosihuzzaman, M.; Nahar, N.; Ali, L.; Rokeya, B.; Azad Khan, A.K.; Nur-e-Alam, M.; & Nandi, R.P. (1994). Hypoglycimic effects of three plants from Eastern Himalayan belt. *Diab Res* , Vol. 26, pp. 127-138.

Murshed, S.; Rokeya, B.; Nahar, N.; Azad Khan, A.K.; Mosihuzzaman, M.; Banerjee, A.; Maiti, S.; & Ali, L. (2005). Hypoglycemic and Hypolipidemic Effect of *Hemidesmus indicus* Root on Diabetic Model Rats. *Diab Res*, Vol. 39, pp. 15-23.

Nagarajan, S.; Jain, H.C.& Aulakh, G.S. (1982). Indigenous plants used in the control of diabetes. In: Cultivation and Utilization of Medicinal Plants (CK Atal, BM Kapur eds), pp. 584-604. *Regional Research Laboratory, Council of Scientific and Industrial Research,* Jammu-tawi, India.

Nahar, N.; Rokeya, B.; Ali, L.; Hassan, Z.; Nur-e-Alam, M.; Chowdhury, N.S.; Azad Khan, A.K. & Mosihuzzaman, M. (2000). Effects of three medicinal plants on blood glucose levels of nondiabetic and diabetic model rats. *Diab Res,* Vol. 35, pp. 41-49.

Nahar, N.; Rokeya, B.; Ali, L.; Hassan, Z.; Nur-E-Alam, M.; Chowdhury, N.S.; Azad Khan, A.K. & Mosihuzzamaan, M. (2000). Effects of three medicinal plants on blood glucose levels of nondiabetic and diabetic model rats. *Diabetes Research,* Vol. 35, pp.041-049.

Rao, P.G. & Kodandaramaiah, J. (1982). Association of Chlorophyll content, phyllotaxy, photosynthesis and B group vitamins in some C_3 and C_4 plants. *Proc. Indian Acad. Sci. (Plant Sci.),* Vol. 91, No 6, pp. 495-500.

Rokeya, B.; Hannan, J.M.A., Rahman, M.H.; Nurun Nabi, A.H.M.; Ali, L.; Mosihuzzaman, M. & Nahar, N. (2000). Chronic effect of cold aqueous extract of *Allium sativum* on glycemic and lipidemic status and platelet aggregation in Type 2 diabetic model rats. *Diab Res Clin Pract,* Vol. 50, No. 1, pp. S393.

Rokeya, B.; Mosihuzzaman, M.; Nahar, N.; Azad Khan, A.K.& Ali, L. (2005). Hypoglycemic effect of PE071 seeds in type 2 diabetic Long-Evens rats. *Diabetologia,* Suppl 1 Vol. 761, pp. A276

Rokeya, B.; Nahar, N.; Ali, L.; Hassan, Z.; Nur-e-Alam, M.; Chowdhury, N.S.; Azad Khan, A.K. & Mosihuzzaman, M. (1999). Effects of five medicinal plants on blood glucose levels in nondiabetic and diabetic model rats. *Diab Res,* Vol. 34, pp. 219-228.

Rokeya, B.; Rahman, M.M.; Hannan, J.M.A.; Akter, M.; Lamin, M.; Azad khan, A.K. (2006). Insulin secretory effect of plant extracts PE080 and PE081 in perfused pancreas and BRIN-BD cells. *Diabetologia,* Vol. 49, suppl 1, pp. 0858.

Simmond, M.S.J & Howes, M.J.R. (2006). Edited by A Soumayanath A. Traditional Medicine for modern times: Antidiabetic plants, Taylor & Francis group, UK.

Singh, K.L.; Rao, J.; Srivastava, V. & Tandon, J.S.; Arborside, D. (1995). A Minor Iridoid Glucoside From *Nyctanthes arbor-tristis. Journal of Natural Products,* Vol. 58, No. 10, pp.1562-1564.

Singh, R.B. & Jindal, V.K. (1985). Polysaccharide from *Nyctanthes arbor-tristis Linn.* Seeds-isolation, Purification and Preliminary Analysis of polysaccharide. *Journal of the Indian Chemical Society* August, Vol. 62, No. 7, pp. 627-628.

Singh, S.; Gupta, S.K.; Sabir, G.; Gupta, M.K. & Seth, P.K. (2009). A database for anti-diabetic plants with clinical/ experimental trials. *Bioinformation.* Vol 4, No. 6, pp. 263 268 © 2009 Biomedical Informatics 263.

Sokeng, S.D.; Rokeya, B.; Hannan, J.M.A.; Junaida, K.; Zitech, P.; Ali, L.; Ngounou, G.; Lontsi, D.& Kamtchouing (2007). Inhibitory effect of *Ipomoea aquatica* extracts on glucose absorption using a perfused rat intestinal preparation. *Fitoterapia;* 78: 526-529.

Sokeng, S.D.; Rokeya, B.; Mostafa, M.; Nahar, N.; Mosihuzzaman, M. Ali, L & Kamtchouing, P. (2005). Antihyperglycemic effect of *Bridelia ndellensis* ethanol extract and fractions in streptozotocin induced diabetic rats. *Afr J Trad CAM,* Vol. 2, pp. 94-102.

Srinivasa, R.M. (2007). Medicinal plant species with potential anti diabeties Properties. *J Sci Food Agric,* Vol. 87, pp. 743-750.

Srivastava, V.; Rathore, A.; Ali, S.M. & Tandon, J.S. (1990). New Benzoic esters of loganin and 6β-Hydroxyloganin from *Nyctanthes arbortristis*. *Journal of Natural Products*. Vol. 53, No. 2, pp. 303-308.

Stamler, J.; Vaccaro, O.; Neaton, J.D. et al. (1993). Diabetes, other risk factors and 12-year cardiovascular mortality for men screened in the Multiple Risk Factor Intervention Trial. *Diabetes Care*, Vol. 16, pp. 434-44.

Subbulakshmi, G. & Naik, M. (2001). Indeginous food in the treatment of diabetes mellitus. Bombay *Hosp Res J*, Vol. 43, pp.548-561.

Tandon, J.S.; Srivastava, V. & Guru, P.Y. (1991). Iridoids: A new class of leishmanicidal agents from *Nyctanthes arbortristis*. Journal of *Natural Products*. Vol. 54, pp. 1102-1104.

Tuomilehto, J.; Lindstrom, J.; Eriksson, J.G.; Valle, T.T.; Hamalainen, H.; Ilanne-Parikka, P.; Keinanen-Kiukaanniemi, S.;, Laakso, M.; Louheranta, A.; Rastas, M.; Salminen, V.; & Uusitupa, M. (2001). Prevention of type 2 diabetes mellitus by changes in lifestyle among subjects with impaired glucose tolerance. *N. Engl. J. Med*, Vol. 344, pp. 1343–1350. [PubMed]

World Health Organization (WHO), (2006). Diabetes Programme, Department of Chronic diseases and Health Promotion; Facts and Figures sheet-Diabetes, Geneva, Switzerland.

21

Nutritional Therapy in Diabetes: Mediterranean Diet

Pablo Pérez-Martínez, Antonio García-Ríos, Javier Delgado-Lista, Francisco Pérez-Jiménez and José López-Miranda
Department of Medicine, IMIBIC, Hospital Universitario Reina Sofía, Universidad de Córdoba and CIBEROBN Instituto de Salud Carlos III, Madrid Spain

1. Introduction

Diabetes mellitus is a chronic illness which has an outstanding impact on public health due to its increasing prevalence, poor prognosis, and due to the high impact on cardiovascular health. Such is its importance, that diabetes is actually considered an independent predictor of cardiovascular disease (which includes coronary heart disease and stroke). Moreover, the cardiovascular risk of individuals with diabetes is considered to be equivalent to the risk of nondiabetic individuals with pre-existing cardiovascular diesease. Therefore, persons with diabetes mellitus have an increased susceptibility to atherosclerosis and an increased prevalence of ahterogenic risk factors, notably hypertension, obesity, and anormal lipids. This compendium of the abnormalities can be found in people with metabolic syndrome (MetS) which is now regarded as a prelude to diabetes and such as diabetes, MetS is a substantial predictor of cardiovascular disease and all-cause mortality(Ford, et al. 2002).

Morbidity and mortality from these chronic diseases in the general population have a multifactorial origin, resulting from the interaction between genetic background and environmental factors. Among the latter, diet is probably the most relevant factor in order to prevent acute complications and to reduce the risk of long-term complications. Thus, it has been demonstrated that medical nutrition therapy is important in preventing diabetes, managing existing diabetes, and preventing, or at least slowing, the rate of development of diabetes complications. The basis of what constitutes optimal nutrition has been the subject of decades of research spanning the whole range of study designs, from ecological studies to in vitro modulation of gene expression. Based on this approach, there is now sufficient evidence supporting the notion that the monounsaturated fatty acids (MUFA) as a nutrient, olive oil as a food, and the Mediterranean diet (MedDiet) as a food pattern are associated with a decreased risk of cardiovascular disease, MetS, and diabetes mellitus.

In the last decade, research in nutritional epidemiology has moved from the single food approach to the dietary pattern, which better reflects the complexity of interactive effects of multiple nutrients on health status(Hu 2002; Trichopoulou, et al. 2003; Trichopoulou, et al. 1995). Thus, the MedDiet pattern is built on the basis of a consumption of fat primarily from foods high in MUFA (olive oil as the principal source of fat), and emphasizes the consumption of fruits, vegetables, legumes, nuts, and fish, as well as a moderate consumption of alcohol. In this regard, the MedDiet pattern has been associated with higher survival due to lower all cause mortality(Knoops, et al. 2004). A recent meta-analysis of prospective studies based on 1.5 million subjects and 40,000 fatal and non-fatal events showed that a greater adherence to this dietary pattern was significantly associated with a reduction of overall mortality, cardiovascular mortality, cancer incidence and cancer mortality, and incidence of Alzheimer's disease and Parkinson's disease(Sofi, et al. 2008). In addition, a recently cross-sectional assessment of baseline data from a cohort of high-risk participants in the PREDIMED study, a large-scale feeding trial of primary cardiovascular prevention(Sanchez-Tainta, et al. 2008), showed that adherence to the MedDiet was inversely associated with the clustering of diabetes mellitus, obesity, hypertension and hypercholesterolemia. The follow-up of large cohorts of healthy populations living in Mediterranean countries, such as the Greek EPIC(Psaltopoulou, et al. 2004; Trichopoulou, et al. 2005a; Trichopoulou et al. 2003; Trichopoulou, et al. 2005b) and ATTICA(Panagiotakos, et al. 2009a; Panagiotakos, et al. 2006) study cohorts and the Spanish EPIC(Agudo, et al. 2007) and SUN(Nunez-Cordoba, et al. 2009) study cohorts, are providing new information suggesting that increasing adherence to the MedDiet relates to a reduced prevalence of risk phenotypes. In this regard, the MedDiet pattern is being reconsidered as the one of the more holistic approaches for the control of metabolic diseases including at the same time salutary and pleasure components.

The principal goals of medical nutrition therapy for subjects with metabolic syndrome, and/or diabetes are to attain and maintain an optimal metabolic control, including blood glucose, lipid profiles, and blood pressure; to prevent and treat obesity and cardiovascular complications; and to improve general health and well-being through food choices that take personal and cultural preferences into consideration. In this regard, pioneering nutritional strategies, such as nutraceuticals, have been developed aimed at reducing the main metabolic risk factors and promoting cardiovascular health. In this context, a growing body of clinical evidence has demonstrated positive cardiovascular effects associated with olive oil, antioxidants, and polyphenols intake.

Traditionally, many beneficial properties associated with olive oil have been ascribed to its high oleic acid content. Olive oil, however, can be considered a functional food that, besides having high-MUFA content, contains other minor components with biological properties(Perez-Jimenez, et al. 2007). Thus, phenolic compounds have shown antioxidant and antiinflammatory properties, prevent lipoperoxidation, induce favorable changes of lipid profile, improve endothelial function, and disclose antithrombotic properties(Lopez-Miranda, et al. 2007; Lopez-Miranda, et al. 2010; Perez-Jimenez, et al. 2005; Perez-Jimenez, et al. 2006; Ruano, et al. 2007; Ruano, et al. 2005). Therefore, all those evidences suggest that MedDiet could serve as an antiinflammatory dietary pattern, which could help fighting diseases that are related to chronic inflammation, such as MetS and type 2 diabetes. In this context, it has been clearly demonstrated that many components of the MedDiet have been considered to be important in the treatment and modulation of cardiometabolic diseases. In the present chapter, we review the state of the art illustrating the relationship between MedDiet rich in olive oil and metabolic diseases, including MetS and diabetes mellitus and to discuss potential mechanisms by which this food can help in disease prevention and treatment.

2. Mediterranean diet and diabetes

In the last decade the incidence of conditions associated with insulin resistance, including metabolic syndrome and diabetes mellitus, is increasing rapidly worldwide. Although pharmacological interventions are available for minimizing or delaying the comorbidities associated with insulin resistance and the metabolic syndrome, as well as diabetes, initial management for the vast majority of the affected population remains focused on lifestyle modification, consisting of sustainable changes in dietary habits and physical activity. Lifestyle modification, in particular recommendations to follow an appropriate dietary pattern, has generally been accepted as a cornerstone of treatment for people with these conditions, with the expectation that an appropriate intake of energy and nutrients will improve glycaemic control and will reduce the risk of complications. The factors that regulate body fat distribution, insulin resistance, and associated metabolic disturbances are not fully understood. Nevertheless, increasing scientific evidence suggests that dietary habits may be an important environmental factor regulating glucose and fat metabolism(Phillips, et al. 2006). Epidemiological studies indicate that Western-style dietary patterns promote the MetS, while diets rich in vegetables, fruits, grains, fish and low-fat dairy products have a protective role(Esmaillzadeh, et al. 2007; Lutsey, et al. 2008; Pereira, et al. 2005). In the same line, two studies in Southern European populations showed that a greater adherence to the MedDiet was associated with reduced prevalence (Panagiotakos, et al. 2004) and incidence (Tortosa, et al. 2007) of MetS. To date, several feeding trials have assessed the effect of dietary patterns on the metabolic syndrome status (Azadbakht, et al. 2005; Esposito, et al. 2004; Orchard, et al. 2005; Salas-Salvado, et al. 2008). These studies used a behavioral program to implement a relatively low-fat MedDiet(Esposito et al. 2004), intensive lifestyle intervention with inclusion of a vegetable-rich diet restricted in animal fat (Orchard et al. 2005), the DASH diet (Azadbakht et al. 2005), and two MedDiets supplemented with virgin olive oil or nuts(Salas-Salvado et al. 2008) in comparison with standard advices. Three studies (Azadbakht et al. 2005; Esposito et al. 2004; Orchard et al. 2005) used energy-restricted diets that led to some degree of weight loss, while one study(Salas-Salvado et al. 2008) used ad libitum diets. In all these studies, a decreased prevalence of metabolic syndrome was shown in the intervention groups. In the PREDIMED study(Salas-Salvado et al. 2008), the MedDiet with nuts significantly reduced MetS prevalence at 1 year, mostly because of increased reversion of prior MetS due to reduction in waist girth in spite of no weight loss, suggesting fat redistribution. Moreover, in a subgroup of this study including the Reus PREDIMED Centre some components of the MedDiet, such as olive oil, legumes and red wine were associated with lower prevalence of MetS (Babio, et al. 2009). On the other hand, results of a study in overweight, insulin-resistant patients also suggest that, by comparison with a low-fat diet, a MUFA-rich diet prevents the redistribution of body fat from peripheral to visceral adipose tissue without affecting total body weight(Paniagua, et al. 2007b). More recently Jimenez-Gomez et al. have demonstrated that postprandial abnormalities associated with MetS can be attenuated with high MUFA diets(Jimenez-Gomez, et al. 2010).

Because diabetes is a frequent outcome in patients with sustained MetS, it is reasonable to assume that the MedDiet might also prevent the development of diabetes in predisposed persons or beneficially influence the metabolic abnormalities associated with the diabetic status(Giugliano and Esposito 2008). In this context, two prospective studies from Southern European cohorts suggest a lower incidence of diabetes with increasing adherence to the MedDiet in previously healthy persons(Martinez-Gonzalez, et al. 2008) or survivors of a myocardial infarction(Mozaffarian, et al. 2007). In contrast, in the absence of weight loss, the low-fat diet used in the Women's Health Initiative trial(Tinker, et al. 2008) was ineffective to prevent the development of diabetes. Furthermore, in the set of the PREDIMED study, it has been tested the effects of two MedDiet interventions versus a low-fat diet on incidence of diabetes. This was a three-arm randomized trial in 418 nondiabetic subjects aged 55–80 years where participants were randomly assigned to education on a low-fat diet (control group) or to one of two MedDiets, supplemented with either free virgin olive oil (1 liter/week) or nuts (30 g/day). Diets were ad libitum, and no advice on physical activity was given. After a median follow-up of 4.0 years, diabetes incidence was 10.1%, 11.0%, and 17.9% in the MedDiet with olive oil group, the MedDiet with nuts group, and the control group, respectively. Multivariable adjusted hazard ratios of diabetes were 0.49 (0.25- 0.97) and 0.48 (0.24–0.96) in the MedDiet supplemented with olive oil and nuts groups, respectively, compared with the control group. Interestingly, when the two MedDiet groups were pooled and compared with the control group, diabetes incidence was reduced by 52%. In all study arms, increased adherence to the MedDiet was inversely associated with diabetes incidence. It is also important to highlight that diabetes risk reduction occurred in the absence of significant changes in body weight or physical activity. These results extend those of prior studies showing that lifestyle interventions can substantially reduce the incidence of diabetes in individuals at high risk(Knowler, et al. 2002; Pan, et al. 1997; Ramachandran, et al. 2006; Tuomilehto, et al. 2001). However, in these studies, the interventions consisted of advice on a calorie-restricted diet plus physical activity and, except for one study(Ramachandran et al. 2006), weight loss was a major driving force in reducing the incidence of diabetes(Salas-Salvado, et al. 2011).

Diets high in SFA consistently impair both insulin sensitivity and blood lipids, while substituting carbohydrates or MUFA for SFA reverts these abnormalities(Riccardi, et al. 2004). Postprandial lipemia and glucose homeostasis are also improved after meals containing MUFA from olive oil compared to meals rich in SFA(Lopez, et al. 2008; Paniagua, et al. 2007a). Thus, an examination of the association of dietary and membrane fatty acids with insulin secretion in the cross-sectional Pizarra study(Rojo-Martinez, et al. 2006) showed that dietary MUFA contributed to the variability of β-cell function, with a favorable relationship of MUFA with β-cell insulin secretion, independently of the level of insulin resistance.

The question as to what was the best nutrient to replace energy sources from SFA in the diabetic diet, carbohydrates or MUFA, was also hotly debated. Since the late 1980's, many feeding trials have compared the effects of isoenergetic high carbohydrates (CHO) and high MUFA diets on insulin sensitivity in healthy subjects and on glycemic and lipid control in diabetic patients(Garg 1998; Ros 2003). Garg's meta-analysis(Garg 1998) favored high MUFA diets, but most of the studies reviewed therein were performed with metabolic diets having wide differences in total fat content between the two experimental diets, ranging from 15% to 25% of energy. The studies reviewed by Ros(Ros 2003) were performed on an outpatient basis with natural foods, olive oil as the main source of MUFA, and <15% energy difference in total fat content between diets; the conclusion was that both dietary approaches provided a similar degree of glycemic control. Nevertheless, high MUFA diets generally had more favorable effects on proatherogenic alterations associated with the diabetic status, such as dyslipidemia, postprandial lipemia, small LDL, lipoprotein oxidation, inflammation, thrombosis, and endothelial dysfunction(Ros 2003). Although we will discuss this point later, of particular interest is the ability of the olive oil-rich MedDiet to improve mild systemic inflammation, as shown by the reduction of C-reactive protein and inflammatory cytokines in the study of Esposito et al.(Esposito et al. 2004) in subjects with MetS and by the PREDIMED study(Estruch, et al. 2006) in diabetic patients and other subjects at high risk for coronary heart disease (CHD). In addition, in a cross-sectional analysis of a population of type 2 diabetic patients, the adherence to a MedDiet was inversely associated with glycosylated haemoglobin and postprandial glucose levels during free living conditions, independent of age, adiposity, energy intake, physical activity and other potential confounders(Esposito, et al. 2009b). This association was apparent even although no strong associations were evident for each of the components of the MedDiet score, except for a modest association with whole grains and the ratio of MUFA to saturated lipids. However its cross-sectional nature does not allow us to make inference about cause and effect. According to these findings, Itsiopoulos et al. have recently demonstrated that a traditional MedDiet improved glycemic control, glycosylated haemoglobin fell from 7.1% to 6.8%, in men and women with well-controlled type 2 diabetes, without adverse effects on weight(Itsiopoulos, et al. 2010). Furthermore a systematic review of the available studies confirmed that adopting a MedDiet may help to prevent type 2 diabetes, and also improve glycaemic control and cardiovascular risk in persons with established diabetes(Esposito, et al. 2010).

Despite the beneficial effect attributed to the MedDiet, the American Diabetes Association (ADA) recommends that patients with newly diagnosed type 2 diabetes be treated with pharmacotherapy as well as lifestyle changes(Nathan, et al. 2006). The rationale for combination therapy is presumably that each form of treatment alone is imperfect. Lifestyle changes are often inadequate because patients do not lose weight or regain weight or their diabetes worsens independent of weight. Pharmacotherapy also often fails with time(Turner, et al. 1999), and some drugs have associated cardiovascular and other risks(Goldfine 2008). In this context Esposito et al. in 2009, conducted a randomized trial to compare the effects of a low-carbohydrate Mediterranean-style or a low-fat diet on the need for antihyperglycemic drug therapy in 215 patients with newly diagnosed type 2 diabetes(Esposito, et al. 2009a). After 4 years, they found that the MedDiet delayed the need for antihyperglycemic drug therapy. There were no differences in the degree to which participants in each group increased their physical activity or decreased their caloric intake, so the effect seems specific to the MedDiet and is probably, although not exclusively, linked to its ability to induce greater weight loss, in accord with results of a recent trial(Shai, et al. 2008). The between-group difference in the proportion of people needing antihyperglycemic drug therapy increased over the course of the trial and favored the MedDiet, whereas the between-group differences in weight loss decreased. Consumption of MUFA is thought to increase insulin sensitivity(Due, et al. 2008; Esposito et al. 2004; Shai et al. 2008), and this component of the diet might explain the favorable effect of the MedDiet on the need for drug therapy. In summary, although more data are mandatory, there is good scientific support for MedDiet diets, especially those based on olive oil, as an alternative approach to low-fat diets for the medical nutritional therapy in MetS and diabetes.

3. Protective mechanisms of mediterranean diet

Several mechanistic links offer potential explanations of protective effect of the MedDiet on type 2 diabetes. Excessive oxidative stress and inflammation are closely associated with the pathogenesis of many human diseases (such obesity, MetS, diabetes, cardiovascular diseases, neurodegenerative diseases and aging). The potential reversal of those conditions can be achieved by reducing the levels of inflammation through the consumption of an anti-inflammatory dietary pattern. Usually this may occur through the reduction of systemic vascular inflammation and endothelium dysfunction without having a drastic effect on body weight. Phenolic compounds are the focus of intense research in the last years, due to the biological properties that they have proven, mainly as potent antioxidants and anti-inflammatory agents; therefore, they can modulate signal transduction pathways to elicit their beneficial effects in human diseases. These mechanisms include modulation of pro-inflammatory gene expression such as cyclooxygenase, lipoxygenase, nitric oxide synthases

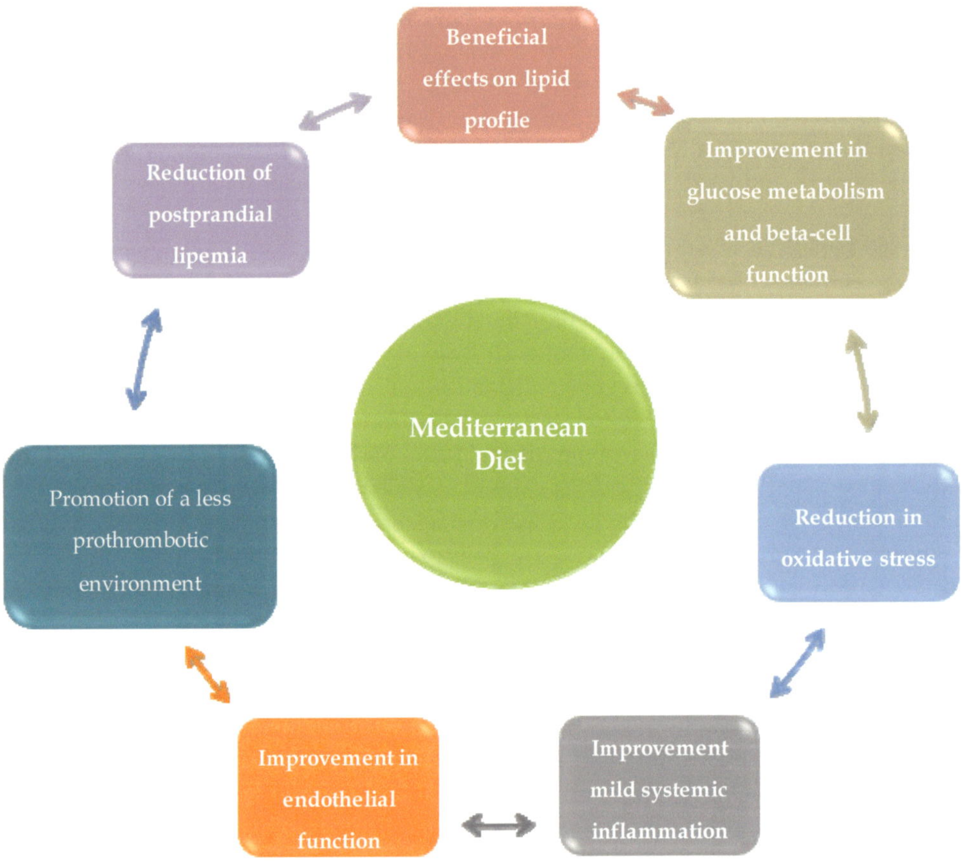

Fig. 1. Health effects of the Mediterranean Diet rich in olive and the potential mechanisms by which this diet can help in disease prevention and treatment.

and several pivotal cytokines, mainly by acting through NF-κb and mitogen-activated protein kinase signaling. It is of note that phenols are not uniquely represented in olive oil in the traditional MedDiet, but also in other classic foods, such as wine, fruits and vegetables. Beyond this, epidemiological and interventional studies have revealed a protective effect of the MedDiet against mild chronic inflammation and its metabolic complications (Chrysohoou, et al. 2004; Dai, et al. 2008; Panagiotakos, et al. 2009b).

3.1 Inflammation and oxidative stress

The origins of heightened inflammatory activity in diabetes are diverse. In type 1 diabetes, islet inflammation is thought to be a local phenomenon driven by a focal autoimmune attack on islet antigens. By contrast, in type 2 diabetes, activation of inflammation results from systemic etiologic factors, such as central obesity and insulin resistance. Ultimately inflammatory mediators activate a series of receptors and transcription factors such as NF-κb, toll-like receptors, c-Jun amino terminal kinase, and the receptor for advanced glycation end products, which lead to β-cell dysfunction and apoptosis, impaired insulin signaling in insulin-sensitive tissues, systemic endothelial dysfunction, and altered vascular flow. In this context inflammation at the cellular level can be described as an increase in the NF-κB in the nucleus and with a concomitant decrease in its inhibitors IκB-alpha and/or IκB-beta(Ghanim, et al. 2004). NF-κB is a pleiotropic transcription factor activated by low levels of reactive oxygen species (ROS) and inhibited by antioxidants(Mantena and Katiyar 2006). This factor regulates the expression of several cytokines, chemokines, cell adhesion molecules, immunoreceptors and inflammatory enzymes(Piva, et al. 2006), molecules that are involved in disease such as atherosclerosis and insulin resistance. In most cells, NF-κB (p50/p65) is present in an inactive form in the cytoplasm, bound to an inhibitor IκB. Certain stimuli result in the phosphorylation, ubiquitination and subsequent degradation of IκB proteins thereby enabling translocation of this transcription factor into the nucleus. In this context, an interesting aspect was the demonstration that supplementing an endothelial cell culture with oleic acid reduces the transcriptional activation of this factor in these cells, similar to what is done by α-linolenic acid, and the opposite of the inflammatory effect of linoleic acid. Hennig et al.(Hennig, et al. 2000) exposed porcine endothelial cells to 18-carbon fatty acids. Both linoleic and stearic fatty acids activated endothelial cells more markedly than did either oleic or linolenic fatty acids. Also, compared with control cultures, treatment with stearic and linoleic acids decreased glutathione concentrations, which suggested an increase in cellular oxidative stress. This increase in oxidative stress with the subsequent activation of NF κB could be one of the mechanisms of the inflammatory properties of 18:0 and 18:2 fatty acids. Previous studies have confirmed that fat consumption induced the activation of inflammatory markers(Jellema, et al. 2004). In this regard, Bellido and Perez-Martinez have previously demonstrated that the MedDiet, enriched in virgin olive oil, attenuated peripheral blood mononuclear cells (PBMCs) NF-κB activation compared with a Western SFA rich diet, and the effect of an n-3 PUFA-enriched diet was intermediate in young healthy population(Bellido, et al. 2004; Perez-Martinez, et al. 2007). These findings suggest that virgin olive oil could be a possible contributor to prevent the activation of NF-κB system, within the frame of the MedDiet. Besides olive oil, the MedDiet contents other source of potentially cardioprotective nutrients from fruits and vegetables which could also enhance this beneficial effect. In contrast, the opposite effect has been observed after the chronic intake of a Western diet rich in saturated fatty acids, corroborating previous data after the acute intake of a butter meal. The effect of a high CHO diet enriched in n-3 fatty acids on the NF-κB activation was intermediate. In this sense, previous data have suggested that n-3 α-linolenic acid found mainly in plants and walnuts may reduce cardiovascular risk through a variety of biological mechanisms, including inhibiting vascular inflammation.

In the same context, Brunelleschi et al.(Brunelleschi, et al. 2007) explored the effects of an extra-virgin olive oil extract, particularly rich in minor polar compounds, on NF-κB translocation in monocytes and monocyte-derived macrophages isolated from healthy volunteers. In a concentration-dependent manner, olive oil extract inhibited p50 and p65 NF-κB translocation in both un-stimulated and phorbol-myristate acetate challenged cells, being particularly effective on the p50 subunit. Interestingly, this effect occurred at concentrations found in human plasma after nutritional ingestion of virgin olive oil and was quantitatively similar to the effect exerted by ciglitazone, a PPAR-γ ligand. However, olive oil extract did not affect PPAR-γ expression in monocytes and monocye-derived macrophages(Brunelleschi et al. 2007). These data suggest the hypothesis of a protective effect of extra-virgin olive oil by indicating its ability to inhibit NF-κB activation in human monocyte/macrophages. On the other hand, NF-κB has been shown to regulate the expression of several adhesion molecules in response to inflammatory stimuli, including P-selectin, E-selectin, intercellular adhesion molecule 1 (ICAM-1) and cell adhesion molecule 1(VCAM-1)(Ghosh, et al. 1998), all implicated in atherosclerosis development. Carluccio et al.(Carluccio, et al. 1999) observed, in an endothelial cell culture model, that the incorporation of oleic acid into cellular membrane lipids reduced the expression of VCAM-1. Furthermore, it has been observed that the expression of VCAM-1 and E-selectin in human umbilical vascular endothelial cells (HUVECs), following the addition of minimally oxidised LDL, was less with LDL obtained from persons who had followed a diet rich in olive oil than from persons whose diet was rich in saturated fat(Bellido, et al. 2006). This anti-inflammatory action of MUFA also explains the fact that the enrichment of LDL particles with oleic acid, during the consumption of different types of diet, reduces their capacity to induce monocyte chemotaxis and adhesion. In accordance with these results, a previous study has shown that LDL obtained from a MUFA-rich diet induced a lower rate of monocyte adhesion to endothelial cells(Mata, et al. 1996).

The mechanism by which LDL from carbohydrate and MedDiets induces a lower expression of VCAM-1 and E-selectin is unknown; however several hypotheses have been suggested, for instance, the interaction of mononuclear leukocytes with vascular endothelial cells is most likely mediated by a complex amalgam of interacting regulatory signals in the inflammatory response characteristic of early atherogenesis. In another study including healthy subjects, virgin olive oil reduced plasma levels of ICAM-1(Bellido et al. 2004). This anti-inflammatory effect has also been observed in MetS patients who modified their diet for two years. In the group that followed a MedDiet model, the prevalence of this syndrome was reduced, improved insulin sensitivity and lowered the levels of C-reactive protein (CRP) and interleukin 6, 7 and 18. Such findings have recently been corroborated by Estruch et al.(Estruch et al. 2006) who evaluated the short-term effects of two ad libitum MedDiets (supplemented with either 1 l/week of virgin olive oil or 30 g/day of nuts) and an ad libitum low-fat diet on intermediate markers of cardiovascular disease. Compared with participants in the low-fat group, after 3 months those in the MedDiet groups had decreased levels of C-reactive protein. In addition, olive oil consumption also reduced levels of IL-6, VCAM-1 and ICAM-1. Moreover, people who eat the MedDiet that includes virgin olive oil reduce their levels of oxidized LDL, as suggested by the results of a subgroup analysis of the PREDIMED study carried out in 372 participants at high risk for cardiovascular disease, including diabetes(Fito, et al. 2007). Furthermore new data suggest that virgin olive oil intake was associated with higher levels of plasma antioxidant capacity after 3 years of intervention(Razquin, et al. 2009). In summary, based in the above evidences presented, we could assume that the MedDiet rich in nutrients with favorable anti-inflammatory properties may protect from metabolic diseases that are related to chronic inflammation and overproduction of reactive oxygen species, such as MetS and diabetes.

3.2 Postprandial state

When explaining possible mechanisms is important to recall that fasting is not the typical physiological state of the modern human being, which spends most the time in the postprandial state. Therefore, the assessment of the postprandial lipemic response may be more relevant to identify disturbances in metabolic pathways related to inflammation and oxidative stress than measures taken in the fasting state. With regard to the postprandial state, several previous studies have demonstrated that a breakfast enriched in saturated fat resulted in an increase in biomarkers of inflammation and oxidative stress(Cardona, et al. 2008; Devaraj, et al. 2008; Ursini, et al. 1998). In this regard, the identification of increased expression of TNF-α, a proinflammatory cytokine, in the adipose tissue of obese mice and humans has been correlated with the degree of adiposity and associated with insulin resistance. This fact is crucial given than insulin resistance will drive towards an increase in oxidative stress, endothelial dysfunction and impairments in lipoprotein metabolism and blood pressure. Therefore, targeting TNF-α and/or its receptors has been suggested as a promising treatment for insulin resistance and type 2 diabetes(Tzanavari, et al. 2010). In this scenario Jimenez-Gomez et al. observed that a breakfast rich in olive oil or walnuts decreased postprandial expression of mRNA TNF-α in PBMCs from healthy men compared with a butter-enriched breakfast(Jimenez-Gomez, et al. 2009). However, the effects of the three fatty breakfasts on the plasma concentrations of these proinflammatory parameters showed no significant differences. The fact that we only found differences in the expression of TNF-α at mRNA levels in PBMCs following the intake of the three breakfasts may be due to that the synthesis and secretion processes of these proteins do not happen simultaneously, and to the short half-life of cytokines(Futterman and Lemberg 2002; Kishimoto 2005).

3.3 Endothelial function

In the last years another interesting observation is that dietary fat may affect the endothelium(Berry, et al. 2008; Fuentes, et al. 2008; Goode, et al. 1997), and factors related to the arterial wall(Perez-Jimenez, et al. 1999). Several studies have shown that the acute administration of a high-fat meal induces a transitory disruption of endothelial function. Moreover, the effect of chronic consumption of a high-fat diet on endothelial function has also been evaluated. One study showed that a Mediterranean-style diet administered during 28 days to healthy subjects, attenuated plasma markers of endothelial activation, suggesting an improvement in endothelial function(Perez-Jimenez et al. 1999). Similarly, the chronic consumption of low-fat diets and Mediterranean-style diets improve endothelial function compared to a high-fat Western-type diet in hypercholesterolemic patients(Fuentes, et al. 2001). In this line, Esposito et al. demonstrated that the consumption of a Mediterranean-style diet by patients with the MetS was associated with improvement of endothelial function, by assessing the vascular responses to L-arginine, the natural precursor of nitric oxide(Esposito et al. 2004). More recently Radillis et al. observed that the close adherence to a MedDiet diet improves endothelial function in subjects with abdominal obesity(Rallidis, et al. 2009). On the other hand, previous studies also demonstrated that postprandial lipemia induces endothelial dysfunction(Anderson, et al. 2001; Bae, et al. 2003). According to this fact, Fuentes et al. studied the chronic effect of three diets with different fat compositions (high-SFA; high-MUFA; and a low-fat diet enriched in alpha-linolenic acid) on postprandial endothelial function and inflammatory biomarkers in twenty healthy men. This study demonstrated that the endothelium-dependent vasodilatory response was greater after the ingestion of the high-MUFA diet. Moreover this diet also induced lower postprandial sVCAM-1 levels and higher bioavailability of NOx compared with the other two diets(Fuentes et al. 2008). In the same line, Perez-Martinez et al. have recently showed that a high-MUFA diet improves endothelial cell, improving vasomotor function, with a higher availability of nitric oxide synthase and decreasing plasma sICAM-1 levels compared with a high-SFA diet and two low-fat, high complex carbohydrate diets, supplemented with 1.24 g/day of long chain n-3 PUFA or placebo, in MetS patients(Perez-Martinez, et al. 2010b). Therefore, those data carried out in the postprandial state support previous evidences suggesting that dietary patterns similar to those of the Mediterranean-style diet exert positive effects on components of the MetS and other conditions associated with, including endothelial dysfunction(Esposito, et al. 2006; Esposito et al. 2004). In the same population, the high-MUFA diet improved postprandial oxidative stress parameters as measured by glutathione levels and the glutathione/oxidized glutathione ratio. In addition, this diet induced lower postprandial plasma levels of lipoperoxides, protein carbonyls concentration and superoxide dismutase activity compared to subjects adhering to the other three diets(Perez-Martinez, et al. 2010a). Furthermore, postprandial plasma hydrogen peroxide levels were unfavourable increased during the high-SFA diet compared to the other three diets(Perez-Martinez et al. 2010a). These findings suggest that the postprandial state is important for understanding possible cardio-protective effects associated with the MedDiet particularly in subject with the MetS. In addition, these findings support recommendations to consume a high MUFA diet as a useful tool to prevent cardiovascular diseases in MetS patients.

3.4 Coagulation

Both endothelial cells and macrophages contribute to the generation of altered vasoreactivity and a procoagulant state through increased expression of plasminogen activator inhibitor (PAI)-1 and tissue factor and through platelet activation and acute phase reactions that increase levels of coagulation factors such as fibrinogen and factor VIII. Many of these molecules enter the circulation at levels that correlate with the degree of inflammatory activity. It has been well stablished that consumption of MedDiet as a dietary pattern, and virgin olive oil as it main fat source, is accompanied by a decrease in thrombogenesis, combining a decrease in coagulation factors and by platelet aggregation (Delgado-Lista, et al. 2008; Lopez-Miranda et al. 2007; Cicerale, et al. 2009; De La Cruz, et al. 2010; Gonzalez-Correa, et al. 2008; Lopez-Miranda et al. 2010; Perez-Jimenez et al. 2006;

Rasmussen, et al. 1994; Thomsen, et al. 1995; Tripoli, et al. 2005; Visioli, et al. 2005). To infer the great value that these facts may have on diabetes, we should have in mind that cardiovascular events are the primary cause of death in these patients, and that, a lowering in their procoagulant/prothrombotic status is, nowadays, the main prophylactic and therapeuthic weapon to avoid cardiovascular events. In other words, adhering to MedDiet may act as a prophylaxis for the appearance of thrombotic driven cardiovascular events. Reinforcing this hypothesis, some authors have recently published in vitro and animal studies in which they show antiaggregant properties of virgin olive oil comparable in efficacy to those of acetylsalicylic acid (ASA). Even more, virgin olive oil and ASA, when in combination, act synergically to further inhibit platelet activation and aggregation(6, 10). Although the cited studies have been realized mostly in healthy persons, diabetic persons may also benefit from the antithrombogenic effects of MedDiet. As an example, Rasmussen et al showed how non-insulin dependent diabetic patients who were fed a MUFA-rich diet for three weeks decreased their von Willebrand factor (an important procoagulant factor) when compared to a carbohydrate-rich diet. The same authors, in an elegant design, compared the effects of two diets similar in carbohydrate and protein content, one rich in MUFA (30 energy %) and one rich in polyunsaturated fatty acids (PUFA) (30 energy %). After three weeks, the diet rich in MUFA reduced the levels of von Willebrand factor, confirming the results of their previous study, and stating the favourable effect that MUFA have on this prothrombotic molecule.

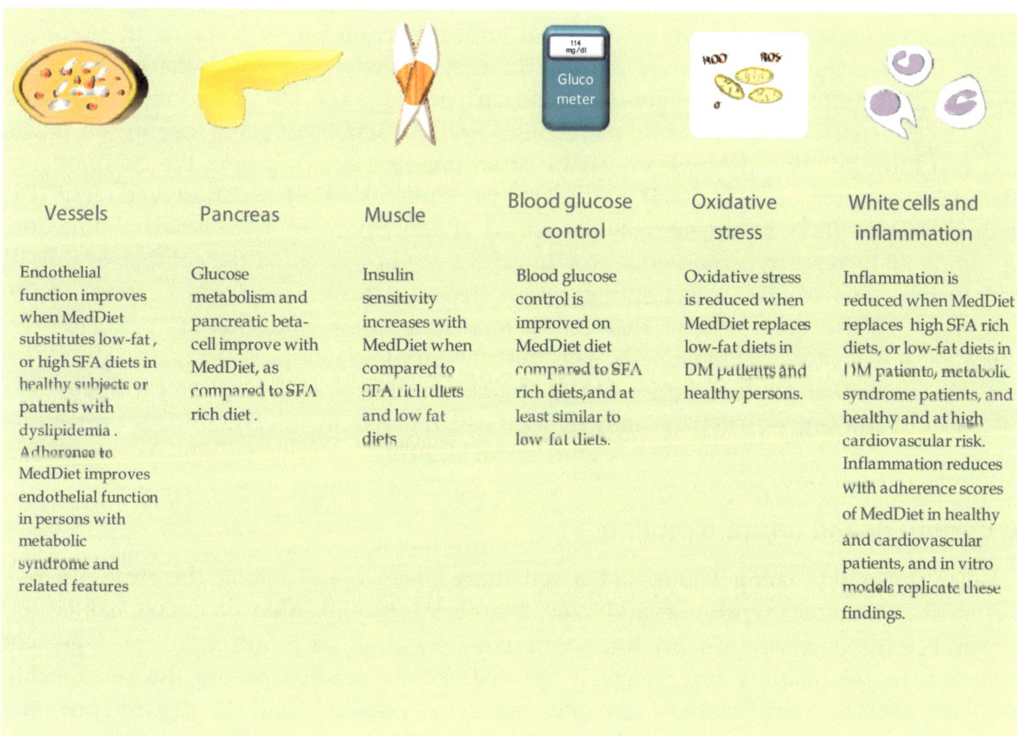

Fig. 2. Effects of Mediterranean diet on key features and organs affected by diabetes mellitus. MedDiet: Mediterranean diet. DM: diabetes mellitus. SFA: saturated fatty acid.

3.5 Nutrigenomics

It has been recently demonstrated the effects that phenolic fraction of olive oil exert at transcriptional level in vivo. In this regard, Camargo et al.(Camargo, et al. 2010) studied postprandial gene expression on peripheral blood mononuclear cells. To this end, two virgin olive oil-based breakfasts with high and low content of phenolic compounds were administered to 20 MetS patients following a double blinded, randomized, crossover design. They demonstrated that intake of virgin olive oil rich in phenol compounds is able to repress in vivo expression of several pro-inflammatory genes, thereby switching activity of peripheral blood mononuclear cells to a less deleterious inflammatory profile. In the same context, the consumption of a MedDiet with virgin olive oil, rich in polyphenols, decreased plasma oxidative and inflammatory status and the gene expression related with both inflammation (INF-gamma, Rho GTPase-activating protein15, and interleukin-7 receptor) and oxidative stress (adrenergic beta(2)-receptor) in PBMCs from healthy volunteers(Konstantinidou, et al. 2010). Moreover the same authors demonstrated the hypothesis that 3 weeks of nutritional intervention with virgin olive oil supplementation, at doses common in the MedDiet, can alter the expression of genes related to atherosclerosis development and progression(Khymenets, et al. 2009). In the same line, Llorente-Cortés et al.(Llorente-Cortes, et al. 2010) have confirmed in a population at high cardiovascular risk, that the MedDiet rich in olive oil influences expression of key genes involved in vascular inflammation, thrombosis and, in general, on atherosclerosis susceptibility. Moreover, it has been previously demonstrated in mice that olive oil up-regulates uncoupling protein (UCP) genes in brown adipose tissue and skeletal muscle(Rodriguez, et al. 2002), which is important given that UCP have been related with the regulation of body fat in mammals across its participation on the system of thermogenesis(Cypess, et al. 2009). It is well reported that mitochondrial biogenesis could, in part, underlie the central role of adipose tissue in the control of whole-body metabolism and the actions of some insulin sensitizers and that mitochondrial dysfunction might be an important contributing the symptoms of MetS(Wilson-Fritch, et al. 2004). In a recent study Hao et al. observed that the hydroxytyrosol (HT) treatment resulted in an enhancement of mitochondrial function, including an increase in activity and protein expression of mitochondrial complexes I, II, III and V; increased oxygen consumption; and a decrease in free fatty acid contents in the adipocytes. These data suggest that HT is able to promote mitochondrial function by stimulating mitochondrial biogenesis. This mitochondrial targeting property may provide a possible mechanism for the efficacy of the MedDiet for lowering the risk of cardiovascular disease and also suggests that HT may be used as a therapeutic intervention for preventing and treating diabetes mellitus and obesity(Hao, et al. 2010).

4. Summary and future direction

Because unhealthy eating habits and a sedentary lifestyle are among the strongest risk factors for metabolic syndrome and type 2 diabetes, modification of eating habits and physical activity constitutes an important component of any successful management program. In this chapter we reviewed the state of the art illustrating the relationship between MedDiet rich in olive oil and metabolic diseases, and to discuss potential mechanisms by which this food can help in disease prevention and treatment. Epidemiological and intervention studies indicate that MedDiet, thanks to its set of benefits, may protect from metabolic diseases that are related to chronic inflammation and overproduction of reactive oxygen species, such as MetS and diabetes. However, despite the significant advances of the last years, the final proof about the specific mechanisms and contributing role of the different dietary models and nutrients to its beneficial effects requires further investigations. In the future, the integrated application of approaches that are becoming available in functional genomics, metabonomics, lipidomics, microbiota, cronobiology, proteomic techniques, and bioinformatics analysis, will lead to a more highly integrated understanding of its positive effects on health. In this context the recent advances in human nutrigenomics and nutrigenetics, two fields with distinct approaches to elucidate the interaction between diet and genes but with a common ultimate goal to optimize health through the personalization of diet, will provide powerful approaches to unravel the complex relationship between nutritional molecules, genetic polymorphisms, and the biological system as a whole. On the other hand efforts should be put into identifying those micronutrients in olive oil that have the greatest beneficial effects on health.

In conclusion after decades of epidemiological, clinical and experimental research, it has become clear that consumption of Mediterranean dietary patterns rich in olive oil have a profound influence on health outcomes. Thus, there is good scientific support for recommend MedDiets, especially those based on olive oil, as an alternative approach for the medical nutritional therapy in obesity, MetS and diabetes.

5. Acknowledgment

Ciber Fisiopatología Obesidad y Nutrición, CIBEROBN, is an initiative of ISCIII government of Spain. This study was supported in part by research grants from the Spanish Ministry of Science and Innovation (AGL2006-01979/ALI, AGL2009-12270 to JL-M , SAF2007/62005 and PI10/02412 to FP-J and PI10/01041 to PP-M), Consejería de Economía, Innovación y Ciencia, Proyectos de Investigación de Excelencia, Junta de Andalucía (CT5015 to FP-J and P06-CTS- 01425 to JL-M); Consejería de Salud, Junta de Andalucía (07/43, PI 0193/09 to JL-M, PI-0252/2009 to JD-L and PI-0058-2010 to PP-M). Also supported by Centro de Excelencia Investigadora en Aceite de Oliva y Salud (CEAS) and FEDER, Fondo Social Europeo. AG-R is supported by a research contract of ISCIII (Programa Río-Hortega). None of the authors had any conflict of interest.

6. References

Agudo A, Cabrera L, Amiano P, Ardanaz E, Barricarte A, Berenguer T, Chirlaque MD, Dorronsoro M, Jakszyn P, Larranaga N, et al. 2007 Fruit and vegetable intakes, dietary antioxidant nutrients, and total mortality in Spanish adults: findings from the Spanish cohort of the European Prospective Investigation into Cancer and Nutrition (EPIC-Spain). *Am J Clin Nutr* 85 1634-1642.

Anderson RA, Evans ML, Ellis GR, Graham J, Morris K, Jackson SK, Lewis MJ, Rees A & Frenneaux MP 2001 The relationships between post-prandial lipaemia, endothelial function and oxidative stress in healthy individuals and patients with type 2 diabetes. *Atherosclerosis* 154 475-483.

Azadbakht L, Mirmiran P, Esmaillzadeh A, Azizi T & Azizi F 2005 Beneficial effects of a Dietary Approaches to Stop Hypertension eating plan on features of the metabolic syndrome. *Diabetes Care* 28 2823-2831.

Babio N, Bullo M, Basora J, Martinez-Gonzalez MA, Fernandez-Ballart J, Marquez-Sandoval F, Molina C & Salas-Salvado J 2009 Adherence to the Mediterranean diet and risk of metabolic syndrome and its components. *Nutr Metab Cardiovasc Dis* 19 563-570.

Bae JH, Schwemmer M, Lee IK, Lee HJ, Park KR, Kim KY & Bassenge E 2003 Postprandial hypertriglyceridemia-induced endothelial dysfunction in healthy subjects is independent of lipid oxidation. *Int J Cardiol* 87 259-267.

Bellido C, Lopez-Miranda J, Blanco-Colio LM, Perez-Martinez P, Muriana FJ, Martin-Ventura JL, Marin C, Gomez P, Fuentes F, Egido J, et al. 2004 Butter and walnuts, but not olive oil, elicit postprandial activation of nuclear transcription factor kappaB in peripheral blood mononuclear cells from healthy men. *Am J Clin Nutr* 80 1487-1491.

Bellido C, Lopez-Miranda J, Perez-Martinez P, Paz E, Marin C, Gomez P, Moreno JA, Moreno R & Perez-Jimenez F 2006 The Mediterranean and CHO diets decrease VCAM-1 and E-selectin expression induced by modified low-density lipoprotein in HUVECs. *Nutr Metab Cardiovasc Dis* 16 524-530.

Berry SE, Tucker S, Banerji R, Jiang B, Chowienczyk PJ, Charles SM & Sanders TA 2008 Impaired postprandial endothelial function depends on the type of fat consumed by healthy men. *J Nutr* 138 1910-1914.

Brunelleschi S, Bardelli C, Amoruso A, Gunella G, Ieri F, Romani A, Malorni W & Franconi F 2007 Minor polar compounds extra-virgin olive oil extract (MPC-OOE) inhibits NF-kappa B translocation in human monocyte/macrophages. *Pharmacol Res* 56 542-549.

Camargo A, Ruano J, Fernandez JM, Parnell LD, Jimenez A, Santos-Gonzalez M, Marin C, Perez-Martinez P, Uceda M, Lopez-Miranda J, et al. 2010 Gene expression changes in mononuclear cells in patients with metabolic syndrome after acute intake of phenol-rich virgin olive oil. *BMC Genomics* 11 253.

Cardona F, Tunez I, Tasset I, Montilla P, Collantes E & Tinahones FJ 2008 Fat overload aggravates oxidative stress in patients with the metabolic syndrome. *Eur J Clin Invest* 38 510-515.

Carluccio MA, Massaro M, Bonfrate C, Siculella L, Maffia M, Nicolardi G, Distante A, Storelli C & De Caterina R 1999 Oleic acid inhibits endothelial activation : A direct vascular antiatherogenic mechanism of a nutritional component in the mediterranean diet. *Arterioscler Thromb Vasc Biol* 19 220-228.

Cicerale S, Conlan XA, Sinclair AJ & Keast RS 2009 Chemistry and health of olive oil phenolics. *Crit Rev Food Sci Nutr* 49 218-236.

Cypess AM, Lehman S, Williams G, Tal I, Rodman D, Goldfine AB, Kuo FC, Palmer EL, Tseng YH, Doria A, et al. 2009 Identification and importance of brown adipose tissue in adult humans. *N Engl J Med* 360 1509-1517.

Chrysohoou C, Panagiotakos DB, Pitsavos C, Das UN & Stefanadis C 2004 Adherence to the Mediterranean diet attenuates inflammation and coagulation process in healthy adults: The ATTICA Study. *J Am Coll Cardiol* 44 152-158.

Dai J, Miller AH, Bremner JD, Goldberg J, Jones L, Shallenberger L, Buckham R, Murrah NV, Veledar E, Wilson PW, et al. 2008 Adherence to the mediterranean diet is inversely associated with circulating interleukin-6 among middle-aged men: a twin study. *Circulation* 117 169-175.

De La Cruz JP, Del Rio S, Lopez-Villodres JA, Villalobos MA, Jebrouni N & Gonzalez-Correa JA 2010 Virgin olive oil administration improves the effect of aspirin on retinal vascular pattern in experimental diabetes mellitus. *Br J Nutr* 104 560-565.

Delgado-Lista J, Lopez-Miranda J, Cortes B, Perez-Martinez P, Lozano A, Gomez-Luna R, Gomez P, Gomez MJ, Criado J, Fuentes F, et al. 2008 Chronic dietary fat intake modifies the postprandial response of hemostatic markers to a single fatty test meal. *Am J Clin Nutr* 87 317-322.

Devaraj S, Wang-Polagruto J, Polagruto J, Keen CL & Jialal I 2008 High-fat, energy-dense, fast-food-style breakfast results in an increase in oxidative stress in metabolic syndrome. *Metabolism* 57 867-870.

Due A, Larsen TM, Mu H, Hermansen K, Stender S & Astrup A 2008 Comparison of 3 ad libitum diets for weight-loss maintenance, risk of cardiovascular disease, and diabetes: a 6-mo randomized, controlled trial. *Am J Clin Nutr* 88 1232-1241.

Esmaillzadeh A, Kimiagar M, Mehrabi Y, Azadbakht L, Hu FB & Willett WC 2007 Dietary patterns, insulin resistance, and prevalence of the metabolic syndrome in women. *Am J Clin Nutr* 85 910-918.

Esposito K, Ciotola M & Giugliano D 2006 Mediterranean diet, endothelial function and vascular inflammatory markers. *Public Health Nutr* 9 1073-1076.

Esposito K, Maiorino MI, Ceriello A & Giugliano D 2010 Prevention and control of type 2 diabetes by Mediterranean diet: a systematic review. *Diabetes Res Clin Pract* 89 97-102.

Esposito K, Maiorino MI, Ciotola M, Di Palo C, Scognamiglio P, Gicchino M, Petrizzo M, Saccomanno F, Beneduce F, Ceriello A, et al. 2009a Effects of a Mediterranean-style diet on the need for antihyperglycemic drug therapy in patients with newly diagnosed type 2 diabetes: a randomized trial. *Ann Intern Med* 151 306-314.

Esposito K, Maiorino MI, Di Palo C & Giugliano D 2009b Adherence to a Mediterranean diet and glycaemic control in Type 2 diabetes mellitus. *Diabet Med* 26 900-907.

Esposito K, Marfella R, Ciotola M, Di Palo C, Giugliano F, Giugliano G, D'Armiento M, D'Andrea F & Giugliano D 2004 Effect of a mediterranean-style diet on endothelial dysfunction and markers of vascular inflammation in the metabolic syndrome: a randomized trial. *JAMA* 292 1440-1446.

Estruch R, Martinez-Gonzalez MA, Corella D, Salas-Salvado J, Ruiz-Gutierrez V, Covas MI, Fiol M, Gomez-Gracia E, Lopez-Sabater MC, Vinyoles E, et al. 2006 Effects of a Mediterranean-style diet on cardiovascular risk factors: a randomized trial. *Ann Intern Med* 145 1-11.

Fito M, Guxens M, Corella D, Saez G, Estruch R, de la Torre R, Frances F, Cabezas C, Lopez-Sabater Mdel C, Marrugat J, et al. 2007 Effect of a traditional Mediterranean diet on lipoprotein oxidation: a randomized controlled trial. *Arch Intern Med* 167 1195-1203.

Ford ES, Giles WH & Dietz WH 2002 Prevalence of the metabolic syndrome among US adults: findings from the third National Health and Nutrition Examination Survey. *JAMA* 287 356-359.

Fuentes F, Lopez-Miranda J, Perez-Martinez P, Jimenez Y, Marin C, Gomez P, Fernandez JM, Caballero J, Delgado-Lista J & Perez-Jimenez F 2008 Chronic effects of a high-fat diet enriched with virgin olive oil and a low-fat diet enriched with alpha-linolenic acid on postprandial endothelial function in healthy men. *Br J Nutr* 100 159-165.

Fuentes F, Lopez-Miranda J, Sanchez E, Sanchez F, Paez J, Paz-Rojas E, Marin C, Gomez P, Jimenez-Pereperez J, Ordovas JM, et al. 2001 Mediterranean and low-fat diets improve endothelial function in hypercholesterolemic men. *Ann Intern Med* 134 1115-1119.

Futterman LG & Lemberg L 2002 High-sensitivity C-reactive protein is the most effective prognostic measurement of acute coronary events. *Am J Crit Care* 11 482-486.

Garg A 1998 High-monounsaturated-fat diets for patients with diabetes mellitus: a meta-analysis. *Am J Clin Nutr* 67 577S-582S.

Ghanim H, Aljada A, Hofmeyer D, Syed T, Mohanty P & Dandona P 2004 Circulating mononuclear cells in the obese are in a proinflammatory state. *Circulation* 110 1564-1571.

Ghosh S, May MJ & Kopp EB 1998 NF-kappa B and Rel proteins: evolutionarily conserved mediators of immune responses. *Annu Rev Immunol* 16 225-260.

Giugliano D & Esposito K 2008 Mediterranean diet and metabolic diseases. *Curr Opin Lipidol* 19 63-68.

Goldfine AB 2008 Assessing the cardiovascular safety of diabetes therapies. *N Engl J Med* 359 1092-1095.

Gonzalez-Correa JA, Navas MD, Munoz-Marin J, Trujillo M, Fernandez-Bolanos J & de la Cruz JP 2008 Effects of hydroxytyrosol and hydroxytyrosol acetate administration to rats on platelet function compared to acetylsalicylic acid. *J Agric Food Chem* 56 7872-7876.

Goode GK, Garcia S & Heagerty AM 1997 Dietary supplementation with marine fish oil improves in vitro small artery endothelial function in hypercholesterolemic patients: a double-blind placebo-controlled study. *Circulation* 96 2802-2807.

Hao J, Shen W, Yu G, Jia H, Li X, Feng Z, Wang Y, Weber P, Wertz K, Sharman E, et al. 2010 Hydroxytyrosol promotes mitochondrial biogenesis and mitochondrial function in 3T3-L1 adipocytes. *J Nutr Biochem* 21 634-644.

Hennig B, Meerarani P, Ramadass P, Watkins BA & Toborek M 2000 Fatty acid-mediated activation of vascular endothelial cells. *Metabolism* 49 1006-1013.

Hu FB 2002 Dietary pattern analysis: a new direction in nutritional epidemiology. *Curr Opin Lipidol* 13 3-9.

Itsiopoulos C, Brazionis L, Kaimakamis M, Cameron M, Best JD, O'Dea K & Rowley K 2010 Can the Mediterranean diet lower HbA1c in type 2 diabetes? Results from a randomized cross-over study. *Nutr Metab Cardiovasc Dis.*

Jellema A, Plat J & Mensink RP 2004 Weight reduction, but not a moderate intake of fish oil, lowers concentrations of inflammatory markers and PAI-1 antigen in obese men during the fasting and postprandial state. *Eur J Clin Invest* 34 766-773.

Jimenez-Gomez Y, Lopez-Miranda J, Blanco-Colio LM, Marin C, Perez-Martinez P, Ruano J, Paniagua JA, Rodriguez F, Egido J & Perez-Jimenez F 2009 Olive oil and walnut breakfasts reduce the postprandial inflammatory response in mononuclear cells compared with a butter breakfast in healthy men. *Atherosclerosis* 204 e70-76.

Jimenez-Gomez Y, Marin C, Peerez-Martinez P, Hartwich J, Malczewska-Malec M, Golabek I, Kiec-Wilk B, Cruz-Teno C, Rodriguez F, Gomez P, et al. 2010 A low-fat, high-complex carbohydrate diet supplemented with long-chain (n-3) fatty acids alters the postprandial lipoprotein profile in patients with metabolic syndrome. *J Nutr* 140 1595-1601.

Khymenets O, Fito M, Covas MI, Farre M, Pujadas MA, Munoz D, Konstantinidou V & de la Torre R 2009 Mononuclear cell transcriptome response after sustained virgin olive oil consumption in humans: an exploratory nutrigenomics study. *OMICS* 13 7-19.

Kishimoto T 2005 Interleukin-6: from basic science to medicine--40 years in immunology. *Annu Rev Immunol* 23 1-21.

Knoops KT, de Groot LC, Kromhout D, Perrin AE, Moreiras-Varela O, Menotti A & van Staveren WA 2004 Mediterranean diet, lifestyle factors, and 10-year mortality in elderly European men and women: the HALE project. *JAMA* 292 1433-1439.

Knowler WC, Barrett-Connor E, Fowler SE, Hamman RF, Lachin JM, Walker EA & Nathan DM 2002 Reduction in the incidence of type 2 diabetes with lifestyle intervention or metformin. *N Engl J Med* 346 393-403.

Konstantinidou V, Covas MI, Munoz-Aguayo D, Khymenets O, de la Torre R, Saez G, Tormos Mdel C, Toledo E, Marti A, Ruiz-Gutierrez V, et al. 2010 In vivo nutrigenomic effects of virgin olive oil polyphenols within the frame of the Mediterranean diet: a randomized controlled trial. *FASEB J* 24 2546-2557.

Lopez-Miranda J, Delgado-Lista J, Perez-Martinez P, Jimenez-Gomez Y, Fuentes F, Ruano J & Marin C 2007 Olive oil and the haemostatic system. *Mol Nutr Food Res* 51 1249-1259.

Lopez-Miranda J, Perez-Jimenez F, Ros E, De Caterina R, Badimon L, Covas MI, Escrich E, Ordovas JM, Soriguer F, Abia R, et al. 2010 Olive oil and health: summary of the II international conference on olive oil and health consensus report, Jaen and Cordoba (Spain) 2008. *Nutr Metab Cardiovasc Dis* 20 284-294.

Lopez S, Bermudez B, Pacheco YM, Villar J, Abia R & Muriana FJ 2008 Distinctive postprandial modulation of beta cell function and insulin sensitivity by dietary fats: monounsaturated compared with saturated fatty acids. *Am J Clin Nutr* 88 638-644.

Lutsey PL, Steffen LM & Stevens J 2008 Dietary intake and the development of the metabolic syndrome: the Atherosclerosis Risk in Communities study. *Circulation* 117 754-761.

Llorente-Cortes V, Estruch R, Mena MP, Ros E, Gonzalez MA, Fito M, Lamuela-Raventos RM & Badimon L 2010 Effect of Mediterranean diet on the expression of pro-atherogenic genes in a population at high cardiovascular risk. *Atherosclerosis* 208 442-450.

Mantena SK & Katiyar SK 2006 Grape seed proanthocyanidins inhibit UV-radiation-induced oxidative stress and activation of MAPK and NF-kappaB signaling in human epidermal keratinocytes. *Free Radic Biol Med* 40 1603-1614.

Martinez-Gonzalez MA, de la Fuente-Arrillaga C, Nunez-Cordoba JM, Basterra-Gortari FJ, Beunza JJ, Vazquez Z, Benito S, Tortosa A & Bes-Rastrollo M 2008 Adherence to

Mediterranean diet and risk of developing diabetes: prospective cohort study. *BMJ* 336 1348-1351.

Mata P, Alonso R, Lopez-Farre A, Ordovas JM, Lahoz C, Garces C, Caramelo C, Codoceo R, Blazquez E & de Oya M 1996 Effect of dietary fat saturation on LDL oxidation and monocyte adhesion to human endothelial cells in vitro. *Arterioscler Thromb Vasc Biol* 16 1347-1355.

Mozaffarian D, Marfisi R, Levantesi G, Silletta MG, Tavazzi L, Tognoni G, Valagussa F & Marchioli R 2007 Incidence of new-onset diabetes and impaired fasting glucose in patients with recent myocardial infarction and the effect of clinical and lifestyle risk factors. *Lancet* 370 667-675.

Nathan DM, Buse JB, Davidson MB, Heine RJ, Holman RR, Sherwin R & Zinman B 2006 Management of hyperglycemia in type 2 diabetes: A consensus algorithm for the initiation and adjustment of therapy: a consensus statement from the American Diabetes Association and the European Association for the Study of Diabetes. *Diabetes Care* 29 1963-1972.

Nunez-Cordoba JM, Valencia-Serrano F, Toledo E, Alonso A & Martinez-Gonzalez MA 2009 The Mediterranean diet and incidence of hypertension: the Seguimiento Universidad de Navarra (SUN) Study. *Am J Epidemiol* 169 339-346.

Orchard TJ, Temprosa M, Goldberg R, Haffner S, Ratner R, Marcovina S & Fowler S 2005 The effect of metformin and intensive lifestyle intervention on the metabolic syndrome: the Diabetes Prevention Program randomized trial. *Ann Intern Med* 142 611-619.

Pan XR, Li GW, Hu YH, Wang JX, Yang WY, An ZX, Hu ZX, Lin J, Xiao JZ, Cao HB, et al. 1997 Effects of diet and exercise in preventing NIDDM in people with impaired glucose tolerance. The Da Qing IGT and Diabetes Study. *Diabetes Care* 20 537-544.

Panagiotakos D, Pitsavos C, Chrysohoou C, Palliou K, Lentzas I, Skoumas I & Stefanadis C 2009a Dietary patterns and 5-year incidence of cardiovascular disease: a multivariate analysis of the ATTICA study. *Nutr Metab Cardiovasc Dis* 19 253-263.

Panagiotakos DB, Chrysohoou C, Pitsavos C & Stefanadis C 2006 Association between the prevalence of obesity and adherence to the Mediterranean diet: the ATTICA study. *Nutrition* 22 449-456.

Panagiotakos DB, Dimakopoulou K, Katsouyanni K, Bellander T, Grau M, Koenig W, Lanki T, Pistelli R, Schneider A & Peters A 2009b Mediterranean diet and inflammatory response in myocardial infarction survivors. *Int J Epidemiol* 38 856-866.

Panagiotakos DB, Pitsavos C, Chrysohoou C, Skoumas J, Tousoulis D, Toutouza M, Toutouzas P & Stefanadis C 2004 Impact of lifestyle habits on the prevalence of the metabolic syndrome among Greek adults from the ATTICA study. *Am Heart J* 147 106-112.

Paniagua JA, de la Sacristana AG, Sanchez E, Romero I, Vidal-Puig A, Berral FJ, Escribano A, Moyano MJ, Perez-Martinez P, Lopez-Miranda J, et al. 2007a A MUFA-rich diet improves posprandial glucose, lipid and GLP-1 responses in insulin-resistant subjects. *J Am Coll Nutr* 26 434-444.

Paniagua JA, Gallego de la Sacristana A, Romero I, Vidal-Puig A, Latre JM, Sanchez E, Perez-Martinez P, Lopez-Miranda J & Perez-Jimenez F 2007b Monounsaturated fat-rich diet prevents central body fat distribution and decreases postprandial adiponectin expression induced by a carbohydrate-rich diet in insulin-resistant subjects. *Diabetes Care* 30 1717-1723.

Pereira MA, Kartashov AI, Ebbeling CB, Van Horn L, Slattery ML, Jacobs DR, Jr. & Ludwig DS 2005 Fast-food habits, weight gain, and insulin resistance (the CARDIA study): 15-year prospective analysis. *Lancet* 365 36-42.

Perez-Jimenez F, Alvarez de Cienfuegos G, Badimon L, Barja G, Battino M, Blanco A, Bonanome A, Colomer R, Corella-Piquer D, Covas I, et al. 2005 International conference on the healthy effect of virgin olive oil. *Eur J Clin Invest* 35 421-424.

Perez-Jimenez F, Castro P, Lopez-Miranda J, Paz-Rojas E, Blanco A, Lopez-Segura F, Velasco F, Marin C, Fuentes F & Ordovas JM 1999 Circulating levels of endothelial function are modulated by dietary monounsaturated fat. *Atherosclerosis* 145 351-358.

Perez-Jimenez F, Lista JD, Perez-Martinez P, Lopez-Segura F, Fuentes F, Cortes B, Lozano A & Lopez-Miranda J 2006 Olive oil and haemostasis: a review on its healthy effects. *Public Health Nutr* 9 1083-1088.

Perez-Jimenez F, Ruano J, Perez-Martinez P, Lopez-Segura F & Lopez-Miranda J 2007 The influence of olive oil on human health: not a question of fat alone. *Mol Nutr Food Res* 51 1199-1208.

Perez-Martinez P, Garcia-Quintana JM, Yubero-Serrano EM, Tasset-Cuevas I, Tunez I, Garcia-Rios A, Delgado-Lista J, Marin C, Perez-Jimenez F, Roche HM, et al. 2010a Postprandial oxidative stress is modified by dietary fat: evidence from a human intervention study. *Clin Sci (Lond)* 119 251-261.

Perez-Martinez P, Lopez-Miranda J, Blanco-Colio L, Bellido C, Jimenez Y, Moreno JA, Delgado-Lista J, Egido J & Perez-Jimenez F 2007 The chronic intake of a Mediterranean diet enriched in virgin olive oil, decreases nuclear transcription factor kappaB activation in peripheral blood mononuclear cells from healthy men. *Atherosclerosis* 194 e141-146.

Perez-Martinez P, Moreno-Conde M, Cruz-Teno C, Ruano J, Fuentes F, Delgado-Lista J, Garcia-Rios A, Marin C, Gomez-Luna MJ, Perez-Jimenez F, et al. 2010b Dietary fat differentially influences regulatory endothelial function during the postprandial state in patients with metabolic syndrome: from the LIPGENE study. *Atherosclerosis* 209 533-538.

Phillips C, Lopez-Miranda J, Perez-Jimenez F, McManus R & Roche HM 2006 Genetic and nutrient determinants of the metabolic syndrome. *Curr Opin Cardiol* 21 185-193.

Piva R, Belardo G & Santoro MG 2006 NF-kappaB: a stress-regulated switch for cell survival. *Antioxid Redox Signal* 8 478-486.

Psaltopoulou T, Naska A, Orfanos P, Trichopoulos D, Mountokalakis T & Trichopoulou A 2004 Olive oil, the Mediterranean diet, and arterial blood pressure: the Greek European Prospective Investigation into Cancer and Nutrition (EPIC) study. *Am J Clin Nutr* 80 1012-1018.

Rallidis LS, Lekakis J, Kolomvotsou A, Zampelas A, Vamvakou G, Efstathiou S, Dimitriadis G, Raptis SA & Kremastinos DT 2009 Close adherence to a Mediterranean diet improves endothelial function in subjects with abdominal obesity. *Am J Clin Nutr* 90 263-268.

Ramachandran A, Snehalatha C, Mary S, Mukesh B, Bhaskar AD & Vijay V 2006 The Indian Diabetes Prevention Programme shows that lifestyle modification and metformin prevent type 2 diabetes in Asian Indian subjects with impaired glucose tolerance (IDPP-1). *Diabetologia* 49 289-297.

Rasmussen O, Thomsen C, Ingerslev J & Hermansen K 1994 Decrease in von Willebrand factor levels after a high-monounsaturated-fat diet in non-insulin-dependent diabetic subjects. *Metabolism* 43 1406-1409.

Razquin C, Martinez JA, Martinez-Gonzalez MA, Mitjavila MT, Estruch R & Marti A 2009 A 3 years follow-up of a Mediterranean diet rich in virgin olive oil is associated with high plasma antioxidant capacity and reduced body weight gain. *Eur J Clin Nutr* 63 1387-1393.

Riccardi G, Giacco R & Rivellese AA 2004 Dietary fat, insulin sensitivity and the metabolic syndrome. *Clin Nutr* 23 447-456.

Rodriguez VM, Portillo MP, Pico C, Macarulla MT & Palou A 2002 Olive oil feeding up-regulates uncoupling protein genes in rat brown adipose tissue and skeletal muscle. *Am J Clin Nutr* 75 213-220.

Rojo-Martinez G, Esteva I, Ruiz de Adana MS, Garcia-Almeida JM, Tinahones F, Cardona F, Morcillo S, Garcia-Escobar E, Garcia-Fuentes E & Soriguer F 2006 Dietary fatty acids and insulin secretion: a population-based study. *Eur J Clin Nutr* 60 1195-1200.

Ros E 2003 Dietary cis-monounsaturated fatty acids and metabolic control in type 2 diabetes. *Am J Clin Nutr* 78 617S-625S.

Ruano J, Lopez-Miranda J, de la Torre R, Delgado-Lista J, Fernandez J, Caballero J, Covas MI, Jimenez Y, Perez-Martinez P, Marin C, et al. 2007 Intake of phenol-rich virgin olive oil improves the postprandial prothrombotic profile in hypercholesterolemic patients. *Am J Clin Nutr* 86 341-346.

Ruano J, Lopez-Miranda J, Fuentes F, Moreno JA, Bellido C, Perez-Martinez P, Lozano A, Gomez P, Jimenez Y & Perez Jimenez F 2005 Phenolic content of virgin olive oil improves ischemic reactive hyperemia in hypercholesterolemic patients. *J Am Coll Cardiol* 46 1864-1868.

Salas-Salvado J, Bullo M, Babio N, Martinez-Gonzalez MA, Ibarrola-Jurado N, Basora J, Estruch R, Covas MI, Corella D, Aros F, et al. 2011 Reduction in the incidence of type 2 diabetes with the Mediterranean diet: results of the PREDIMED-Reus nutrition intervention randomized trial. *Diabetes Care* 34 14-19.

Salas-Salvado J, Fernandez-Ballart J, Ros E, Martinez-Gonzalez MA, Fito M, Estruch R, Corella D, Fiol M, Gomez-Gracia E, Aros F, et al. 2008 Effect of a Mediterranean diet supplemented with nuts on metabolic syndrome status: one-year results of the PREDIMED randomized trial. *Arch Intern Med* 168 2449-2458.

Sanchez-Tainta A, Estruch R, Bullo M, Corella D, Gomez-Gracia E, Fiol M, Algorta J, Covas MI, Lapetra J, Zazpe I, et al. 2008 Adherence to a Mediterranean-type diet and reduced prevalence of clustered cardiovascular risk factors in a cohort of 3,204 high-risk patients. *Eur J Cardiovasc Prev Rehabil* 15 589-593.

Shai I, Schwarzfuchs D, Henkin Y, Shahar DR, Witkow S, Greenberg I, Golan R, Fraser D, Bolotin A, Vardi H, et al. 2008 Weight loss with a low-carbohydrate, Mediterranean, or low-fat diet. *N Engl J Med* 359 229-241.

Sofi F, Cesari F, Abbate R, Gensini GF & Casini A 2008 Adherence to Mediterranean diet and health status: meta-analysis. *BMJ* 337 a1344.

Thomsen C, Rasmussen OW, Ingerslev J & Hermansen K 1995 Plasma levels of von Willebrand factor in non-insulin-dependent diabetes mellitus are influenced by dietary monounsaturated fatty acids. *Thromb Res* 77 347-356.

Tinker LF, Bonds DE, Margolis KL, Manson JE, Howard BV, Larson J, Perri MG, Beresford SA, Robinson JG, Rodriguez B, et al. 2008 Low-fat dietary pattern and risk of treated diabetes mellitus in postmenopausal women: the Women's Health Initiative randomized controlled dietary modification trial. *Arch Intern Med* 168 1500-1511.

Tortosa A, Bes-Rastrollo M, Sanchez-Villegas A, Basterra-Gortari FJ, Nunez-Cordoba JM & Martinez-Gonzalez MA 2007 Mediterranean diet inversely associated with the incidence of metabolic syndrome: the SUN prospective cohort. *Diabetes Care* 30 2957-2959.

Trichopoulou A, Bamia C & Trichopoulos D 2005a Mediterranean diet and survival among patients with coronary heart disease in Greece. *Arch Intern Med* 165 929-935.

Trichopoulou A, Costacou T, Bamia C & Trichopoulos D 2003 Adherence to a Mediterranean diet and survival in a Greek population. *N Engl J Med* 348 2599-2608.

Trichopoulou A, Kouris-Blazos A, Wahlqvist ML, Gnardellis C, Lagiou P, Polychronopoulos E, Vassilakou T, Lipworth L & Trichopoulos D 1995 Diet and overall survival in elderly people. *BMJ* 311 1457-1460.

Trichopoulou A, Orfanos P, Norat T, Bueno-de-Mesquita B, Ocke MC, Peeters PH, van der Schouw YT, Boeing H, Hoffmann K, Boffetta P, et al. 2005b Modified Mediterranean diet and survival: EPIC-elderly prospective cohort study. *BMJ* 330 991.

Tripoli E, Giammanco M, Tabacchi G, Di Majo D, Giammanco S & La Guardia M 2005 The phenolic compounds of olive oil: structure, biological activity and beneficial effects on human health. *Nutr Res Rev* 18 98-112.

Tuomilehto J, Lindstrom J, Eriksson JG, Valle TT, Hamalainen H, Ilanne-Parikka P, Keinanen-Kiukaanniemi S, Laakso M, Louheranta A, Rastas M, et al. 2001 Prevention of type 2 diabetes mellitus by changes in lifestyle among subjects with impaired glucose tolerance. *N Engl J Med* 344 1343-1350.

Turner RC, Cull CA, Frighi V & Holman RR 1999 Glycemic control with diet, sulfonylurea, metformin, or insulin in patients with type 2 diabetes mellitus: progressive requirement for multiple therapies (UKPDS 49). UK Prospective Diabetes Study (UKPDS) Group. *JAMA* 281 2005-2012.

Tzanavari T, Giannogonas P & Karalis KP 2010 TNF-alpha and obesity. *Curr Dir Autoimmun* 11 145-156.

Ursini F, Zamburlini A, Cazzolato G, Maiorino M, Bon GB & Sevanian A 1998 Postprandial plasma lipid hydroperoxides: a possible link between diet and atherosclerosis. *Free Radic Biol Med* 25 250-252.

Visioli F, Bogani P, Grande S & Galli C 2005 Mediterranean food and health: building human evidence. *J Physiol Pharmacol* 56 Suppl 1 37-49.

Wilson-Fritch L, Nicoloro S, Chouinard M, Lazar MA, Chui PC, Leszyk J, Straubhaar J, Czech MP & Corvera S 2004 Mitochondrial remodeling in adipose tissue associated with obesity and treatment with rosiglitazone. *J Clin Invest* 114 1281-1289.

22

Pharmacogenetics for T2DM and Anti-Diabetic Drugs

Qiong Huang[1] and Zhao-qian Liu[2]
[1]*Institute of Clinical Pharmacology, Anhui Medical University, Key Laboratory of Anti-inflammatory and Immunopharmacology of Education Ministry, Hefei, Anhui*
[2]*Institute of Clinical Pharmacology, Hunan Key Laboratory of Pharmacogenetics, Central South University, Changsha, Hunan*
[1,2]*P. R. China*

1. Introduction

1.1 Genes associated with T2DM

1.1.1 Genes associated with ion transport

1.1.1.1 KCNJ11

The potassium inwardly rectifying channel subfamily J member 11 (*KCNJ11*) gene encodes Kir6.2 protein, the inwardly rectifying potassium channel, which is a complex of two subunits [2]. ATP-sensitive K^+ (K_{ATP}) channels critically control insulin secretion by coupling metabolism to electrical activity [3]. The β-cell channels are assembled, with tetradimeric stoichiometry, from two structurally distinct subunits. inwardly rectifying K-channel subunit (KIR6.2) and the regulatory sulfonylurea receptor subunit-1 (SUR1). Some studies showed that the *KCNJ11* E23K (Lys23Glu, 67 G>A, rs5219) polymorphism could affect insulin secretion and T2DM susceptibility by influencing the sensitivity of the K_{ATP} channel to ATP [4-6]. E23K promotes development of T2DM by increasing the threshold ATP concentration, thus inducing over activity of pancreatic β-cell K_{ATP} channels and inhibiting insulin secretion [7]. E23K markedly affected channel gating, significantly reduced the time spent in long inter burst closed states. Meta-analysis of all case-control data showed that the E23K allele was associated with T2DM [8]. The E23K variant was associated with a reduction in estimates of glucose-induced serum insulin levels in middle-aged glucose-tolerant subjects. This result is in accordance with the recent *in vitro* finding that the E23K variant is associated with a reduced ATP sensitivity of the Kir6.2/SUR1channel complex [4, 7]. T2DM patients with one A allele of the *KCNJ11* E23K polymorphism seem to be more sensitive to repaglinide as compared with individuals with the GG genotype [9].

1.1.1.2 KCNQ1

KCNQ1 (potassium voltage-gated channel, KQT-like subfamily, member 1) gene, locates on 11p15.5, encodes a voltage-gated K^+ channel with six transmembrane regions and is expressed in the heart, stomach, small and large intestine, kidney and pancreas [10]. Two independent GWA studies identified that SNPs rs2237892, rs2237895, and rs2237897 located in intron 15 of the *KCNQ1* gene were strongly associated with T2DM [6,7]. The association of rs2237892, rs2237897, and rs2283228 with T2DM was confirmed in populations of Korean, Singaporean, Chinese, European ancestry and Japanese. The risk allele of rs2237892, rs2237895, and rs2237897 were associated with impairment of insulin secretion according to the homeostasis model assessment of β-cell function or the corrected insulin response [11, 12]. In a Chinese study, SNP rs2237892 was significantly associated with increasing fasting plasma glucose, while rs2237892 and rs2237897 were associated with HbA1c. The SNP rs2237897 was associated with both acute insulin and C-peptide response after arginine stimulation in T2DM group. The SNP rs2237895 was associated with both first- and second-phase insulin secretions in the controls. For rs2237892, rs2237895 and rs2237897 polymorphisms, homozygous carriers of the diabetes-associated allele had significantly decreased BMI (body mass index) and waist circumferences [13]. In German population, the rs2237892, rs2237895 and rs2237897 were nominally associated with OGTT (oral glucose tolerance test)-derived insulin secretion indexes [14]. It has been reported that SNP rs2237892 affected repaglinide and rosiglitazone therapeutic response. Individuals who were rs2237892 TT homozygote carriers treated with repaglinide for 48 weeks exhibited lower 2-h glucose levels and significantly higher cumulative attainment rates of target 2-h glucose levels than the C allele carriers; patients with a greater number of rs2237892 C alleles showed larger augmentations in both fasting insulin and HOMA-IR. The rs2237895 C allele was also associated with greater increments in both fasting insulin and HOMA-IR. SNP rs2237897 associated with decrease in 2-h glucose levels in the rosiglitazone 48-week therapy [15]. The minor C-allele of rs2237895 of *KCNQ1* gene, which had a prevalence of about 42% among Caucasians was associated with reduced measures of insulin release following an oral glucose load suggesting that the increased risk T2DM [16]. Another SNP rs151290 was associated with 30-min C-peptide levels during OGTT, first-phase insulin secretion, and insulinogenic index after adjustment in the dominant model in the population of mainland China [17]. And rs151290 was associated with glucose-stimulated gastric inhibitory polypeptide and GLP-1 increase after adjustment in the dominant model [14]. The molecular mechanism of KCNQ1 SNPs in the intron affects insulin secretion is unclear [6,8,9], suggesting the important role of KCNQ1 in insulin secretion by pancreatic β-cells. The increased risk for T2DM associated with KCNQ1 is likely to be caused by a reduction in insulin secretion. Further studies will be needed to verify these findings and to fully delineate the role of KCNQ1 and its related pathways in disease pathogenesis [18] .

1.1.1.3 SLC30A8

GWA studies also identified that the zinc transporter solute carrier family 30 member 8 gene (*SLC30A8*) polymorphism was a risk of T2DM in several populations [19-25]. The *SLC30A8* gene is an especially interesting candidate gene because of its exclusive expression in the pancreas and major in β-cell [25, 26]. *SLC30A8* gene encodes ion channel zinc transporter protein member 8 (ZnT-8), which is thought to be the β-cell zinc concentration regulator. ZnT-8 is a critical molecule during the insulin maturation and release process that carries zinc from the cytoplasm into insulin secretory vesicles [26]. Therefore, its polymorphisms may affect its activity, which in turns correlates with T2DM susceptibility and therapeutic efficacy. SNP rs13266634 polymorphism (973C>T) in *SLC30A8* gene is a non synonymous SNP that causes an amino acid change from arginine (R) to tryptophan (W) at position 325 (Arg325Trp). This SNP is associated with T2DM onset and development in several populations [19-25]. It has been reported that the genetic polymorphism of *SLC30A8* was associated with impaired proinsulin conversion involved in the production and secretion pathway [27]. Fu *et al.* found that reduced ZnT-8 expression in cultured pancreatic β cells gives rise to reduced insulin response to hyperglycemia and that *SLC30A8* polymorphism could affect insulin secretion and glycemic response [28]. Another two studies indicated that patients with the rs13266634 C allele showed decreased first-phase insulin release following an intravenously administered glucose load [29, 30]. Furthermore, it has been found that the C alleles of rs13266634 at *SLC30A8* were associated with increased FPG and decreased insulin during the OGTT. An investigation also showed SNP rs13266634 increased the risk for T2DM by 1.24-fold in Chinese Han population [30]. A Chinese population study explored SLC30A8 is one susceptibility gene for T2DM and influences response to repaglinide. T2DM patients with T allele showed a better repaglinide response on FINS and PINS compared with CC wild-type homozygote [31].

1.1.1.4 WSF1

Wolfram syndrome 1 (*WFS1*) gene encodes wolframin, a 100 kDa transmembrane glycoprotein that maintains calcium homeostasis of the endoplasmic reticulum, which is expressed in neurons and pancreatic β-cells and regulates calcium fluxes in the endoplasmic reticulum [32]. *WFS1* is critical for survival and function of insulin-producing pancreatic β-cells [33]. *WFS1* gene polymorphism rs10010131 was confirmed with T2DM in several GWA studies [19-25]. In the Diabetes Prevention Program, it is noted a trend towards increased insulin secretion in carriers of the protective rs10010131 variants [34]. Rare mutations in *WFS1* cause Wolfram syndrome, variation in *WFS1* also predisposes to common T2DM. It has been reported that *WFS1* gene variants were associated with reduced insulin response to oral but not intravenous glucose [35-39]. *WFS1* gene was associated with estimates of a decreased pancreatic β-cell function among middle-aged individuals with abnormal glucose regulation [37]. *WFS1* gene was also associated with impaired incretin signaling, the level of glycemia determines SNP effects on insulin secretion. This indicated the increasing relevance of these SNPs during the progression of prediabetes stages toward clinically overt T2DM [10].

1.1.2 Genes involved in cell cycles

1.1.2.1 CDKAL1

A variant in the cyclin-dependent kinase 5 (CDK5) regulatory subunit associated protein 1-like 1 (*CDKAL1*) gene was associated with T2DM in individuals of European ancestry and individuals from Hong Kong of Han Chinese ancestry [22]. SNP rs7756992 is located in intron 5 of the *CDKAL1*. It resides in a large LD block of 201.7 kb that includes the *CDKAL1* gene exons 1-5 and the minimal promoter region but no other known genes. It has been proposed that polymorphism rs7756992 confers risk of T2DM through reduced insulin secretion because the insulin response for heterozygote was approximately 20% lower than for heterozygote or non carriers. The function of the CDKAL1 gene product is still unknown. But the CDKAL1 gene product is similar to CDK5 regulatory subunit-associated protein 1 (CDK5RAP1) gene product. CDK5RAP1 is expressed in neuronal tissues and inhibits CDK5 activity by binding to the CDK5 regulatory subunit p35. In pancreatic β-cells, CDK5 shows to act in the loss of β-cell function under glucotoxic conditions [41]. Inhibition of the CDK5/p35 complex prevents a decrease of insulin gene expression and glucotoxicity [42]. It is proposed that CDKAL1 may act in the inhibition of the CDK5/p35 complex in β-cells similar to CDK5RAP1 in neuronal tissue. Reduced

CDKAL1 expression or inhibitory function could lead to an impaired response to glucotoxicity. The association of CDKAL1 rs7756992 with T2DM was replicated in Japanese [43], Chinese [30] and Indians populations [44]. And variants in *CDKAL1* were strongly associated with β-cell function estimated by HOMA-β (Homeostasis model assessment for β cell function) [30]. Evidence from previous GWA studies implicating variants in *CDKAL1* and near *CDKN2A/B* implies that cell cycle dysregulation may be a common pathogenetic mechanism in T2DM [19, 20, 24].

1.1.2.2 CDKN2A/B

Cyclin-dependent kinase inhibitor-2A/B (CDKN2A/B) gene encode $p15^{INK4b}$ and $p16^{INK4a}$ protein which are tumor suppressors that inhibit cyclin-dependent kianse 6 (CDK6) and CDK4, respectively. CDKN2B and CDKN2A are expressed in pancreatic islets and adipocytes [19, 20, 24]. CDKN2A/2B (rs10811661) was associated with T2DM [45]. SNP rs10811661 located 125 kb upstream of the CDKN2B and CDKN2A genes, has been associated with T2DM in three of the GWA studies (OR for pooled studies 1.20 [95% CI 1.14–1.25], $P=5\times10^{-15}$) [19, 20, 24]. And the association was confirmed in Danish, Norwegian, French, Korean, Japanese and Chinese participants [10–15]. In murine models studies suggest that the rs10811661 polymorphism located upstream of the CDKN2B and CDKN2A genes may confer increased risk for T2DM by affecting β cell function [46-48].

1.1.2.3 CDC123/CAMK1D

SNP rs12779790 is located ~90 kb from cell division cycle 123 homolog [S. cerevisiae] (*CDC123*) gene and~63.5kb from calcium/calmodulin-dependent protein kinase I delta (*CAMK1D*) gene. *CDC123* gene encodes a protein involved in cell cycle regulation and nutritional control of gene transcription [23, 49]. CAMK1D regulates granulocyte function [50], it is also possible that a causative variant in this region is related to CAMK1D and affects pancreatic β-cell function through increased apoptosis. SNP rs12779790 is found associated with T2DM in several studies. G risk allele of rs12779790 was associated with a lower insulin genic index, corrected insulin response, and area under the insulin/glucose curve during OGTTs and a lower DI in carriers of the G allele [51]. In Asian Indian descent subjects also found the β-cell defect [34]. Trend toward lower β-cell function could be observed in Caucasians population [35, 38, 52]. SNP rs12779790 variation carriers showed a lower insulin response to glucose stimulation and noted a trend toward a reduced insulin response after arginine stimulation. Arginine stimulation during hyperglycemia is a measure of (near) maximal insulin secretion and has been suggested as a proxy for β-cell mass. This gene variant affected β-cell function by causing reduced β-cell mass due to enhanced apoptosis [50].

1.1.3 Genes involved in gene transcription

1.1.3.1 TCF2

The SNPs rs7501939 and rs4430796 on 17q12 are located in the first and second intron of the transcription factor 2 isoform b (*TCF2*) gene, respectively [53]. One of the variants is in *TCF2* (*HNF-1β*), a gene known to be mutated in individuals with maturity-onset diabetes of the young type 5 [54]. SNPs in *TCF2* are also associated with both T2DM and prostate cancer [53, 54]. Three genes with common variants that influence risk of T2DM were first discovered based on rare Mendelian mutations (*KCNJ11*, *WSF1* and *TCF2*). This is particularly interesting given the recent finding that SNPs in *TCF2* are also associated both with T2DM and prostate cancer [53, 54].

1.3.2 TCF7L2

Transcription factor 7-like 2 (*TCF7L2*) gene encodes a transcription factor (Tcf-4) which involved in the regulation of cellular proliferation and differentiation [55]. TCF7L2 plays an important role in the Wnt signaling pathway. TCF7L2 is involved in the growth, differentiation, proliferation, and insulin secretion of pancreatic β-cells [56]. GWA studies found variants in the *TCF7L2* showed to be associated with an increased risk for T2DM [19, 20, 22, 23, 25, 57]. The strongest associations with T2DM with a clear gene dose effect were reported for the rs7903146 variant [58]. *TCF7L2* was found to be associated with less weight loss in response to lifestyle intervention [59]. Genetic variants in the exon 4 (including rs7903146) block of *TCF7L2* were associated with impaired insulin secretion and incident diabetes in a prospective Chinese cohort [60]. *TCF7L2* gene polymorphism also affected the drug response for T2DM therapy which was the only predictor of sulfonylureas treatment failure [61]. The rs7903146 T-allele conferred a higher risk for sulfonylurea treatment failure [61]. It has been observed that homozygous carriers of the *TCF7L2* risk alleles (rs1225372 and rs7903146) were twice as likely not to respond to sulfonylureas as patients homozygous for the non-risk alleles [62].

1.1.3.3 HHEX

GWA studies identified that the haematopoietically expressed homeobox (*HHEX*) gene polymorphism was a risk of T2DM in several populations [19-25]. *HHEX* encodes the transcription factor hematopoietically expressed homeobox protein, which is expressed in the embryonic ventral-lateral foregut that causes the ventral pancreas and the liver [63]. It has been confirmed the significant association of *HHEX* with T2DM in the Japanese population [64]. *HHEX* was a common T2DM-susceptibility gene across different ethnic groups. The OR values of the three SNPs rs1111875, rs5015480 and rs7923837 genotyped in *HHEX* (1.20–1.46) were higher in Japanese than those of the European population (1.20) [64]. *HHEX* variant was associated with impaired proinsulin conversion [38]. SNP rs1111875 and rs7923837 was associated with T2DM independent of body fat [65]. SNP rs7923837 in the 3′-flanking region of the HHEX locus was associated with altered glucose-stimulated insulin release. This SNP's major allele represented a risk allele for β-cell dysfunction and might confer increased susceptibility of β-cells toward adverse environmental factors [66] Knockout of *HHEX* gene showed impair proliferation of endodermal epithelial cells, positioning of ventral foregut endoderm cells relative to the mesoderm, and budding and morphogenesis of the ventral pancreas [63]. This genetic manipulation finally provoked lethality during midge station [63].

1.1.3.4 JAZF1

The juxtaposed with another zinc finger gene 1 (*JAZF1*) gene encodes a transcriptional repressor of nuclear receptor subfamily 2, group C, member 2 (NR2C2) with three C2H2-type zinc fingers [67]. Mice deficient in Nr2c2 exhibit growth retardation, low IGF1 serum levels, and perinatal and early [53, 54] stnatal hypoglycaemia [68]. JAZF1 is expressed in pancreas, brain, thalamus, liver, uterus, endometrial and prostate. In a meta-analysis in East Asians, it has been found that the variant of *JAZF1* rs864745 was significantly associated with T2DM [69]. SNP rs864745 is in intron 1 of the JAZF1 gene. The major T-allele of the rs864745 conferring increased diabetes risk was associated with increased 2nd phase serum insulin release during an IVGTT, and an increased fasting serum insulin level [69]. Carriers of the diabetes-associated T-allele of rs864745 had an allele dependent 3% decrease in BIGTT-AIR. JAZF1 is expressed in the pancreas [67], one might speculate that a gain-of-function variant in JAZF1 may lead to postnatal growth restriction also affecting pancreatic β-cell mass and function [51]. SNP rs864745 in JAZF1 were significantly associated with traits of insulin secretion in a glucose-tolerant Danish population [51].

1.1.4 Others

1.1.4.1 PPAR-γ2

Peroxisome proliferator-activated receptor-γ2 (PPAR-γ2) is one of PPAR-γ isoforms and is a member of the nuclear hormone receptor subfamily of transcription factors, which regulates transcription of various genes [70]. *PPAR-γ* plays an important role in adipocyte differentiation, regulating glucose, and lipid homeostasis [70]. Pro12Ala is one of important polymorphism in codon 12 of exon B causing proline-to-alanine change [71]. The Ala allele reduces the transcriptional activity of PPAR-γ2 and may protect against T2DM compared with the more common Pro/Pro genotype [72, 73]. The effects of the PPAR-γ2 Pro12Ala polymorphism on glucose and insulin metabolism may be modified by prenatal exposure to famine during midge station [74]. Patients with the Pro12Ala genotype had a better therapeutic response to rosiglitazone than the Pro12Pro genotype subjects. The genetic variations in the PPAR-γ2 gene can affect the response to rosiglitazone therapeutic efficacy in T2DM patients [75].

1.1.4.2 IGF2BP2

Insulin-like growth factor 2 mRNA-binding protein 2 (IGF2BP2) belongs to an mRNA-binding protein family that plays role in RNA localization, stability and translation [76]. IGF2BP2 is highly expressed in pancreatic islets and binds to insulin-like growth factor 2 (IGF-2), which is an important growth and insulin signaling molecule [24]. IGF2BP2 is a homolog of IGF2BP1, which binds to the 5'UTR of IGF2 mRNA and regulates IGF2 translation [77]. Several GWA studies have found that subjects carrying mutant alleles of SNPs rs1470579 and rs4402960 in *IGF2BP2* gene showed a moderately increased risk of T2DM. Several studies have confirmed this result in Asian populations [30, 57, 78, 79]. T2DM patients with different *IGF2BP2* genotypes showed various levels of insulin secretion. It has been demonstrated that variants in *IGF2BP2* gene affect first-phase insulin secretion and the disposition index detected by hyperglycemic clamps [80].

Interactions between genetic variation in *IGF2BP2* and T2DM maybe exerted through this IGF2 pathway and through the insulin pathway. The *IGF2BP2* gene is located at chromosome 3q27.2. Intron 2 is the longest intron among mammalian species. SNPs rs1470579 and rs4402960 are located in a 50-kb region of this intron. Diabetes-predisposing variants may affect regulation of IGF2BP2 expression [20]. The *IGF2BP2* gene variant (rs4402960) was associated with insulin sensitivity, FPG, glucose AUC, and FPG [81]. SNP rs4402960 was also associated with reductions in first-phase insulin secretion and in the disposition index, which reflected the failing adaptive capacity of pancreatic β-cells [80] resulting in hyperglycemia including FPG and PPG. SNP rs4402960 has also been shown to be associated with the disposition index in Hispanic Americans [82], HOMA-β in non-diabetic Japanese individuals and lower acute insulin release and tolerance [64]. SNP rs4402960 is strongly associated with an increased risk of T2DM and increased AUC of glucose in individuals of Dutch descent [83]. Wu et al observed a significant association of SNPs (rs1470579 and rs4402960) in *IGF2BP2* [1.17 (1.03–1.32); *P*=0.014] with combined IFG (impaired fasting glycemia)/T2DM group. The association of these SNPs with HOMA-β reduction suggested that *IGF2BP2* gene confers T2DM risk through a reduction of β-cell function [30]. Another study in Chinese T2DM population according with these results and found *IGF2BP2* variations effect on the therapeutic efficacy of repaglinide treatment in Chinese T2DM patients. Patients with the rs1470579 AC+CC genotypes had poor responses to repaglinide treatment with respect to FPG and PPG compared with individuals with the AA genotype. Patients with the GT+TT genotypes of rs4402960 also showed a better repaglinide therapeutic effect on PINS compared with individuals with the GG genotype. Replication of this research has indicated that *IGF2BP2* variants were more likely to be associated with reduced β-cell function [80, 84]. IGF2BP2 was shown to affect insulin secretion in a previous study. Understanding the biological mechanism by which variants in *IGF2BP2* could mediate these effects on the biphasic pattern of insulin secretion will require further investigation.

1.1.4.3 FTO

Fat mass and obesity associated (*FTO*) gene was found in a GWA study for T2DM susceptibility genes identified and showed to predispose to diabetes through an effect on BMI [85]. SNPs rs9939609 in the *FTO* gene region on chromosome 16 was strongly associated with T2DM [85]. A number of SNPs in tight linkage disequilibrium with rs9939609, and residing in the first intron of the *FTO* gene, had been associated with obesity in large populations of adults and children. It had been showed that common variation rs9939609 was reproducibly associated with BMI and obesity from childhood into old age [86]. And recently it has been identified T2DM risk variants only the risk variant of the FTO gene (rs8050136) showed statistically significant association with BMI, FMI, and Waist Circumferences [87] .Some data indicated that *FTO* SNP rs9939609 was associated with differences in BMI, with the presence of the A allele linked to a greater risk of increased BMI and increased values for specific measures of adiposity, such as the sum of skin fold values and total body water as assessed by isotope analysis [88].

1.1.4.4 THADA

THADA (thyroid adenoma associated) gene encodes thyroid adenoma–associated protein may involve in the death receptor pathway and apoptosis [89]. Disruption of THADA by chromosomal rearrangements (including fusion with intronic sequence from PPAR-γ) is observed in thyroid adenomas [90]. The function of THADA has not been well-characterized, but there is some evidence to suggest that it may be involved in the death receptor pathway and apoptosis [89, 91]. The THADA gene variant was also associated with lower β-cell response to GLP-1 and arginine, suggested lower β-cell mass as a possible pathogenic mechanism [92]. SNP rs7578597 was a non-synonymous SNP causing threonine to alanine in 1187 position which strongly associated with T2DM (combined OR [95%CI] of 1.15[1.10-1.20], $P=1.1\times10^{-9}$) resided in exon 24 of *THADA* gene[23]. Subjects with the rs7578597 (T1187A) gene variant in *THADA* had a reduced β-cell mass due to increased apoptosis [92]. Analyses in the control subjects showed that THADA SNP rs7578597 was association with 2-h insulin during oral glucose tolerance tests [93].

1.1.4.5 TSPAN8/ LGR5

Tetraspanin 8 is a cell-surface glycoprotein, widely expressed cell surface glycoprotein known to form complexes with integrins to regulate cell motility in cancer cell lines [23, 94]. Tetraspanin 8 gene (TSPAN8) polymorphism rs7961581 was one of the strongest statistical signals associated with T2DM. SPAN8/LGR5 rs7961581 was significantly associated with T2DM in a meta-analysis in East Asians [69]. SNP rs7961581 associated with decreased levels of CIR, of AUC-insulin/AUC-glucose ratio, and of the insulinogenic index [51]. SNP rs7961581 resided ~110 kb upstream of *TSPAN8* gene. Because 6-integrin binding to laminin had been shown to negatively affect pancreatic β-cell mass maintenance [95], it was possible that variation in TSPAN8 influenced pancreatic β-cell function.

1.1.4.6 ADAMTS9

ADAMTS9 is a member of the ADAMTS (a disintegrin and metalloproteinase with thrombospondin motifs) protein family which has been implicated in the cleavage of proteoglycans [96], the control of organ maturation, development [97] and inhibition of angiogenesis [98]. ADAMTS9 is a secreted metalloprotease that cleaves the proteoglycans versican and aggrecan, and is expressed in skeletal muscle and pancreas [23]. SNP rs4607103 in *ADAMTS9* gene representing a cluster of associated SNPs, resides ~38 kb upstream of the *ADAMTS9* gene, and also associated with T2DM susceptibility [52]. It has been found common diabetes-related C allele of rs4607103 at chromosome 3p14.3-2 upstream of ADAMTS9 was associated with a decrease in insulin sensitivity of peripheral tissues, as estimated from a euglycemichy perinsulinemic clamp [69]. And impairment of insulin sensitivity occurred in the presence of an increase in serum insulin levels in response to intravenous and oral glucose loads [69]. The major C-risk allele of rs4607103 near ADAMTS9 conferred increased risk of T2DM, associated with increased fasting plasma glucose levels and reduced insulin-stimulated glucose uptake during a euglycemic-hyperinsulinemic clamp. The C-risk allele also showed statistically significant associations with increased levels of serum insulin at 30 min after oral ingestion of glucose as well as with increased first and second phase serum insulin release as estimated from an IVGTT [99].

1.1.4.7 NOTCH2

Notch 2 (Notch homolog 2 [Drosophila]) expresses when pancreatic buds branch and is restricted to embryonic ducts, should be the source for endocrine and exocrine stem cells in mice [23, 100]. Notch pathway plays key role in dictating endocrine differentiation. Activation of this pathway is critical for the maintenance of the progenitor pool between the first and second transitions of pancreatic development [101]. NOTCH2 is a type 1 transmembrane receptor. The SNP rs10923931 residing in intron 5 of the NOTCH2 gene strongly associate with T2DM susceptibility. SNP rs10923931 is near complete linkage disequilibrium with SNP rs2641348 in the ADAM30 gene [23]. Rs2641348, a non-synonymous SNP (L359P) within the neighboring ADAM metallo-peptidase domain 30 gene (ADAM30) represented the same signal (r^2=0.92 based on HapMap CEU data) and was also followed-up.

1.1.4.8 PTPRD

A GWA study in Chinese population identified two genes, PTPRD and SRR, which were not previously described to be involved in diabetes or glucose metabolism [102]. PTPRD is the protein tyrosine phosphatase receptor type D gene and widely expressed in skeletal muscle, pancreas, and brain which belong to the receptor type IIA (R2A) subfamily of protein tyrosine phosphatases (PTPs). The R2A PTP subfamily comprises leukocyte common antigen-related (LAR), protein tyrosine phosphatase sigma (PTPRS), and PTPRD. The R2A family has been implicated in neural development, cancer, and diabetes [103]. PTPRD-deficient mice exhibited impaired learning and memory, early growth retardation, neonatal mortality, posture and motor defects [104]. LAR- and PTPRS-deficient mice showed defected glucose homeostasis and insulin sensitivity [105-107]. Transgenic mice over expressing LAR in skeletal muscle showed whole-body insulin resistance [108]. R2A subfamily members have similar structure [109]. PTPRD could act in T2DM pathogenesis and affect insulin signaling on its target cells. But it need further

Gene	SNP	Position	Effect	References	Chromosome
KCNJ11	rs5219	Exon	E23K	[25]	11p15.1
PPAR-γ2	rs1801282	Exon B	P12A	[74]	3p25
TCF2	rs7501939	Intron 1	/	[53]	17q12
	rs4430796	Intron 2	/	[53]	
WSF1	rs10010131	Intron	/	[40]	4p12
	rs752854	Intron	/	[37]	
	rs6446482	Intron	/	[37]	
	rs734312	Exon	H61R	[37]	
TCF7L2	rs7903146	Exon 4		[58]	10q25.3
HHEX	rs1111875	3'-UTR	/	[20]	
	rs5015480	?	/	[20]	
	rs7923837	?	/	[20]	
SLC30A8	rs13266634	Exon 8	R325W	[25]	8q24.11
CDKAL1	rs7756992	Intron 5	/	[22]	6p22.3
	rs7754840	?	/	[118]	
	rs9465871	?	/	[30]	
	rs10946398	?	/	[30]	
CDKN2A-2B	rs10811661	?	/	[19]	9p21
IGF2BP2	rs1470579	Intron 2	/	[20]	3q27.2
	rs4402960	Intron 2	/	[20]	
FTO	rs8050136	Intron	/	[87]	16q12.2
	rs9939609	Intron 1		[86]	
JAZF1	rs864745	Intron 1	/	[23]	7p15.2-p15.1
CDC123/CAMK1D	rs12779790	?	/	[23]	10p13
THADA	rs7578597	Exon 24	T1187A	[23]	2p21
TSPAN8	rs7961581	?	/	[23]	12q14.1-q21.1
ADAMTS9	rs4607103	near	/	[23]	3p14.3-2
NOTCH2	rs 10923931	Intron 5	/	[23]	1p13-p11
PTPRD	rs17584499	Intron 10	/	[102]	9p24.1-p23
SRR	rs391300			[102]	17p13.3
	rs4523957			[102]	
KCNQ1	rs2237892	Intron 15	/	[23]	11p15.5
	rs2237895	Intron 15	/	[23]	
	rs2237897	Intron 15	/	[23]	
	rs2283228	Intron 15	/	[11]	
	rs151290	Intron 15	/	[17]	

Table 1.1 Summary of associated genes

characterize. *PTPRD* gene polymorphism rs17584499 showed significant association with T2DM ($P = 8.54610^{-10}$; odds ratio [OR] = 1.57; 95% confidence interval [CI] = 1.36–1.82) [102]. This SNP locates in intron 10.

1.1.4.9 SRR

SRR (serine racemase) gene encodes aserine racemase that synthesizes D-serine from L-serine [110, 111]. D-serine (co-agonist) and the neurotransmitter glutamate bind to the N-methyl Daspartate (NMDA) receptors and trigger excitatory neurotransmission in the brain [102, 112, 113]. NMDA receptor activation requires binding of glutamate and D-serine, which plays a neuromodulatory role in NMDA receptor transmission, synaptic plasticity, cell migration, and neurotoxicity [62]. D-serine and SRR express in the pancreas [114]. Glutamate signaling has function involved in positively regulates insulin and glucagon secretion in pancreatic islets [115-117]. Thus, SRR and D-serine may play roles in the etiology of T2DM. SNPs rs391300 and rs4523957 in the SRR gene were associated with T2DM in a Han Chinese GWA study. SNPs rs391300 and rs4523957 were in tight LD with each other (r^2 = 0.942 in HapMap HCB)[102]. The nearby SNP rs216193 also showed significant association; this SNP resides 3.8 kb upstream from SRR. SNP rs216193 was in tight LD with rs391300 (r^2 = 0.942 in HapMap HCB) [102].

2. Anti-diabetic drugs pharmacogenetics

2.1 Insulin secretagogue agents ------sulfonylureas (SUs)

The sulfonylurea anti-diabetic agents are insulin secretogogues including the first generation sulfonylureas (acetohexomide, chlorpropamide, tolazamide and tolbutamide) and second generation sulfonylureas (glibenclamide (glyburide), glipizide, gliclazide, and glimepiride) which are most widely used for T2DM treatment by closing the pancreatic β-cell potassium channels and stimulation insulin secretion [119].

2.1.1 Cytochrome P450

Sulfonylurea hypoglycemic agents are metabolized by cytochrome P450 2C9 (CYP2C9) enzyme. Genetic polymorphisms Arg144Cys (*CYP2C9*2*) and Ile359Leu (*CYP2C9*3*) could affect the safety and efficacy of sulphanylureas drugs in T2DM patients [120]. *CYP2C9* genotypes significantly affected glyburide pharmacokinetics. Carriers with *CYP2C9* variant *3 had decreased oral clearances [121]. Suzuki *et al* reported the subjects with *CYP2C9*3* alleles showed the metabolic activity decrease of glimepiride hydroxylation and a marked elevation in the plasma concentrations of glimepiride, compared with subjects with a *CYP2C9*1/*1*(wild type). The elevated glimepiride concentrations in subject with *CYP2C9*1/*3* may increase the pharmacological effects [122]. Zhang *et al* reported the pharmacokinetics of gliclazide modified release were affected mainly by *CYP2C19* genetic polymorphism in healthy Chinese subjects [123].

2.1.2 Sulfonylurea receptor

The sulphonylurea receptor is a subunit of the ATP-sensitive potassium channel located in pancreatic β-cell. The variants in the exon 16 -3C/T variant (rs1799854) of *SUR1* (Sulfonylurea Receptor 1) was associated with T2DM and 25% reduction in second-phase insulin secretion in -3T allele carriers in Dutch subjects with normal glucose tolerance (NGT) and impaired glucose tolerance (IGT) [124]. The association also found in Japanese [125] and

Finnish population [126]. A recent publication reported genotyped 25 SNPs from 661 Chinese T2DM patients who received 8 weeks of gliclazide therapy. The subjects with GG genotype in SUR exon 33(S1369A, rs757110) had a 7.7% greater decrease in FPG and 11.9% greater decrease in HbA1c after 8 weeks of gliclazide therapy [127].

2.1.3 Others

It was described that the exon 33 of the ABCC8 (rs757110) and KCNJ11 (rs5210) genes were associated with gliclazide antidiabetic efficacy [127]. SNPs of TCF7L2 had been consistently associated with T2DM in different ethnic descent and also had great impact on the T2DM patients' response to sulfonylureas [128]. The Go-DARTS2 study reported that the T allele of rs7903146 was associated with increased HbA1c in both cases and controls [129]. The same study group revealed that carriers of TCF7L2 variants were more likely to fail sulfonylurea therapy but not metformin (HbA1c > 7 %) within 3-12 months of treatment initiation [62].

Hepatocyte nuclear factor-1α (HNF-1α) is a homeodomain-containing transcription factor that expressed in the pancreatic β-cell and HNF-1α SNPs have been associated with β-cell dysfunction and maturity onset diabetes of the young (MODY) [130]. Variations in HNF-1α polymorphisms of T2DM were reported to be more sensitive to the hypoglycaemic effects of sulfonylureas [131-133]. *Pearson et al* reported that patients with HNF-1α polymorphisms (P129T, E132K, R159W, R229P, W267R and P291fsinsC) had a 5.2-fold greater response to gliclazide than to metformin and 3.9-fold greater response to gliclazide than patients without HNF-1α mutations [134].

2.2 Insulin secretagogue agents ------ Non-sulfonylureas

Meglitinides (repaglinide and nateglinide) represent a new class of insulin secretagogue, structurally unrelated to sulphanylureas by very rapid onset and abbreviated duration of action [135]. Meglitinides stimulate first-phase insulin release in a glucose-sensitive manner and reduce the risk of hypoglycemic events.

2.2.1 Cytochrome P450 and transporters

Repaglinide is metabolized by CYP2C8 and CYP3A4 [136]. The *CYP2C8*3* variant (Arg139Lys, Lys399Arg) allele was associated with reduced plasma concentrations of repaglinide [137]. Repaglinide mean AUC and maximium plasma concentration (C_{max}) were 45 and 39 lower, respectively, in subjects with the *CYP2C8*1/*3* genotype compared with wild-type homozygotes. Repaglinide AUC was also 13% lower in subjects with the *CYP2C8*1/*4* genotype compared with wild-type homozygotes, although this was not statistically significant [137]. Genetic polymorphisms of *CYP3A4*, specifically *CYP3A4*18*, played a major role in contributing to the inter-individual variability in repaglinide's pharmacokinetics [138].

The oral bioavailability of nateglinide is about 73%, and it is rapidly absorbed and extensively metabolized primarily by CYP2C9 in the liver and a smaller fraction by CYP3A4 and CYP2D6 [139]. Nateglinide is confirmed as a substrate of CYP2C9. A previous report showed that the *CYP2C9*3* allele was associated with significantly reduced oral nateglinide clearance and pharmacokinetic parameters, which seemed to be unaffected by *CYP2C9*2* and *CYP2D6*4* or *5 carriers [140].

The meglitinide class drug nateglinide is metabolized by CYP2C9. According to pharmacokinetic data, moderate dose adjustments based on CYP2C9 genotypes may help in reducing interindividual variability in the anti hyperglycemic effects of nateglinide [173]. Carriers of the *CYP2C9*3/*3* genotype may be at a slightly higher risk of hypoglycemia compared to carriers of *CYP2C9*1*, particularly when taking nateglinide doses above 120 mg [140].

Polymorphic organic anion transporting polypeptide 1B1 (SLCO1B1) is a major determinant of repaglinide pharmacokinetics [141]. SLCO1B1 (which codes the *OATP1B1* gene, also known as OATP-C, OATP2) polymorphisms are important predictors of repaglinide pharmacokinetics [141]. Repaglinide AUC was 60–110% greater in participants with the c.521CC genotype than in those with the c.521TT genotype after ingestion of single repaglinide doses ranging from 0.25 to 2mg [142]. Haplotypes of SLCO1B1*1b/*1b (c.388 G–c.521 T) was associated with reduced pharmacokinetic exposure after a single dose oral administration of 2 mg repaglinide, including decreased AUC0-∞ and increased clearance of repaglinide [143].

2.2.2 Others

An association of (*IGF2BP2*) rs1470579 and rs4402960 polymorphisms and development of T2DM and therapeutic efficacy of repaglinide in Chinese T2DM patients was reported. The effects of the repaglinide treatment on FPG ($P<0.05$) and PPG ($P<0.05$) were reduced in patients with the rs1470579 AC+CC genotypes compared with AA genotype carriers. Patients with the rs4402960 GT+TT genotypes exhibited an enhanced effect of repaglinide treatment on PINS ($P<0.01$) compared with GG genotype subjects [144]. *SLC30A8* rs13266634 and rs16889462 polymorphisms were associated with repaglinide therapeutic efficacy in Chinese T2DM patients. There were significantly augmented repaglinide effects in patients with rs13266634 CT+TT genotypes on FINS and PINS compared with rs13266634 CC genotype. And patients with rs16889462 GA genotype showed enhanced repaglinide effects on FPG, PPG, and HbAlc compared with GG genotype [31]. Variations in the neural nitric oxide synthase adaptor protein (NOS1AP) involved in insulin secretion and insulin signal pathway may explain some of the variability in response to anti-diabetic drug. A common variant in rs10494366 was associated with repaglinide monotherapy efficacy on insulin resistance in newly diagnosed Shanghai Chinese T2DM patients [145]. And *sheng et al* study suggested that NAMPT -3186C>T polymorphism was significantly associated with plasma levels of PINS and CHO in Chinese T2DM patients with repaglinide monotherapy [146]. KCNQ1 polymorphism rs2237892 was associated with repaglinide's efficacy on improving insulin sensitivity in Chinese patients with T2DM [15].

2.3 Biguanides

Metformin (a biguanide) is among the most widely prescribed drugs and has a gluco-regulator effect in the presence of endogenous insulin by reducing gastrointestinal glucose absorption, decreasing endogenous glucose production and reducing peripheral resistance to insulin [147].

2.3.1 Transporters

Organic cation transporter 1 (OCT1, gene name SLC22A1) is the major mechanism for metformin entry into hepatocytes and enterocytes [148]. Human OCT1 is highly polymorphic. Shu' study provided proof of concept that genetic variation in OCT1 may be associated with variation in response to metformin OCT1 Met420del had reduced activity for metformin [149]. Another study in healthy subjects also confirmed polymorphisms in OCT1 were associated with the renal clearance of metformin [150]. Low-function OCT1 amino acid substitutions Arg61Cys, Ser401Gly, Met420del, and Gly465Arg, and the OCT1 promoter-linked variant rs1867351, were associated with an increase in the renal clearance of metformin by~20% and ~30%, respectively. These data suggested that a reduction in OCT1 expression or activity may increase renal excretion of metformin [150]. But in T2DM patients, the OCT1 loss-of-function variants, Arg61Cys and Met420del, did not attenuate the HbA1C reduction achieved by metformin [151].

2.3.2 Others

Recently, serine-threonine kinase 11 (*STK11*), which phosphorylates AMPK, has also been reported to be involved in metformin effects. The *STK11* rs8111699 SNP influenced insulin sensitivity and metformin efficacy [152]. Schroner et al showed that the degree of reduction in HbA1c and FPG after ulphonylurea treatment in addition to previous metformin monotherapy was related to *TCF7L2* gene polymorphisms [153]. ATM, a gene known to be involved in DNA repair and cell cycle control, played a role in the effect of metformin upstream of AMP-activated protein kinase, and variation in this gene altered glycemic response to metformin [154].

2.4 Euglycemic agents

Thiazolidinediones (pioglitazone, rosiglitazone) are insulin sensitizing agents and have glucose and lipid lowering activity. They are selective agonists for the PPAR-γ and decrease insulin resistance and enhance the biological response to endogenously produced insulin.

2.4.1 Cytochrome P450

Both rosiglitazone and pioglitazone are extensively metabolized in the liver by CYP2C8 [155, 156]. Kirchheiner and colleagues considered the influence of the *CYP2C8*3* polymorphism on single dose and multiple-dose rosiglitazone (8 mg) pharmacokinetics in German healthy volunteers [157]. Tornio et al evaluated the effects of the *CYP2C8*3* allele on single-dose pioglitazone (15 mg) pharmacokinetics in healthy volunteers [158]. The weight-adjusted pioglitazone AUC was 34% lower in *CYP2C8*3* homozygotes and 26% lower in heterozygotes compared with wild-type homozygotes ($P < 0.05$, both comparisons). The half-life of pioglitazone was significantly shorter in heterozygotes (3.4 h) and *CYP2C8*3* homozygotes (3.3 h) compared with wild-type homozygotes (4.5 h). Daily et al reported following a single dose of rosiglitazone 4 mg, mean AUC was 29% lower and weight-adjusted oral clearance was 39% higher in heterozygotes compared with wild-type homozygotes [159].

2.4.2 Others

Rosiglitazone improves insulin sensitivity by reducing plasma glucose levels and serum insulin, NEFA and triglyceride and by increasing HDL cholesterol levels [160, 161]. *Vestergaard et al* reported rosiglitazone treatment, in combination with insulin and metformin, of patients with severe primary insulin resistance due to IR mutations and diabetes mellitus, had no impact on the measured estimates of glucose and lipid metabolism [162]. It was found that variations SNP45 and SNP276 in the *adiponectin* gene could affect the rosiglitazone treatment response to the serum adiponectin level and blood glucose control [158]. *Sun et al* reported that the adiponectin allele 45T/G and -11377C/G polymorphisms were significantly associated with the therapeutic efficacy of multiple-dose rosiglitazone in Chinese patients with T2DM [163]. And *TNF-a* G-308A polymorphism might be associated with the therapeutic efficacy of rosiglitazone in T2DM patients [164]. Genetic variations 11482G/A in the perilipin gene could affect weight gain associated with rosiglitazone treatment in patients with T2DM [165]. *Brunham et al* demonstrated that the ATP-binding cassette transporter subfamily A number 1 (ABCA1) probably had an effect on islet cholesterol homeostasis, and influencing glucose tolerance and insulin secretion [166]. The 219K variant of *ABCA1* gene was associated with the therapeutic effect of rosiglitazone. The RR homozygotes had a better response to rosiglitazone treatment in terms of insulin sensitivity improvement than minor K allele carriers [167]. The genetic variations in the *PPAR-γ2* gene could affect the response to rosiglitazone treatment in patients with T2DM. Patients with the Pro12Ala genotype in the *PPAR-γ2* gene had a better therapeutic response to rosiglitazone than did patients with the Pro12Pro genotype [75]. *LPIN1* genetic variations rs10192566 could affect rosiglitazone treatment response in T2DM [168]. Zhang et al reptored carriers of A allele of Thr394Thr or Ser allele of Gly482Ser in *PGC-1a* gene showed a trend for poor therapeutic efficacy to rosiglitazone for A allele of Thr394Thr but a significant improvement in its effectiveness for Gly482Ser. Variants in PGC-1α gene might impair the therapeutic efficacy of rosiglitazone [169].

Himelfarb et al investigated TNF-α and IL-6 expression in leukocytes and their association with polymorphisms and bone markers in diabetic individuals treated with pioglitazone. *TNF-a* -308G>A polymorphism appeared to be involved in regulation of gene expression independently of hyperglycemia and its interaction with pioglitazone might modify tALP, a important bone marker. *IL6* -174G>C variant was related with reduced risk of postprandial hyperglycemia but not with mRNA expression or bone markers [170]. The *PPAR-γ* Pro12Ala gene polymorphism was associated with the response to pioglitazone in Chinese patients with T2DM [171]. Pioglitazone treatment had significantly beneficial effects on serum lipid profile and blood pressure in S447S genotype carriers. The S447X variant in lipoprotein lipase (LPL) gene might be a cause for therapy modification by pioglitazone [172].

3. Conclusion

The rapidly increasing prevalence of T2DM is becoming a tremendous public health problem that affects more than 170 million patients worldwide. T2DM is a complex metabolic disorder with two major pathophysiological features: insulin resistance and pancreatic β-cell dysfunction. The mechanism of this disease remains unknown; however, environmental factors and genetic variations are considered two major contributors to onset and development of T2DM. In this chapter, we introduced gene associated with T2DM, such as: KCNJ11, KCNQ1, SLC30A8, WSF1, CDKAL1, CDKN2A/B, TCF2, TCF7L2, HHEX, JAZF1, PPAR-γ2, IGF2BP2, FTO, THADA, TSPAN8/ LGR5, ADAMTS9, NOTCH2, PTPRD, and SRR. Meanwhile, we described four anti-diabetic drugs pharmacogenetics, including insulin secretagogue agent sulfonylureas (SUs) and meglitinides, biguanides, and euglycemic agents. Genetic polymorphisms in drug-metabolizing enzymes, transporters, receptors, and other drug targets have been linked to interindividual differences in the efficacy and toxicity of a number of medications. Mutations in genes important in drug absorption, distribution, metabolism and excretion (ADME) play critical role in pharmacogenetics of diabetes. Numerous genes that influence pharmacogenetics of oral antidiabetics have been described. The investigations of genes associated with T2DM benefits of personalized medicine. And different types of genetic mutations and their influence on the response to therapy with oral antidiabetics are needed future study.

4. References

[1] Permutt, M.A., Wasson, J., Cox, N. (2005) Genetic epidemiology of diabetes. *J Clin Invest* 115, 1431-9.

[2] Clement, J.P.t., Kunjilwar, K., Gonzalez, G., Schwanstecher, M., Panten, U., Aguilar-Bryan, L., Bryan, J. (1997) Association and stoichiometry of K(ATP) channel subunits. *Neuron* 18, 827-38.

[3] Koster, J.C., Marshall, B.A., Ensor, N., Corbett, J.A., Nichols, C.G. (2000) Targeted overactivity of beta cell K(ATP) channels induces profound neonatal diabetes. *Cell* 100, 645-54.

[4] Nielsen, E.M., Hansen, L., Carstensen, B., Echwald, S.M., Drivsholm, T., Glumer, C., Thorsteinsson, B., Borch-Johnsen, K., Hansen, T., Pedersen, O. (2003) The E23K variant of Kir6.2 associates with impaired post-OGTT serum insulin response and increased risk of type 2 diabetes. *Diabetes* 52, 573-7.

[5] Love-Gregory, L., Wasson, J., Lin, J., Skolnick, G., Suarez, B., Permutt, M.A. (2003) E23K single nucleotide polymorphism in the islet ATP-sensitive potassium channel gene (Kir6.2) contributes as much to the risk of Type II diabetes in Caucasians as the PPARgamma Pro12Ala variant. *Diabetologia* 46, 136-7.

[6] Barroso, I., Luan, J., Middelberg, R.P., Harding, A.H., Franks, P.W., Jakes, R.W., Clayton, D., Schafer, A.J., O'Rahilly, S., Wareham, N.J. (2003) Candidate gene association study in type 2 diabetes indicates a role for genes involved in beta-cell function as well as insulin action. *PLoS Biol* 1, E20.

[7] Schwanstecher, C., Meyer, U., Schwanstecher, M. (2002) K(IR)6.2 polymorphism predisposes to type 2 diabetes by inducing overactivity of pancreatic beta-cell ATP-sensitive K(+) channels. *Diabetes* 51, 875-9.

[8] Gloyn, A.L., Weedon, M.N., Owen, K.R., Turner, M.J., Knight, B.A., Hitman, G., Walker, M., Levy, J.C., Sampson, M., Halford, S., McCarthy, M.I., Hattersley, A.T., Frayling, T.M. (2003) Large-scale association studies of variants in genes encoding the pancreatic beta-cell KATP channel subunits Kir6.2 (KCNJ11) and SUR1 (ABCC8) confirm that the KCNJ11 E23K variant is associated with type 2 diabetes. *Diabetes* 52, 568-72.

[9] Yu, M., Xu, X.J., Yin, J.Y., Wu, J., Chen, X., Gong, Z.C., Ren, H.Y., Huang, Q., Sheng, F.F., Zhou, H.H., Liu, Z.Q. KCNJ11 Lys23Glu and TCF7L2 rs290487(C/T) polymorphisms affect therapeutic efficacy of repaglinide in Chinese patients with type 2 diabetes. *Clin Pharmacol Ther* 87, 330-5.

[10] Robbins, J. (2001) KCNQ potassium channels: physiology, pathophysiology, and pharmacology. *Pharmacol Ther* 90, 1-19.

[11] Unoki, H., Takahashi, A., Kawaguchi, T., Hara, K., Horikoshi, M., Andersen, G., Ng, D.P., Holmkvist, J., Borch-Johnsen, K., Jorgensen, T., Sandbaek, A., Lauritzen, T., Hansen, T., Nurbaya, S., Tsunoda, T., Kubo, M., Babazono, T., Hirose, H., Hayashi,

M., Iwamoto, Y., Kashiwagi, A., Kaku, K., Kawamori, R., Tai, E.S., Pedersen, O., Kamatani, N., Kadowaki, T., Kikkawa, R., Nakamura, Y., Maeda, S. (2008) SNPs in KCNQ1 are associated with susceptibility to type 2 diabetes in East Asian and European populations. *Nat Genet* 40, 1098-102.

[12] Yasuda, K., Miyake, K., Horikawa, Y., Hara, K., Osawa, H., Furuta, H., Hirota, Y., Mori, H., Jonsson, A., Sato, Y., Yamagata, K., Hinokio, Y., Wang, H.Y., Tanahashi, T., Nakamura, N., Oka, Y., Iwasaki, N., Iwamoto, Y., Yamada, Y., Seino, Y., Maegawa, H., Kashiwagi, A., Takeda, J., Maeda, E., Shin, H.D., Cho, Y.M., Park, K.S., Lee, H.K., Ng, M.C., Ma, R.C., So, W.Y., Chan, J.C., Lyssenko, V., Tuomi, T., Nilsson, P., Groop, L., Kamatani, N., Sekine, A., Nakamura, Y., Yamamoto, K., Yoshida, T., Tokunaga, K., Itakura, M., Makino, H., Nanjo, K., Kadowaki, T., Kasuga, M. (2008) Variants in KCNQ1 are associated with susceptibility to type 2 diabetes mellitus. *Nat Genet* 40, 1092-7.

[13] Hu, C., Wang, C., Zhang, R., Ma, X., Wang, J., Lu, J., Qin, W., Bao, Y., Xiang, K., Jia, W. (2009) Variations in KCNQ1 are associated with type 2 diabetes and beta cell function in a Chinese population. *Diabetologia* 52, 1322-5.

[14] Mussig, K., Staiger, H., Machicao, F., Kirchhoff, K., Guthoff, M., Schafer, S.A., Kantartzis, K., Silbernagel, G., Stefan, N., Holst, J.J., Gallwitz, B., Haring, H.U., Fritsche, A. (2009) Association of type 2 diabetes candidate polymorphisms in KCNQ1 with incretin and insulin secretion. *Diabetes* 58, 1715-20.

[15] Yu, W., Hu, C., Zhang, R., Wang, C., Qin, W., Lu, J., Jiang, F., Tang, S., Bao, Y., Xiang, K., Jia, W. Effects of KCNQ1 polymorphisms on the therapeutic efficacy of oral antidiabetic drugs in Chinese patients with type 2 diabetes. *Clin Pharmacol Ther* 89, 437-42.

[16] Holmkvist, J., Banasik, K., Andersen, G., Unoki, H., Jensen, T.S., Pisinger, C., Borch-Johnsen, K., Sandbaek, A., Lauritzen, T., Brunak, S., Maeda, S., Hansen, T., Pedersen, O. (2009) The type 2 diabetes associated minor allele of rs2237895 KCNQ1 associates with reduced insulin release following an oral glucose load. *PLoS One* 4, e5872.

[17] Liu, Y., Zhou, D.Z., Zhang, D., Chen, Z., Zhao, T., Zhang, Z., Ning, M., Hu, X., Yang, Y.F., Zhang, Z.F., Yu, L., He, L., Xu, H. (2009) Variants in KCNQ1 are associated with susceptibility to type 2 diabetes in the population of mainland China. *Diabetologia* 52, 1315-21.

[18] Tan, J.T., Nurbaya, S., Gardner, D., Ye, S., Tai, E.S., Ng, D.P. (2009) Genetic variation in KCNQ1 associates with fasting glucose and beta-cell function: a study of 3,734 subjects comprising three ethnicities living in Singapore. *Diabetes* 58, 1445-9.

[19] Saxena, R., Voight, B.F., Lyssenko, V., Burtt, N.P., de Bakker, P.I., Chen, H., Roix, J.J., Kathiresan, S., Hirschhorn, J.N., Daly, M.J., Hughes, T.E., Groop, L., Altshuler, D., Almgren, P., Florez, J.C., Meyer, J., Ardlie, K., Bengtsson Bostrom, K., Isomaa, B., Lettre, G., Lindblad, U., Lyon, H.N., Melander, O., Newton-Cheh, C., Nilsson, P., Orho-Melander, M., Rastam, L., Speliotes, E.K., Taskinen, M.R., Tuomi, T., Guiducci, C., Berglund, A., Carlson, J., Gianniny, L., Hackett, R., Hall, L., Holmkvist, J., Laurila, E., Sjogren, M., Sterner, M., Surti, A., Svensson, M., Tewhey, R., Blumenstiel, B., Parkin, M., Defelice, M., Barry, R., Brodeur, W., Camarata, J., Chia, N., Fava, M., Gibbons, J., Handsaker, B., Healy, C., Nguyen, K., Gates, C., Sougnez, C., Gage, D., Nizzari, M., Gabriel, S.B., Chirn, G.W., Ma, Q., Parikh, H.,

Richardson, D., Ricke, D., Purcell, S. (2007) Genome-wide association analysis identifies loci for type 2 diabetes and triglyceride levels. *Science* 316, 1331-6.

[20] Scott, L.J., Mohlke, K.L., Bonnycastle, L.L., Willer, C.J., Li, Y., Duren, W.L., Erdos, M.R., Stringham, H.M., Chines, P.S., Jackson, A.U., Prokunina-Olsson, L., Ding, C.J., Swift, A.J., Narisu, N., Hu, T., Pruim, R., Xiao, R., Li, X.Y., Conneely, K.N., Riebow, N.L., Sprau, A.G., Tong, M., White, P.P., Hetrick, K.N., Barnhart, M.W., Bark, C.W., Goldstein, J.L., Watkins, L., Xiang, F., Saramies, J., Buchanan, T.A., Watanabe, R.M., Valle, T.T., Kinnunen, L., Abecasis, G.R., Pugh, E.W., Doheny, K.F., Bergman, R.N., Tuomilehto, J., Collins, F.S., Boehnke, M. (2007) A genome-wide association study of type 2 diabetes in Finns detects multiple susceptibility variants. *Science* 316, 1341-5.

[21] Scuteri, A., Sanna, S., Chen, W.M., Uda, M., Albai, G., Strait, J., Najjar, S., Nagaraja, R., Orru, M., Usala, G., Dei, M., Lai, S., Maschio, A., Busonero, F., Mulas, A., Ehret, G.B., Fink, A.A., Weder, A.B., Cooper, R.S., Galan, P., Chakravarti, A., Schlessinger, D., Cao, A., Lakatta, E., Abecasis, G.R. (2007) Genome-wide association scan shows genetic variants in the FTO gene are associated with obesity-related traits. *PLoS Genet* 3, e115.

[22] Steinthorsdottir, V., Thorleifsson, G., Reynisdottir, I., Benediktsson, R., Jonsdottir, T., Walters, G.B., Styrkarsdottir, U., Gretarsdottir, S., Emilsson, V., Ghosh, S., Baker, A., Snorradottir, S., Bjarnason, H., Ng, M.C., Hansen, T., Bagger, Y., Wilensky, R.L., Reilly, M.P., Adeyemo, A., Chen, Y., Zhou, J., Gudnason, V., Chen, G., Huang, H., Lashley, K., Doumatey, A., So, W.Y., Ma, R.C., Andersen, G., Borch-Johnsen, K., Jorgensen, T., van Vliet-Ostaptchouk, J.V., Hofker, M.H., Wijmenga, C., Christiansen, C., Rader, D.J., Rotimi, C., Gurney, M., Chan, J.C., Pedersen, O., Sigurdsson, G., Gulcher, J.R., Thorsteinsdottir, U., Kong, A., Stefansson, K. (2007) A variant in CDKAL1 influences insulin response and risk of type 2 diabetes. *Nat Genet* 39, 770-5.

[23] Zeggini, E., Scott, L.J., Saxena, R., Voight, B.F., Marchini, J.L., Hu, T., de Bakker, P.I., Abecasis, G.R., Almgren, P., Andersen, G., Ardlie, K., Bostrom, K.B., Bergman, R.N., Bonnycastle, L.L., Borch-Johnsen, K., Burtt, N.P., Chen, H., Chines, P.S., Daly, M.J., Deodhar, P., Ding, C.J., Doney, A.S., Duren, W.L., Elliott, K.S., Erdos, M.R., Frayling, T.M., Freathy, R.M., Gianniny, L., Grallert, H., Grarup, N., Groves, C.J., Guiducci, C., Hansen, T., Herder, C., Hitman, G.A., Hughes, T.E., Isomaa, B., Jackson, A.U., Jorgensen, T., Kong, A., Kubalanza, K., Kuruvilla, F.G., Kuusisto, J., Langenberg, C., Lango, H., Lauritzen, T., Li, Y., Lindgren, C.M., Lyssenko, V., Marvelle, A.F., Meisinger, C., Midthjell, K., Mohlke, K.L., Morken, M.A., Morris, A.D., Narisu, N., Nilsson, P., Owen, K.R., Palmer, C.N., Payne, F., Perry, J.R., Pettersen, E., Platou, C., Prokopenko, I., Qi, L., Qin, L., Rayner, N.W., Rees, M., Roix, J.J., Sandbaek, A., Shields, B., Sjogren, M., Steinthorsdottir, V., Stringham, H.M., Swift, A.J., Thorleifsson, G., Thorsteinsdottir, U., Timpson, N.J., Tuomi, T., Tuomilehto, J., Walker, M., Watanabe, R.M., Weedon, M.N., Willer, C.J., Illig, T., Hveem, K., Hu, F.B., Laakso, M., Stefansson, K., Pedersen, O., Wareham, N.J., Barroso, I., Hattersley, A.T., Collins, F.S., Groop, L., McCarthy, M.I., Boehnke, M., Altshuler, D. (2008) Meta-analysis of genome-wide association data and large-scale replication identifies additional susceptibility loci for type 2 diabetes. *Nat Genet* 40, 638-45.

[24] Zeggini, E., Weedon, M.N., Lindgren, C.M., Frayling, T.M., Elliott, K.S., Lango, H., Timpson, N.J., Perry, J.R., Rayner, N.W., Freathy, R.M., Barrett, J.C., Shields, B., Morris, A.P., Ellard, S., Groves, C.J., Harries, L.W., Marchini, J.L., Owen, K.R., Knight, B., Cardon, L.R., Walker, M., Hitman, G.A., Morris, A.D., Doney, A.S., McCarthy, M.I., Hattersley, A.T. (2007) Replication of genome-wide association signals in UK samples reveals risk loci for type 2 diabetes. *Science* 316, 1336-41.

[25] Sladek, R., Rocheleau, G., Rung, J., Dina, C., Shen, L., Serre, D., Boutin, P., Vincent, D., Belisle, A., Hadjadj, S., Balkau, B., Heude, B., Charpentier, G., Hudson, T.J., Montpetit, A., Pshezhetsky, A.V., Prentki, M., Posner, B.I., Balding, D.J., Meyre, D., Polychronakos, C., Froguel, P. (2007) A genome-wide association study identifies novel risk loci for type 2 diabetes. *Nature* 445, 881-5.

[26] Chimienti, F., Devergnas, S., Favier, A., Seve, M. (2004) Identification and cloning of a beta-cell-specific zinc transporter, ZnT-8, localized into insulin secretory granules. *Diabetes* 53, 2330-7.

[27] Kirchhoff, K., Machicao, F., Haupt, A., Schafer, S.A., Tschritter, O., Staiger, H., Stefan, N., Haring, H.U., Fritsche, A. (2008) Polymorphisms in the TCF7L2, CDKAL1 and SLC30A8 genes are associated with impaired proinsulin conversion. *Diabetologia* 51, 597-601.

[28] Fu, Y., Tian, W., Pratt, E.B., Dirling, L.B., Shyng, S.L., Meshul, C.K., Cohen, D.M. (2009) Down-regulation of ZnT8 expression in INS-1 rat pancreatic beta cells reduces insulin content and glucose-inducible insulin secretion. *PLoS One* 4, e5679.

[29] Boesgaard, T.W., Zilinskaite, J., Vanttinen, M., Laakso, M., Jansson, P.A., Hammarstedt, A., Smith, U., Stefan, N., Fritsche, A., Haring, H., Hribal, M., Sesti, G., Zobel, D.P., Pedersen, O., Hansen, T. (2008) The common SLC30A8 Arg325Trp variant is associated with reduced first-phase insulin release in 846 non-diabetic offspring of type 2 diabetes patients--the EUGENE2 study. *Diabetologia* 51, 816-20.

[30] Wu, Y., Li, H., Loos, R.J., Yu, Z., Ye, X., Chen, L., Pan, A., Hu, F.B., Lin, X. (2008) Common variants in CDKAL1, CDKN2A/B, IGF2BP2, SLC30A8, and HHEX/IDE genes are associated with type 2 diabetes and impaired fasting glucose in a Chinese Han population. *Diabetes* 57, 2834-42.

[31] Huang, Q., Yin, J.Y., Dai, X.P., Wu, J., Chen, X., Deng, C.S., Yu, M., Gong, Z.C., Zhou, H.H., Liu, Z.Q. Association analysis of SLC30A8 rs13266634 and rs16889462 polymorphisms with type 2 diabetes mellitus and repaglinide response in Chinese patients. *Eur J Clin Pharmacol* 66, 1207-15.

[32] Inoue, H., Tanizawa, Y., Wasson, J., Behn, P., Kalidas, K., Bernal-Mizrachi, E., Mueckler, M., Marshall, H., Donis-Keller, H., Crock, P., Rogers, D., Mikuni, M., Kumashiro, H., Higashi, K., Sobue, G., Oka, Y., Permutt, M.A. (1998) A gene encoding a transmembrane protein is mutated in patients with diabetes mellitus and optic atrophy (Wolfram syndrome). *Nat Genet* 20, 143-8.

[33] Sandhu, M.S., Weedon, M.N., Fawcett, K.A., Wasson, J., Debenham, S.L., Daly, A., Lango, H., Frayling, T.M., Neumann, R.J., Sherva, R., Blech, I., Pharoah, P.D., Palmer, C.N., Kimber, C., Tavendale, R., Morris, A.D., McCarthy, M.I., Walker, M., Hitman, G., Glaser, B., Permutt, M.A., Hattersley, A.T., Wareham, N.J., Barroso, I. (2007) Common variants in WFS1 confer risk of type 2 diabetes. *Nat Genet* 39, 951-3.

[34] Sanghera, D.K., Been, L., Ortega, L., Wander, G.S., Mehra, N.K., Aston, C.E., Mulvihill, J.J., Ralhan, S. (2009) Testing the association of novel meta-analysis-derived

diabetes risk genes with type II diabetes and related metabolic traits in Asian Indian Sikhs. *J Hum Genet* 54, 162-8.

[35] Lyssenko, V., Jonsson, A., Almgren, P., Pulizzi, N., Isomaa, B., Tuomi, T., Berglund, G., Altshuler, D., Nilsson, P., Groop, L. (2008) Clinical risk factors, DNA variants, and the development of type 2 diabetes. *N Engl J Med* 359, 2220-32.

[36] Florez, J.C., Jablonski, K.A., McAteer, J., Sandhu, M.S., Wareham, N.J., Barroso, I., Franks, P.W., Altshuler, D., Knowler, W.C. (2008) Testing of diabetes-associated WFS1 polymorphisms in the Diabetes Prevention Program. *Diabetologia* 51, 451-7.

[37] Sparso, T., Andersen, G., Albrechtsen, A., Jorgensen, T., Borch-Johnsen, K., Sandbaek, A., Lauritzen, T., Wasson, J., Permutt, M.A., Glaser, B., Madsbad, S., Pedersen, O., Hansen, T. (2008) Impact of polymorphisms in WFS1 on prediabetic phenotypes in a population-based sample of middle-aged people with normal and abnormal glucose regulation. *Diabetologia* 51, 1646-52.

[38] Stancakova, A., Kuulasmaa, T., Paananen, J., Jackson, A.U., Bonnycastle, L.L., Collins, F.S., Boehnke, M., Kuusisto, J., Laakso, M. (2009) Association of 18 confirmed susceptibility loci for type 2 diabetes with indices of insulin release, proinsulin conversion, and insulin sensitivity in 5,327 nondiabetic Finnish men. *Diabetes* 58, 2129-36.

[39] Schafer, S.A., Mussig, K., Staiger, H., Machicao, F., Stefan, N., Gallwitz, B., Haring, H.U., Fritsche, A. (2009) A common genetic variant in WFS1 determines impaired glucagon-like peptide-1-induced insulin secretion. *Diabetologia* 52, 1075-82.

[40] Heni, M., Ketterer, C., Thamer, C., Herzberg-Schafer, S.A., Guthoff, M., Stefan, N., Machicao, F., Staiger, H., Fritsche, A., Haring, H.U. Glycemia determines the effect of type 2 diabetes risk genes on insulin secretion. *Diabetes* 59, 3247-52.

[41] Wei, F.Y., Nagashima, K., Ohshima, T., Saheki, Y., Lu, Y.F., Matsushita, M., Yamada, Y., Mikoshiba, K., Seino, Y., Matsui, H., Tomizawa, K. (2005) Cdk5-dependent regulation of glucose-stimulated insulin secretion. *Nat Med* 11, 1104-8.

[42] Ubeda, M., Rukstalis, J.M., Habener, J.F. (2006) Inhibition of cyclin-dependent kinase 5 activity protects pancreatic beta cells from glucotoxicity. *J Biol Chem* 281, 28858-64.

[43] Omori, S., Tanaka, Y., Takahashi, A., Hirose, H., Kashiwagi, A., Kaku, K., Kawamori, R., Nakamura, Y., Maeda, S. (2008) Association of CDKAL1, IGF2BP2, CDKN2A/B, HHEX, SLC30A8, and KCNJ11 with susceptibility to type 2 diabetes in a Japanese population. *Diabetes* 57, 791-5.

[44] Chidambaram, M., Radha, V., Mohan, V. Replication of recently described type 2 diabetes gene variants in a South Indian population. *Metabolism* 59, 1760-6.

[45] Xu, M., Bi, Y., Xu, Y., Yu, B., Huang, Y., Gu, L., Wu, Y., Zhu, X., Li, M., Wang, T., Song, A., Hou, J., Li, X., Ning, G. Combined effects of 19 common variations on type 2 diabetes in Chinese: results from two community-based studies. *PLoS One* 5, e14022.

[46] Moritani, M., Yamasaki, S., Kagami, M., Suzuki, T., Yamaoka, T., Sano, T., Hata, J., Itakura, M. (2005) Hypoplasia of endocrine and exocrine pancreas in homozygous transgenic TGF-beta1. *Mol Cell Endocrinol* 229, 175-84.

[47] Rane, S.G., Dubus, P., Mettus, R.V., Galbreath, E.J., Boden, G., Reddy, E.P., Barbacid, M. (1999) Loss of Cdk4 expression causes insulin-deficient diabetes and Cdk4 activation results in beta-islet cell hyperplasia. *Nat Genet* 22, 44-52.

[48] Tsutsui, T., Hesabi, B., Moons, D.S., Pandolfi, P.P., Hansel, K.S., Koff, A., Kiyokawa, H. (1999) Targeted disruption of CDK4 delays cell cycle entry with enhanced p27(Kip1) activity. *Mol Cell Biol* 19, 7011-9.

[49] Bieganowski, P., Shilinski, K., Tsichlis, P.N., Brenner, C. (2004) Cdc123 and checkpoint forkhead associated with RING proteins control the cell cycle by controlling eIF2gamma abundance. *J Biol Chem* 279, 44656-66.

[50] Verploegen, S., Ulfman, L., van Deutekom, H.W., van Aalst, C., Honing, H., Lammers, J.W., Koenderman, L., Coffer, P.J. (2005) Characterization of the role of CaMKI-like kinase (CKLiK) in human granulocyte function. *Blood* 106, 1076-83.

[51] Grarup, N., Andersen, G., Krarup, N.T., Albrechtsen, A., Schmitz, O., Jorgensen, T., Borch-Johnsen, K., Hansen, T., Pedersen, O. (2008) Association testing of novel type 2 diabetes risk alleles in the JAZF1, CDC123/CAMK1D, TSPAN8, THADA, ADAMTS9, and NOTCH2 loci with insulin release, insulin sensitivity, and obesity in a population-based sample of 4,516 glucose-tolerant middle-aged Danes. *Diabetes* 57, 2534-40.

[52] Staiger, H., Machicao, F., Kantartzis, K., Schafer, S.A., Kirchhoff, K., Guthoff, M., Silbernagel, G., Stefan, N., Fritsche, A., Haring, H.U. (2008) Novel meta-analysis-derived type 2 diabetes risk loci do not determine prediabetic phenotypes. *PLoS One* 3, e3019.

[53] Gudmundsson, J., Sulem, P., Steinthorsdottir, V., Bergthorsson, J.T., Thorleifsson, G., Manolescu, A., Rafnar, T., Gudbjartsson, D., Agnarsson, B.A., Baker, A., Sigurdsson, A., Benediktsdottir, K.R., Jakobsdottir, M., Blondal, T., Stacey, S.N., Helgason, A., Gunnarsdottir, S., Olafsdottir, A., Kristinsson, K.T., Birgisdottir, B., Ghosh, S., Thorlacius, S., Magnusdottir, D., Stefansdottir, G., Kristjansson, K., Bagger, Y., Wilensky, R.L., Reilly, M.P., Morris, A.D., Kimber, C.H., Adeyemo, A., Chen, Y., Zhou, J., So, W.Y., Tong, P.C., Ng, M.C., Hansen, T., Andersen, G., Borch-Johnsen, K., Jorgensen, T., Tres, A., Fuertes, F., Ruiz-Echarri, M., Asin, L., Saez, B., van Boven, E., Klaver, S., Swinkels, D.W., Aben, K.K., Graif, T., Cashy, J., Suarez, B.K., van Vierssen Trip, O., Frigge, M.L., Ober, C., Hofker, M.H., Wijmenga, C., Christiansen, C., Rader, D.J., Palmer, C.N., Rotimi, C., Chan, J.C., Pedersen, O., Sigurdsson, G., Benediktsson, R., Jonsson, E., Einarsson, G.V., Mayordomo, J.I., Catalona, W.J., Kiemeney, L.A., Barkardottir, R.B., Gulcher, J.R., Thorsteinsdottir, U., Kong, A., Stefansson, K. (2007) Two variants on chromosome 17 confer prostate cancer risk, and the one in TCF2 protects against type 2 diabetes. *Nat Genet* 39, 977-83.

[54] Winckler, W., Weedon, M.N., Graham, R.R., McCarroll, S.A., Purcell, S., Almgren, P., Tuomi, T., Gaudet, D., Bostrom, K.B., Walker, M., Hitman, G., Hattersley, A.T., McCarthy, M.I., Ardlie, K.G., Hirschhorn, J.N., Daly, M.J., Frayling, T.M., Groop, L., Altshuler, D. (2007) Evaluation of common variants in the six known maturity-onset diabetes of the young (MODY) genes for association with type 2 diabetes. *Diabetes* 56, 685-93.

[55] Clatworthy, J.P., Subramanian, V. (2001) Stem cells and the regulation of proliferation, differentiation and patterning in the intestinal epithelium: emerging insights from gene expression patterns, transgenic and gene ablation studies. *Mech Dev* 101, 3-9.

[56] Grant, S.F., Thorleifsson, G., Reynisdottir, I., Benediktsson, R., Manolescu, A., Sainz, J., Helgason, A., Stefansson, H., Emilsson, V., Helgadottir, A., Styrkarsdottir, U.,

Magnusson, K.P., Walters, G.B., Palsdottir, E., Jonsdottir, T., Gudmundsdottir, T., Gylfason, A., Saemundsdottir, J., Wilensky, R.L., Reilly, M.P., Rader, D.J., Bagger, Y., Christiansen, C., Gudnason, V., Sigurdsson, G., Thorsteinsdottir, U., Gulcher, J.R., Kong, A., Stefansson, K. (2006) Variant of transcription factor 7-like 2 (TCF7L2) gene confers risk of type 2 diabetes. *Nat Genet* 38, 320-3.

[57] Takeuchi, F., Serizawa, M., Yamamoto, K., Fujisawa, T., Nakashima, E., Ohnaka, K., Ikegami, H., Sugiyama, T., Katsuya, T., Miyagishi, M., Nakashima, N., Nawata, H., Nakamura, J., Kono, S., Takayanagi, R., Kato, N. (2009) Confirmation of multiple risk Loci and genetic impacts by a genome-wide association study of type 2 diabetes in the Japanese population. *Diabetes* 58, 1690-9.

[58] Zeggini, E., McCarthy, M.I. (2007) TCF7L2: the biggest story in diabetes genetics since HLA? *Diabetologia* 50, 1-4.

[59] Haupt, A., Thamer, C., Heni, M., Ketterer, C., Machann, J., Schick, F., Machicao, F., Stefan, N., Claussen, C.D., Haring, H.U., Fritsche, A., Staiger, H. Gene variants of TCF7L2 influence weight loss and body composition during lifestyle intervention in a population at risk for type 2 diabetes. *Diabetes* 59, 747-50.

[60] Chang, Y.C., Chiu, Y.F., Ho, L.L., Ting, C.T., Shih, K.C., Curb, J.D., Chen, Y.D., Li, H.Y., Chuang, L.M. TCF7L2 genetic variants and progression to diabetes in the Chinese population: pleiotropic effects on insulin secretion and insulin resistance. *J Mol Med* 88, 183-92.

[61] Holstein, A., Hahn, M., Korner, A., Stumvoll, M., Kovacs, P. TCF7L2 and therapeutic response to sulfonylureas in patients with type 2 diabetes. *BMC Med Genet* 12, 30.

[62] Pearson, E.R., Donnelly, L.A., Kimber, C., Whitley, A., Doney, A.S., McCarthy, M.I., Hattersley, A.T., Morris, A.D., Palmer, C.N. (2007) Variation in TCF7L2 influences therapeutic response to sulfonylureas: a GoDARTs study. *Diabetes* 56, 2178-82.

[63] Bort, R., Martinez-Barbera, J.P., Beddington, R.S., Zaret, K.S. (2004) Hex homeobox gene-dependent tissue positioning is required for organogenesis of the ventral pancreas. *Development* 131, 797-806.

[64] Horikoshi, M., Hara, K., Ito, C., Shojima, N., Nagai, R., Ueki, K., Froguel, P., Kadowaki, T. (2007) Variations in the HHEX gene are associated with increased risk of type 2 diabetes in the Japanese population. *Diabetologia* 50, 2461-6.

[65] Schulze, M.B., Al-Hasani, H., Boeing, H., Fisher, E., Doring, F., Joost, H.G. (2007) Variation in the HHEX-IDE gene region predisposes to type 2 diabetes in the prospective, population based EPIC-Potsdam cohort. *Diabetologia* 50, 2405-7.

[66] Staiger, H., Stancakova, A., Zilinskaite, J., Vanttinen, M., Hansen, T., Marini, M.A., Hammarstedt, A., Jansson, P.A., Sesti, G., Smith, U., Pedersen, O., Laakso, M., Stefan, N., Fritsche, A., Haring, H.U. (2008) A candidate type 2 diabetes polymorphism near the HHEX locus affects acute glucose-stimulated insulin release in European populations: results from the EUGENE2 study. *Diabetes* 57, 514-7.

[67] Nakajima, T., Fujino, S., Nakanishi, G., Kim, Y.S., Jetten, A.M. (2004) TIP27: a novel repressor of the nuclear orphan receptor TAK1/TR4. *Nucleic Acids Res* 32, 4194-204.

[68] Collins, L.L., Lee, Y.F., Heinlein, C.A., Liu, N.C., Chen, Y.T., Shyr, C.R., Meshul, C.K., Uno, H., Platt, K.A., Chang, C. (2004) Growth retardation and abnormal maternal behavior in mice lacking testicular orphan nuclear receptor 4. *Proc Natl Acad Sci U S A* 101, 15058-63.

[69] Zhou, D.Z., Liu, Y., Zhang, D., Liu, S.M., Yu, L., Yang, Y.F., Zhao, T., Chen, Z., Kan, M.Y., Zhang, Z.F., Feng, G.Y., Xu, H., He, L. Variations in/nearby genes coding for JAZF1, TSPAN8/LGR5 and HHEX-IDE and risk of type 2 diabetes in Han Chinese. *J Hum Genet* 55, 810-5.

[70] Auwerx, J. (1999) PPARgamma, the ultimate thrifty gene. *Diabetologia* 42, 1033-49.

[71] Yen, C.J., Beamer, B.A., Negri, C., Silver, K., Brown, K.A., Yarnall, D.P., Burns, D.K., Roth, J., Shuldiner, A.R. (1997) Molecular scanning of the human peroxisome proliferator activated receptor gamma (hPPAR gamma) gene in diabetic Caucasians: identification of a Pro12Ala PPAR gamma 2 missense mutation. *Biochem Biophys Res Commun* 241, 270-4.

[72] Buzzetti, R., Petrone, A., Ribaudo, M.C., Alemanno, I., Zavarella, S., Mein, C.A., Maiani, F., Tiberti, C., Baroni, M.G., Vecci, E., Arca, M., Leonetti, F., Di Mario, U. (2004) The common PPAR-gamma2 Pro12Ala variant is associated with greater insulin sensitivity. *Eur J Hum Genet* 12, 1050-4.

[73] Deeb, S.S., Fajas, L., Nemoto, M., Pihlajamaki, J., Mykkanen, L., Kuusisto, J., Laakso, M., Fujimoto, W., Auwerx, J. (1998) A Pro12Ala substitution in PPARgamma2 associated with decreased receptor activity, lower body mass index and improved insulin sensitivity. *Nat Genet* 20, 284-7.

[74] de Rooij, S.R., Painter, R.C., Phillips, D.I., Osmond, C., Tanck, M.W., Defesche, J.C., Bossuyt, P.M., Michels, R.P., Bleker, O.P., Roseboom, T.J. (2006) The effects of the Pro12Ala polymorphism of the peroxisome proliferator-activated receptor-gamma2 gene on glucose/insulin metabolism interact with prenatal exposure to famine. *Diabetes Care* 29, 1052-7.

[75] Kang, E.S., Park, S.Y., Kim, H.J., Kim, C.S., Ahn, C.W., Cha, B.S., Lim, S.K., Nam, C.M., Lee, H.C. (2005) Effects of Pro12Ala polymorphism of peroxisome proliferator-activated receptor gamma2 gene on rosiglitazone response in type 2 diabetes. *Clin Pharmacol Ther* 78, 202-8.

[76] Christiansen, J., Kolte, A.M., Hansen, T.O., Nielsen, F.C. (2009) IGF2 mRNA-binding protein 2: biological function and putative role in type 2 diabetes. *J Mol Endocrinol* 43, 187-95.

[77] Nielsen, J., Christiansen, J., Lykke-Andersen, J., Johnsen, A.H., Wewer, U.M., Nielsen, F.C. (1999) A family of insulin-like growth factor II mRNA-binding proteins represses translation in late development. *Mol Cell Biol* 19, 1262-70.

[78] Hinohara, K., Nakajima, T., Sasaoka, T., Sawabe, M., Lee, B.S., Ban, J., Park, J.E., Izumi, T., Kimura, A. (2009) Replication studies for the association of PSMA6 polymorphism with coronary artery disease in East Asian populations. *J Hum Genet* 54, 248-51.

[79] Ng, M.C., Park, K.S., Oh, B., Tam, C.H., Cho, Y.M., Shin, H.D., Lam, V.K., Ma, R.C., So, W.Y., Cho, Y.S., Kim, H.L., Lee, H.K., Chan, J.C., Cho, N.H. (2008) Implication of genetic variants near TCF7L2, SLC30A8, HHEX, CDKAL1, CDKN2A/B, IGF2BP2, and FTO in type 2 diabetes and obesity in 6,719 Asians. *Diabetes* 57, 2226-33.

[80] Groenewoud, M.J., Dekker, J.M., Fritsche, A., Reiling, E., Nijpels, G., Heine, R.J., Maassen, J.A., Machicao, F., Schafer, S.A., Haring, H.U., t Hart, L.M., van Haeften, T.W. (2008) Variants of CDKAL1 and IGF2BP2 affect first-phase insulin secretion during hyperglycaemic clamps. *Diabetologia* 51, 1659-63.

[81] Ruchat, S.M., Elks, C.E., Loos, R.J., Vohl, M.C., Weisnagel, S.J., Rankinen, T., Bouchard, C., Perusse, L. (2009) Association between insulin secretion, insulin sensitivity and type 2 diabetes susceptibility variants identified in genome-wide association studies. *Acta Diabetol* 46, 217-26.

[82] Palmer, N.D., Goodarzi, M.O., Langefeld, C.D., Ziegler, J., Norris, J.M., Haffner, S.M., Bryer-Ash, M., Bergman, R.N., Wagenknecht, L.E., Taylor, K.D., Rotter, J.I., Bowden, D.W. (2008) Quantitative trait analysis of type 2 diabetes susceptibility loci identified from whole genome association studies in the Insulin Resistance Atherosclerosis Family Study. *Diabetes* 57, 1093-100.

[83] van Hoek, M., Langendonk, J.G., de Rooij, S.R., Sijbrands, E.J., Roseboom, T.J. (2009) Genetic variant in the IGF2BP2 gene may interact with fetal malnutrition to affect glucose metabolism. *Diabetes* 58, 1440-4.

[84] Grarup, N., Rose, C.S., Andersson, E.A., Andersen, G., Nielsen, A.L., Albrechtsen, A., Clausen, J.O., Rasmussen, S.S., Jorgensen, T., Sandbaek, A., Lauritzen, T., Schmitz, O., Hansen, T., Pedersen, O. (2007) Studies of association of variants near the HHEX, CDKN2A/B, and IGF2BP2 genes with type 2 diabetes and impaired insulin release in 10,705 Danish subjects: validation and extension of genome-wide association studies. *Diabetes* 56, 3105-11.

[85] (2007) Genome-wide association study of 14,000 cases of seven common diseases and 3,000 shared controls. *Nature* 447, 661-78.

[86] Frayling, T.M., Timpson, N.J., Weedon, M.N., Zeggini, E., Freathy, R.M., Lindgren, C.M., Perry, J.R., Elliott, K.S., Lango, H., Rayner, N.W., Shields, B., Harries, L.W., Barrett, J.C., Ellard, S., Groves, C.J., Knight, B., Patch, A.M., Ness, A.R., Ebrahim, S., Lawlor, D.A., Ring, S.M., Ben-Shlomo, Y., Jarvelin, M.R., Sovio, U., Bennett, A.J., Melzer, D., Ferrucci, L., Loos, R.J., Barroso, I., Wareham, N.J., Karpe, F., Owen, K.R., Cardon, L.R., Walker, M., Hitman, G.A., Palmer, C.N., Doney, A.S., Morris, A.D., Smith, G.D., Hattersley, A.T., McCarthy, M.I. (2007) A common variant in the FTO gene is associated with body mass index and predisposes to childhood and adult obesity. *Science* 316, 889-94.

[87] Pecioska, S., Zillikens, M.C., Henneman, P., Snijders, P.J., Oostra, B.A., van Duijn, C.M., Aulchenko, Y.S. Association between type 2 diabetes loci and measures of fatness. *PLoS One* 5, e8541.

[88] Wardle, J., Carnell, S., Haworth, C.M., Farooqi, I.S., O'Rahilly, S., Plomin, R. (2008) Obesity associated genetic variation in FTO is associated with diminished satiety. *J Clin Endocrinol Metab* 93, 3640-3.

[89] Rippe, V., Drieschner, N., Meiboom, M., Murua Escobar, H., Bonk, U., Belge, G., Bullerdiek, J. (2003) Identification of a gene rearranged by 2p21 aberrations in thyroid adenomas. *Oncogene* 22, 6111-4.

[90] Drieschner, N., Belge, G., Rippe, V., Meiboom, M., Loeschke, S., Bullerdiek, J. (2006) Evidence for a 3p25 breakpoint hot spot region in thyroid tumors of follicular origin. *Thyroid* 16, 1091-6.

[91] Drieschner, N., Kerschling, S., Soller, J.T., Rippe, V., Belge, G., Bullerdiek, J., Nimzyk, R. (2007) A domain of the thyroid adenoma associated gene (THADA) conserved in vertebrates becomes destroyed by chromosomal rearrangements observed in thyroid adenomas. *Gene* 403, 110-7.

[92] Simonis-Bik, A.M., Nijpels, G., van Haeften, T.W., Houwing-Duistermaat, J.J., Boomsma, D.I., Reiling, E., van Hove, E.C., Diamant, M., Kramer, M.H., Heine, R.J., Maassen, J.A., Slagboom, P.E., Willemsen, G., Dekker, J.M., Eekhoff, E.M., de Geus, E.J., t Hart, L.M. Gene variants in the novel type 2 diabetes loci CDC123/CAMK1D, THADA, ADAMTS9, BCL11A, and MTNR1B affect different aspects of pancreatic beta-cell function. *Diabetes* 59, 293-301.

[93] Hu, C., Zhang, R., Wang, C., Wang, J., Ma, X., Lu, J., Qin, W., Hou, X., Bao, Y., Xiang, K., Jia, W. (2009) PPARG, KCNJ11, CDKAL1, CDKN2A-CDKN2B, IDE-KIF11-HHEX, IGF2BP2 and SLC30A8 are associated with type 2 diabetes in a Chinese population. *PLoS One* 4, e7643.

[94] Gesierich, S., Paret, C., Hildebrand, D., Weitz, J., Zgraggen, K., Schmitz-Winnenthal, F.H., Horejsi, V., Yoshie, O., Herlyn, D., Ashman, L.K., Zoller, M. (2005) Colocalization of the tetraspanins, CO-029 and CD151, with integrins in human pancreatic adenocarcinoma: impact on cell motility. *Clin Cancer Res* 11, 2840-52.

[95] Kilkenny, D.M., Rocheleau, J.V. (2008) Fibroblast growth factor receptor-1 signaling in pancreatic islet beta-cells is modulated by the extracellular matrix. *Mol Endocrinol* 22, 196-205.

[96] Somerville, R.P., Longpre, J.M., Jungers, K.A., Engle, J.M., Ross, M., Evanko, S., Wight, T.N., Leduc, R., Apte, S.S. (2003) Characterization of ADAMTS-9 and ADAMTS-20 as a distinct ADAMTS subfamily related to Caenorhabditis elegans GON-1. *J Biol Chem* 278, 9503-13.

[97] Jungers, K.A., Le Goff, C., Somerville, R.P., Apte, S.S. (2005) Adamts9 is widely expressed during mouse embryo development. *Gene Expr Patterns* 5, 609-17.

[98] Clark, M.E., Kelner, G.S., Turbeville, L.A., Boyer, A., Arden, K.C., Maki, R.A. (2000) ADAMTS9, a novel member of the ADAM-TS/ metallospondin gene family. *Genomics* 67, 343-50.

[99] Boesgaard, T.W., Gjesing, A.P., Grarup, N., Rutanen, J., Jansson, P.A., Hribal, M.L., Sesti, G., Fritsche, A., Stefan, N., Staiger, H., Haring, H., Smith, U., Laakso, M., Pedersen, O., Hansen, T. (2009) Variant near ADAMTS9 known to associate with type 2 diabetes is related to insulin resistance in offspring of type 2 diabetes patients--EUGENE2 study. *PLoS One* 4, e7236.

[100] Lammert, E., Brown, J., Melton, D.A. (2000) Notch gene expression during pancreatic organogenesis. *Mech Dev* 94, 199-203.

[101] Apelqvist, A., Li, H., Sommer, L., Beatus, P., Anderson, D.J., Honjo, T., Hrabe de Angelis, M., Lendahl, U., Edlund, H. (1999) Notch signalling controls pancreatic cell differentiation. *Nature* 400, 877-81.

[102] Tsai, F.J., Yang, C.F., Chen, C.C., Chuang, L.M., Lu, C.H., Chang, C.T., Wang, T.Y., Chen, R.H., Shiu, C.F., Liu, Y.M., Chang, C.C., Chen, P., Chen, C.H., Fann, C.S., Chen, Y.T., Wu, J.Y. A genome-wide association study identifies susceptibility variants for type 2 diabetes in Han Chinese. *PLoS Genet* 6, e1000847.

[103] Chagnon, M.J., Uetani, N., Tremblay, M.L. (2004) Functional significance of the LAR receptor protein tyrosine phosphatase family in development and diseases. *Biochem Cell Biol* 82, 664-75.

[104] Uetani, N., Kato, K., Ogura, H., Mizuno, K., Kawano, K., Mikoshiba, K., Yakura, H., Asano, M., Iwakura, Y. (2000) Impaired learning with enhanced hippocampal long-term potentiation in PTPdelta-deficient mice. *EMBO J* 19, 2775-85.

[105] Ren, J.M., Li, P.M., Zhang, W.R., Sweet, L.J., Cline, G., Shulman, G.I., Livingston, J.N., Goldstein, B.J. (1998) Transgenic mice deficient in the LAR protein-tyrosine phosphatase exhibit profound defects in glucose homeostasis. *Diabetes* 47, 493-7.

[106] Chagnon, M.J., Elchebly, M., Uetani, N., Dombrowski, L., Cheng, A., Mooney, R.A., Marette, A., Tremblay, M.L. (2006) Altered glucose homeostasis in mice lacking the receptor protein tyrosine phosphatase sigma. *Can J Physiol Pharmacol* 84, 755-63.

[107] Batt, J., Asa, S., Fladd, C., Rotin, D. (2002) Pituitary, pancreatic and gut neuroendocrine defects in protein tyrosine phosphatase-sigma-deficient mice. *Mol Endocrinol* 16, 155-69.

[108] Zabolotny, J.M., Kim, Y.B., Peroni, O.D., Kim, J.K., Pani, M.A., Boss, O., Klaman, L.D., Kamatkar, S., Shulman, G.I., Kahn, B.B., Neel, B.G. (2001) Overexpression of the LAR (leukocyte antigen-related) protein-tyrosine phosphatase in muscle causes insulin resistance. *Proc Natl Acad Sci U S A* 98, 5187-92.

[109] Pulido, R., Serra-Pages, C., Tang, M., Streuli, M. (1995) The LAR/PTP delta/PTP sigma subfamily of transmembrane protein-tyrosine-phosphatases: multiple human LAR, PTP delta, and PTP sigma isoforms are expressed in a tissue-specific manner and associate with the LAR-interacting protein LIP.1. *Proc Natl Acad Sci U S A* 92, 11686-90.

[110] Wolosker, H., Blackshaw, S., Snyder, S.H. (1999) Serine racemase: a glial enzyme synthesizing D-serine to regulate glutamate-N-methyl-D-aspartate neurotransmission. *Proc Natl Acad Sci U S A* 96, 13409-14.

[111] Wolosker, H., Sheth, K.N., Takahashi, M., Mothet, J.P., Brady, R.O., Jr., Ferris, C.D., Snyder, S.H. (1999) Purification of serine racemase: biosynthesis of the neuromodulator D-serine. *Proc Natl Acad Sci U S A* 96, 721-5.

[112] De Miranda, J., Panizzutti, R., Foltyn, V.N., Wolosker, H. (2002) Cofactors of serine racemase that physiologically stimulate the synthesis of the N-methyl-D-aspartate (NMDA) receptor coagonist D-serine. *Proc Natl Acad Sci U S A* 99, 14542-7.

[113] Mothet, J.P., Parent, A.T., Wolosker, H., Brady, R.O., Jr., Linden, D.J., Ferris, C.D., Rogawski, M.A., Snyder, S.H. (2000) D-serine is an endogenous ligand for the glycine site of the N-methyl-D-aspartate receptor. *Proc Natl Acad Sci U S A* 97, 4926-31.

[114] Imai, K., Fukushima, T., Santa, T., Homma, H., Huang, Y., Shirao, M., Miura, K. (1998) Whole body autoradiographic study on the distribution of 14C-D-serine administered intravenously to rats. *Amino Acids* 15, 351-61.

[115] Inagaki, N., Kuromi, H., Gonoi, T., Okamoto, Y., Ishida, H., Seino, Y., Kaneko, T., Iwanaga, T., Seino, S. (1995) Expression and role of ionotropic glutamate receptors in pancreatic islet cells. *FASEB J* 9, 686-91.

[116] Gonoi, T., Mizuno, N., Inagaki, N., Kuromi, H., Seino, Y., Miyazaki, J., Seino, S. (1994) Functional neuronal ionotropic glutamate receptors are expressed in the non-neuronal cell line MIN6. *J Biol Chem* 269, 16989-92.

[117] Bertrand, G., Gross, R., Puech, R., Loubatieres-Mariani, M.M., Bockaert, J. (1993) Glutamate stimulates glucagon secretion via an excitatory amino acid receptor of the AMPA subtype in rat pancreas. *Eur J Pharmacol* 237, 45-50.

[118] Stancakova, A., Pihlajamaki, J., Kuusisto, J., Stefan, N., Fritsche, A., Haring, H., Andreozzi, F., Succurro, E., Sesti, G., Boesgaard, T.W., Hansen, T., Pedersen, O., Jansson, P.A., Hammarstedt, A., Smith, U., Laakso, M. (2008) Single-nucleotide polymorphism rs7754840 of CDKAL1 is associated with impaired insulin secretion in

nondiabetic offspring of type 2 diabetic subjects and in a large sample of men with normal glucose tolerance. *J Clin Endocrinol Metab* 93, 1924-30.
[119] Groop, L.C. (1992) Sulfonylureas in NIDDM. *Diabetes Care* 15, 737-54.
[120] Niemi, M., Cascorbi, I., Timm, R., Kroemer, H.K., Neuvonen, P.J., Kivisto, K.T. (2002) Glyburide and glimepiride pharmacokinetics in subjects with different CYP2C9 genotypes. *Clin Pharmacol Ther* 72, 326-32.
[121] Kirchheiner, J., Brockmoller, J., Meineke, I., Bauer, S., Rohde, W., Meisel, C., Roots, I. (2002) Impact of CYP2C9 amino acid polymorphisms on glyburide kinetics and on the insulin and glucose response in healthy volunteers. *Clin Pharmacol Ther* 71, 286-96.
[122] Suzuki, K., Yanagawa, T., Shibasaki, T., Kaniwa, N., Hasegawa, R., Tohkin, M. (2006) Effect of CYP2C9 genetic polymorphisms on the efficacy and pharmacokinetics of glimepiride in subjects with type 2 diabetes. *Diabetes Res Clin Pract* 72, 148-54.
[123] Zhang, Y., Si, D., Chen, X., Lin, N., Guo, Y., Zhou, H., Zhong, D. (2007) Influence of CYP2C9 and CYP2C19 genetic polymorphisms on pharmacokinetics of gliclazide MR in Chinese subjects. *Br J Clin Pharmacol* 64, 67-74.
[124] Hart, L.M., Dekker, J.M., van Haeften, T.W., Ruige, J.B., Stehouwer, C.D., Erkelens, D.W., Heine, R.J., Maassen, J.A. (2000) Reduced second phase insulin secretion in carriers of a sulphonylurea receptor gene variant associating with Type II diabetes mellitus. *Diabetologia* 43, 515-9.
[125] Yokoi, N., Kanamori, M., Horikawa, Y., Takeda, J., Sanke, T., Furuta, H., Nanjo, K., Mori, H., Kasuga, M., Hara, K., Kadowaki, T., Tanizawa, Y., Oka, Y., Iwami, Y., Ohgawara, H., Yamada, Y., Seino, Y., Yano, H., Cox, N.J., Seino, S. (2006) Association studies of variants in the genes involved in pancreatic beta-cell function in type 2 diabetes in Japanese subjects. *Diabetes* 55, 2379-86.
[126] Rissanen, J., Markkanen, A., Karkkainen, P., Pihlajamaki, J., Kekalainen, P., Mykkanen, L., Kuusisto, J., Karhapaa, P., Niskanen, L., Laakso, M. (2000) Sulfonylurea receptor 1 gene variants are associated with gestational diabetes and type 2 diabetes but not with altered secretion of insulin. *Diabetes Care* 23, 70-3.
[127] Feng, Y., Mao, G., Ren, X., Xing, H., Tang, G., Li, Q., Li, X., Sun, L., Yang, J., Ma, W., Wang, X., Xu, X. (2008) Ser1369Ala variant in sulfonylurea receptor gene ABCC8 is associated with antidiabetic efficacy of gliclazide in Chinese type 2 diabetic patients. *Diabetes Care* 31, 1939-44.
[128] Xu, H., Murray, M., McLachlan, A.J. (2009) Influence of genetic polymorphisms on the pharmacokinetics and pharmaco-dynamics of sulfonylurea drugs. *Curr Drug Metab* 10, 643-58.
[129] Kimber, C.H., Doney, A.S., Pearson, E.R., McCarthy, M.I., Hattersley, A.T., Leese, G.P., Morris, A.D., Palmer, C.N. (2007) TCF7L2 in the Go-DARTS study: evidence for a gene dose effect on both diabetes susceptibility and control of glucose levels. *Diabetologia* 50, 1186-91.
[130] Winter, W.E., Nakamura, M., House, D.V. (1999) Monogenic diabetes mellitus in youth. The MODY syndromes. *Endocrinol Metab Clin North Am* 28, 765-85.
[131] Hathout, E.H., Cockburn, B.N., Mace, J.W., Sharkey, J., Chen-Daniel, J., Bell, G.I. (1999) A case of hepatocyte nuclear factor-1 alpha diabetes/MODY3 masquerading as type 1 diabetes in a Mexican-American adolescent and responsive to a low dose of sulfonylurea. *Diabetes Care* 22, 867-8.

[132] Pearson, E.R., Liddell, W.G., Shepherd, M., Corrall, R.J., Hattersley, A.T. (2000) Sensitivity to sulphonylureas in patients with hepatocyte nuclear factor-1alpha gene mutations: evidence for pharmacogenetics in diabetes. *Diabet Med* 17, 543-5.

[133] Sovik, O., Njolstad, P., Folling, I., Sagen, J., Cockburn, B.N., Bell, G.I. (1998) Hyperexcitability to sulphonylurea in MODY3. *Diabetologia* 41, 607-8.

[134] Pearson, E.R., Starkey, B.J., Powell, R.J., Gribble, F.M., Clark, P.M., Hattersley, A.T. (2003) Genetic cause of hyperglycaemia and response to treatment in diabetes. *Lancet* 362, 1275-81.

[135] Glamoclija, U., Jevric-Causevic, A. Genetic polymorphisms in diabetes: influence on therapy with oral antidiabetics. *Acta Pharm* 60, 387-406.

[136] Bidstrup, T.B., Bjornsdottir, I., Sidelmann, U.G., Thomsen, M.S., Hansen, K.T. (2003) CYP2C8 and CYP3A4 are the principal enzymes involved in the human in vitro biotransformation of the insulin secretagogue repaglinide. *Br J Clin Pharmacol* 56, 305-14.

[137] Niemi, M., Leathart, J.B., Neuvonen, M., Backman, J.T., Daly, A.K., Neuvonen, P.J. (2003) Polymorphism in CYP2C8 is associated with reduced plasma concentrations of repaglinide. *Clin Pharmacol Ther* 74, 380-7.

[138] Ruzilawati, A.B., Gan, S.H. CYP3A4 genetic polymorphism influences repaglinide's pharmacokinetics. *Pharmacology* 85, 357-64.

[139] McLeod, J.F. (2004) Clinical pharmacokinetics of nateglinide: a rapidly-absorbed, short-acting insulinotropic agent. *Clin Pharmacokinet* 43, 97-120.

[140] Kirchheiner, J., Meineke, I., Muller, G., Bauer, S., Rohde, W., Meisel, C., Roots, I., Brockmoller, J. (2004) Influence of CYP2C9 and CYP2D6 polymorphisms on the pharmacokinetics of nateglinide in genotyped healthy volunteers. *Clin Pharmacokinet* 43, 267-78.

[141] Niemi, M., Backman, J.T., Kajosaari, L.I., Leathart, J.B., Neuvonen, M., Daly, A.K., Eichelbaum, M., Kivisto, K.T., Neuvonen, P.J. (2005) Polymorphic organic anion transporting polypeptide 1B1 is a major determinant of repaglinide pharmacokinetics. *Clin Pharmacol Ther* 77, 468-78.

[142] Kalliokoski, A., Neuvonen, M., Neuvonen, P.J., Niemi, M. (2008) The effect of SLCO1B1 polymorphism on repaglinide pharmacokinetics persists over a wide dose range. *Br J Clin Pharmacol* 66, 818-25.

[143] He, J., Qiu, Z., Li, N., Yu, Y., Lu, Y., Han, D., Li, T., Zhao, D., Sun, W., Fang, F., Zheng, J., Fan, H., Chen, X. Effects of SLCO1B1 polymorphisms on the pharmacokinetics and pharmacodynamics of repaglinide in healthy Chinese volunteers. *Eur J Clin Pharmacol* 67, 701-7.

[144] Huang, Q., Yin, J.Y., Dai, X.P., Pei, Q., Dong, M., Zhou, Z.G., Huang, X., Yu, M., Zhou, H.H., Liu, Z.Q. IGF2BP2 variations influence repaglinide response and risk of type 2 diabetes in Chinese population. *Acta Pharmacol Sin* 31, 709-17.

[145] Qin, W., Zhang, R., Hu, C., Wang, C.R., Lu, J.Y., Yu, W.H., Bao, Y.Q., Xiang, K.S., Jia, W.P. A variation in NOS1AP gene is associated with repaglinide efficacy on insulin resistance in type 2 diabetes of Chinese. *Acta Pharmacol Sin* 31, 450-4.

[146] Sheng, F.F., Dai, X.P., Qu, J., Lei, G.H., Lu, H.B., Wu, J., Xu, X.J., Pei, Q., Dong, M., Liu, Y.Z., Zhou, H.H., Liu, Z.Q. NAMPT -3186C/T polymorphism influences repaglinide response in Chinese patients with type 2 diabetes mellitus. *Clin Exp Pharmacol Physiol.*

[147] Kirpichnikov, D., McFarlane, S.I., Sowers, J.R. (2002) Metformin: an update. *Ann Intern Med* 137, 25-33.

[148] Wang, D.S., Jonker, J.W., Kato, Y., Kusuhara, H., Schinkel, A.H., Sugiyama, Y. (2002) Involvement of organic cation transporter 1 in hepatic and intestinal distribution of metformin. *J Pharmacol Exp Ther* 302, 510-5.

[149] Shu, Y., Sheardown, S.A., Brown, C., Owen, R.P., Zhang, S., Castro, R.A., Ianculescu, A.G., Yue, L., Lo, J.C., Burchard, E.G., Brett, C.M., Giacomini, K.M. (2007) Effect of genetic variation in the organic cation transporter 1 (OCT1) on metformin action. *J Clin Invest* 117, 1422-31.

[150] Tzvetkov, M.V., Vormfelde, S.V., Balen, D., Meineke, I., Schmidt, T., Sehrt, D., Sabolic, I., Koepsell, H., Brockmoller, J. (2009) The effects of genetic polymorphisms in the organic cation transporters OCT1, OCT2, and OCT3 on the renal clearance of metformin. *Clin Pharmacol Ther* 86, 299-306.

[151] Zhou, K., Donnelly, L.A., Kimber, C.H., Donnan, P.T., Doney, A.S., Leese, G., Hattersley, A.T., McCarthy, M.I., Morris, A.D., Palmer, C.N., Pearson, E.R. (2009) Reduced-function SLC22A1 polymorphisms encoding organic cation transporter 1 and glycemic response to metformin: a GoDARTS study. *Diabetes* 58, 1434-9.

[152] Lopez-Bermejo, A., Diaz, M., Moran, E., de Zegher, F., Ibanez, L. A single nucleotide polymorphism in STK11 influences insulin sensitivity and metformin efficacy in hyperinsulinemic girls with androgen excess. *Diabetes Care* 33, 1544-8.

[153] Schroner, Z., Javorsky, M., Tkacova, R., Klimcakova, L., Dobrikova, M., Habalova, V., Kozarova, M., Zidzik, J., Rudikova, M., Tkac, I. Effect of sulphonylurea treatment on glycaemic control is related to TCF7L2 genotype in patients with type 2 diabetes. *Diabetes Obes Metab* 13, 89-91.

[154] Zhou, K., Bellenguez, C., Spencer, C.C., Bennett, A.J., Coleman, R.L., Tavendale, R., Hawley, S.A., Donnelly, L.A., Schofield, C., Groves, C.J., Burch, L., Carr, F., Strange, A., Freeman, C., Blackwell, J.M., Bramon, E., Brown, M.A., Casas, J.P., Corvin, A., Craddock, N., Deloukas, P., Dronov, S., Duncanson, A., Edkins, S., Gray, E., Hunt, S., Jankowski, J., Langford, C., Markus, H.S., Mathew, C.G., Plomin, R., Rautanen, A., Sawcer, S.J., Samani, N.J., Trembath, R., Viswanathan, A.C., Wood, N.W., Harries, L.W., Hattersley, A.T., Doney, A.S., Colhoun, H., Morris, A.D., Sutherland, C., Hardie, D.G., Peltonen, L., McCarthy, M.I., Holman, R.R., Palmer, C.N., Donnelly, P., Pearson, E.R. Common variants near ATM are associated with glycemic response to metformin in type 2 diabetes. *Nat Genet* 43, 117-20.

[155] Baldwin, S.J., Clarke, S.E., Chenery, R.J. (1999) Characterization of the cytochrome P450 enzymes involved in the in vitro metabolism of rosiglitazone. *Br J Clin Pharmacol* 48, 424-32.

[156] Jaakkola, T., Laitila, J., Neuvonen, P.J., Backman, J.T. (2006) Pioglitazone is metabolised by CYP2C8 and CYP3A4 in vitro: potential for interactions with CYP2C8 inhibitors. *Basic Clin Pharmacol Toxicol* 99, 44-51.

[157] Kirchheiner, J., Thomas, S., Bauer, S., Tomalik-Scharte, D., Hering, U., Doroshyenko, O., Jetter, A., Stehle, S., Tsahuridu, M., Meineke, I., Brockmoller, J., Fuhr, U. (2006) Pharmacokinetics and pharmacodynamics of rosiglitazone in relation to CYP2C8 genotype. *Clin Pharmacol Ther* 80, 657-67.

[158] Tornio, A., Niemi, M., Neuvonen, P.J., Backman, J.T. (2008) Trimethoprim and the CYP2C8*3 allele have opposite effects on the pharmacokinetics of pioglitazone. *Drug Metab Dispos* 36, 73-80.

[159] Daily, E.B., Aquilante, C.L. (2009) Cytochrome P450 2C8 pharmacogenetics: a review of clinical studies. *Pharmacogenomics* 10, 1489-510.

[160] Saltiel, A.R., Olefsky, J.M. (1996) Thiazolidinediones in the treatment of insulin resistance and type II diabetes. *Diabetes* 45, 1661-9.

[161] Keen, H. (1994) Insulin resistance and the prevention of diabetes mellitus. *N Engl J Med* 331, 1226-7.

[162] Vestergaard, H., Lund, S., Pedersen, O. (2001) Rosiglitazone treatment of patients with extreme insulin resistance and diabetes mellitus due to insulin receptor mutations has no effects on glucose and lipid metabolism. *J Intern Med* 250, 406-14.

[163] Sun, H., Gong, Z.C., Yin, J.Y., Liu, H.L., Liu, Y.Z., Guo, Z.W., Zhou, H.H., Wu, J., Liu, Z.Q. (2008) The association of adiponectin allele 45T/G and -11377C/G polymorphisms with Type 2 diabetes and rosiglitazone response in Chinese patients. *Br J Clin Pharmacol* 65, 917-26.

[164] Liu, H.L., Lin, Y.G., Wu, J., Sun, H., Gong, Z.C., Hu, P.C., Yin, J.Y., Zhang, W., Wang, D., Zhou, H.H., Liu, Z.Q. (2008) Impact of genetic polymorphisms of leptin and TNF-alpha on rosiglitazone response in Chinese patients with type 2 diabetes. *Eur J Clin Pharmacol* 64, 663-71.

[165] Kang, E.S., Cha, B.S., Kim, H.J., Kim, S.H., Hur, K.Y., Lee, H.J., Shim, W.S., Ahn, C.W., Lee, H.C. (2006) The 11482G >A polymorphism in the perilipin gene is associated with weight gain with rosiglitazone treatment in type 2 diabetes. *Diabetes Care* 29, 1320-4.

[166] Brunham, L.R., Kruit, J.K., Pape, T.D., Timmins, J.M., Reuwer, A.Q., Vasanji, Z., Marsh, B.J., Rodrigues, B., Johnson, J.D., Parks, J.S., Verchere, C.B., Hayden, M.R. (2007) Beta-cell ABCA1 influences insulin secretion, glucose homeostasis and response to thiazolidinedione treatment. *Nat Med* 13, 340-7.

[167] Wang, J., Bao, Y.Q., Hu, C., Zhang, R., Wang, C.R., Lu, J.X., Jia, W.P., Xiang, K.S. (2008) Effects of ABCA1 variants on rosiglitazone monotherapy in newly diagnosed type 2 diabetes patients. *Acta Pharmacol Sin* 29, 252-8.

[168] Kang, E.S., Park, S.E., Han, S.J., Kim, S.H., Nam, C.M., Ahn, C.W., Cha, B.S., Kim, K.S., Lee, H.C. (2008) LPIN1 genetic variation is associated with rosiglitazone response in type 2 diabetic patients. *Mol Genet Metab* 95, 96-100.

[169] Zhang, K.H., Huang, Q., Dai, X.P., Yin, J.Y., Zhang, W., Zhou, G., Zhou, H.H., Liu, Z.Q. Effects of the peroxisome proliferator activated receptor-gamma coactivator-1alpha (PGC-1alpha) Thr394Thr and Gly482Ser polymorphisms on rosiglitazone response in Chinese patients with type 2 diabetes mellitus. *J Clin Pharmacol* 50, 1022-30.

[170] Himelfarb, S.T., Silva, F.A., Arazi, S.S., Farjado, C.M., Garofalo, A., Bertolami, M.C., Bertolami, A., Faludi, A., Sampaio, M.F., Rezende, A.A., Hirata, R.D., Hirata, M.H. Tumor necrosis factor-alpha and interleukin-6 expression in leukocytes and their association with polymorphisms and bone markers in diabetic individuals treated with pioglitazone. *Drug Metabol Drug Interact* 26, 37-40.

[171] Hsieh, M.C., Lin, K.D., Tien, K.J., Tu, S.T., Hsiao, J.Y., Chang, S.J., Lin, S.R., Shing, S.J., Chen, H.C. Common polymorphisms of the peroxisome proliferator-activated receptor-gamma (Pro12Ala) and peroxisome proliferator-activated receptor-gamma

coactivator-1 (Gly482Ser) and the response to pioglitazone in Chinese patients with type 2 diabetes mellitus. *Metabolism* 59, 1139-44.
[172] Wang, G., Wang, X., Zhang, Q., Ma, Z. (2007) Response to pioglitazone treatment is associated with the lipoprotein lipase S447X variant in subjects with type 2 diabetes mellitus. *Int J Clin Pract* 61, 552-7.
[173] Rosenkranz, B., Brockmoller, J. (2005) Effect of genetic polymorphisms in cytochrome p450 (CYP) 2C9 and CYP2C8 on the pharmacokinetics of oral antidiabetic drugs: clinical relevance. *Clin Pharmacokinet* 44, 1209-25.